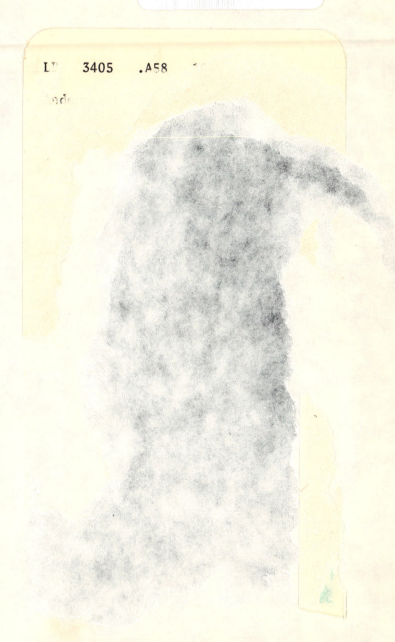

SCHOOL HEALTH PRACTICE

SCHOOL HEALTH PRACTICE

C. L. ANDERSON, B.S., M.S., Dr.P.H.

Emeritus Professor of Health,
Oregon State University, Corvallis, Oregon

WILLIAM H. CRESWELL, Jr., A.B., M.S., Ed.D.

Professor and former Head,
Department of Health Education and Safety,
University of Illinois, Champaign, Illinois

SEVENTH EDITION

With 135 illustrations

The C. V. Mosby Company

ST. LOUIS • TORONTO • LONDON   1980

Cover photographs by David S. Strickler

Seventh edition

Copyright © 1980 by The C. V. Mosby Company

Previous editions copyrighted 1956, 1960, 1964, 1968, 1972, 1976

Printed in the United States of America

The C. V. Mosby Company
11830 Westline Industrial Drive, St. Louis, Missouri 63141

Library of Congress Cataloging in Publication Data

Anderson, Carl Leonard, 1901-
    School health practice.

    Bibliography: p.
    Includes index.
    1. School hygiene.   I. Creswell, William H.,
1920- joint author.   II. Title.
[DNLM: 1. School health services.   WA350 A545s]
LB3405.A58 1980   371.7'1   79-27664
ISBN 0-8016-0216-5

GW/VH/VH 9 8 7 6 5 4 3   02/C/241

Preface to seventh edition

The history of health education may someday record that the period of the 1970s marked the emergence of health education into the public consciousness, as evidenced by a general awareness of and interest in health and the concept of living the healthy life. The public is now beginning to accept the idea that many of today's major health problems in the United States such as heart disease, cancer, and stroke are related to the population's habits of living. The effect of certain life-styles and the importance of disease prevention are being recognized. Health education is seen not only as the means for achieving a healthier life, but also as an economic benefit that contributes to disease control and the containment of the rising costs of health care.

Since the publication of the sixth edition, new federal, state, and local programs have been developed and several of the recommendations contained in the 1971 *President's Committee Report on Health Education* have been implemented. The Bureau of Health Education has been created within the federal government and, in the private sector, a National Center for Health Education has been established. At the federal level, the U.S. Department of Health, Education and Welfare has adopted a Forward Plan for Health, which outlines the government's role in preventing disease and promoting health. Recently enacted federal laws, such as the Health Planning and Resources Development Act and Consumer Health Information and Health Promotion Act, have given new impetus to health education. Perhaps most significant for schools is the Health Education Act of 1978. This law makes funds available to states and to local school systems for the purpose of strengthening health instruction programs.

Paralleling these events are other developments of significance to school health education. Nearly every state in the union has mandated some type of health instruction in schools. Several professional organizations have issued statements on the professional training of health educators. It is recognized that health educators are employed to perform a number of different roles and to work in a variety of settings, including hospitals, clinics, industries, health departments, and voluntary agencies as well as in schools. Efforts are now under way to determine the areas of professional training that are common and essential to all health educators. In this regard, the National Center for Health Education has undertaken a project, which has as its purpose the development of nationally recognized standards to guide the preparation and certification of health educators and the accreditation of training programs in health education.

Although Americans in general enjoy a high standard of health and health care, a significant number of school children are not receiving needed health care. This is particularly true of children of low-income families who suffer a disproportionately large share of dental, nutritional, and mental health problems and exposure to the dangers of accidents and violence. Efforts are being made through the Early Periodic Screening Diagnosis and Treatment Program to provide the needed care.

Accidents continue to be the leading cause of death among all school children. The marked increase in deaths from motor vehicle accidents is of special concern to school officials. This, plus the growing threat of violence including child abuse, homicide, and suicide among school-age children, deserves the attention of all school and community leaders. The Block Program described in Chapter 9 illustrates a home-school-community effort to provide increased protection for young children.

Also included in this edition are recently developed growth charts that portray the growth trends for height and weight of children between 2 and 18 years old. The data for these charts were collected by the National Center for Health Statistics and are representative of children and youth in the United States.

In this seventh edition, Chapter 11 has been completely rewritten to help provide health educators with a greater understanding of the theoretical and scientific bases for health instruction. The chapter includes a comprehensive review of the definitions and statements of purpose developed for health education and a discussion of two major theories of learning. Included are the health belief model, self-management behavior modification, and Fishbein's behavioral intentions model. Examples are given of health education applications to health behavior change theory including the School Health Education Study's conceptual approach to curriculum design, the School Health Curriculum project, and a self-management behavior modification approach for school health instruction.

In an effort to help teachers relate learning theory to curriculum practice, new examples of curriculum materials have been provided, including two risk factor units selected from the Know Your Body Program of the American Health Foundation of New York City and a dental health unit developed by the American Dental Association. A new evaluative instrument, a self-appraisal checklist for school health programs developed by the state of Ohio, has been included in Appendix C.

Many persons and organizations have contributed to this edition, and to all of them we express our sincere thanks. This includes all of the children in the various classrooms we visited and the teachers who so generously provided samples of health learning activities. Special thanks are extended to the American Dental Association, the American Health Foundation of New York City, the Bureau of Health Education, the Ohio State Departments of Health and Education, and Ross Laboratories of Ohio for generously providing us with educational materials for this edition.

C. L. Anderson
William H. Creswell, Jr.

Far best is he who is himself all-wise,
And he, too, good who listens to wise words;
And whoso is not wise nor lays to heart
Another's wisdom is a useless man.

Hesiod (800 B.C.)

Preface to first edition

Health promotion is a recognized component of present-day functional public school education, which is designed to prepare each youngster to deal with life's academic, cultural, and practical needs. No phase of the school's activities has more to contribute to the student than does the health program. Closely interwoven with all phases of school life, the health program aims to develop each student in terms of his present and future needs. As an achievement in living, health is integrated with all aspects of school life which contribute to the effectiveness and enjoyment of life for each youngster.

Primary responsibility for the health of the child rests with the parents, but the school is in a strategic position to contribute effectively to the health of every school-age child. The school does not assume the role of parent nor substitute for the parent. Rather, the school health program is planned to fortify and supplement the efforts of the parents.

The *what*, the *how*, and the *why* of the functional school health program are the substance of this publication. Special attention is given to the practical considerations of everyday school life. The approach has been that of presenting a clear, unified, composite picture of school health as represented by the most valuable contributions of the many health educators who have devoted their talents to the school health movement. So far as possible, superfluous material has been discarded and the truly essential substance has been presented. Material of an older vintage has been refreshed to fit the modern school situation. Much of the material is new but nevertheless bears the label of having been tried and found to be effective.

A self-contained textbook designed to serve the optimum preprofessional and in-service health preparation needs of teachers must be based upon actual experienced needs and practices. Successful educators in the field represent a fertile source of information on the health preparation needs of teachers. An extensive survey of the experience and thinking of successful teachers served as one guide in determining the content of this manuscript. College faculties, preparing teachers in health, were further consulted for suggestions on the desirable content of a comprehensive school health textbook. With the recommendations of these various professional groups as a guide, the organization and content of the manuscript were developed.

Because the child is the concern of all school health work, attention is given to an understanding of normal child growth, development, and health. Common departures from health are introduced to enable teachers to understand their proper role in contributing to the needs of the child who falls outside of the normal range. The complete school health program is developed so the material can be applied to the model health program of the large school system or adapted to the needs of the system or school with a minimum health program. Teachers with a modicum of resourcefulness can adapt the instructional materials to their particular classroom needs.

The school health field has attained that level of maturity where it has its own terminology, expressions, picturesque passages, and even shibboleths. Anyone writing in the health field today will use expressions that are the creations of others and the accepted tools of the profession. Maeterlinck, in his essay on *Literary Manners,* commented, "I have at times been twigged for using sentences and phrases that had a familiar ring or were identical with what others had written before me. No writer who loves words, their flair, nuances and beauty can escape such impeachment. We are struck with some beautiful line or paragraph reread many times and lo! later we may find it has popped into our heads as something original. Our only excuse is our utter innocence."

Acknowledgments must begin with an expression of gratitude to that vast number of public school teachers who have expressed their health preparation needs and have thus contributed to the form and substance of the manuscript. These people represent a segment of that legion of unheralded and unsung classroom teachers who are the institution of education in America. An expression of appreciation must be addressed to several individuals: Dr. Rex Putnam, Oregon Superintendent of Public Instruction, for making all of his department's health resources available; Professor Lucille Hall Jones, Walla Walla College, for her work in developing the School Health Program Evaluation Scale; Dr. Helen G. Smith, State College of Washington, for her constructive review and appraisal of the entire manuscript; Dr. Bernice Moss, University of Utah; Dr. Charles J. Hart, Brigham Young University; Dr. Franklin B. Haar, University of Oregon; Professor L. J. Sparks, Willamette University; Professor I. E. Langstaff, Saskatchewan Teachers College; Professor Warren Smith, Lewis and Clark College; Professor Betty J. Owen, Pacific University; Professor Anna Pavlov and Professor L. J. Carmody, Central Washington College; and Dr. C. F. Shockey, Seattle Pacific College.

C. L. Anderson
Corvallis, Oregon

Contents

1 Introduction: Development of school health and health education, 1

The quest for health, 1
The school health movement, 6
Modern school health era, 6
Current developments in school health education, 14
Today's school health program, 15
Essential terminology, 18

PART ONE

The school-age child

2 Health of the normal child, 25

Concept of normal, 26
The healthy child, 27
Outward indices of physical health, 27
Attributes of mental health, 30
Levels of health, 31
Individual variations, 32
Building up and maintaining health, 33
Conservation of human resources, 33
Promoting the health of students, 34

3 Physical growth and development, 37

Growth—cellular and intercellular, 37
Development or maturation, 38
Biological determination, 39
Environmental factors, 40
Full-term infant, 40

Prematurity and growth retardation, 41
Characteristics of the preschool child, 42
The elementary school-age child, 43
Puberty and adolescence, 45
Male-female differences, 50
Height, 54
Weight, 55
Developmental profiles, 56
National Center for Health Statistics growth charts, 58
Heart function and blood pressure, 61

4 Emotional development, 66

Biosocial development, 66
Concept of emotions, 66
Physical bases of emotions, 67
Genesis of emotional responses, 68
Preschool years, 69
Early elementary school years, 69
Later elementary school years, 70
Junior high school years, 70
Puberty, 71
Senior high school years, 72
Unrest of high school youths, 73
Individual differences, 76

5 Departures from normal health, growth, and development, 78

Responsibility of the school, 78
Low vitality, 79
Malnutrition, 80

Endocrine disturbances, 82
Rheumatic fever, 83
Cardiovascular disorders, 84
Anemia, 86
Disorders of posture, 87
Deviations of the respiratory
  system, 88
Disorders of the oral cavity, 90
Disorders of vision, 91
Hearing disability, 92
Neurological disorders, 93
Delayed maturation and growth, 94
Accelerated maturation and growth, 94
Deviations in mental health, 94
Mental health promotion, 97
Appraisal, 99

PART TWO

Organization of the school health program

6 Basic plan of the health program, 103

Authorization of school health
  programs, 104
Basic divisions of the health
  program, 106
School health services, 107
Health instruction, 110
Healthful school living, 111
School health personnel, 112

PART THREE

School health services

7 Appraisal aspect of health
services, 127

Fundamental objectives, 127
Health examination, 128
Dental examination, 139
Health assessment by the teacher, 142
Conservation of vision, 144
Conservation of hearing, 148
Height and weight measures, 152
Health guidance and supervision, 153
Health and the teacher, 158

8 Preventive aspects of health
services—control of communicable
diseases, 161

Communicable disease, 161
Infection and disinfection, 161
Contamination and decontamination, 162
Causative agents, 162
Classification of communicable
  diseases, 162
Transmission of infectious disease, 164
Blocking routes of transmission, 164
Resistance and immunity, 165
Cycle of respiratory infectious
  diseases, 166
Infectious respiratory diseases, 167
Common skin infections and
  infestations, 172
Responsibility for control of
  communicable diseases, 174
Immunization program, 177
School-parent-health department
  practices, 181
Detection of communicable diseases, 181
Isolation of a child at school, 185
Exclusions, 185
Readmissions, 186
Epidemics and school policies, 187

9 Preventive aspects of health
services—safety, emergency care,
and first aid, 190

School safety program, 190
Block home program, 200
Emergency care, 202
First aid at school, 203
General conditions and injuries, 205
Localized conditions and injuries, 210
First aid supplies, 214

10 Remedial aspects of health
services, 218

Importance of follow-up programs, 218
Defects that are the province of the
  physician or orthodontist, 223
Corrective work of the school, 228
Modified program for the
  handicapped, 235

PART FOUR

Health instruction

11 Health education and health behavior: the foundation of health instruction, 241

Purpose and ethics of health education, 242

Code of ethics, 244

The contribution of health education to health, 244

A theoretical basis for health education, 247

Health education application: theories and models, 252

Guidelines for the health instruction program, 271

12 Elementary school health instruction, 274

Organizing for effective health instruction, 274

Classroom instruction, 276

Integrated living as health instruction, 277

Planned direct instruction, 280

Grade-to-grade integrated resource units—grades K, 1, 2, 3, 284

Kindergarten, 286

Grade 1, 286

Grade 2, 288

Grade 3, 289

Resource unit—grade 2, 290

Resource unit—grade 3, 293

Learning about your oral health, level II: 4-6, 294

Resource unit—grade 6, 305

Incidental instruction, 309

Correlated health instruction, 310

13 Junior high or middle school health instruction, 314

Basic objectives of health instruction, 314

Areas of primary interest, 315

Correlation of health and other subject fields, 316

Integrated and incidental health learning, 316

Organizing for health instruction, 316

Instructional personnel, 320

Methods of instruction, 320

Know Your Body (KYB) risk factor units, levels I and II, 320

Resource unit—tobacco, alcohol, and other harmful drugs, 336

Resource unit—mental health, 342

Evaluation, 343

14 Senior high school health instruction, 346

Basic objectives of health instruction, 346

Areas of primary interest, 348

Correlation of health and other subject areas, 350

Integrated and incidental health learning, 351

Organizing for health instruction, 351

Teacher preparation, 354

Methods of instruction, 356

Know Your Body (KYB) risk factor unit, level II, 356

Physical and emotional growth issues and interpersonal relationships, 369

Methodology, 375

Evaluation, 378

15 Health contributions of high school subject fields, 381

Health preparation of the secondary school staff, 381

Health responsibilities of all instructors, 382

Essential safeguards, 385

Health in English or communication fields, 387

Physical education, 387

Biological science, 388

Social studies, 388

Home economics, 389

Physics, 389

Chemistry, 389

Mathematics, 390

Summary, 390

PART FIVE

Healthful school living

16   Healthful school environment, 395

Responsibility for healthful school
  environment, 396
Location and plan of school
  building, 399
Heating and ventilation, 399
Illumination, 401
Water supply, 405
General toilet room, 408
Special toilet rooms, 410
Food service, 410
Gymnasium and activity room, 412
Locker rooms, 415
Shower rooms, 415
Swimming pool, 416
Housekeeping, 416
Healthful mental environment, 416

PART SIX

Appraisal in school health practice

17   Evaluation, 423

Purposes of evaluation, 423
Evaluation procedures, 425
Evaluation devices, 425
Evaluation of change in health status
  of child, 428
Evaluation of administrative
  practices, 428
Evaluation of the school health
  program, 429
Evaluation of health services, 430
Evaluation of healthful school
  living, 430
Evaluation and health instruction, 431
Summary, 440

Appendices

A   Resources in health
  instruction, 445
B   Record and report forms, 448
C   School health program evaluation
  scale, 459
D   Self-appraisal checklist for school
  health programs, 468

SCHOOL HEALTH PRACTICE

In darkness dwells the people which
knows its annals not.
Ullrich Phillips

CHAPTER 1

Introduction: Development of school health and health education

Paraphrasing Ralph Waldo Emerson, "We think the practice of school health is near its meridian but we are yet only at the cock-crowing, and the morning star." Although humanity's attempt to promote health is of ancient vintage, only in relatively recent times has the school been incorporated into the general program of health promotion. Even more recently has the school health program demonstrated a positive, measurable effect on the health of citizens. However, the present-day school health program falls short of realizing the opportunities afforded it, and new concepts are developing rapidly.

Health in the school is an outgrowth of the universal search for more effective and more enjoyable living. This has been the central, dominant purpose of humanity from the beginning of recorded history. To attain this goal, individuals have studied the phenomena of the universe, controlled the forces of nature, developed languages, invented various devices, instituted new practices, written laws and regulations, established institutions, and even sought to improve genetic endowment.

Civilization has advanced most during those periods in which major progress has been made in the promotion of health. Progress in health has always been associated with advancement in the various pursuits of learning and with improvement in providing for material needs. When health has been neglected, civilization has declined and humanity has retrogressed.

THE QUEST FOR HEALTH

Certain periods in the history of the health movement serve as landmarks of progress in health promotion. Increased understanding of health and changing concepts of health promotion are reflected in the pertinent contributions of the various periods. The school became one of the principal agencies for health promotion, and health education developed a history of its own. To understand the role and position of the school in the health field, it is necessary to understand the background from which school health emerged.

Egyptian health practice. Before the year 1000 B.C. the Egyptians stressed personal cleanliness, compounded pharmaceutical preparations, built earth closets, and laid public drainage pipes—all in the interest of better health.

Hebrew health code. The Hebrews extended the Egyptian health ideas when they formulated the first formal health code in the Mosaic law. Of interest to the health student of today are nine of the basic areas covered by the law:

1. Personal and community responsibility for health
2. Maternal health
3. Control of communicable diseases
4. Isolation of lepers (*Leviticus,* Chapter XIII, gives an interesting account of procedures for control of leprosy)
5. Sanitation of camp sites
6. Fumigation
7. Disposal of wastes
8. Protection of water supplies
9. Protection of food

Reasons based on health and cleanliness were secondary to the basic approach of a system of taboos and a philosophy of holiness. However, the Jewish practice of considering pork unclean probably grew out of the observation that people became ill from eating pork. Trichinosis doubtless existed then as it does today.

Greek approach to health. At the height of Corinthian prosperity and achievement, primary emphasis was placed on the individual, and secondary emphasis on the state. In this philosophy the state existed to serve the individual. Consequently, stress was placed on individual grace, beauty, dexterity, skill, and ability. It was believed that the development of the individual depended on good health and a sound body, which were attained through exercise. Using but the one factor of exercise for the promotion of health, the Greeks attained but a limited level of health. General requirements, such as control of disease, proper nutrition, protection of water supplies, proper waste disposal, and other community health measures, were of no concern to them. For example, each family, or group of families, had its own supply of well water. Because of the lack of a com-

munity responsibility or concept, none of the cities of illustrious Greece was large. Corinth had a population of only 35,000. This civilization produced the renowned Hippocrates (460-377 B.C.), whose observations on health and whose teaching and practice of medicine have influenced the science and practice of health knowledge for more than 2,000 years. He is still considered to be the father of medicine (Fig. 1-1).

Roman health promotion. During the time of Julius Caesar the state was paramount and the individual was subservient to the state. The Romans provided public water supplies by constructing aqueducts that carried water from distant points to the cities. Sewerage systems provided for disposal of community waste. Street pavement and street cleaning were regarded as health measures. Their emphasis on the community approach to problems enabled the Romans to build large cities. At the time of Julius Caesar, Rome had a population of 800,000. Yet, because of their restricted approach to health matters, the Romans did not enjoy a high level of health.

Dark ages. From about A.D. 400 to 1000, the influence of the church caused all emphasis to be placed on the spiritual aspects of life. The physical was neglected; the body was ignored or abused in order to stress the spiritual values. In such an atmosphere the level of health was low.

Middle Ages. Between the years A.D. 1096 and 1248, during the time of the six great Crusades, the soldiers and followers of the Crusades had to be physically strong to withstand the rigors of the expeditions. For military purposes, the sound body again became esteemed. Disease and malnutrition took their toll, and general knowledge concerning health promotion was lacking.

Health from 1500 to 1800. Even with the revival of learning, health knowledge and the promotion of health practices were limited.

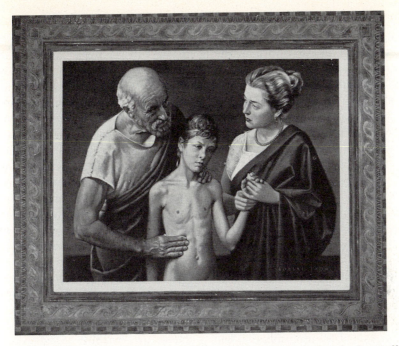

Fig. 1-1. Hippocrates. His aphorism "Where there is love for mankind, there is love for the art of healing" is reflected in the face of this revered physician, scientist, and teacher. (Copyright, Parke, Davis & Company, and reproduced by special permission of Parke, Davis & Company, who commissioned the original oil paintings for the series "A History of Medicine," a project written and directed by George A. Bender and painted by Robert A. Thom.)

The mysticism that had surrounded health survived, and sickness was believed to be of demoniacal origin. In the middle of the seventeenth century, in western Europe 75% of the infants born failed to reach the age of 10 years. Pandemics wiped out large segments of the population. The cyclical waves of the great killer, bubonic plague, illustrate this. It had attacked the Philistines and was the first great pandemic in the sixth century in Europe. It reappeared in the 1300s and afflicted two thirds of the population in Europe and then smoldered until the 1600s. In September 1665, during the Great Plague of London, the City of London's weekly Bills of Mortality showed that more than 30,000 people had died. The bubonic plague changed age-old attitudes toward disease. Since the plague infected all it touched, young and old, good or evil, it became clear that sickness was something more than God's punishment. The first concepts of contagion appeared, and such terms as "poisonous vapors," and "pestilential air" began to be blamed for disease rather than a lack of faith.

Although no concerted, unified program of health promotion distinguished this period, certain scientists made discoveries fundamental to health progress. During the later portion of this period, William Harvey traced the circulation of blood, and Edward Jenner introduced scientific vaccination. The invention of the microscope was to play an important part in the development of the scientific approach to health.

Modern era of health (1850 to present). The modern era of health began in the middle of the nineteenth century. Interest in sanitation of the general environment marked its beginnings. Although launched on a misconception, it expanded into a program that progressively has reduced the incidence of disease, increased the expectation of life, and extended the general well-being.

The *miasma phase* (1850 to 1880), the first of four phases of the modern era, was based on the erroneous theory that disease was caused by noxious odors. Emphasis was placed on the cleanliness of the general environment. Garbage and refuse disposal, street cleaning, fumigation, and cleanliness of home surroundings were considered important to an odor-free atmosphere. The term *malaria* (ill air) is but descriptive of the original belief that this disease was caused by the damp evening air. Interpreting mere coincidence as a cause-and-effect relationship is a frequent mistake of the public's attempt to explain health problems. In the thinking of the period, the fact that the *Anopheles* mosquito preferred dusk for its flight activities was not associated with the disease.

Although ineffective in terms of disease control, measures for general cleanliness devised during this health phase were not without merit. They laid the groundwork for the more specific measures that were to follow.

The *bacteriological phase* (1880 to 1920) of this era was ushered in by the research work of Louis Pasteur and Robert Koch. The discovery that a specific organism causes a specific disease transferred attention from the general environment to specific things in the environment. It quickly was recognized that spread of disease could be prevented by blocking the routes over which the disease

traveled. Emphasis was placed on the sanitation of water, milk, and other foods, the elimination of insects, and the disposal of sewage. Sanitary engineers, sanitary inspectors, bacteriologists, and laboratory technicians became essential to the health program.

Control of the ill person, who was the source of the disease, became an established practice. Isolation and quarantine measures were enforced by quarantine officers who posted placards on homes warning others of reported cases of the common communicable diseases that were within. Progress in the prevention and control of infectious diseases included immunization, antiseptic procedures, and chemical treatment. Immunization was a natural outcome of the interest in bacteriology. In 1883 Pasteur developed the inoculation against rabies. Von Behring's development of diphtheria antitoxin was first put to use in 1894. Wright developed the typhoid inoculations in 1904. Lord Lister's development of the use of carbolic acid (phenol) and Ehrlich's discovery of the value of arsenic compounds in the treatment of syphilis aided in the decline in the death rate from communicable diseases.

The *positive health phase* (1920 to 1960) resulted from the discovery that more than 34% of the men reporting for military service in World War I had to be rejected because of health disabilities, most of which were correctable. It was apparent that, although the United States had been successful in preventing deaths from infectious disease, the quality of health of its individual citizens had been neglected. To survive is not enough. To develop and to maintain a high level of health in each person also is important. While sanitation and control measures, including immunization, were still important in the nation's health program, the center of interest shifted to the individual—to human beings. This required new services and new types of trained personnel.

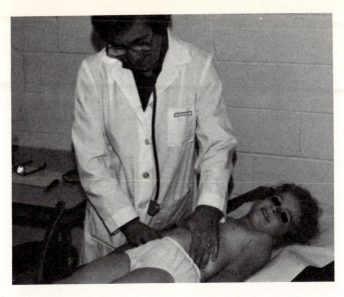

Fig. 1-2. The experience the child has with the physician through school health examinations helps to influence positive attitudes toward health care.

In addition to sanitarians, sanitary engineers, and laboratory technologists, a vast number of skilled health specialists were employed, primarily for the purpose of promoting the health of the individual citizen. Among these were health educators, nutritionists, industrial hygienists, nurses, pediatricians, vision conservationists, audiometrists, epidemiologists, statisticians, and administrators.

The *social engineering phase* (1960 to present) describes today's public health approach. With the increase in health discoveries and developments, it became clear that, if these advances were to be of use to the public, measures must be taken to bring this health knowledge into the lives of the populace. In the attempt to bring discoveries and citizens together, analysis of the situation uncovered a number of significant factors.

As society becomes more complex, a larger portion of the public appears to be incapable of adjusting to that increasing complexity. Consequently, the public must be prepared

if it is to utilize health developments. This means dealing with groups, neighborhoods, and even the entire population of a community. Public health education has become of special importance in preparing the public for the broad programs of sanitation, health promotion, disease prevention, and all other public health services available today. An understanding of human beings is basic to today's public health service. Ethnic backgrounds; neighborhood forces; personal, family, and group purposes and values; and economic, educational, and religious factors must all be considered if services are to be adjusted to people and if the public in turn is to adjust to the growing health complex.

Modern public health does not seek to control the populace. It seeks to bring together available health services and the people who need these services by making these people receptive to and able to utilize the services in a way that would be most beneficial to them (Fig. 1-2). This requires a form of social engineering not previously demanded of the public health profession. It has become the essential ingredient of modern public health promotion.

The school's role has become increasingly important as the nature of health and the measures that must be taken to achieve it have become better understood. Recognition of the school as an important agency for the promotion of health has increased equally with the emphasis on health promotion for the individual. The extent to which the school health movement has grown out of advances in health science, health application, and health advancement is as interesting as it is important.

THE SCHOOL HEALTH MOVEMENT

Health of children has long been a concern of the public, and history is replete with individual and group efforts to improve their lot. A century or more ago a lack of organization and a lack of understanding of the fundamentals of health prevented any semblance of an organized, continuous program directed primarily to the health needs of the child. Yet some of these early sporadic efforts were forerunners of child health programs that eventually developed into a school health program.

It is logical that the early contributions to the school health movement should come from Europe. Many of the contributors were nonprofessional people who sought to improve the lot of the growing child. In their efforts to find a way to promote child health, several of these pioneers recognized the possible role of the school in the promotion of children's well-being.

European heritage of school health. As early as 1790 Bavaria provided free school lunches for the underprivileged. This program was fostered by Benjamin Thompson, a transplanted New Englander. The eminent European scientist Johann Peter Frank

(1745-1821) published a series of papers dealing with the general subject of school health. In 1832 Edwin Chadwick was an assistant commissioner to study the operation of the poor laws of England. A year later he became Secretary of the Factory Commission. From his studies of the conditions of child employment came reforms that recognized the health needs of children.

In 1833 France passed a law that held public school authorities responsible for the health of schoolchildren and the sanitation of school buildings. This law was extended 9 years later to require that physicians inspect all schools at regular intervals.

Physicians were placed on public school staffs in Sweden in 1868, Germany in 1869, Russia in 1871, and Austria in 1873. In Brussels, Belgium, the first organized, regular medical inspection system was instituted in 1874. Every 3 months all schools were inspected by a physician. Later, dentists and vision specialists were added to the inspection staff.

It is significant that all these early school health activities in Europe were directed toward doing something *for* the child. The concept of preparing the child to do something for him- or herself had not yet evolved because the essentials for health education were not in existence. An extensive knowledge of health, plus universal education, is the essential for health education.

MODERN SCHOOL HEALTH ERA

The modern era of school health was launched on the fundamental concept that the school can prepare a person to do what is necessary for the protection, preservation, and promotion of his or her own health. Not only has this era retained the school's responsibility for supervising the child's health and for promoting school sanitation, which it inherited from Europe, but it also has added the all-important objective of preparing each child to make the decisions necessary for his or her health.

Period of recognition (1850 to 1880). It was no accident that the modern era of public health and the modern era of school health should date from the same year. A consciousness of the need for doing something about the health of human beings brought the natural question, What can the school do? A combination of fortuitous developments and certain cause-and-effect relationships accounts for the twin birth.

Prior to 1850 the schools in the United States were dominated by the church. This type of imposed pedagogy, which prevailed before 1850, did not lend itself to health education. However, in 1850 tax-supported public schools became a reality in most of the United States, particularly in the northern section.

A second fortunate development of 1850 was the publication of the *Report of the Sanitary Commission of Massachusetts.* The awakening interest in health promotion had led to the appointment of this commission to study and make recommendations on matters affecting the public health. The report dealt with several health topics, but significantly included a plan for school health instruction. A layman, Lemuel Shattuck, wrote the report, which included the following, one of the classic concepts of education:

Every child should be taught, early in life, that to preserve his own life and his own health and the lives and health of others, is one of his most important and constantly abiding duties. Some measure is needed which shall compel children to make a sanitary examination of themselves and their associates, and thus elicit a practical application of the lessons of sanitary science in the everyday duties of life. The recommendation now under consideration is designed to furnish this measure. It is to be carried into operation in the use of a blank schedule, which is to be printed on a letter sheet, in the form prescribed in the appendix, and furnished to the teacher of each school. He is to appoint a sanitary committee of the scholars, at the commencement of school, and on the first day of each month, to fill it out under his superintendence. . . . Such a measure is simple, would take but a few minutes each day, and cannot operate otherwise than usefully upon the children, in forming habits of exact observation, and in making a personal application of the laws of health and life to themselves. This is education of an eminently practical character, and of the highest importance.*

Because the report was the most important health pronouncement in that day of health awakening, it commanded the respect necessary for its perpetuation. It gave recognition to the school as an agency for the promotion of health. For the next 20 years this seed of recognition was nourished by the influence of European leaders in education such as Rousseau, Pestalozzi, and Froebel. This influence cannot be overemphasized because it stressed education as growth from within, not imposed from without, and growth from within is necessary for health education. This influence stimulated an interest in understanding children, their needs, and the best means to meet these needs.

Period of exploration (1880 to 1920). Beginning in 1880, pioneer work in the problems relating to the health of the child was inaugurated. A diversity of concepts developed concerning what body of information constituted school health and what the school's responsibilities were in regard to the health of the child.

The *child study movement* began at the outset of this period in the history of school health. Educators studied the physical and psychological characteristics of child development as the basis for planning the school program. Before the end of this period, child study was an established basis for all school planning and activities.

---

*From Report of the Sanitary Commission of Massachusetts, 1850, Dutton & Wentworth, p. 178.

Physical education experienced a robust expansion during the first 20 years of this period. In the interest of promoting physical conditioning and efficiency, calisthenics comprised a considerable part of the program. Kansas City, Missouri, had a director of physical education as early as 1885, and during the next 10 years physical education was widely adopted by schools in the middle west. Schools in other sections of the nation were slower in accepting physical education. As early as 1892, Ohio law *required* that physical education be taught in the schools of all first and second class cities.* In 1899, North Dakota law *required* the teaching of physical education in all public schools.

Physical education and health were held to be identical; apparently not until 1910 was there a change in this point of view. In that year the seventeenth meeting of the American Physical Education Association had "School Hygiene and Physical Education" as its theme. Not until 1937 did the American Physical Education Association become the American Association for Health and Physical Education and thus recognize a distinction between health and physical education in schools.

Instruction concerning the effects of alcohol and narcotics was required of all schools in every state by 1890. The drive for this requirement came from the temperance forces. In more than half of the states the law also required instruction in physiology and hygiene. As early as 1842 Horace Mann had advocated that the schools carry out health instruction, and hygiene had been taught in a few places in the nation. However, the first concerted health instruction in schools grew out of the statutes requiring instruction in physiology and hygiene. Although at the outset the hygiene instruction was heavily

*Rogers, J. F.: State-wide trends in school hygiene and physical education, Washington, D.C., 1930, United States Office of Education, Pamphlet No. 5.

weighted with anatomy and physiology, with emphasis on memorization of factual material, it did create interest in the subject of personal health.

In 1904 the National Association for the Study and Prevention of Tuberculosis was formed to combat the greatest single cause of death in the United States. In the absence of a specific treatment for tuberculosis, the association selected education of the public as its approach. In 1915 the association conducted a program, called Modern Health Crusade, which made effective use of posters, stories, plays, and ceremonies as motivating devices. The success of this approach supports the value of health education.

In 1909 the American Association for the Study and Prevention of Infant Mortality was formed, which developed programs of education for better child care. Later the association changed its name to American Child Hygiene Association.

The end of the first decade of the 1900s marked two important developments affecting the school health movement. The First White House Conference on Child Health and Protection was held in 1910, and in 1911 the Joint Committee of the National Education Association and the American Medical Association was appointed. The committee, representing the official position of the two parent bodies on health problems affecting schools, became recognized as an authoritative source of recommended policies and practices for school health programs.

The Baltimore, Maryland, school health demonstration of 1914 revealed that health instruction could alter health behavior. During World War I, concern for the health of the nation's children led to the formation in 1918 of the Child Health Organization to promote health instruction in the schools. In 1920 fellowships in health education were awarded. In 1923 the organization merged with the American Child Hygiene Association to form the American Child Health Association which was dissolved in 1935.

Health examinations in schools began in 1894 when Dr. Samuel Durgin, Health Commissioner of Boston, introduced the first regular program for medical inspection in the United States. A similar program was instituted in Chicago in 1895, New York in 1897, Philadelphia in 1898, and Massachusetts in 1906. As early as 1899, Connecticut law required teachers to test the vision of schoolchildren. Reading, Pennsylvania employed a school dentist in 1903, and in 1904 the state of Vermont initiated compulsory eye, ear, nose, and throat examinations in the public schools. By 1910 more than 300 cities required medical inspections in their schools.

In 1918 the Commission on the Reorganization of Secondary Education named health as the first of the seven cardinal objectives of education.

These several enterprises were independent efforts to deal with the problem of health through the medium of the school. Each effort, in its particular way, contributed to the emerging school health program. The need for combining efforts was becoming apparent.

Period of synthesis (1920 to 1935). By 1920 the need for a positive, individual approach to personal health was recognized nationally. Mere survival was only a part of the issue. The quality of a person's health also was important.

The special role of the school in the nation's program for health was not simple to delineate in precise terms. There was general agreement that the school was one of many agencies contributing to health and that its activities must be synchronized with the overall program. Its unique contribution was that of preparing citizens to make the necessary decisions relating to their health. The questions of the responsibility of the school for the present health of the child and the role of the school in the correction of physical defects were to receive intensive study and were eventually crystallized into accepted policies at the close of this period.

Field research in school health during this period provided the foundation for the school health program in the United States. Application of the scientific approach to the problem gave stature to the findings and to the recommendations that resulted. Setting up a demonstration type of study in the field is equivalent to setting up a laboratory study in a social situation. In dealing with social phenomena, precise measurement is not often possible, nor is it always necessary. Observable data that lend themselves to comparison can be highly meaningful. The less precise the data in research, the more important is the interpretative skill of the investigator.

In 1922 in Malden, Massachusetts, under the direction of Dr. C. E. Turner and with the support of the Massachusetts Institute of Technology, a 2-year school health demonstration program was conducted. Incorporating what were considered the best activities in school health, Dr. Turner developed a relatively complete program. At the termination of the demonstration, a crital analysis of the results showed that not only had the health behavior of the youngsters been improved, but the health, growth, and development of the children had also been affected favorably.

From 1922 to 1925, under the sponsorship of the American Red Cross, a similar demonstration with similar results was conducted in Mansfield and Richland counties in Ohio. In Fargo, North Dakota, the Commonwealth Fund conducted a school health demonstration from 1923 to 1927. With the Milbank Memorial Fund assisting financially, Cattaraugus County, New York, conducted a school health demonstration program. Each of these studies contributed to the school health movement by pointing out strengths and weaknesses, suggesting methods and techniques, explaining the procedures that could and could not be used, and showing the results to be obtained from a school health program.

In 1930, the Second White House Conference on Child Health and Protection grappled with the task of synthesizing the various aspects of child health and its concomitant problems. The report of the conference served as a guide for 2 decades, although the Midcentury White House Conference on Children and Youth in 1950 submitted a further report.

Period of integration (1935 to present). By 1935 the principal task of the school health movement was that of integration—of the school health program itself, of health with the entire school program, and of school health with the overall health program of the home, the community, the state, and the nation.

Integration of health activities was inevitable in the development of the school health program. In the process of integration, school health has merged from a multiphased program of seven or more divisions into an integrated program of three phases. In 1935 the program included health examination, health guidance, prevention and correction of physical defects, control of communicable diseases, study of mental health, health instruction, and maintenance of school sanitation. As the program matured, it was integrated into three phases—health services, health instruction, and healthful living. With integration the program became more functional in terms of actual life needs, procedures, and situations. Promotion of each child's health and emphasis on functional health knowledge resulted. As school health became more functional, the static concept of sanitation evolved into healthful school living, in which all aspects of environmental interaction were incorporated. Such a program naturally became an integrated part of the total school program, not an isolated segment of it.

Integration with home and community resulted. It was apparent that the school health program could not be wholly effective unless it was integrated with the home and the community and with the forces in both that contribute to the health of the schoolchild. Services of the personnel of public health departments and staff members of voluntary health agencies were utilized as a regular part of the activities of the school.

Suggested School Health Policies, a publication that has had great influence on school health programs in the United States, was first issued in 1940 by the American Public Health Association. A second edition was published in 1946 by the National Conference for Cooperation in Health Education. This national conference was important because it included representatives from all the leading educational, health, and medical organizations concerned with school health. The fact that the publication was endorsed by all the organizations established it as a charter for school health. *Suggested School Health Policies* was eventually taken over and published by the Joint Committee on Health Problems in Education of the National Education Association and the American Medical Association.*

In 1941 the Joint Committee on Health Problems in Education of the National Education Association and the American Medical Association developed a complete volume titled *Health Education* that, with revisions, has been a standard reference for the school health profession. This book, plus other joint

---

*The American Medical Association Medical and Education Committee on School and College Health has now accepted responsibility for publishing *Suggested School Health Policies*.

publications of the two associations, presented the then current practices in school health.

Beginning in 1942 and continuing for 6 years, a school-community health project sponsored by the W. K. Kellogg Foundation was extended to several hundred schools in 24 states. This project established the value and importance of cooperation of professional personnel of school and community health agencies. It demonstrated that effective health education requires community understanding and support.

In 1944 the American Council on Education issued objectives of general education in its publication, *A Design for General Education.* Special attention was given to health objectives.

A problem that continues to challenge leaders in the school health movement is the professional training of personnel. Beginning in 1948, a series of national conferences sponsored by professional groups and the Office of Education was held for the purpose of defining functions and competencies needed by the school health educator. These conferences were held in Jackson's Mill, Weston, West Virginia, in 1948 and Pere Marquette State Park, Illinois, in 1950; a series of related conferences were held in Washington, D.C. in 1949, 1953, and 1955. The interest in professional preparation was also evident during the decade of the 1960s when the American Association for Health, Physical Education, and Recreation sponsored national conferences for the purpose of developing standards to serve as the basis for accrediting colleges and universities offering training in health education (Means, 1975).

In recent years, several national professional organizations have issued reports on the guidelines or recommended standards of preparation for health education. In 1974 the American Association for Health, Physical Education, and Recreation issued a report on competencies for school health and safety education (AAHPER, 1974), in 1976 a committee of the American School Health Association issued a report on professional preparation (Bruess, 1976), and in 1977 the Society for Public Health Education (SOPHE) published its guidelines for professional practice. Whereas the SOPHE report does not specifically address the preparation of teachers, its recently adopted guidelines reflect the common elements essential for professional training, whether the health educator is working in a school, community, or health care institution. Schaller (1978), in summarizing several of these reports, called attention to the common areas of professional preparation in health education as follows: (1) the fundamental areas of physical and biological sciences, (2) the behavioral sciences, (3) a core of health content courses, and (4) the skills of professional practice. Moreover, the preamble of the SOPHE guidelines report contains an appropriate statement of the purposes and methodologies of the health educator:

Health education is concerned with the health-related behavior of people. Therefore, it must take into account the forces that affect those behaviors and the role of human behavior in the prevention of disease. As a profession, it uses educational processes to stimulate desirable change or to reinforce health practices of individuals, families, groups, organizations, communities, and larger social systems. Its intent is the development of health knowledge, the exploration of behavior change options, and the consequence of these changes.*

In 1978 the Bureau of Health Manpower of the United States Public Health Service sponsored a workshop on the preparation and practice of professional health educators. The purpose of the workshop was to identify the roles and functions of health educators in

*From Society for Public Health Education Ad Hoc Task Force on Professional Preparation and Practice of Health Education. Guidelines for the preparation and practice of professional health educators, SOPHE Health Education Monographs, **5**(1):75-89, Spring, 1977.

their various occupational settings. Conclusions from the conference held that the commonalities of professional preparation and practice in health education would serve as the basis for developing national standards to establish the credentials for health educators. Such an action is believed to be essential in establishing quality control in professional training programs and the future success of health education.

Thus far the training of school administrators and special personnel in health education has been given insufficient attention. However, the maximum effectiveness of a school health program can be attained only when all the personnel related to the program have an adequate understanding of school health in general and their roles in particular.

Current legislative developments in health education. As is sometimes the case, relatively unknown and unpublicized events can lead to developments of major historical significance. In 1970 a governor's steering committee on social problems on health and hospital services (Report from the Governor, 1971) was created by the late Governor Nelson A. Rockefeller. Following submission of its report, delivered to Governor Rockefeller in June 1971, a new and unprecedented level of interest in health education developed.

One of the five major factors determining the level of the nation's personal health as recognized in the committee's report was the necessity of consumer responsibility and public participation. In this regard the report stated:

The responsibility of the individual for his own health and well-being is a vital factor to any rational approach to health. The fact is, the nation does not have the resources, no matter how great a portion of GNP it allocated for health, to provide sufficient services after the patient becomes ill.*

*From Report from the Governor's Steering Committee on Social Problems on Health and Hospital Services and Cost, New York, 1971, State of New York.

This powerful statement created a new awareness of health education among the leaders of government, business, and industry, as well as the general public. Health education began to be considered in terms of national health policy. The report pointed out that disease prevention and sound health maintenance are as much a responsibility of the individual as they are of the medical profession. The difficulties and the level of effort required in taking an active role in protecting and promoting the individual's own well-being were recognized in the report, which states: "Insofar as health education efforts are concerned, this will require a massive, creative, multi-faceted effort with continuity —to awaken and sustain interest in one's own health."*

In 1971 President Nixon appointed the National Committee on Health Education, including several members of Governor Rockefeller's committee. Earlier that year, in his health message to Congress, the President had stated that there was no national instrument, no central force to stimulate and coordinate a comprehensive health program (Report of the President, 1973). Accordingly, the charge to the committee was as follows:

1. Describe the state of the art in health education.
2. Define the nation's need for health education.
3. Establish goals, priorities and objectives for health education.
4. Determine the most appropriate structure, organization, and function for a national health education foundation.

The President's report led directly to the establishment of the Bureau of Health Education in 1974 as a part of the United States Public Health Service. Creation of the bu-

*From Report from the Governor's Steering Committee on Social Problems on Health and Hospital Services and Cost, New York, 1971, State of New York.

reau provided a focal point for health education within the federal government and served as a model to encourage industry to build health education into existing programs. Another purpose for the bureau was to provide funds for the training of health education specialists (Ogden, 1978).

As a further outgrowth of the President's report, a study was conducted by the National Health Council concerning the feasibility of establishing a center for health education. Subsequently, the National Center for Health Education was created in 1975 and established permanent headquarters in San Francisco. As stated in its 1978 brochure, the primary mission of the center is "Improving and increasing the education of the American public about health matters, encouraging people to place greater value on their health, emphasizing health rather than sickness, . . . and (creating) better understanding of how to shape those forces which influence our health." The center also serves in an advocacy role for health education in the development of national health policy. For example, it issues statements on patient education and research and evaluation of health education. The Center has also served in a convening role to bring together leaders to discuss important as well as controversial views affecting health education, and has recognized the need to develop practical approaches for measuring progress in health education in order to assure the future success of programs.

In addition to the creation of the Bureau of Health Education, the Report of the President's Committee on Health Education triggered a number of other federal activities, including publications, legislative initiatives, and organizational developments in which health education has become increasingly recognized as a necessary part of the government's public health policy. For example, Congress has written new charters for the National Cancer Institute and the National

Heart, Lung and Blood Institute. In addition to their traditional biomedical research missions, it is now mandated that more attention be given to prevention, education, and control measures. Federal legislation has authorized establishment of the Health Maintenance Organization, the Health Planning and Development Act of 1974, and the National Consumer Health Information and Health Promotion Act of 1976. This new legislation specifically addresses health education as an aspect of the law.

The national Forward Plan for Health, FY 1978-1982 issued in 1976 by the Chief Health Officers of HEW, stated that the administration should address itself to the improvement and expansion of health education as a fundamental method for achieving the goal of disease prevention (U.S. Department of Health, Education and Welfare, 1976). The 1975 edition of this report offered several recommendations directly related to school health education. Public Health Service was charged to give priority attention to the following:

1. To foster research and pilot programs aimed at improving health education principles and techniques.
2. To conduct specific health education activities in accident prevention.
3. To conduct research to determine the best methods of teaching children about the harmful effects of smoking, alcohol, drug abuse, and careless driving.
4. To determine ways in which the school health education programs can most effectively be used to deliver health information.
5. To emphasize the development of life-long attitudes toward health and the improvement of health in later years as a major goal of child health. Health activities concerning schools given attention in this report were immunizations, nutrition, dental health, and mental health.

Perhaps one of the most important statements to be issued on health education was the report of the Task Force on Consumer Health Education of 1976 (Preventive Medicine USA, 1976). This was one of eight major task force reports issued under the joint sponsorship of the Fogarty International Center, the National Institutes of Health, and the American College of Preventive Medicine. This report summarized the current status of health education, including an assessment of the problems facing the field as well as the future promise of health education. It concluded with a series of recommendations that are intended to serve as a basis for future action and provided the background information and support necessary for the passage of Public Law 94-317, The Consumer Health Information and Health Promotion Act of 1976. The law created the Office of Health Information and Health Promotion within the Office of the Assistant Secretary for Health and emphasized the importance of educational and health promotional activities.

CURRENT DEVELOPMENTS IN SCHOOL HEALTH EDUCATION

The curriculum reform of the late 1960s, set in motion by the launching of the Russian *Sputnik* in 1957, created a new interest in the school curriculum and curriculum planning. In addition to national curriculum projects in science and mathematics, the nation-wide *School Health Education Study: A Conceptual Design for Curriculum Development* was developed. The first phase of this study was launched in 1962 with a national survey of health instruction in the elementary and secondary schools of the United States. The second phase of this study involved the development of a comprehensive curriculum covering the full range of health topics with appropriate instructional materials for the various grade levels.

This influence plus the issuance of the 1964 *Surgeon General's Report on Smoking and Health* and the resulting concern over youth smoking helped to kindle a new interest in school health education. The trend toward mandating health instruction at the state level has been in evidence over the past decade. According to a 1976 survey by the American School Health Association (Castile and Jerrick, 1976), all but three states require some health instruction. Some states have offered local school districts the option of providing a comprehensive health education curriculum. Such a curriculum has been widely advocated by such groups as the American Association of School Administrators and the National Congress of Parents and Teachers, as well as a number of professional organizations in the fields of health and medicine.

New York, Florida, Illinois, and Oregon have implemented development. New York was one of the first, with the enactment of its Critical Health Problems Act of 1967. Although California did not pass such a law, the State Department of Education did publish in 1972 a *Framework for Health Instruction*, providing the structure for comprehensive health education in keeping with this trend.

National legislation in 1978 resulted in the passage of the health education amendment to the Elementary and Secondary Education Act that was originally passed in 1965. The purpose of this amendment, The Health Education Act of 1978, is, as a part of the regular education program, to encourage and to support programs that prepare students to maintain their physical health and well-being and to prevent illness and disease. Specifically, the amendment will award grants to state and local educational agencies for the purpose of establishing and supporting programs of health education. This is a significant development, since by enacting this amendment the federal government is now on record as supporting health education as an integral part of elementary and secondary education.

Teacher preparation and certification. In 1974 the American School Health Association conducted a national survey of state school health programs in order to determine the status of teacher certification for health education. Results of the survey showed that 30 states required special certification in health education, 10 states offered dual certification in health and physical education, two states plus the District of Columbia offered only dual certification in health and physical education, one state offered certification in physical education only, and one state offered certification in health and safety education. The remaining 16 states either do not have a requirement or simply impose a general teacher certification requirement as qualification for health education teaching. Most of the health teaching in today's secondary schools is being done by physical education teachers who have a minor preparation in health education. Typically such teachers will have satisfied a minimum requirement of 24 to 30 hours of designated course work in health education.

Typically, elementary school teaching candidates take a limited number of health course hours. Usually 6 to 9 hours of course work in health are required. Later, as a teacher, on-the-job guidance from a health coordinator combined with in-service training for the teacher can produce an effective health educator.

TODAY'S SCHOOL HEALTH PROGRAM

It is essential to view the present-day school health program in the context of the overall change in American education. Because the American concept has been changing from a traditional, classical education to a functional education in terms of life re-

quirements, health has become a natural concern of the school. Health is a functional activity, dealing with the process of living and its needs. It thus has an obvious place in a curriculum based on a functional philosophy.

Philosophy. Primary responsibility for the health of the school-age child rests with the parents, but the school should assist the parents in establishing and maintaining the highest possible level of health in each child. The role of the school is to supplement the efforts of the parents to develop the competence in each child to deal with the health problems of life.

Although legally the school has the authority of a parent, a school would err to assume the complete role of a parent. The classical decision of the Supreme Court of the State of Nebraska in 1933 is considered the legal authority on the principle of the school *in loco parentis* (in place of the parent) in matters of school health.

During school hours general education and control of pupils are in the hands of school boards, superintendents, principals and teachers, which control extends to health while parental authority is temporarily superseded.*

Yet a school health program based on the ultimate in legal authority is suspect. Not legal authority but child needs, parental support, and professional service are the bases of today's school health program. Although the school accepts the responsibilities of the parent during school hours, it does so in the spirit of service, not in the role of an enforcement officer.

The United States population can be proud of their generally high level of health and the medical care that they receive. However, it is important that school officials have an accurate and complete picture of the health

*From *Richardson* v. *Braham*, 249 N.W. 557, 125 Neb. 142; *Haffner* v. *Braham*, 249 N.W. 560, 125 Neb. 147.

needs of all today's school-age children. For health problems do exist, despite the great progress that has been made in controlling the acute infectious diseases of childhood that took such a heavy toll in the past. Elementary school-age children still suffer an average of three episodes of illness per year and 4.5 days absent from school. Accidents for the group age 1 through 14 years claimed over 12,000 lives in 1973; nearly half of these deaths were caused by motor vehicle accidents. Of even greater concern is the fact that those deaths caused by motor vehicles have increased markedly during the period since 1960, while the overall accidental death rate has been declining (U.S. Department of Health, Education and Welfare, 1976b). In addition, deaths by violence have been increasing rapidly since 1950, with accidents, homicides, and suicides taking their greatest toll among male students.

Other health problems that call for special consideration in the modern era of school health are those relating to the dental, nutritional, and mental health needs of school children. The problems of malocclusion and decayed or missing teeth are especially widespread. The potential benefits to be derived from good dental care and proper diet provide the school health program with a unique opportunity to prevent disease through effective dental health education.

An analysis of health data points to a paradox in American society. While many schoolchildren enjoy an excellent standard of health and health care, a significant number of schoolchildren are not receiving the health care that they need. For too many American children, health status and the amount of the health care received are related to socioeconomic status. For example, there is an inch difference in the average heights of children of the same age between those who come from homes in the lower socioeconomic range and those who come from homes in the upper socioeconomic range. With respect to dental care, a study (U.S. Department of Health, Education and Welfare, 1976a) in 1973 revealed that children of families with more than $15,000 income had an average of one decayed and four filled teeth. Children from families having less than $3,000 had just the reverse—four decayed teeth and one filled tooth. Children from poverty-level homes make, on the average, only one fourth as many visits to the dentist each year.

When children do not receive needed health care, not only is their health threatened, but they also begin to incur educational and economic handicaps that affect them the rest of their lives. The school should not usurp the responsibilities of the family, but what should be the role of the school in securing needed health care for schoolchildren? One possible approach being considered (U.S. Department of Health, Education and Welfare, 1975) is the establishment of a school-based health care delivery system. As envisioned, the focus of such a service would be primary health care and preventive medicine, including dentistry and accident prevention.

At the very least, schools must contact the family to explain the child's health problem and to aid the family in securing the needed health care. The health program is not something apart from the general school program, but an integrated phase of it. Health activities are interwoven with all phases of the school program in doing everything practical to develop each child to the fullest possible extent in terms of his or her basic endowment. Health is an integral part of education.

Such a philosophy should be examined in the light of the recognized objectives of general education. Perhaps the best statement of these objectives is contained in a report entitled *A Design for General Education*, issued by the American Council on Education. The report contains 10 major objectives, with the first one pertaining directly to health education. In the committee's judgment, general education should lead the student: *to improve and maintain his own health and take his share of responsibility for protecting the health of others. In order to accomplish this purpose, the student should acquire the following:*

A. Knowledge and understanding
  1. Of normal body functions in relation to sound health practice
  2. Of the major health hazards, their prevention and control
  3. Of the interrelation of mental and physical processes in health
  4. Of reliable sources of health information
  5. Of scientific methods in evaluating health concepts
  6. Of the effect of socioeconomic conditions on health
  7. Of community health problems, such as problems related to sanitation, industrial hygiene, and school hygiene
  8. Of community organization and services for health maintenance and improvement
B. Skills and abilities
  1. The ability to organize time to include planning for food, work, recreation, rest, and sleep
  2. The ability to improve and maintain good nutrition
  3. The ability to attain and maintain good emotional adjustment
  4. The ability to select and engage in recreative activities and healthful exercises suitable to individual needs
  5. The ability to avoid unnecessary exposure to disease and infection
  6. The ability to utilize medical and dental services intelligently
  7. The ability to participate in measures for the protection and improvement of community health
  8. The ability to evaluate popular beliefs critically
C. Attitudes and appreciations
  1. Desire to attain optimum health
  2. Personal satisfaction in carrying out sound health practices
  3. Acceptance of responsibility for his own health and for the protection of the health of others
  4. Willingness to make personal sscrifices for the health of others

  5. Willingness to comply with health regulations and to work for their improvement*

The philosophy of the present-day school health program is to assist all students in attaining their maximum potential in mental, physical, and emotional capacities. Students should live effectively and enjoyably, and be prepared to meet the many health problems they will encounter in their lives. Living is very much a matter of solving one problem after another. An understanding of health not only helps in solving problems related to it, but is also an asset of infinite value.

Evaluation of health. An adage goes, "The healthy know not their health, only the sick." Of all their assets, normal people would rate health as the most important. It is one of the necessities that makes possible the acquisition and enjoyment of other benefits. The cardinal challenge to the school health program is to develop in healthy children a lasting appreciation of this magnificent asset.

The individual's state of health determines the capacity for performance, endurance, and even interest. Efficiency in accomplishment is determined both by interest and by endurance. Accomplishment is the true source of enjoyment. Performance and enjoyment during childhood and youth set the pattern for an effective and enjoyable life— the dominant purpose of normal persons. A pleasant disposition, wholesome attitudes, and radiant personality are the products of effective and enjoyable living that good health makes possible.

General objective. The goal toward which all school health work is directed is well-adjusted, physically vigorous children free from remediable defects, with practices, attitudes, and knowledge that will assure them a high level of well-being and the ability to make the necessary decisions that will

---

*From A design for general education, Washington, D.C., 1944, American Council on Education.

affect their own health and that of their families.

Specific objectives. To an educator, the general objective of the school health program is like a star to a mariner—it sets the direction and the destination. Charting the navigation requires an orderly, planned, definite course. Such a course is laid out by determining specific markers, or objectives, that will lead to the desired goal when they are attained. The purposes of today's school health program can be stated by 18 specific objectives:

1. Continuing appraisal of each child's health status
2. Understanding of each youngster's health needs
3. Supervision and guidance of the health of the children
4. Development of the highest possible level of health for each child
5. Prevention of defects and disorders
6. Detection and correction of all defects and disorders
7. Special health provisions for the exceptional youngster
8. Reduction in the incidence of communicable and noncommunicable diseases
9. Positive health awareness and a desire for a high level of health in each child
10. Development of wholesome health attitudes
11. Development of healthful personal practices
12. Acquisition of scientific and functional knowledge of personal and community health
13. Development of an appreciation of esthetic factors related to health
14. Development of a high level of self-esteem in each youngster
15. Effective social adjustment
16. Hygienic mental environment at school
17. Establishment and maintenance of sanitary practices and surroundings
18. Provision of emergency measures

To serve the particular needs of its students and the community, a school may find it advisable to set up other objectives than those listed, but it would be difficult to visualize an effective school health program that rejects any of them. This is presented as an optimum, and in matters of health the optimum should be the minimum.

ESSENTIAL TERMINOLOGY

A definition is a concise statement of the essentials of a word or a term. It does not include all the connotations, shadings, and variations inherent in the term, yet, as a framework, a definition provides a common structure from which each person builds his or her concept.

Since words are the medium used to convey ideas to each other, effort should be exercised to make primary terminology as meaningful as possible. Despite the most earnest efforts in the interest of clarity, misunderstandings will occur. To improve understanding, certain key terms in school health work should be explained. These will be the most important tools of expression the health instructor will use.

Health is that quality of physical, emotional, and mental well-being that enables one to live effectively and enjoyably. In appraising the possible health value of an activity, one can employ the criterion, Does it contribute to a person's effectiveness and enjoyment in living? Quality is a relative term, and youngsters in the normal range of health can vary in terms of the quality of well-being. The noun *hygiene* has fallen into disuse, but the adjective *hygienic* is employed extensively in health literature.

Normal is that which is regarded as the usual, not in terms of an absolute, but in terms of a range. Although each child in a classroom is unique, different from all others, all the children may be normal within the usual range as accepted by society.

Education comes from the Latin *educo*, meaning to lead out. It can be applied to the institution that, through organization and the utilization of experience, provides the opportunities and the stimulation for individual learning. Education as an institution illuminates knowledge and develops the science and art of utilizing knowledge. It deals in academic and cultural explorations as well as in practical and vocational experience. It gives a child knowledge, concepts, techniques, and esthetic appreciation, each illuminated by the others. Perhaps most important 's the influence of an instructor's personality on the personality of a child.

Applied to the student, education is a process of self-growth, a process within the student, and not something imposed from without. It is the leading out of self-growth. Education implies the ability to utilize knowledge and apply meaning and value to it. Education is an expression of a person's capacity to penetrate and deal relevantly with significant problems. It relates what we know to what we need and want. It is represented in our capacity for reflection and analysis and in our ability to examine basic assumptions and make valid distinctions and interpretations. It enables us to discriminate, to appraise, and to evaluate people as well as material things and concepts. Thus a teacher is not just a conveyor of knowledge, but an expeditor of learning and a tiller of dreams.

Public health program encompasses all of society's organized efforts to deal with the problems of prevention of disease, extension of life, and the promotion of well-being. This concept was first advanced by C.-E. A. Winslow,* one of America's revered leaders in public health. This definition conceives or-

*Winslow, C.-E. A.: The untilled fields of public health, Science **51**:23, 1920.

ganized, voluntary health work as an integral part of the public health program.

School health program means the prepared course of action taken by the school in the interest of the health of the schoolchild and school personnel. It includes health services, health instruction, and healthful school living.

School health services include all school activities and procedures designed to affect the present health status of the youngster. This encompasses appraisal of student health, prevention and control of disease, prevention and correction of physical defects, health guidance and supervision, and emergency care.

Guidance is the organized process of helping children to understand and direct their abilities into the channels of life that will be most fruitful in terms of their interest, abilities, and opportunities.

Health guidance is concerned with acquainting individuals with ways in which they may discover and use their natural endowments so that they may live to their maximum capacities to the benefit of themselves and society. Guidance means accepting each pupil as an independent personality.

Guidance services consist of analysis of individual students, availability of information service and counseling, and follow-up. As members of the school guidance team, health personnel can contribute effectively to these services. Organized health guidance makes health instruction more effective through focusing the students' interest on the appraisal of their own health status and thus making health knowledge personally identifiable and more meaningful to them.

Counseling is a guidance procedure that is a mutual deliberation consisting of an exchange of ideas that will aid a child to comprehend his or her problem and understand its solution. Whether directive or nondirective, counseling is essentially a matter of mutual advisement—of deliberating together.

Health instruction is the planned and incidental imparting of formal and informal health information. It may be a lecture, a class discussion, a laboratory situation, or individual tutoring. It carries the connotation of something from the outside directed to children for their understanding.

Health education means the growth within a child of his or her ability to develop health knowledge and to utilize and apply meaning to it. Health education implies the growth of a child's ability to discriminate, appraise, and evaluate health knowledge and experience. The best health instruction in the world can result in education only when there is a candle of interest in the child that can be lit. Motivation sparks education.

Correlation means mutual relationship, and the task of health instruction in school health is to connect those various aspects of the school curriculum that have a relation to health. Home economics, biological science, social studies, and other disciplines have health contributions that should be utilized.

Integration denotes the unification of different elements into a whole. Ideally, there should be but one subject in school—life itself—but educators have not yet devised the procedure nor developed the skill for a complete integration of the school program. Yet integration is possible to a considerable degree. Many activities include health aspects as well as other factors, and opportunities for experience in health are afforded in many of the daily school experiences of children. Health is usually more than a by-product, but even as a by-product the health experience can be valuable.

Sanitation denotes the health of the physical environment. Its derivation from the Latin *sanitas* (health) maintains the aura of the emphasis the Romans gave to environ-

mental health. Formerly sanitation was limited primarily to the prevention of the spread of disease. Today sanitation goes beyond water purification, sewage disposal, and insect control and includes positive factors such as lighting and ventilation, as well as esthetic factors such as attractive school premises and community housekeeping.

Healthful school living means conditions and manners of existing and experiencing that permit effective accomplishment and joy in the experience. It means a safe, sanitary, esthetic, and wholesome physical environment in which children can participate in normal activity with a minimum of interference, disturbance, and frustration.

A *mentally healthful school environment* is one in which all the children are at ease, have a high level of self-esteem, feel their classmates and instructor hold them in high regard, feel they can succeed, do succeed, and enjoy their success.

QUESTIONS AND EXERCISES

1. Why are the nations with the highest level of health in the vanguard in political, economic, social, and other advances, and, conversely, why are nations in the vanguard of political, economic, and social advances also the nations with the highest level of health?
2. What persons or programs in the school and in the general community contribute to the school health program?
3. What is the relationship between a civilization's philosophy and its health practices?
4. How do you account for the fact that in the United States the modern public health movement, the public education movement, and the modern school health movement date from the same period?
5. What was the significance of Shattuck's 1850 *Report of the Sanitary Commission of Massachusetts* with respect to the development of school health in the United States?
6. Evaluate the statement, Where or when the benefits of the school health program end, no one knows.
7. Why did the early interest in child study hasten the promotion of the school health movement?
8. Evaluate the statement, There is less need for

school health programs today than there was 50 years ago.

9. Why was the National Association for the Study and Prevention of Tuberculosis of great importance to the school health movement?

10. What are the advantages in having school health education recognized as an academic discipline in its own right?

11. What characteristics of the United States make it a natural place or environment in sich school health programs may flourish?

12. Give some illustrations of field research in school health.

13. What developments in the past decade do you consider to be of major importance to health education?

14. What is meant by the integration of health activities in schools?

15. What does the term "social engineering" mean to you?

16. To what extent has the school health program development been a revolutionary movement, and to what extent has it been an evolutionary one?

17. What are the purposes on which a school health program should be based?

18. What has been the effect of regulation in the development of health education?

19. Distinguish between health education, health teaching, and health instruction.

20. To what extent is health counseling also health education?

21. What is your reaction to the statement, Health education is synonymous with disease prevention.

REFERENCES

American Alliance for Health, Physical Education, and Recreation: Professional preparation in safety education and school health education, Washington, D.C., 1974, The Association.

Bruess, C. E., editor: Professional Preparation of the Health Educator. Report of the ASHA Committee on Professional Preparation and College Health Education Conference at Towson State University, January 29-30, 1976, J. School Health 46(7):418-421, Sept., 1976.

Castile, A. S., and Jerrick, S. J.: School health in America: a survey of state school health programs, Kent, Ohio, 1976, American School Health Association.

Means, R. K.: Historical perspectives on school health, Thorofare, N. J., 1975, Charles B. Slack, Inc.

National Center for Health Education: Brochure, San Francisco, 1978, National Center for Health Education.

Ogden, H. G.: Recent developments in health education policy, SOPHE Health Education Monographs (suppl. 1) **6**:67-73, 1978.

Preventive Medicine USA: Health promotion and consumer health education, New York, 1976, Prodist.

Report from the Governor's Steering Committee on Social Problems on Health and Hospital Services and Cost, New York, 1971, State of New York.

Report of the President's Committee on Health Education, Washington D.C., 1973, U.S. Government Printing Office.

Schaller, W. E.: Professional preparation and curriculum planning, J. School Health 48(4):236-240, April, 1978.

Society for Public Health Education Ad Hoc Task Force on Professional Preparation and Practice: Guidlines for the preparation and practice of professional health educators, SOPHE Health Education Monographs, 5(1):75-89, Spring, 1977.

U.S. Department of Health, Education and Welfare: Forward plan for health, 1977-1981, Washington, D.C., 1975, U.S. Government Printing Office.

U.S. Department of Health, Education and Welfare: Forward plan for health, 1978-1982, Washington, D.C., 1976a, U.S. Government Printing Office.

U.S. Department of Health, Education and Welfare: Health in America: 1776-1976, Washington, D.C., 1976b, U.S. Government Printing Office.

SELECTED READINGS

Alder, S.: Health and education of the economically deprived child, St. Louis, 1968, Warren H. Green, Inc.

American Council on Education, Commission on Teacher Education (Armstrong, W. E., editor): A design for general education, Washington, D.C., 1944, American Council on Education.

American Medical Association: Suggested school health policies, ed. 5, Chicago, 1966, American Medical Association.

Barrett, M.: Health education guide, ed. 2, Philadelphia, 1974, Lea & Febiger.

Birel, L., and Bay, J., editors: Health and leisure, West Haven, Conn., 1973, Pendulum Press, Inc.

Calder, R.: The lamp is lit: the story of WHO, Geneva, Switzerland, 1951, WHO Division of Public Information.

A design for general education, Washington, D.C., 1944, American Council on Education.

Flook, E. E., and Sanazaro, P., editors: Health services research and research and development, New York, 1973, Health Administrative Press.

Garrison, F. H.: An introduction to the history of medicine, ed. 4, Philadelphia, 1929, W. B. Saunders Co.

Health in schools, 20th yearbook, ed. 2, Washington, D.C., 1951, American Association of School Administrators.

Jefcoate, A.: Health and human values: an ecological approach, New York, 1972, John Wiley & Sons, Inc.

Kozh, R. C., et al., editors: Health information systems evaluation, Boulder, 1974, Colorado Associated University Press.

Leff, S., and Leff, V.: From witchcraft to world health, New York, 1957, The Macmillan Co.

Leff, S., and Leff, V.: Health and humanity, New York, 1962, International Publishers Co., Inc.

Lerner, M., and Anderson, W. W.: Health progress in the United States 1900-1960: a report of the Health Information Foundation, Chicago, 1963, University of Chicago Press.

Means, R. K.: A history of health education in the United States, Philadelphia, 1962, Lea & Febiger.

Paul, B. D., editor: Health, culture and community, New York, 1955, Russell Sage Foundation.

Pollock, M. B., and Oberteuffer, D.: Health science and the young child, New York, 1974, Harper & Row, Publishers.

Ravenel, M. P.: A half century of public health, New York, 1951, American Public Health Association.

Real, D. A., et al. In Zulch, J. C., editor: Concept of health, ed. 3, New York, 1973, The Macmillan Co.

School Health Education Study (Sliepcevich, E. M., Director): A summary report, Washington, D.C., 1967, National Education Association Publications.

Sigerist, H. E.: History of medicine, vols. I (1951) and II (1961), London, Oxford University Press, Inc.

Sigerist, H. E.: Landmarks in the history of hygiene, London, 1956, Oxford University Press, Inc.

Spiegelman, M.: Introduction to demography, Philadelphia, 1974, Lea & Febiger.

Ulich, R.: Three thousand years of educational wisdom, ed. 2, Cambridge, 1954, Harvard University Press.

Ulich, R.: History of educational thought, ed. 2, New York, 1968, American Book Co.

Winslow, C.-E. A.: The untilled fields of public health, Science **51**:23, 1920.

PART ONE

The school-age child

Health is a crown on the well person's head
but only the sick seem to see it.

Arab proverb

CHAPTER 2

Health of the normal child

The most important thing on earth is life, the most important form of life is human life, and the most important human life is one's own. Yet to the teacher the life of each child can be as precious as his or her own life. Certainly to the conscientious teacher, a child's health is as important as the teacher's health. No teaching service can yield greater results or provide greater personal gratification than what the teacher does to protect, maintain, and further the health of schoolchildren. Here is a professional opportunity for the teacher who understands children and their health and who applies this knowledge effectively.

While it is not necessary for all teachers to have a high level of health expertise, it is desirable that some teachers in key positions on the staffs of elementary schools have an intensive in-service program. In addition, a comprehensive health planning authority is recommended. Each school district should consider an organization of health teachers, nurses, parents, and students. These people should be expected to identify health problems and recommend solutions to these problems. Perhaps some schools would benefit by having health aides who can relieve regular teachers of the tasks of making teaching devices and preparing materials.

"Understand the child" is an admonition that applies equally to the prospective teacher and the teacher in the classroom. It is both logical and imperative that the teacher responsible for school health possess a sound understanding of children, their growth process, their health, and their health problems. It is the health of children that is the concern of the school's health program, and children themselves are the object of all health activity. More than this, professional preparation should develop in the teacher an attitude toward health that immediately focuses primary attention on the child and from this point proceeds to evolve an approach to any existing health problem. Just as the law student must develop a certain frame of mind and approach to problems of law, the health educator must develop an approach to problems of health that is founded on an understanding and appreciation of the individual child's health.

Health science is both a collective and an applied discipline. It integrates and utilizes the contributions of several fields of knowledge. There is nothing mystical about true health science, although there probably are more misconceptions about health than about any other sphere of human thought. For the person responsible for health in schools, certain fundamental concepts and essential knowledge can serve as the base of the pyra-

25

mid of competence in health promotion. The broader and more substantial the base, the higher and sturdier will be the pyramid. College preparation provides the base; growth on the job completes the structure.

A teacher does not have to attain the stature of the final authority—the general of the health army. Rather, the teacher is the frontline officer who comes in direct contact with the situation. The more accomplished the frontline health worker is, the more readily the true problems and situations are recognized and their immediate solution initiated. Extremely difficult or special problems are the responsibilities of specialists, who are available to deal with those problems requiring special tactics and techniques.

To be a competent health educator, the teacher does not need to be an expert. Experience has indicated that certain basic knowledge is adequate for the position the teacher rightfully should hold on the health team. Primarily, that basic knowledge is an understanding of normal growth and development, normal health status, and common deviations from the normal. A study of deviations does not imply that the educator is to be a diagnostician, but rather a "suspectitian." As an officer in the forefront of health, the teacher may well be in the best position to recognize first that a particular child does not appear to be normal in some respect.

In a book on school health, a discussion of the essentials of normal growth, mental development, and health should be concise and cogent, rather than comprehensive.

CONCEPT OF NORMAL

Normal is that which is accepted as the usual. It must be conceived of as encompassing a range of concepts, rather than a single entity. It includes the average, but extends considerably on both sides of average. No two persons are exactly alike; each is unique. Yet both persons may be considered within the normal range.

What constitutes the normal, or usual, is easy to determine in some instances, but extremely difficult to ascertain in others. To say with assurance that the normal range of glucose in human blood is between 0.08 and 0.14 mg/100 ml is easy because in more than 96% of analyzed blood samples the glucose content will fall in this range. Many physiological norms are well established; yet the normal range for certain physical measurements is not so easily set down. For example, what is the normal range of height for the American adult male? Should one arbitrarily say it is between 5 feet 4 inches and 6 feet 4 inches? What of the man who is 6 feet 5 inches in height? Should he be considered abnormal? This suggests the need for criteria. Should normal height be that which seems to be all right? Is the outer 10% or the outer 5% on each end of the array of heights for man to be considered as outside the normal? Very quickly it is recognized that for many physiological and physical phenomena there are no definite, prescribed normal ranges. Normal for the same factor may mean one thing at a time and a very different thing at another time.

If normal for physical factors is not a precise quantity, consider how variable it can be when applied to social and psychological phenomena. What is the normal range of emotional responsiveness of junior high school girls in situations involving frustrations such as failure of election to an office or to a group? Thus standards of normal social acceptance may vary from community to community, from school to school, and from family to family. Yet determining what is normal usually does not pose too difficult a problem.

In actual school practice, most cases fall definitely in the normal range, whether a physical, a psychological, or a social phenomenon is being considered. In the relatively few instances that are borderline, the decision of an expert or the collective judgment of several competent teachers can serve the needs of the school for that particular case. Even more important, many deviations from the normal are of little significance in terms of effective and enjoyable living. Every human being has imperfections, most of which go unnoticed or are accepted by this imperfect world of imperfect people. To be abnormal in some respects, perhaps, is normal.

THE HEALTHY CHILD

When health is regarded as that quality of well-being that enables one to live effectively and enjoyably, it must be considered a means to an end. To a person who is ill, health may be an end to be gained, but to the person who possesses health, it is a means to an end—a vehicle for effective and enjoyable living.

It is germane to the best interests of the youngsters in a schoolroom that the teacher be conscious of the health status of every child, whether the child has normal health or is ill or indisposed. The teacher must have a positive attitude or frame of mind and think in terms of the attributes or qualities of health each child possesses. It requires an evaluation of the native constitutional endowment of each child. The constitutional makeup of one child may be such that he or she has great vitality and almost unlimited energy, endurance, and ability to recover, even though neither the child nor the parents follow the accepted practices of good health promotion. Another child may possess a constitution that is adequate for typical living, but so near to inadequacy that every principle of health promotion must be practiced to maintain a normal level of health. Intergrades between these two types require thoughtful discrimination by the teacher who strives to understand the native health capacity of each child, just as he or she seeks to understand the native intellectual capacity of each child.

Normal health is to be appraised neither in terms of physical size nor in terms of muscular strength. The little fellow who appears to be underweight may possess an adequate level of health. Often these wiry little fellows seem to possess boundless energy, are on the go constantly, and recover quickly from fatigue. It may be desirable to add to such a child's weight, but he may be healthy "for a' that." It is more likely that the level of health of a grossly overweight child is lowered because of the excessive overweight.

In appraising a schoolchild's health in terms of the capacity to carry on the activities he or she wishes to and has a right to engage in, personality dynamics of the individual youngster must be given consideration. A student who is not aggressive, driving, and extremely active physically nevertheless may possess a high level of health, both physical and mental. The studious, industrious, methodical child may possess a level of health as adequate as that of the athletic child whose activity is so obvious.

It is the overall capacity of a child to measure up to life's demands that should be the cardinal criterion used by a teacher who attempts to appraise the health of a child. Health is one overall condition of well-being, and it encompasses the physical, mental, emotional, and social aspects of well-being.

OUTWARD INDICES OF PHYSICAL HEALTH

A clinical examination by a physician, supplemented by laboratory tests, would be necessary for a thorough inventory of a person's precise status of health, but for practical purposes a teacher can observe certain outward indices as a general gauge of health. These landmarks of health are of special significance in the school situation in which the teacher can observe the child 5 days a week and get a day-to-day inventory of

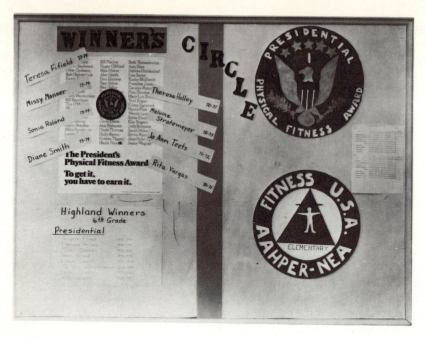

Fig. 2-1. Winner's circle. Promotion of physical fitness through recognition of students who have attained a high level of fitness. (Courtesy Salem Public Schools, Salem, Ore.)

each child's general pattern of health. Being thus familiar with the child's normal condition, the teacher readily will become aware of any deviation from the normal pattern. The teacher does not deal in the specifics of the diagnostician, but in the overall condition of the child.

When they are observed individually but evaluated collectively, certain outward indices or characteristics can convey a meaning of child health that is adequate for the needs of the teacher in guiding the child (Fig. 2-1). They can also be used to adapt the school program to the child and the child to his or her school needs. Of necessity, these indices are interpreted in relative terms, as follows.

1. *Buoyancy*. The healthy child possesses bounce or a feeling of lightness. Perhaps a concept of this attribute can be attained by visualizing the converse, the lack of buoyancy, which accompanies old age. The aged

feel heavy, associated with a feeling of chronic fatigue. However, healthy children convey the impression that they carry no weight, and they actually feel as though they have no particular physical restriction to movement.

2. *Unaware of the body*. Healthy children are not conscious of the existence of their bodies. This is somewhat true of healthy adults, but through various experiences adults have attained some awareness of their normal bodily existence. However, only in a diseased or disordered condition do children display any recognition of the existence of any part of their physical being.

3. *Pleasure in activity*. Every normal child delights in physical action. Restraint—physical or psychological—is both irritating and frustrating to the child. Teachers soon recognize that the solution to most restlessness in the classroom is an opportunity for physical action. A child who prefers not to be

active usually suggests a child not well physically or mentally.

4. *Sufficient vigor.* Healthy children possess the energy to do the things they want to do and can be expected to do in a normal day. This does not imply that children have a great deal of muscular power, but that they have a feeling of muscular power equal to the normal demands of their regimen of living.

5. *Zest.* A day's activity should be more stimulating than fatiguing. That children do not want to stop what they are doing though they have been at it for a long time and should be tired out is a very normal situation. They get tired but are so occupied with their very gratifying experiences that they are not conscious of any fatigue.

6. *Sleeps well and recovers from the day's fatigue.* Not all children function maximally at 9 o'clock in the morning. Some have a constitutional makeup that is slow to accelerate; others have been socially conditioned by the home or other influence to a slow pace in the morning. An alert teacher will quickly identify these types and will aid each child in acquiring a faster tempo of activity.

More serious are youngsters who come to school dragging one foot after the other. These children may come from homes in which they do not go to bed at a desirable hour.

Another type of child goes to bed at a proper hour, but sleeps poorly and comes to school looking and acting like a person who has had no sleep. This child needs the counsel of a physician to determine if there is a physical basis for the condition. Usually a low level of general function is the basic factor, rather than a specific disorder. The shuttled picture of poor health–inadequate rest, inadequate rest–poor health is frequent in these cases.

Although most children occasionally may show indications of inadequate rest, continued week-by-week indications of inadequate rest merit a study of basic causes and a constructive program of readjustment.

7. *Relaxation.* Being at ease in the school situation is necessary for good health and is an indication of good health. An occasional short-lived display of tension is to be expected in most children, but a child who is constantly tense is not a healthy child of today or a healthy adult of tomorrow. Tenseness must be displaced by ease and relaxation in the normal channels of life.

8. *Appetite steady and not capricious.* A finicky appetite may be the product of improper or negligent rearing in the home, but more often it is associated with a low level of health. Which is cause and which is effect are for a physician to determine, but a poor appetite is a symptom of the need for constructive attention by the school.

Occasionally, any normal youngster will have a transitory loss of appetite. It may be the result of such a simple thing as an inopportune sampling of sweets. Or it may be the result of fatigue, a cold, other mild infection, or special concern about some situation—real or imagined. However, the teacher should be concerned about a child with a chronically poor appetite.

9. *No appreciable variation in weight.* During his or her school-age years, a child experiences a steady increase in weight. Variation in the rate of increase is to be expected and is normal, but a child whose weight fluctuates appreciably is in need of a thorough physical checkup. Included in this category are children who lose 3 or 4 pounds in a week for no discernible cause and may regain the weight just as mysteriously, only to go through the same down-and-up cycle again. Failure to maintain a stabilized body weight is a symptom of a lack of constitutional stability. While the normal body is in a delicate state of equilibrium, constantly shifting slightly away from center then back again,

a balance, or homeostasis, is maintained. A small degree of fluctuation in bodily phenomena is normal; pronounced fluctuation is not normal.

10. *Absence of disabling remediable defects.* Freedom from defects that limit the effectiveness of one's activities is essential to optimum health. Some defects are not disabling. Even the loss of a finger or toe may not be disabling. Some defects are not remediable, and thus the health potential of a child must be weighed accordingly. Fortunately, many defects can be corrected or compensated for. Hearing aids can give normal hearing to persons with some hearing defects.

Most defects that are overlooked in school-children are minor ones that in their present state are not noticeably disabling. However, through the years their cumulative effect can be considerable, even though they do not become more aggravated. The presence of a so-called minor disabling defect lowers the child's health level, perhaps even to subnormal levels.

ATTRIBUTES OF MENTAL HEALTH

Since every child is unique, it would seem that an evaluation of mental health would have to be an individual matter, applied to each particular child. Strictly speaking, perhaps this would be true for detailed or specialized purposes, but children, although different, are not so tremendously different. For the purposes of the school, certain optimum attributes should be identifiable in every child. Although each child in his or her normal maturation exhibits variations in emotional responsiveness, the same fundamental attributes provide the framework or timber of mentally healthy persons. By the same token these are the qualities the school should strive to develop in each child to assure a high level of adjustment during both childhood and adulthood.

1. *High level of self-esteem.* Every child should have a feeling of worthiness, that others regard him or her highly. A child who knows he or she has something to live up to rather than something to live down has a first essential for a high level of adjustment.

2. *Obtain self-gratification through avenues approved by society.* Every child is self-centered and seeks to gratify his or her ego. Society recognizes this desire for self-gratification, but lays down rules by which this gratification may be attained. By precept and example children learn the ways of the world.

3. *Security.* No person attains absolute security, but normal children seek and need acceptance by their own group.

4. *Confidence.* All children have a feeling of inferiority, but through the acquisition of skill and experience much of this feeling can be displaced by confidence.

5. *Courage.* Children with the courage to face new situations and difficult tasks have a valuable asset for effective and enjoyable living. In contrast, fear of failure is a liability in childhood as well as in adulthood.

6. *Stability.* No person is perfectly stable, but mood and conduct should fluctuate within a relatively narrow range.

7. *Orderliness.* Some degree of order is essential for both efficient and gratifying living.

8. *Adaptability.* Life changes constantly, and good mental health requires flexibility to adjust to changes with a minimum of friction and disturbance.

9. *Self-discipline.* Perhaps no one is perfectly self-disciplined, but the mentally healthy person is usually master of his or her actions, rather than a slave to whim, caprice, or indolence.

10. *Self-reliance.* Although interdependence typifies the complex society of our country, within that framework, well-adjusted persons depend on their own resources and rely on others as a last resort.

They have both stamina and the ability to mobilize their resources under stress.

11. *Sincerity.* Everyone appreciates and even admires a sincere person.

12. *Emotional control.* When the self is frustrated, negative emotions naturally are aroused, but to attain the highest levels of mental health, a person must learn to restrain these emotions and substitute reasoned conduct. Although this practice will not enable one to reach a stage at which negative emotions will never arise, the control one acquires will conceal their existence and display the poise of a well-integrated personality.

13. *Quick recovery from disturbing experiences.* All persons encounter disturbing experiences and even tragedies, but a well-integrated person, although he or she is disturbed emotionally, recovers rather quickly. A high degree of sensitivity hardly furnishes the child with the necessary timber for this rugged life.

14. *Confidence in the ability to succeed and enjoyment of success.* No person enjoys a situation in which he or she is failing. Occasional failure is the lot of all, but constant failure is injurious to mental health. Children who feel they can succeed, do succeed, and fully appreciate and enjoy their success have valuable ingredients for mental health.

15. *Moderation in daydreaming.* Every normal person enjoys the luxury of daydreaming, and in moderation daydreaming can contribute to mental health. The child who is submerged in excessive daydreaming and rarely lives in the world of reality needs to be brought into the world of doing.

16. *Congeniality.* Whereas happiness is a level of elation that a normal person acquires only occasionally and retains but a short period of time, the normal emotional mold or temperament should be cheerful and congenial.

17. *Perception of humor.* Normal chil-

dren learn that some things in life are incongruous or funny. From these they get an enjoyable experience whether their laughter is a response to frustration or a feeling of superiority because they see the unusual aspects of the situation. Humor is an excellent buffer for the rigors of life. To achieve the highest expression of humor in terms of mental health, children should learn to laugh at themselves. Persons who can look at themselves as objectively as that have the antidote for their inherent egocentricity. It is an attribute of children with the highest level of mental health.

18. *Sincere interest in other persons.* Basic to good social adjustment is an active, sincere interest in other people. A child who likes other persons intensely will experience no self-consciousness, embarrassment, or loneliness. Altercentricity (self-gratification through interest in others) is the key to successful social adjustment because an interest in people telegraphs itself. People who know that a particular person likes them usually hold that person in high regard. A sincere liking for people is an acquired attribute, one that makes conversation more easy and enhances one's social activities.

LEVELS OF HEALTH

Almost all the children in classrooms fall within the range of normal health. Yet the teacher knows that the quality of these students' health varies. As a practical guide for the teacher and the student, a grading system can be devised to designate various levels of health. Although such a scale, like any other appraisal system, does not provide for refined discriminations, it does provide a workable means for evaluating the general quality of a child's health.

A level. A high level of health, but not perfect health, is indicated by this classification. A person with this quality of health may have an occasional cold or other minor infection, perhaps an occasional headache or other mild disturbance. Freedom from disabling remediable defects is an obvious requirement. Youngsters in this category display pronounced vigor and buoyancy and sufficient vitality to carry on the demands of life. This does not connote great muscular power and endurance, but more than enough strength and endurance for any likely eventuality. It does not include physical size. A child of small physical stature as well as a child with average or large stature can have an A level of health. The child in this health category enjoys life, participates wholesomely in normal activities, and adjusts well to social situations.

B level. Freedom from disabling defects is a primary requirement in this category. Persons in this group do not have quite the vigor and buoyancy of the A level. Many in this classification can attain the higher level of health by conscientious application of health principles.

C level. Persons in this classification pass as well, but lack the vitality for a dynamic mode of living. They go through life functioning at a minimum—not sick, but draggy, rather than buoyant like people with good health. Many can attain an A level of health, and most can attain at least a B level of health. There should be no school child with a C level of health.

D level. Children in this classification attend school regularly, but are not well. A chronic infection or some other apparent or concealed factor or factors are the basic cause of the low level of health. Until the cause is discovered and remedied, the child is not likely to improve his or her level of health. The teacher or other school personnel should be aware of the state of health of these children and take the proper steps to safeguard their welfare. School obviously is not the place for them. Even children with a low level of vitality, but without specific de-

fects or diseases, should be under the supervision of a physician.

E level. Children in this classification are obviously ill and should not be in school; usually they are not.

INDIVIDUAL VARIATIONS

Not all children will be tall and not all will be short; the fact that a child is small for his or her age does not indicate a low level of health. An elementary school principal relates an experience with a third-grade youngster who was much below the height of his classmates. A health conference was held in which the boy's teacher, the school nurse, and the principal developed a special program to help Tony to grow. Nutrition (adding midmorning and midafternoon lunches) included a noonday lunch high in proteins, vitamins, and minerals. A half hour rest period following a moderate exercise period completed the program for Tony's growing up.

Just before the Christmas vacation the school held its annual program to which all parents were invited and even urged to attend. Among the parents were a father just over 5 feet tall and his wife, who was 2 inches less than 5 feet tall. Unknowingly, Tony's parents taught the school staff that their best intentions may be useless without full knowledge of all the factors involved.

That variations exist from person to person and from day to day for a given person are common observations. When the concept of variations is applied to child health, the important task is to identify the particular differences by having a unified, almost catalogued concept of the status of each child's health. Each child is unique and has a particular constitution with which he or she functions. The teacher should identify the particular health entity in each child and thus immediately recognize any deviations from the established pattern.

Children with a constitutional makeup of decidedly marked limitations will exhibit more fluctuations in health than other children and may be the cause of special concern to the teacher. Yet all children are susceptible to variation in their state of well-being—all the way from a slight indisposition to serious disorders. Each child merits the best efforts of the teacher in appraising his or her health status and any deviation from this health state.

School-age youngsters with chronic disabilities of varying severity may require special measures. It is desirable that these children feel they are normal members of the class. If the impression that they are abnormal is created, they may feel stigmatized by both themselves and their classmates. School-age children who have had rheumatic fever or have diabetes mellitus, asthma, or epilepsy do pose problems for the school, but knowledge and planning will enable the school staff to deal satisfactorily with these problems. The school should insist that a physician, perferably the family physician, determine the needs of the child and, in consultation with the school, outline the school's course of action in providing for the child's best interests.

BUILDING UP AND MAINTAINING HEALTH

For the normal school-age child, the primary health consideration is to build up and maintain the highest possible level of health. No child has a quality of health beyond improvement, and no child can be expected to maintain the health he or she has attained without following the course of living necessary for the conservation of the dynamic processes of life itself. A program designed to promote health will both build up and maintain health at one and the same time. Such a program of health promotion is one in which the person adapts established health principles to his or her specific needs and assiduously applies these principles in everyday practice. This would include principles of nutrition, activity, rest, sleep, safety, oral health, vision, hearing, cleanliness, control of communicable diseases, prevention of degenerative diseases, and social adjustment.

Because the benefits that accrue from sound health practices are not spectacular, children (and adults) are prone to be doubtful of the value of these practices. The long-range effects are the real sources of health dividends, and long-range vision is needed to see the total results. Although the specific manner in which certain recognized practices promote health is not scientifically established, the general cause-and-effect relationship has been ascertained sufficiently to warrant their use with assurance of health benefits. As more refined aspects of these principles are worked out or as new principles are developed, they will be profitably incorporated into the matrix of health practices.

CONSERVATION OF HUMAN RESOURCES

The school deals in futures. While it concerns itself with the children of today, it always projects its goals to the young man and woman of tomorrow, the mature man and woman of the following day, on to late adulthood.

Surely the most important thing in the universe is life, the most important form of life is human life, and the most important human life is one's own. Humans are the most restless and most widely dispersed living form and have the greatest adaptive capacity. Humans have a remarkable ability to bend nature to their will, but frequently they find that when they solve one problem, they actually create another. The school must remember that, while it is interested in advancing health practices in the young that will postpone death, it must also consider health problems that relate to the process of aging and the aged, along with measures to promote health during the early years of life. Certainly the school can play a vital role in the conservation of human resources.

The conservation of human resources means the husbanding of all factors that will help to (1) postpone death, (2) increase the quality of health, and (3) extend the prime of life.

Death cannot be prevented, but it can be postponed. In our present-day complex society, survival is not just an individual matter. One must rely on the collective efforts of the community to deal with those factors that he or she, as an individual, cannot cope with alone. In their school experiences children learn the community agencies and forces that exist to aid them in their quest for survival. A well-informed person profits most from the services of community health agencies. Since a reciprocal relationship exists between personal and community health, the way in which each person lives affects the community both directly and indirectly.

PROMOTING THE HEALTH OF STUDENTS

Generally speaking, most school teachers recognize a professional responsibility to safeguard and promote the health of all schoolchildren. Unfortunately, many teachers handicap themselves because they feel inadequate to provide students with meaningful opportunities for self-development. Teachers ask, How does one recognize opportunities for effective teaching? Or, How does one create situations that are ripe for learning? How can a teacher involve students in the diversity of health experiences that occur in the daily school life and make these experiences into health opportunities?

A structured, didactic health instruction program has merit as the basic plan of teaching procedure, but such learning does not produce the most meaningful and lasting health education. Teachers recognize their responsibility for preparing children to guide their own health. But teachers who are conscientious encounter frustrations in filling the gap between recognized health principles and the application of these principles to the life-style of the students. How does one create situations and a diversity of experiences for children so that health knowledge can be most applicable and most meaningful? The following suggestions are offered to give the teacher an insight into means by which health principles can be related to pupil needs and comprehension.

Giving attention to the health status of school youngsters is the first and most valuable contribution a teacher can make toward children's health. Complimenting youngsters who carry on good health practices will fortify the benefits students derive from their health activities. Using the motivation of all children in a class will add to the health promotion of every child. Such a program day in and day out will have some eventual health benefits largely because of the child's own motivation, developed as a by-product of the atmosphere in his or her schoolroom.

Thus it is apparent that all teachers can assist all normal youngsters to further their health status. An ongoing awareness of the value of health and its promotion is a service all teachers can contribute to all normal children.

Fortunately no normal schoolchild knows what his or her particular cause of death will be, but from records he or she can learn which are the most numerous causes of death at various ages. Armed with this knowledge, which should be acquired in school health education, the child can be better prepared to survive. The guiding force in life for a prospective adult is the positive approach of what to do to survive, rather than the negative approach of what causes death.

Not how long one lives, but how well one lives is important. A high level of health in childhood, based on established sound health practices, is the best possible prologue to a high level of health in adulthood. Proper nutrition, proper rest, and other essential health practices during childhood yield their greatest dividends in later years.

To extend the prime of life is a more recent goal of health science. The normal aging process involves a multitude of changes. Normal for one age or period of life is not normal for another. Normal is a series of variables and changes from age period to age period. The United States has made tangible progress in the conservation of the vigor and efficient function of young adults. The typical 60-year-old person of today possesses about the same health index as did a person 50 years of age at the turn of the century. If during early years he or she avoided health practices injurious to his or her well-being and followed the principles that conserve and promote good health, a person 60 years of age need not feel old. Studies reveal that chronic, low-grade infections, unattended over extended periods of time, have an adverse effect on the level of health of middle-age persons. The same effect results from gross overweight or undue tension. On the positive side, persons who have lived well-regulated, moderate lives and who have relaxed regularly rather than succumbed to the tensions of life enjoy a long youth and an extended prime of life. How well does my motor idle? is a question young and old alike should ask themselves.

QUESTIONS AND EXERCISES

1. To what extent is the field of health both a science and an art?
2. Why is homeostasis an important indicator of the level of physical health?
3. What, if any, attention should th
   program give to the subject of dea
4. What should the school do about
   viously is of the D level of health
   ents nevertheless keep sending th
5. What is the difference between go
   good health?
6. Appraise the contention that the real health dividends of the school health program will accrue to the youngster 25 years after he or she is out of school.
7. What is meant by the extension of the prime of life, and why do modern health scientists regard this highly as an objective of the health program?
8. What is the responsibility of the school to understand the present health of each child?
9. "Youngsters are all different but not so greatly different." What are the implications of this quotation?
10. "The most difficult task in health education is to develop an appreciation of health in a child who already has good health." Appraise this quotation.
11. How will the physical health of a pupil affect his or her mental health?
12. When a teacher has reason to believe that a certain student under his or her supervision does not have normal health, who should the teacher contact?
13. Why do we say that for the normal child health is a means to an end?
14. What is normal in one situation may not be normal in another situation. How do you appraise this statement?
15. What would you regard as the best single index of normal mental health?
16. Why is it important that all teachers have a basic knowledge of health?
17. What significance do you place on the health of the teacher?
18. Differentiate between optimum and maximum health.
19. In your judgment, which is of greater importance to schoolchildren—their education or their health, and what is the basis for your conclusion?
20. Is it sound educational policy to treat a child with a defect as you treat other children?

REFERENCES AND SELECTED READINGS

American Alliance for Health, Physical Education, and Recreation: Completed research in health, physical education and recreation, vol. 16, Washington, D.C., 1974, The Alliance.

American Association for Health, Physical Education, and Recreation and National Association of Secondary School Principals: Fitness for secondary school youth,

Washington, D.C., 1956, American Association for Health, Physical Education and Recreation.

American Association for Health, Physical Education, and Recreation: School health services, Washington, D.C., 1964, The Association.

American Association for Health, Physican Education, and Recreation: Suggested school health policies, revised ed., Washington, D.C., 1966, The Association.

American Association for Health, Physical Education, and Recreation: Healthful school environment, 1969, Washington, D.C., The Association.

American Association for Health, Physical Education, and Recreation: Health appraisal of school children, ed. 4, Washington, D.C., 1970, The Association.

American Council on Education, Commission on Teacher education: Helping teachers understand children, Washington, D.C., 1965, The Council.

Babcock, D. E.: Introduction to growth, development and family life, ed. 3, Philadelphia, 1972, F. A. Davis Co.

Bach, M.: The power of total living, New York, 1977, Dodd, Mead & Co.

Beyer, M. K., et al.: Positive health: designs for action, ed. 2, Philadelphia, 1976, Lea & Febiger.

Clark, R. L., and Cumley, R. W.: The book of health, ed. 3, New York, 1977, Harcourt Brace Jovanovich, Inc.

Crawford, C. D., editor: Health and the family, New York, 1972, The Macmillan Co.

Ellis, R. B.: Child health and development, New York, 1966, Grune & Stratton, Inc.

English, O. S., and Pearson, G. H. J.: Emotional problems of living, ed. 3, New York, 1976, W. W. Norton & Co., Inc.

Haag, J. H.: School health program, ed. 3, New York, 1972, Holt, Rinehart & Winston.

Haag, J. H.: Consumer health products and services, Philadelphia, 1976, Lea and Febiger.

Haggerte, R. J., et al.: Child health and the community, New York, 1975, John Wiley & Sons, Inc.

Hall, G. S.: Aspects of child life and education, New York, 1975, Arno Press, Inc.

Harvard Child Health Project: Developing a better health care system for children, vol. 3, Philadelphia, 1977, Ballinger Publishing Co.

Hurlock, E. B.: Child development, ed. 6, New York, 1978, McGraw-Hill Book Co.

Illingworth, R. S.: The normal child, ed. 6, Atlanta, 1975, Churchill Livingston.

Jenne, F. H., and Greene, W. H.: Turner's school health and health education, ed. 7, St. Louis, 1976, The C. V. Mosby Co.

Johnson, W.: Health in action, New York, 1977, Holt, Rinehart & Winston.

Joint Committee on Health Problems in Education: Health appraisals of school children, ed. 3, Washington, D.C., 1961, National Education Association.

Jones, K. et al.: Health science, ed. 3, New York, 1975, Harper & Row, Publishers.

Knotts, G. R., and McGovern, J. P.: School health, Springfield, Ill., 1974, Charles C Thomas, Publisher.

Nemir, A., and Shaller, W. E.: The school health program, ed. 4, New York, 1975, W. B. Saunders Co.

Pollock, M. B., and Oberteuffer, D.: Health science and the young child, New York, 1974, Harper & Row, Publishers.

Tanner, L. N., and Lindgren, H. C.: Classroom teaching and learning: a mental health approach, New York, 1971, Holt, Rinehart & Winston.

Wallis, E. L., and Logan, G.: Exercise for children, Englewood Cliffs, N. J., 1966, Prentice-Hall, Inc.

Wheatley, G. M., and Hallock, G. T.: Health observation of school children, ed. 3, New York, 1965, McGraw-Hill Book Co.

Growth is always more and more but can be
better and better when properly nurtured.

Anonymous

CHAPTER 3

Physical growth and development

The school deals in futures. How the child develops into the mature adult is a concern of the school. Physical growth and development are no less important than other phases of the evolving youngster. Physical growth and development represent a special phase in the maturing process, but are entwined in the total pattern of maturation. Understanding physiological change and the rate of change enables the teacher to understand each youngster in terms of his or her own particular development and relationship to the normal pattern. It is fascinating to watch the development of a child. It is most fascinating when one has a scholarly understanding of the developmental process.

Growth and development are individual matters, each child being distinctive. However, there are typical or recognized ranges of growth into which most children fall. A conscientious teacher is eager to understand each child in terms of his or her patterns of growth and development. Perhaps the teacher should think of the child as a "human becoming." After all, human beings require one-third of their life span to reach maturity, and the school deals in that future.

GROWTH—CELLULAR AND INTERCELLULAR

Growth occurs at the cellular level in three different ways: (1) increase in the size of the cells, (2) increase in the number of cells by cell division or multiplication, and (3) increase of the substance between the cells (intercellular).

This cellular growth consists of the addition of proteins, carbohydrates, fat, water, and minerals to the cell substance. Although vitamins are not directly involved, their regulatory function is also necessary. At least 45 nutrients are needed for healthy growth. However, recent research has led to the conclusion that the most important elements required are proteins and calories. Growth is work, and calories are the units providing the fuel for the energy needed to grow.

Calories are needed for cell multiplication, whereas protein is related primarily to increase in the size of cells. Elements of the major food groups, including carbohydrates, fats, and proteins, can be oxidized and used for energy. However, food must also provide the necessary raw materials for the growth and replacement of cells and cell products.

37

All the molecules of the body must either be obtained directly from the food that is eaten or must be synthesized from other compounds in the diet.

Some molecules are needed in great numbers because they form the structural material making up the tissues of muscle, bone, and cell membranes. Other molecules, such as vitamins, are required in lesser amounts because they are involved in the activities of the enzymes of the body. Although enzymes control chemical reactions, they are not used up in the reaction but can be used repeatedly.

Intercellular growth consists of the addition of organic and inorganic materials between cells. Fat, calcium, phosphate, or other substances retained between cells, although having a relation to the cells, must be considered a part of body growth if they are added to the total mass. Intercellular calcium is the principal constituent of bone growth. The noncellular part of tissue undergoes considerable increase in mass during the stage of physical growth of life.

DEVELOPMENT OR MATURATION

Development or maturation is an increase in the complexity and effectiveness of bodily functions, whereas growth usually refers to an increase in size. For example, there is relatively little difference in the physical size of the head of a 3-month-old infant and that of a 16-year-old adolescent. But obviously, the changes that have occurred over this period in the nature and complexity of the brain and its capacity to function are enormous.

In comparing the maturational differences between infancy and childhood, a comparatively shorter period of time, the 3-month-old infant is still a bundle of reflexes dominated by the need for food, warmth, and rest, whereas the child of 5 years, about to enter school, has already developed a wide range of abilities and skills.

As Krogman expresses it, "The postnatal growth period of twenty years is like a race: we all run it, but some run it fast and some run it slow." Thus at any point in time during this period some are biologically ahead and some are behind.

An individual's pattern of growth and development is unique. Because of this uniqueness of individual development, the concept of biological age has come into use. Standards have now been established for determining an individual's maturity by using x-ray examinations of the wrist or knee joints. Experimental investigations using standards of skeletal age are able to establish the degree of maturity quite accurately. Skeletal age (SA) is determined by the number of ossification centers and the amount of cartilage material separating those centers from the main body of bony structure in the extremity. Separation means that the epiphysis is open and that the limb or bone is still growing. Gradually these bony centers grow together, converting the cartilaginous material into bone and concluding growth in adult maturity.

Fig. 3-1, which is based on x-ray films taken by J. Roswell Gallagher, M.D., former Chief of Adolescent Medicine of Children's Hospital in Boston, illustrates the growth maturity or skeletal age differences between two adolescent boys who are of the same chronological age, 14 years and 11 months. The illustration on the left reveals a skeletal age rating of 13 years and 6 months, whereas the bone development pictured on the right is considered to be 16 years and 10 months. This represents a maturational difference of nearly 3½ years, thus demonstrating the necessity for school officials to consider more than chronological age when classifying students for athletic competition or evaluating age group performances. Tables portraying averages in growth and development are useful, but so-called normal development encompasses a very wide range of differences.

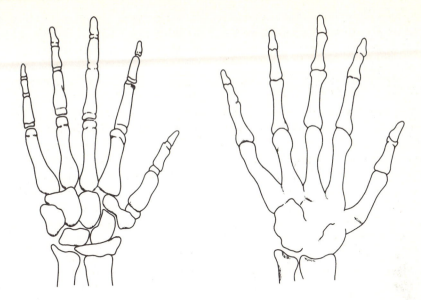

Fig. 3-1. Variations in skeletal age.

In addition to these differences in growth patterns of normal children, there are variations caused by calorie and protein deprivation. Such malnourished children may never attain their normal complement of cells. Lack of protein in the diet will cause their cell growth to be limited, resulting in smaller stature throughout their growth period and into adulthood.

Since the various systems of the body develop at differing rates, it is desirable that a teacher have an understanding of the patterns of maturation of the various systems. Their separate as well as composite developmental patterns can be the avenue through which the teacher may better understand each child and thus better serve his or her interests.

BIOLOGICAL DETERMINATION

Potential biological growth and development are determined at fertilization. The genetic combinations at that moment set the biological potential and limit for both.

Inheritance. Growth and development are governed or regulated primarily by the hor-

mones of the body, and a child's genetic endocrine endowment is the is the principal asset for both growth and development. General body size depends on the output of *somatotropin*, the principal growth hormone, which is produced by the anterior pituitary gland. Carbohydrate, fat, and water balance are affected by other secretions from this gland. Thyroxin from the thyroid gland governs the growth of long bones, the rate at which energy is used, and the rate at which the body matures. Sex hormones affect maturation as well as determine secondary sex characteristics. *Cortin*, the principal secretion of the adrenal cortex, which is located at the tip of the kidneys, markedly affects the rate of maturation. An overactive adrenal cortex produces precocious children.

Considering the hormones alone, geneticists calculate at least 40 million possible patterns of genetic endocrine endowment. The particular combination of factors that a child inherits appears to be a matter of mere chance. Once fertilization takes place, nothing can be done to change the inherited characteristics. Therefore a teacher who appreciates that there are many possible genetic combinations will likely have a better understanding and appreciation of each child in the class.

ENVIRONMENTAL FACTORS

No one attains the absolute genetic maximum in growth and development because environmental factors retard or obstruct normal processes. If it were possible to provide the perfect environment for all life processes, the individual doubtless would develop more rapidly than he or she presently does and would attain greater growth. This would entail a better internal bodily environment through scientifically perfected nutrition and respiration, as well as freedom from infection, and an external environment of temperature, humidity, and other factors that best permit processes to function.

A study of growth trends over the past century provides information on the effects of improved health care, improved nutrition, and a more healthful environment on the growth and development of the young. Data collected throughout this period have shown an increasingly earlier age of maturation and an increasing size with each succeeding generation. According to health officials, this universal trend among the young of the Western world has served as a good biological index of the effects of the environment. Although it is not likely that the perfect environment will ever be created to enable the individual to reach his or her maximum genetic growth potential, there are indications that humankind may be nearing this growth ceiling. For example, after observing several generations of Harvard youth, Damon (1968) has concluded that the growth trend has stabilized. The average heights of Harvard students are no longer increasing and, in fact, have leveled off and are now remaining at a consistent average height.

Damon's findings have been confirmed by a recent analysis of growth trends conducted by the National Center for Health Statistics (NCHS) (1976). A comparative analysis of the growth measurements taken from representative samples of children and youth from ages 2 to 18 years in the earlier 1960s shows that the average heights are essentially the same as those taken in the 1970s. It would seem that the average heights of children and youth have stabilized over the past 10 to 15 years. However, children in the lower end of the distribution of heights provide an exception. Those of the 5th and 10th percentile levels have continued to show slight increases in heights, whereas the heights of children at the twenty-fifth percentile levels and above have stabilized. A possible explanation of this fact is that more children from lower socioeconomic backgrounds constitute the 5th and 10th percentile levels of height. Therefore it would follow that these children have not had the full benefits of good nutrition and health care and would have a greater potential for improvement in health. A resulting increase in their heights would be more likely than would an increase in height in children from the upper socioeconomic levels.

Children from disadvantaged backgrounds become a special concern to the school. Although the school represents only a part of their total environmental influences, it can play a vital role in their healthy development. The school health services can protect and supervise the child's healthy growth by promoting the child's health through effective nutrition and health education. As was expressed in the NCHS report, "When the stragglers will finally achieve their genetic potential to full stature can probably be better predicted by economic and social factors than by biologic ones."

FULL-TERM INFANT

If the normal gestation period is estimated at 280 days after the beginning of the last menstruation, it is interesting to note that

35% of all births occur within one week on either side of this estimate and 65% of births occur within two weeks of it. A child who is born at 37 weeks of gestation (within 3 weeks of the 280 days) is considered a full-term infant.

Medical research has revealed that the early stages of pregnancy, between the second and tenth weeks, constitute the most important growth period of life. During this time cell differentiation takes place, and the special tissues of the limbs, eyes, ears, and vital organs are formed. Special emphasis should be given to protecting the mother's health during this period, because an illness or adverse condition may affect the intrauterine environment and damage the developing tissues of the fetus. For example, many childhood defects of hearing, vision, and vital function have been traced to an incident of German measles contracted by the mother during this first trimester.

Antibodies passing from the mother through the placenta to the developing fetus give the child an infantile immunity until about 6 months of age. The immunity may be against diphtheria, smallpox, tetanus, measles, and poliomyelitis. This does not give the child the ability to produce antibodies. Thus when the antibodies received from the mother disintegrate, the immunity ceases unless the child, in the meantime, has been immunized by other means.

Although usually smaller at birth, girls are about 1 month in advance of boys according to bone development or skeletal age measures. Girls entering school continue to be more mature in terms of skeletal age than are boys. (This advantage increases progressively to 12 years of age.)

PREMATURITY AND GROWTH RETARDATION

Until recently, all infants weighing less than 5½ pounds were classified as premature. However, results from medical research have shown that low birth weight may be caused by two distinct conditions: (1) prematurity or (2) growth retardation. Prematurity means that such infants are born before completing the normal period of intrauterine life (37 weeks). Therefore premature infants weigh less because they have not had enough time to grow and develop fully. On the other hand, growth-retarded infants may have been born after a full-term pregnancy of 40 weeks but still be far below average weight at birth. As many as one third to one half of the incidents of low birth weight are believed to be caused by conditions that retard normal growth. Among the factors believed to be responsible are inadequate placental development, insufficient blood supply to the uterus, genetic defects, the mother's health, and other environmental conditions.

A number of techniques are employed to distinguish between the premature and the growth-retarded infant. The ultrasonic sound device is used to measure fetal size, and a precise measure of the duration of pregnancy can be obtained by amniocentesis. Standards describing the various neuromuscular reflexes typical of the neurological behavior of the different stages of development are used. For example, the growth-retarded infant would be expected to demonstrate behavior patterns similar to those of the full-term infant with normal swallowing and sucking reflexes, whereas the premature infant would not display fully developed reflexes. In general, the premature infant would be expected to be behind the full-term infant in development.

At this time no one has been able to determine precisely what the long-term effects of low birth weight are on the individual. With proper medical care and supervision the premature infant may be expected to reach the developmental level of the full-term infant. However, research on identical twins shows that the smaller individual rarely reaches the same size as the other sibling.

CHARACTERISTICS OF THE PRESCHOOL CHILD

The period from infancy to the school years is a critical one for the child's growth and development. Recently, worldwide attention has been focused on the health and nutrition of very young children and the dramatic effects brought about by extreme malnutrition. Pictures of children from underdeveloped countries of the world suffering from marasmus or kwashiorkor stir a sense of concern and compassion in the viewer. But malnutrition is not restricted to distant lands. Actually the breast-fed infant from an underdeveloped country may be better nourished than an infant from the United States who is not breast-fed and fails to get an adequate diet from bottle feedings. It is after weaning that the infant from an underdeveloped nation suffers from malnutrition and diarrheal infection from unhygienically prepared food. As a result, these children suffer the severe effects of kwashiorkor, which retards their growth and leaves them dull and listless with the possibility of permanent brain damage. Research has shown that nutritionally deprived children may have brain cell counts 20% lower than those of normal children.

Recent surveys of child nutrition in the United States show that malnutrition exists in this country to a far greater extent than had been realized, and it is not restricted to poor children who do not get enough food or suffer from dietary deficiencies. Malnutrition also refers to the state of "overnutrition" that can be found in many children from financially stable families. They may suffer from a form of malnutrition that involves taking in too many calories. Overfed children may develop into obese children and adults. Some researchers believe that the consumption of too many calories causes the body to develop an excess of fat cells, thus predisposing the individual to a lifelong tendency to obesity and perhaps to the chronic diseases associated with that condition.

The preschool period marks a transition from the very rapid growth of infancy to the slower but steady, continuous growth of childhood. By the time children reach the age of 5 months, they will have doubled their birth weight. Moreover, their bodies will have changed from the rounded, plump appearance of infancy to the longer-limbed body type characteristic of childhood.

During this preschool period certain normal growth characteristics predispose children to upper respiratory illnesses. Tonsils and adenoidal tissue grow very rapidly, reaching full adult size by the time the child is 5 years old. This large growth of tissue in the relatively small nose and throat area of the child often encourages an infection in the middle ear. Since the child of this age has a shorter eustachian tube leading from the throat to the middle ear, bacterial infections often invade the middle ear. Such infections should receive prompt treatment in order to avoid a possible hearing loss. Teachers and parents should be alert to identify those children with hearing difficulty and a pattern of mouth breathing. Such a condition may indicate the presence of infection.

During the first 2½ years of the child's life, the cerebellum portion of the brain influences to a large extent the child's posture, coordination, and ability to perform certain movements. Efforts to teach neuromotor skills such as those that are involved in walking or in toilet training will be of no avail until such time as the child is "ready" developmentally, that is to say, until the neural pathways have been established. After a child has attained sufficient physical maturity, it has been demonstrated that preschool programs have a significant and positive effect on the child's development.

Among so-called normal children, there is a variation in physical, social, and intellectual maturity. Some lag behind, some are on schedule, and some race ahead. In a group of preschoolers a variation in maturation of

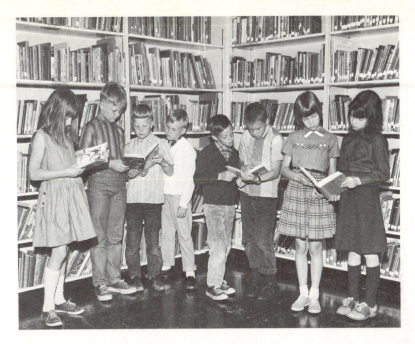

Fig. 3-2. Constitutional types. Only 3 months separate the ages of the oldest and youngest in the group. All are in the same grade and all have excellent health, although they are different.

6 months is not unusual (Fig. 3-2). This seemingly short period of time can represent, however, the equivalent of nearly one fourth of a young child's life span. Children whose birthdays occur in late summer or early fall may be as much as 10 to 11 months behind, chronologically. Such children may not be ready for school simply because of this lack of maturation. Pushing them ahead can lead to difficulty.

THE ELEMENTARY SCHOOL-AGE CHILD

Technically the elementary school growth period includes the time span from kindergarten up to and including the preadolescent growth spurt of puberty. However, since the timing of the growth spurt varies widely and often extends well into the middle or junior high school years, pubertal growth will be discussed with adolescence.

The growth stage of the early elementary school years has often been described as undramatic, as compared to the rapid growth changes that characterize both the earlier and later growth periods. The gradual and steady rate of growth that began in preschool continues well into the elementary school years. Children tend to become heavier in relation to their height. The tendency toward lower back curvature or lordosis ends, creating a more erect posture. During this period children lose all their primary teeth with the exception of the second and third molars, while acquiring their permanent teeth. These children may continue to have problems because of the abundance of lymphatic tissue that makes up the tonsils and adenoids. The presence of these disproportionately large tissues frequently blocks the child's eustachian tubes, causing middle ear infection and a temporary loss of hearing.

The preschool child usually is farsighted, which he or she does not outgrow until about the sixth year of age. At this time both the involuntary and voluntary muscles of accommodation mature to give the child the visual apparatus necessary for reading. At the 6-year level of visual maturity, a child can read large type (12 point), but not without sustained effort.

If a child is nearsighted, the condition usually appears early.

Eyestrain in school is not necessarily a deficiency in visual acuity, but may be a tendency of the relatively immature muscles of accommodation to fatigue very easily.

The normal eye reaches its maximum growth and acuity at the age of 12 years. It is the first organ to mature.

At 7 years of age children tend to become daring, adventuresome, boisterous, and vigorous in their play. Running, chasing, skating, jumping rope, bicycle riding, and swimming appeal to them. Joy, as an expression of self, motivates the child to master a skill that actually becomes a means to an end.

Manipulative skills begins to improve markedly at age 8 years. The child normally becomes progressively stronger and sturdier. Legs lengthen rather rapidly, but the rate of general body growth is slower. Considerable variation in muscular development and co-ordination occurs. The child fatigues quite easily, but recovers just as readily. At 8 years of age, the smaller muscles begin to be used, although not too skillfully. Marked improvement in manipulative skill and eye-hand co-ordination results in a surprisingly high level of dexterity.

By the age of 11 years rapid muscular growth has begun, particularly in the girl. At age 12 years a child attains a near-adult level of perfection in control of the shoulder, arm, and wrist muscles. Finger control is slower. Development of large muscle skills first and then small muscle skills is a sound practice.

Handedness becomes noticeable by the time a child enters school. Neurologically most persons are right-handed or left-handed. This marked preference is inherited; right-handedness is a dominant trait and left-handedness is a simple recessive trait. About 7% of all males and 6% of all females are strongly left-handed. About 20% of the members of both sexes are mix-handed and can use either hand about equally well. The hand that is used more depends on training. These persons can be truly ambidextrous.

These early years of the schoolchild's life, coming between two periods of rapid change, are often termed the healthiest period of the entire human growth span. Children at this age have the lowest death rates and the lowest rates of serious illness of the entire society.

But children of this age group do have health problems. Their leading cause of death is accidents. A common example is the tendency to dash suddenly across the street. Certain forms of cancer, principally leukemia, constitute a major cause of death. The most common illnesses are episodes of infection causing respiratory illness and digestive upsets. Vaccines have been developed for many of the so-called childhood diseases, such as measles, mumps and German measles, and have brought these diseases under control.

In recent years, health authorities have become concerned over the increasing use of cigarettes by elementary school children. The community and social pressures to smoke have persisted despite major efforts to inform children about the hazards of smoking. The tendency of children to experiment with drug usage and alcoholic beverages has caused many school systems to strengthen and extend health education in the schools.

Although the emphasis of this chapter is on the child's physical growth and development, a number of emotional health problems have a direct and important effect on physical development and well-being. The child's adjustment to school, his or her fear of separation from mother, the effect of broken homes or incomplete families, and the tendency to become too involved and stimulated in academic, athletic, and social activities are often the sources of difficulties that affect both health and school progress.

PUBERTY AND ADOLESCENCE

With the exception of the growth period of infancy, the pubertal growth spurt, which precedes adolescence, is perhaps the most dramatic stage of human development. It is widely discussed, but a great deal of misunderstanding still continues about this phase of growth. Puberty marks the time in life when a person is first capable of sexual reproduction, whereas adolescence is designated as that period of transition between puberty and maturity. Researchers designate pubescence as the period extending from the first evidence of sexual maturation (breast development in girls and changes in the genitals of boys) to the onset of menstruation in girls and the production of spermatozoa in boys. Adolescence is defined as the period in an individual's life extending from menstruation or spermatogenesis to the time of physical growth maturity. Maturity in this sense means the culmination of linear growth when the epiphyses have closed and the individual has reached his or her maximum height.

To appreciate the magnitude of the growth change that takes place during puberty, the amount of growth during this time should be compared with that of other periods. Fig. 3-3 depicts the velocity curves (amount gain in height at various age levels) from infancy to puberty. The amount of gain, while steady, gradually declines until the sharp upsurge takes place at puberty. This spurt of growth occurs at approximately age 12 years for girls and age 14 years for boys. Extensive study and research of the pubertal growth phenomena have revealed that more is involved than simply an abrupt change in linear growth. Instead, puberty consists of a complex sequence of interrelated events. The mechanisms, which are not yet fully understood, involve an orchestration of interrelationships between the endocrine gland system and the various other body systems.

The research by Dr. Li at the University of California has helped to explain the role of the endocrine glands in growth. His studies have provided more information about the pituitary gland and its production of the human growth hormone (HGH), which causes an increase in size. In addition to the growth-promoting qualities of HGH, it also is believed to serve an important regulatory function in many metabolic processes. For example, the pituitary gland is thought to initiate the secretion of *gonadotropins*, after which the gonads or sex glands begin to secrete sex hormones. These sex hormones, in turn, promote such effects as protein synthesis, muscle development, bone growth, and the development of secondary sex characteristics.

The female sex hormones *estrogen* and *progesterone* are responsible for inducing the menarche. According to Tanner, the male sex hormone, testosterone, which is also stimulated by a hormone from the anterior pituitary gland, is responsible for much of the adolescent growth spurt in boys. The presence of testosterone leads to the development of the male reproductive cell spermatozoa in the testes. This event of sexual maturation or spermatogenesis in the male usually occurs some 2 to 3 years after the onset of puberty.

Charts developed by Tanner (Figs. 3-4 and 3-5) from the Institute of Child Health in London illustrate the sequence of major events occurring at puberty for boys and girls. The symbols on the charts represent

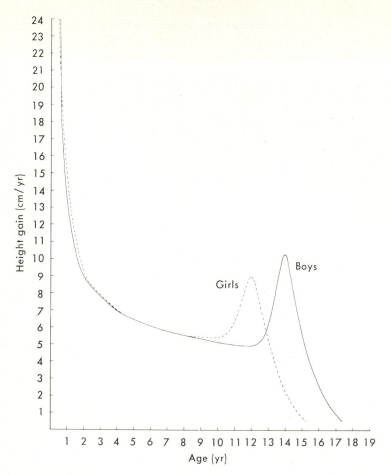

Fig. 3-3. Typical individual velocity curves for supine length or height in boys and girls. These curves represent the velocity of the typical boy and girl at any given instant. (From Tanner, J. M., Whitehouse, R. H., and Takaishi, M.: Arch. Dis. Child. 41:455-471, 1966.)

the typical ages at which these changes occur. The timing and coordination of these various events, which include height gain, breast development, and menarche in girls and changes in the sex organs along with height gain in boys, demonstrate the interrelationship of growth and glandular functions discussed in Li's research.

Based on a number of longitudinal studies, researchers at the Harvard School of Public Health describe the variations in physical growth patterns as characteristic of "early"

and "late" maturers. In Fig. 3-6 the concept of velocity curves (yearly increments in growth) is again used to illustrate the differences in the timing of the growth spurt among girls and boys. Although this dramatic increase usually occurs at ages 12 and 14 years, respectively, individual growth patterns may vary greatly from these norms. Tanner speaks of these variations as the individual's "tempo of growth." Variations are present at all ages; however, these differences are more dramatic during adolescence.

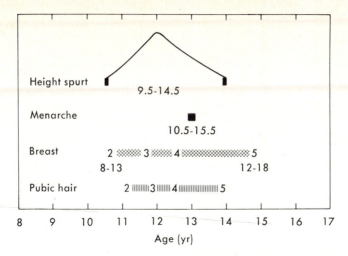

Fig. 3-4. Sequence of events of puberty in girls at various ages is diagramed for the average child. The hump in the bar labeled "height spurt" represents the peak velocity of the spurt. The bars represent the beginning and completion of the events of puberty. Although the adolescent growth spurt for girls typically begins at age 10.5 years and ends at age 14 years, it can start as early as age 9.5 years and end as late as age 15 years. Similarly, menarche (the onset of menstruation) can come at any time between the ages of 10 and 16.5 years and tends to be a late event of puberty. Some girls begin to show breast development as early as age 8 years and have completed it by age 13 years; others may not begin it until age 13 years and complete it at age 18 years. First pubic hair appears after the beginning of breast development in two-thirds of all girls. (From Tanner, J. M.: In Forfar, J. O., and Arneil, G. C., editors: Textbook of paediatrics, Edinburgh, 1962, Churchill Livingstone.)

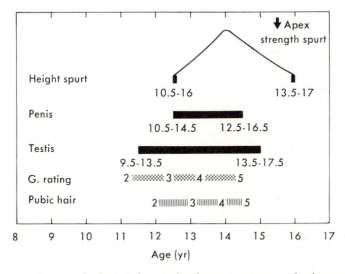

Fig. 3-5. Sequence of events of puberty in boys is also shown at various ages for the average child. The adolescent growth spurt of boys can begin as early as age 10.5 years or as late as age 16 years and can end anywhere from age 13.5 years to age 17.5 years. Elongation of the penis can begin from age 10.5 to 14.5 years and can end from age 12.5 to 16.5 years. Growth of the testes can begin as early as age 9.5 years or as late as age 13.5 years and end at any time between the ages of 13.5 and 17 years. (From Tanner, J. M.: In Forfar, J. O., and Arneil, G. C., editors: Textbook of paediatrics, Edinburgh, 1962, Churchill Livingstone.)

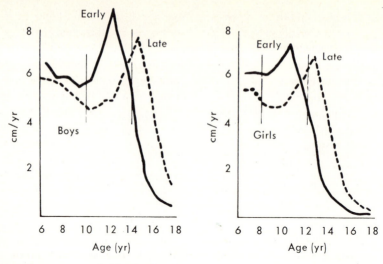

Fig. 3-6. Annual increments in height of early and late maturing boys and girls (means of 20 in each group). (From Valadian, I.: Proceedings of the National Nutrition Conference, U.S. Department of Agriculture, November 1971.)

For example, the range of chronological ages within which menarche may normally fall is approximately 10 to 16½ years of age. For boys, differences in the chronological age when the growth of the penis begins may also vary widely, from 10½ to 14½ years of age. This means that some boys and girls have finished their pubescent growth before others of their same chronological age have started.

Because of these variations, growth authorities recommend the use of other measures in addition to chronological age in order to make a more accurate assessment of maturity. Bone growth or skeletal age correlates much more closely with growth changes. Evidently the physiological processes controlling the ossification and growth of bones is also rather closely related to the other events that occur during this spurt of growth. Early maturing girls start the growth spurt at 9 years of age, whereas late maturing girls start at the age of 11 years. Early maturing boys start at 11 years of age and late maturing boys at age 13 years. In addition to

the difference between early and late maturers of both sexes, there is also a difference in the amount of incremental gain or height increases. In each instance those entering the growth spurt earliest also achieved the greatest amount of gain. This would seem to indicate that those who enter this growth cycle first not only have an early advantage in but also maintain their height advantage in later life. However, this is not always the case. Some late maturing boys may have a longer growing period and eventually catch up with and in some instances achieve greater height than their age-mates.

Because individual growth characteristics loom so important to the adolescent and to his or her self-image, being an early or late maturer can have lasting personality effects. Since girls begin their growth spurt first, they may suddenly find themselves taller than boys in the same classroom and become very concerned about being "too tall." Boys, on the other hand, especially the late maturing, are greatly concerned about their lack of height and size. Boys are said to be at greater risk than girls, since their changes in strength and size are correspondingly greater. Teachers need to understand the effects of these changes on students. Patterns of growth should be explained, as should the differences between male and female growth rates. Physicians and counselors can help to allay what, in most instances, is an unnecessary concern about growth. Also, for those relatively few adolescents who have medically diagnosed growth problems, medical science has made great strides in treating growth abnormalities, so that even these boys and girls may be able to grow to heights similar to those of their peers.

Girls begin to taper off in motor performance at the age of 15 years. Boys taper off at about 18 years of age. Although both will develop further skills after these ages, the rate of improvement will be much slower, and the maximum skill attained will not be appreciably higher. Biological maturity is a stage at which motor skill approaches the maximum potential. The girl's maximum potential will be attained at about 20 years of age, and the boy's maximum potential will be attained at about 23 years of age. Girls generally fall far below their potential skill, largely because of inadequate educational programs.

However, with the recent developments in girls' athletics, new records and higher levels of performance from the older, more mature girls and adult women can be expected in the future. In fact, there are several examples of women athletes in their mid- to late twenties competing successfully at world class competition levels in track and skating events.

A question that is often posed today is, Are we becoming bigger and taller than our ancestors? A frequently made observation, although not based on scientific data, is that today's college football and basketball players are much larger and taller than their predecessors. In this respect, the age-height-weight tables of some 25 years ago are now outdated. The scientifically based data that provide an answer to this question are drawn from what are called secular trend studies. Tanner cites such trend studies of English boys in which he has compared the heights of boys in the mid-nineteenth century with those of English boys in 1965. These data suggest that the differences result from the effects of environment and nutrition. Although today's youth tend to be taller and heavier than their predecessors, this may result from the differences in their rates of development and maturation rather than from true differences in height. For example, records based on nineteenth century English working boys revealed that they continued their growth in height until well into their middle twenties. By comparison, such boys would be shorter in height during their teens, but because of their continued growth might eventually be as tall as the earlier maturing boys of the twentieth century. At the same time, there is little doubt that the advantages of superior medical care, nutrition, and environmental conditions have contributed to greater average heights and weights among the youth of today. Figs. 3-7 and 3-8 illustrate such secular trend differences in average heights and weights of North American white boys between 1880 and 1960. However, it is of interest to note the narrowing of the height differences at age 20 years. This may indicate a delayed maturation or slower growth for the 1880 sample and a continuation of height gain that would eventually catch up to the 1960 comparison sample of boys.

Researchers in the fields of growth and development and in early childhood education point to some of the skills and abilities that can be expected of the nursery school-child. For example, most of these children

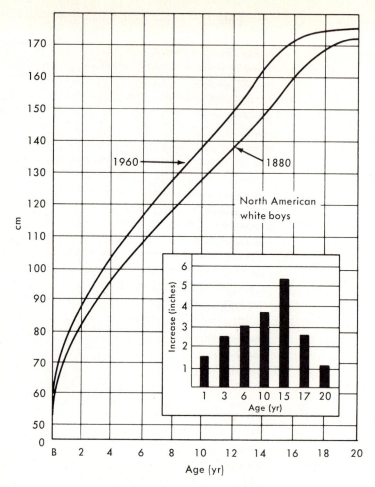

Fig. 3-7. Secular trend in height, 1880 to 1960. (From Lipsett, L. P., and Spiker, C. C.: Advances in child development and behavior I, New York, 1963, Academic Press, Inc.)

will be able to feed and dress themselves, with certain qualifications, of course, as teachers and mothers of children this age can attest. Tying shoe laces and donning heavy winter clothing present special problems. Most children will have established bowel control by the age of 3 years, but bladder control will come later. These behavior patterns respond to emotional pressures, and teachers working with preschool children must be alert to the fact that stresses may cause temporary loss of these controls and re-

gression to previous levels of behavior. The adult's ability to handle these situations with sensitivity and understanding is of paramount importance to the child's satisfactory adjustment and continuing development.

MALE-FEMALE DIFFERENCES

One of the major outcomes of the civil rights movement of the 1960s was legal enforcement of the constitutional right of every individual, regardless of race, age, sex, or religious preference, to receive fair and equal

North American white boys

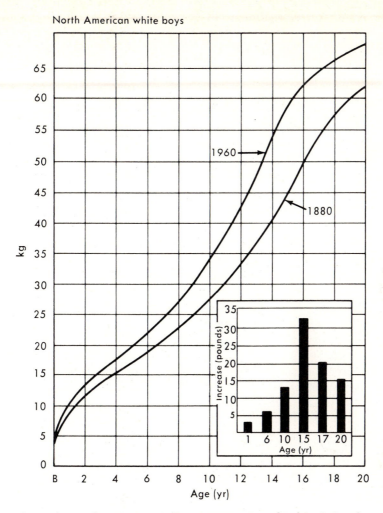

Fig. 3-8. Secular trend in weight, 1880 to 1960. (From Lipsitt, L. P., and Spiker, C. C.: Advances in child development and behavior I, New York, 1963, Academic Press, Inc.)

treatment as well as the opportunity to participate fully in all aspects of American life. This has led to major changes in society and in the public school programs. In the past, female students were rarely given the same opportunity as male students to enter certain fields of study, to practice the professions, or to participate in certain activities included in interschool athletics. Many of these restrictions were based on misconceptions and stereotyped attitudes about female interests, mental and physical capacities, and athletic capabilities in particular. Now that these barriers are being removed, many high schools are giving girls an opportunity to participate in school athletics. However, the fact that few secondary schools have the budget, staff, or facilities to provide such an expanded program has, in numerous instances, forced girls to compete with boys "to make the team." Although this effort to give girls opportunities in athletics is commendable, a single, combined sports program for boys and girls cannot be justified. On the basis of their physical growth characteristics, such programs place girls at a distinct disadvantage.

Because girls have a 1- to 2-year maturational advantage over boys that lasts from infancy through childhood, many observers have reached the false conclusion that girls can compete favorably with boys. However, with puberty comes the emergence of the male-female sex differences in height, weight, strength, and speed. A number of these developing characteristics are highly correlated with success in sports activities. For example, males have the advantage of greater size, both in height and in weight, in addition to having an inherited capacity for speed and endurance. Although the female's maturational advantages during childhood are well known, the fact that males have a muscle cell advantage over the female is not generally appreciated. Studies have revealed that as early as 3 weeks of age, the male already has a larger complement of muscle cells than does the female. This advantage continues throughout childhood, and adolescent growth increases the difference. By the time a girl has reached the age of 10 years, she has undergone a fivefold increase in the number of muscle cells. However, at this stage, the girl's muscle growth has just about reached its maximum. For boys, however, the adolescent growth spurt means an increase in the number of muscle cells, which may increase by as much as 14 times by the age of 18 to 20 years.

Other well-known findings have established the fact that females have a greater proportion of fatty tissue to muscle cells than do males. Moreover, adolescent growth causes girls to develop an even greater proportion of fatty tissue.

Until the age of 8 years, there is a slight difference between the basal metabolic rate (BMR) of males and females. From that age until the age of 20 years, the BMR of both sexes is equal. From the age of 20 years onward, a male's basal requirement is 10% greater than a female's of the same height, weight, and age.

Males, however, in addition to possessing greater amounts of muscle cells (which determine the development of strength and power) also develop larger hearts and lungs in relation to their size. This means that they develop higher systolic blood pressure and lower resting pulse rate, with a greater capacity for carrying oxygen in the blood. As a result, males have a greater capacity for neutralizing the waste products or lactic acid accumulating from physical exertion. As a consequence, they enjoy a more rapid recovery from fatigue. The comparatively greater oxygen-carrying capacity of the blood of the male is a result of the greater number of red cells and hemoglobin present in the blood, caused by the presence of the male sex hormone *testosterone*. This marked difference can be observed in Fig. 3-9.

Another difference reported by Tanner shows that males develop larger forearms than do females. This difference is undoubtedly reflected in the greater arm strength of the male as illustrated in Fig. 3-10.

As a direct result of the anatomical and physiological differences that develop in the adolescent period, athletic ability increases greatly in boys during this period. Public schools have a responsibility to provide a girls' sports program that gives them an equal opportunity to develop to their maximum potential. The unusually gifted girl may be able to compete successfully with boys of her peer group, especially during childhood, but the male-female differences that develop during adolescence necessitate a separate program for average girls, in order that they be able to develop athletic skills to their individual level of excellence.

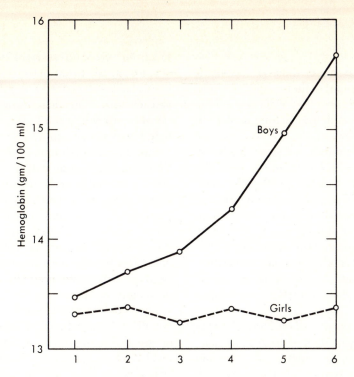

Fig. 3-9. Blood hemoglobin level in girls and boys according to stage of puberty; cross-sectional data. (From Young, H. B.: Dev. Med. Child Neurol. **5:**451-460, 1963.)

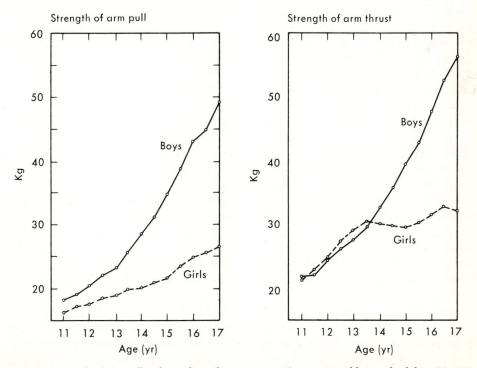

Fig. 3-10. Strength of arm pull and arm thrust from age 11 to 17 years. Mixed longitudinal data, 65 to 95 boys and 66 to 93 girls in each age group. (From Tanner, J. M.: Growth at adolescence, ed. 2, Oxford, 1962, Blackwell Scientific Publications; data from Jones, H. E.: Motor performance and growth, Berkeley, 1949, University of California Press.)

HEIGHT

Teachers have more than an academic interest in the height of their pupils. Besides their personal interest, they will need to help children understand the factors related to growth in height.

Inheritance of stature and size. Height is a multiple factor. The length of the legs, the trunk, the neck, and the head collectively determine the height of a person. Several genes are influential in determining these structures. Genes that affect size also affect other characteristics. The endocrine glands affect both size and other characteristics. Therefore the genes that produce these glands will also have an effect on various other factors.

A child may inherit all of the relatively long or short segment lengths of both parents and thus may be taller or shorter than the parents. Because of the many possible combinations, uniformity is hardly to be expected. Tallness is a recessive trait that represents a high output of the growth hormone somatotropin, which comes from the anterior pituitary gland, and of thyroxin, which comes from the thyroid gland. Shortness is a dominant trait. Thus tall parents, having only genes for tallness, will have tall children. Short parents may have tall children if both parents have genes for both shortness and tallness. Parents of medium height tend to have children who vary widely in height. Generally speaking, the prospective tallness shows early in the child, and, as will be pointed out later, it is possible to predict in childhood the approximate height a person will be in adulthood.

Dwarfism, an example of abnormal growth, is believed to be caused by a combination of genetic and endocrine factors. In the case of an endocrine disorder, there is an insufficient amount of the growth hormone secreted by the pituitary gland. The shortness in stature results from the premature ossification or closing of the epiphyses of the long bones.

When the growth lines ossify early in life instead of at about 20 years of age, the long bones fail to attain their normal length. Short and irregular bones may show some retardation in growth, but not to the extent that the long bones are affected.

Simple gigantism is an inherited condition that is a chance combination of height-giving genes, abnormal endocrine secretions, and other attributes, which produces an extremely large stature. Gigantism is an anomaly in which the epiphyses do not close, and the eosinophil cells of the anterior pituitary gland secrete excessive amounts of the principal growth hormone. About 90% of all giants are in this category.

Preschool years. The mean for height is not all-important, but does serve as a marker of the midstream of height for various age levels. One standard deviation includes 66⅔% of the total, and two standard deviations include 95% of the total.

Children of normal term will be 20 inches long at birth. At 1 year of age they will have added 10 inches to their height and at 4 years of age will be twice their height at birth. More precise figures can be tabulated.

School-age children. From Table 3-1 it is apparent that up to 10 years of age, school-age boys gain about 2¼ inches a year. The gain drops at 2 inches a year for the next 2 years and then increases to about 3 inches a year to 15 years, when the leveling off begins. School girls have a gain of about 2¼ inches a year to 11 years of age. The gain steps up to 2½ inches for the next 2 years until 12 to 13 years of age, and then begins to level off. Full height is reached by 16 years of age.

Individual variations from this pattern are to be expected; statistics in Table 3-1 serve merely as an index of the general tendency. Some boys will grow an inch a year for 2 years after the seventeenth birthday. However, the statistics have predictive value. A boy who is 55.2 inches tall at 10 years of age

Table 3-1. Height of American children in inches*

Age (yr)	Boys		Girls	
	Mean	Standard deviation	Mean	Standard deviation
1	29.7	1.1	29.3	1.0
2	34.5	1.2	34.1	1.2
3	37.8	1.3	37.5	1.4
4	40.8	1.9	40.6	1.6
5	43.7	2.0	43.8	1.7
6	46.7	2.07	46.4	2.15
7	49.0	2.13	48.6	2.33
8	51.2	2.33	50.9	2.45
9	53.3	2.64	53.3	2.71
10	55.2	2.67	55.5	2.86
11	57.4	2.75	58.1	3.08
12	59.3	3.35	60.5	2.63
13	61.2	3.39	61.8	2.79
14	64.4	3.40	63.0	2.53
15	66.7	3.13	63.8	2.47
16	68.2	2.68	63.9	2.53
17	69.0	2.78	64.2	2.53

*Data for this table are taken from the National Health Examination Survey (HES). Data for children 1 to 5 years of age represent pooled data, USPHS, 1960; data for children 6 to 11 years of age are from Cycle II, 1963-1965; and data for children 12 to 17 years of age are from Cycle III, 1966-1970. NCHS Series II, Numbers 104 and 124, Department HEW PHS.

and 57.4 inches tall at 11 years of age will not vary appreciably from 69 inches in height at 17 years of age. The standard deviations can be helpful in charting the likely future growth curve of those children above or below the mean curve.

It is significant that with the onset of biological maturity, height growth slows down because of the decline in the output of the growth hormone from the anterior pituitary gland. It thus is understandable why persons who mature early have a growth curve that starts to level off sooner than the normal curve.

WEIGHT

From a practical standpoint, for use in the school, weight is not a satisfactory index of growth (Fig. 3-11). Obese children would rate highly if weight were used as the sole index of growth.

Indices of growth. When a child is assessed in terms of a table of mean weights, the constitutional makeup of the child must be taken into consideration if weight is to be of any value as an index to growth. Even then, height must be considered in the assessment.

Inherited factors. Weight is determined by body conformation or proportions as well as by adipose tissue. The person who inherits a conformation of long torso and short legs will tend to weigh above the mean, although he or she appears to be about normal in weight. If a tendency toward obesity is inherited, a sluggish thyroid or pituitary gland may be the inherited factor. Yet if this person reduces food intake, the obesity need not develop. A person is not a helpless victim of heredity. Medical science can help individuals, and they can help themselves.

The misconception that large bones account for excess weight should be dispelled.

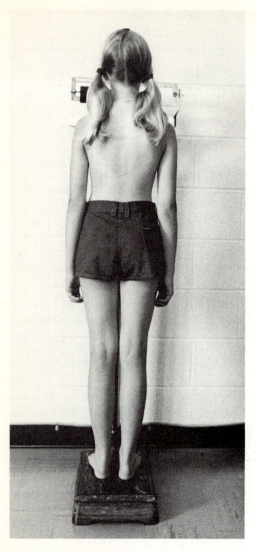

Fig. 3-11. Weight measurement. Appraisal of a child's height and weight by a nurse at the time of measurement can be an effective means of health education for both the parent and the child.

In two men six feet tall, the skeleton of the one with large bones will not weigh in excess of three pounds more than that of the one with small bones.

Preschool years. At birth the average boy weighs about 7.6 pounds, the girl, 7.5 pounds. Blacks are slightly smaller at birth than whites. At 5 months the weight at birth has doubled, and at 12 months it has trebled. In the next 4 years the child will have an average gain of about 5 pounds a year.

School-age children. From Table 3-2 we observe that school-age boys gradually increase their yearly gain in weight from 6 pounds to about 18 pounds between 13 and 14 years of age. The annual gain then declines progressively, being only 6 pounds between the ages of 16 and 17 years. Weight gain will continue to 30 years of age. School-age girls gain from 4 to 8 pounds a year until 11 years of age. Then a gain of 11.6 pounds is followed by a gradual decline in the increment of gain.

Standard deviations of the magnitude indicated in Table 3-2 suggest a wide range of variation in a group of children. Persons who regularly record the weights of children are surprised at the number of them below the mean. This contrasts with the fallacy that, in terms of the mean, a higher proportion of children are overweight.

DEVELOPMENTAL PROFILES

Height and weight are significant, but busy teachers need a device that gives a quick, reliable picture of a child's development. Several practical devices have been produced, a few of which can be of practical value to the school.

Denver Developmental Screening Test (DDST).* This test serves a limited purpose for the school, since it screens preschool children only. However, its value lies in detecting delayed or deviant development, and at no time in the school life of children is this more important than on the day when they begin school (Fig. 3-12). Many cases of delayed or deviant development are not detected before children enter school, and unfortunately, not even then unless an orga-

---

*Manual and kit distributed by Mead Johnson Laboratories, Evansville, Ind. 47721.

Table 3-2. Weight of American children in pounds*

Age (yr)	Boys		Girls	
	Mean	Standard deviation	Mean	Standard deviation
1	23.0	3.0	21.6	3.0
2	28.0	3.0	27.0	3.0
3	32.0	3.0	31.0	4.0
4	37.0	5.0	36.0	5.0
5	42.0	5.0	41.0	5.0
6	48.4	7.65	47.4	8.20
7	54.3	8.94	53.2	9.26
8	61.1	10.68	60.6	12.06
9	68.6	15.00	69.1	15.04
10	74.2	14.58	77.4	17.93
11	84.4	18.51	88.0	20.42
12	91.6	21.16	99.6	20.7
13	100.3	21.5	107.2	22.6
14	118.1	27.2	115.0	21.3
15	130.9	27.9	120.9	20.8
16	140.2	24.7	125.1	21.6
17	146.6	24.1	128.5	26.2

*Data for this table are taken from the National Health Examination Survey (HES). Data for children 1 to 5 years of age represent pooled data, USPHS, 1960; data for children 6 to 11 years of age are from Cycle II, 1963-1965; and data for children 12 to 17 years of age are from Cycle III, 1966-1970. NCHS Series II, Numbers 104 and 124, Department HEW PHS.

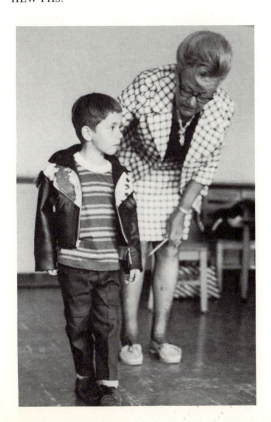

Fig. 3-12. Developmental screening test. Administration of the Denver Developmental Screening Test (DDST) gives the school an index of each child's level of growth and development at the time of admission. (Courtesy Tillamook County Health Department, Tillamook, Ore.)

nized test program is in operation. It is highly important that the school have knowledge of a child's developmental level and any associated problems of adjustment. This is essential not only if the school is to be most helpful in the child's progress but also in bringing delayed development to the attention of parents, advising them to seek professional services.

The test has been developed for use by people without special training in testing. A child at a certain age is given only about 20 items; some of them are sequential and require only a single administration. The DDST evaluates four aspects of the child's functioning: gross motor, fine motor–adaptive (i.e., the use of hands and the ability to solve nonverbal problems), language (i.e., the ability to hear and talk), and personal-social (i.e., the ability to perform tasks of self-care and to relate to others).

This test is designed to alert people working with children to the possibility of developmental delays so that appropriate measures can be pursued in the best interests of the children. It is not designed to derive a developmental or mental age nor a developmental or intelligence quotient. The relative simplicity of the test and its practical application are its merits.

NATIONAL CENTER FOR HEALTH STATISTICS GROWTH CHARTS

The two factors of height and weight in these charts can be used as a practical growth profile for students. These charts are based on data collected by the National Center for Health Statistics (NCHS). The charts show percentile distribution for males and females for height (in centimeters) by age and for weight (in kilograms) by age. These height and weight curves make it possible to compare an individual youth or group with the height and weight of all others in the United States who have the same characteristics

(Figs. 3-13 and 3-14). Children should be weighed without shoes and with sweater or jacket removed. Height is also measured with the shoes removed. As a minimum procedure, each child should be measured in September, January, and May. At each measuring period, the point, or child's location on the chart, is determined by the intersection of two lines formed by a vertical line extended from the base or age line and a horizontal line from the weight or height (stature) portions of the chart. After successive measurements over a period of 2 or 3 years have been recorded, curves of progress can be traced.

The graphs outline six percentile levels: very tall, moderately tall, average, moderately short, short, and very short. The particular zone in which a child's weight point falls indicates his or her position with reference to the weights of other children of the same age and sex. The same principle applies to the location of height points. The height and weight points of most children fall in corresponding zones; for example, if the weight falls in the average zone (at the 50th percentile level), the height also falls in the average zone for height (at the 50th percentile level). The child is of average size in terms of both height and weight.

When a youngster's weight and height points do not fall in corresponding zones, two possible interpretations may explain the dissimilarity: (1) it may indicate natural slenderness or stockiness or (2) it may reflect a poor quality of health. Any child with dissimilar height and weight percentile zones may be in need of medical evaluation. Once the child is established in a particular growth zone, there should be a consistent pattern of growth. Any variation from this pattern or zone should be carefully evaluated. It thus is apparent that the physical growth record can indicate possible health deficiencies, as well as portray normal growth progress.

NAME _____   RECORD # _____

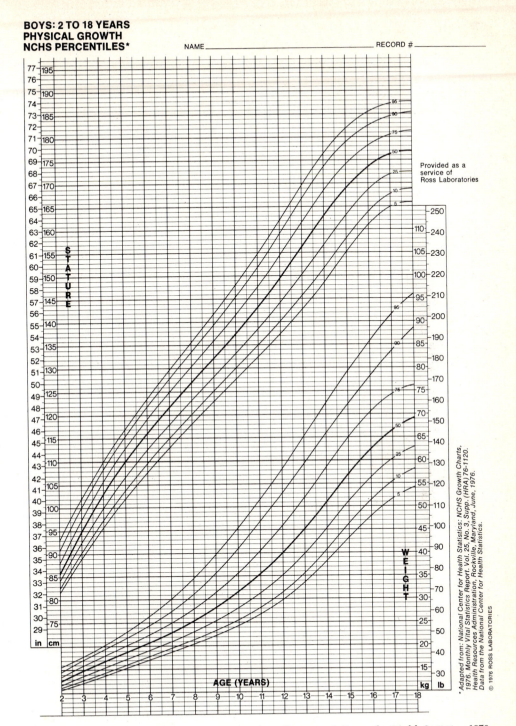

Fig. 3-13. NVHS growth chart for boys. (Modified from the National Center for Health Statistics, 1976. Monthly Vital Statistics Report, vol. 25, No. 3, Suppl. (HRA) 76-1120; courtesy Ross Laboratories, Columbus, Ohio.)

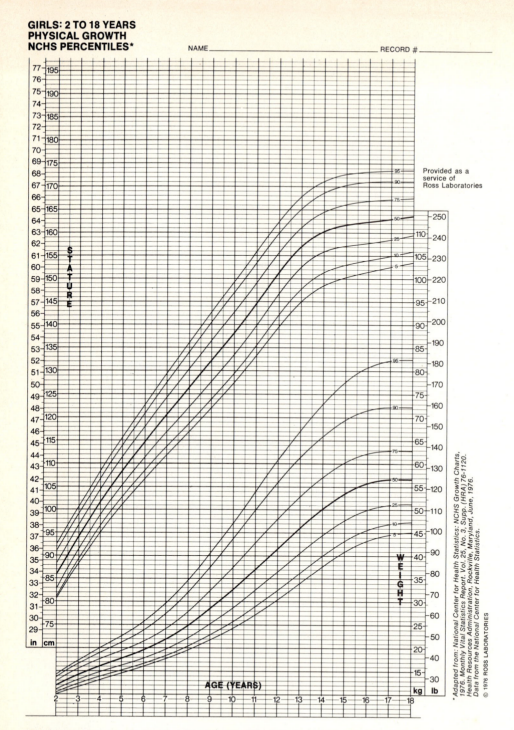

GIRLS: 2 TO 18 YEARS
PHYSICAL GROWTH
NCHS PERCENTILES*

NAME _____ RECORD # _____

Provided as a service of Ross Laboratories

* Adapted from: National Center for Health Statistics: NCHS Growth Charts, 1976. Monthly Vital Statistics Report. Vol. 25, No. 3, Supp. (HRA) 76-1120. Health Resources Administration, Rockville, Maryland, June, 1976. Data from the National Center for Health Statistics.

© 1976 ROSS LABORATORIES

Fig. 3-14. NCHS growth chart for girls. (Modified from the National Center for Health Statistics, 1976; courtesy Ross Laboratories, Columbus, Ohio.)

Graphs and tables. For practical use in the school it might be well to assess the use of graphs and tables in determining physical growth and development.

Advantages of growth and developmental graphs and tables are the following:

1. Implement teacher's observations
2. Aid in understanding a child
3. May indicate the general health level of the child
4. Afford better parental understanding of a child's status
5. Point up abnormalities of growth
6. Help in making comparisons between groups

Disadvantages of growth and developmental graphs and tables are as follows:

1. May be too complex for everyday use
2. Normal may be misleading
3. Optimums not included
4. Many standards needed
5. Measurement of height and weight may become the end, not a means
6. Not a substitute for personal history and physical examination

When the teacher or some other person in the school has an adequate understanding of a growth index such as the NCHS charts, these instruments can be used to advantage. All children should have their growth evaluated periodically at the time of their general health appraisal by a physician. The school then is governed by the physician's recommendation. The NCHS figures are important because they are the most current and the only truly representative growth standards available for the United States. They may be used in the same manner as the Meredith physical growth record. For example, a 7-year-old boy who is 122 cm (48 inches) tall is of average height, or at the 50th percentile level for his age. If that same boy weighs 20 kg (44 pounds), his relative weight for age is below average or at about the 15th percentile in comparison to other boys of his age.

In other words, he is of average height but below average in weight. If he is in good health, as determined by a physician, we can assume that he has a naturally slender build. By keeping a record of his growth over a period of years, a much more accurate assessment can be made of his body type and projection of his ultimate height and weight at maturity.

HEART FUNCTION AND BLOOD PRESSURE

Although adult heart size is 12 times that of the newborn infant, the pattern of operation and the electrocardiograms, or graphs, are similar. When a child is 5 years of age, the heart is four times as large as it was at birth. When he or she is 16 years of age, the heart may be small in comparison to skeletal muscle because heart growth between 14 and 16 years of age lags behind general muscle growth. Since endurance basically is cardiac output, observation of a child who fatigues (is winded) quickly will indicate that circulatory capacity probably lags behind muscular capacity (Table 3-3). This frequently occurs in children who are large for their age, but may occur in youngsters of normal stature.

Heart rate. While the minute volume of the heart depends on both the heart rate and the output per beat, the rate increases as output decreases and decreases as output increases. Thus if the rate is recorded, it gives a satisfactory index of the heart's capacity and level of functioning.

It must be recognized that the heart rate of a person may be altered by many factors, and a person's state of rest is an important aspect. For that reason the pulse rate should be recorded several times if it appears to deviate markedly from the average. Further, a rate within 10 beats on either side of the average may well be within the normal range. Usually a low heart rate indicates a proficient heart (Table 3-4).

Table 3-3. Respiratory minute volume

Age (yr)	Breathing rate (per min)	Tidal air (ml)	Minute volume (air in liters)
Newborn infant	30 (45)* 60	20	1
6	20 (30)* 35	125	3¾
12	20	250	5
14	18	350	6¼
18 (adult level)	16	500	8

*Mode in parentheses; minimum and maximum outside parentheses.

Table 3-4. Average heart rate for persons sitting at rest

Age (yr)	Girls	Boys
Newborn infant	140	135
6	100	95
8	95	88
10	90	83
11	86	80
12	83	81
13	79	77
14	80	78
15	78	77
16	77	73
17	76	71
17½	76	71

Table 3-5. Average blood pressure for persons sitting at rest (mm Hg)

Age (yr)	Girls			Boys		
	Systolic	Diastolic	Pulse	Systolic	Diastolic	Pulse
6	98	62	36	98	62	36
8	104	63	41	105	65	40
10	106	64	42	108	66	42
11	107	64	43	110	68	42
12	108	65	43	112	69	43
13	110	66	44	114	70	44
14	112	66	46	116	70	46
15	112	66	46	118	71	47
16	112	66	46	120	72	48

Table 3-6. Constituents of blood for persons at various ages

Age (yr)	Sex	Red corpuscles (million/mm³)	Hemoglobin (g/100 ml whole blood)	W (
Newborn infant	Male and female	5.5	21	20,000
5	Male and female	4.7	13	8,000
10	Male and female	4.7	13	8,000
14	Male	5.0	14	7,000
	Female	4.7	13	7,000
17	Male	5.3	15.6	7,000
	Female	4.7	13.6	7,000
18	Male	5.3	15.6	7,000
	Female	4.7	14	7,000

Blood pressure. Systolic pressure figures usually represent the pressure exerted by the blood against the wall of the main arm (brachial) artery when the heart is in contraction. Diastole is the pressure in the vessel while the heart is relaxed; pulse pressure is the difference between systolic and diastolic pressures. Pulse pressure indicates the degree of elasticity of the vessels.

Blood pressure is a great deal like a cork in water and can vary considerably in a person. However, a general tendency in pressure can be obtained when a series of readings is taken (Table 3-5). Deviations from the average are to be expected, but more than a 15% deviation from the average for a given age is certainly sufficient indication that the child will need medical supervision. The child's physician will provide the school with the information and instruction necessary to promote the child's best interest.

Blood. From birth to adulthood the blood constitutes about one thirteenth of the total body weight. Since a quart of blood weighs about 2 pounds, one can estimate the blood volume roughly. In persons from 12 to 18 years of age, the rate of increase in blood volume is slightly more rapid in the male than in the female. Final blood volume in the adult is about 4,200 ml in the female and about 5,500 ml in the male.

Quality of the blood as well as volume is important. Table 3-6 shows the average constituents of the blood for persons at various ages.

QUESTIONS AND EXERCISES

1. What is meant by the statement that the school deals in futures?
2. Distinguish between physical growth and physical development.
3. Why do we say physical growth and development are both independent and interdependent?
4. Does health education have a role to play in preventing congenital malformations? Please explain.
5. Why is it that girls at age 11 years can often successfully compete with boys in athletics when they cannot at age 15 years?
6. What health education implications do you draw from the early maturing girls and later maturing boys?
7. Of what value can the Meredith physical growth record be to the school?
8. When a child who was born prematurely enters school, why should the school disregard the fact of prematurity and treat the child as normal?
9. How do you explain that some swimming records are held by girls 13 and 14 years of age?
10. How would you determine whether a child is mixhanded?
11. Why is knowledge of the visual maturity of a child of importance to the school?
12. In schoolchildren abnormalities of upper respiratory tract are relatively rare; then why should the school be concerned about the respiratory system of the children?

13. Why may youngsters be at a disadvantage if they are large for their age?
14. School-age girls have a more rapid heart rate than do boys of the same age; then how would one explain why girls will live longer than boys?
15. Why is it important that a teacher know that different organs reach their maturity at different times?
16. What is your reaction to the following statement: "Children often need glasses in elementary school because of eyestrain from reading?"
17. How do you explain the correspondingly greater height and weight among today's adolescents when compared with the adolescents of 40 to 50 years ago?
18. How can a child benefit by knowing his or her developmental levels?
19. Why do many athletic coaches contend that ninth-grade boys should not be permitted to compete with twelfth-grade boys, particularly in contact sports?
20. How can growth and development be used to motivate students in health education?

REFERENCES AND SELECTED READINGS

American Academy of Pediatrics: School health: a guide for health professionals, Evanston, Ill., 1977, American Academy of Pediatrics.

Boehm, W. W., editor: Maler's three theories of child development, New York, 1965, Harper & Row, Publishers.

Breckenridge, M. E., and Murphy, M. N.: Growth and development of the young child, ed. 8, Philadelphia, 1969, W. B. Saunders Co.

Breckenridge, M. E., and Vincent, E. L.: Child development, physical and psychologic growth through the school years, ed. 5, Philadelphia, 1966, W. B. Saunders Co.

Brisbane, H. E.: Developing child, Peoria, Ill., 1965, Charles A. Bennett Co., Inc.

Damon, A.: Secular trend in height and weight within old American families at Harvard, 1870-1965, Am. J. Phys. Anthropol. 29(1):45-50, 1968.

Falkner, F., editor: Human development, Philadelphia, 1966, W. B. Saunders Co.

Gallagher, J. R.: Medical care of the adolescent, New York, 1960, Appleton-Century-Crofts.

Gardner, D. B.: Development in early childhood, Evanston, Ill., 1964, Elhi Textbook Division, Harper & Row, Publishers.

Gesell, A., Ilg, F. L., and Ames, L. B.: Youth—the years from ten to sixteen, New York, 1956, Harper & Row, Publishers.

Height and weight of children in the United States, Vital and Health Statistics Series, Number 104, NCHS, DHEW Publication No. 1000, Washington, D.C., 1970, U.S. Government Printing Office.

Height and weight of youths 12-17 years in the United States, Vital and Health Statistics Series, Number 124, NCHS, DHEW Publication No. (HSM) 73-1606, Washington, D.C., 1973, U.S. Government Printing Office.

How children grow, DHEW Publication No. (NIH) 72-166, General Clinical Research Centers Branch, Division of Research Resources, National Institutes of Health, Bethesda, Md., June 1972.

Illingworth, R. S.: Development of the infant and young child, ed. 4, Baltimore, 1970, The Williams & Wilkins Co.

Kaplan, S. A.: Growth disorders in children and adolescents, New York, 1964, Twayne Publishers.

Krogman, W. M.: Child growth, Ann Arbor, 1972, The University of Michigan Press.

Krogman, W. M.: A handbook of the interpretation of height and weight in the growing child, Child Development Publications, Urbana, 1950, University of Illinois Press.

McCammon, R. W.: Human growth and development, Springfield, Ill., 1970, Charles C Thomas, Publisher.

McNeil, E. B.: Concept of human development, Belmont, Calif., 1966, Brooks Cole Publishing Co.

Meredith, H. V.: Growth, physical, Encyclopedia Americana, pp. 449-502b, 1953.

Meredith, H. V.: A physical growth record for use in elementary and high schools, Am. J. Public Health 39:878, 1949.

NCHS growth charts. 1976 Monthly vital statistics report USDHEW (HRA) 76-1120, vol. 25, no. 3, Supplement, June 22, 1976.

Sears, R. R., and Feldman, S. S., editors: The seven ages of man, ed. 3, Los Altos, Calif., 1973, William Kaufmann, Inc.

Stott, L. H.: Child development: an individual longitudinal approach, New York, 1967-1968, Holt, Rinehart & Winston.

Stuart, H. C., and Prugh, D. G., editors: The healthy child, his physical, psychological and social development, Cambridge, Mass., 1960, Harvard University Press.

Sussman, M.: Growth and development, ed. 2, Englewood Cliffs, N.J., 1964, Prentice-Hall, Inc.

Tanner, J. M.: Growing up, Sci. Am. 229:35-43, 1973.

Tanner, J. M.: Growth at adolescence, ed. 2, Philadelphia, 1962, F. A. Davis Co.

Tanner, J. M.: Sequence, tempo, and individual variation in the growth and development of boys and girls aged twelve to sixteen, Daedalus, Fall 1971. Issued as Proceedings of the American Academy of Arts and Sciences 100(4):904-930.

Tanner, J. M., and Taylor, G. R.: Growth, Morristown, N.J., 1965, Silver Burdett Co.

Tuddenham, R. D.: Physical growth of California boys and girls from birth to 18 years, Berkeley, 1954, University of California Press.

Valadian, I.: The adolescent—his growth and development. In Proceedings of National Nutrition Education Conference, November 2-4, 1971, U.S. Department of Agriculture, Miscellaneous Publication No. 1254, Washington, D.C., 1973, U.S. Government Printing Office, pp. 21-37.

Watson, E. H., and Lowrey, G. H.: Growth and development of children, ed. 5, Chicago, 1967, Year Book Medical Publishers, Inc.

Wetzel, N. C.: The treatment of growth failure in children, Cleveland, 1948, NEA Service, Inc.

Whipple, D. V.: Dynamics of human development, New York, 1967, McGraw-Hill Book Co.

CHAPTER 4

Emotional development

Teachers recognize that the maturation process of the human being involves the development of many factors and aspects of a child's makeup. Knowledge of intellectual and physical development is vital to the teacher, but knowledge of emotional development is equally important. Many children sufficiently mature physiologically and mentally have difficulty adjusting to their social environment. What commonly is spoken of as mental health is basically emotional adjustment.

An understanding of various levels of emotional maturation enables a teacher to understand each child more fully. The informed teacher not only will know what to expect in emotional responses from children, but will also be able to interpret unusual emotional behavior in terms of the level of emotional maturity it represents.

BIOSOCIAL DEVELOPMENT

Developmental tasks of life contribute to emotional stability. The influence of peers is recognized. The student has to learn how to get along with people because of the human need to communicate with others. While youngsters learn to cooperate in order to communicate with others, they also strive to achieve personal independence. Children must learn the standards of conduct that guide them in interpersonal relations.

A pupil's peers strongly influence the child's development, but it is also important to recognize the value of teachers and the role of the parents in shaping the developing personality of each child. It is true that some parents contribute very little to their child's development, and this can reflect itself in the child's conduct at school.

It is healthy for children to understand the nature of emotions and their control so they can then strive toward a better understanding of their own mental health.

CONCEPT OF EMOTIONS

Emotions are intense feelings accompanied by bodily reactions. A person gets angry physically as well as mentally. One experiences joy physically as well as in other conscious respects. Emotions are highly complex and vary in degrees of intensity. They represent patterns of interaction between neurons, endocrine glands, and other parts of the body. While they arise from a conscious experience that originates in the central nervous system, they produce a reaction of the glandular system, which in turn affects neural function and practically all the rest of the body.

Some authorities maintain that there are only two emotions, the negative emotion of anger and the positive emotion of love. Such a broad, even rough, classification is not satisfactory for the practical needs of the teacher. Therefore a further classification of the negative and positive emotions is in order.

Negative emotions. Feelings that are unpleasant or disagreeable are not entirely distinct, but tend to have certain things in common. There is the further difficulty that words must be used to express the feeling, and words themselves can be an obstacle to understanding, since they convey different things to different people. However, for practical use a classification of negative emotions can be made as follows:

1. Anger—fury, rage, hate, annoyance, irritation, and displeasure
2. Fear—fright and alarm
3. Distress—helplessness and futility
4. Envy—jealousy
5. Humility—submission, inferiority, and insecurity
6. Loneliness—isolation

Positive emotions. Feelings that are pleasant or acceptable are even more subtle than the others, and grades of distinction necessarily are difficult to classify. A classification of positive emotions includes the following:

1. Tenderness—love, affection, and kindness
2. Elation—pride, mastery, confidence, and assertive self-feeling
3. Possession—security and ownership
4. Amusement—jollity and relaxation

PHYSICAL BASES OF EMOTIONS

All overt human conduct arises from a physical source, the protoplasm of the body's cells. Each person possesses a particular constitutional endowment from which emotions arise. When stimuli from the external environment produce an emotional response, virtually all the body is involved, but two systems—the neural and the endocrine—play major roles. These systems function in all coordination and adjustment and are particularly involved in emotional responsiveness. The responses of the neural system are immediate and quick acting. Endocrine functions are slower. A relationship between the two may be visualized by picturing the endocrine hormones as the soil in which the neuronal impulses function. Neurons function in an endocrine soil of a particular kind, perhaps affected by the internal secretions as natural soil is affected by fertilizers.

Since a person is conscious of emotional states, the cortex of the brain, where consciousness is located, obviously is involved. Original external stimuli reach the cortex of the brain and are relayed to the thalamus, from which autonomic nerves originate.

Autonomic neuron system. The autonomic system is particularly important in emotional responses. It is often referred to as the vegetative system, since it maintains the functions necessary to sustain life. It is an involuntary system and has two divisions, the sympathetic nervous system that tends to speed up action and the parasympathetic nervous system that has the opposite effect. All organs of the thoracic and abdominal cavities have a dual supply of autonomic nerves—sympathetics, which speed up the function of the organ, and parasympathetics, which have the opposite action. Thus balance of function is maintained. During emotional states these nerves are stimulated, at times the sympathetics arousing the organs, at other times the parasympathetics reducing the activity of the organs.

The emotional center is in the thalamus, a large ovoid mass of gray matter located toward the center and base parts of the brain. It also is the location of the pain and temperature-regulating centers. That some people are emotionally highly responsive and others much less so is understandable in biological terms. Sensitivity may be inherent in the nerve structure and may be further sensitized by particular endocrine influences. However, social conditioning must not be discounted; neither should training possibilities be discarded. Perhaps all degrees of biological response can be affected by training of the right type.

Endocrine nature of temperament. Generally, temperament is regarded as the emotional mold that distinguishes a person. Each person's temperament is greatly affected by his or her particular endocrine endowment. Most endocrine influences are rather subtle, but there are some manifestations that are more definite. Irritability, fatigability, apathy, enthusiasm, depression, indifference, and aggressiveness are all understandable in terms of the endocrine secretions.

The term *endocrine type* presumes a great deal. Persons whose basic makeup is due entirely to extreme or true endocrine malfunction are rare, but examples do exist. Individuals with an overproduction of thyroxin (hyperthyroidism), in addition to a tendency to lose weight and be thin, are restless, energetic, active, impatient, easily upset, impulsive, and alert. At the other pole are persons with an underproduction of thyroxin (hypothyroidism). For individuals of this type it is an effort, almost, to live. They go along at a low level of function, react slowly, fatigue easily, are usually behind in everything, rarely are enthusiastic about anything, are not easily disturbed or upset, and are usually easygoing and easily pleased.

Most persons represent various intergrades of endocrine balances. Yet in school practice a teacher must recognize that children react as they do, at least in part, because of each one's particular biological makeup. They can be changed some by training, although perhaps some children can be

changed but little. A wise teacher will try to understand children's conduct in terms of their basic constitutional makeup.

GENESIS OF EMOTIONAL RESPONSES

What motivates human conduct? What gives force and direction to what one does? Why does a person become angry or elated? Through what channels are emotions mediated and in what manner? These are questions of significance to all persons. They are of special importance to teachers who, if they are to be of the greatest value in guiding children in self-development, must understand why children act as they do.

Human beings are biologically self-centered, self-interested, and selfish. Knowingly and unknowingly they seek to gratify this self. The ego requires gratification. They seek status. So it is necessary that the teacher, observing overt behavior in a child, go behind the scene and understand just *why* the child acts in this way.

Physiological patterns. Children are born with certain physiological patterns such as hunger, thirst, and pain. A newborn child is a biological being and not a social being. The infant's self is gratified by satisfying such physiological patterns as hunger and thirst, by relieving pain, permitting activity, and eliminating discomfort. If the infant is in pain or hungry or restrained, it responds emotionally by exhibiting the negative emotion of anger. The newborn infant seems to exhibit no positive emotions.

All through life, gratification of these physiological patterns is a factor in the emotional responsiveness of a person. However, as one matures emotionally, control over the emotions rises accordingly. Although teen-age children may not cry or show the intense emotional response of an infant, their responses are different when they are hungry from when they are not hungry, different when they are active from when they are not active.

Universal socially conditioned motives. Although children are born biological beings, they become social beings and learn to obtain self-gratification through certain socially conditioned motives that are universally accepted. All normal persons want attention, affection, approval, applause, praise, and security. They seek mastery, superiority, and achievement. When they display positive emotions, they are getting the attention or approval the self seeks, or a goal has been achieved that has been a source of gratification. If negative emotions are displayed, they have failed to achieve this goal or have not had the approval or praise sought or the self has been thwarted or hurt.

Individualized patterns of motivation. Teachers should be aware of the fact that some children get special gratification through interests or means that are neither universally practiced nor accepted. Children who are gratified by playing harmful pranks are in need of special attention. Perhaps they are not getting attention from the normal, more wholesome avenues of school life. They need to understand which avenues of self-gratification our society recognizes. Somewhere in the school program there must be means and opportunities for wholesome self-gratification for all children.

PRESCHOOL YEARS

By the time children first appear at school, their emotional mold already has been subjected to many influences. What has happened to their emotional makeup is of extreme importance to the school. While the 6-year-old child is pliable and can be modified, the task of the school in rehabilitating a child with marked emotional deviation is an assignment to frustration for the teacher who does

not have an understanding of the factors that characterize normal emotional function and maturation.

Egocentricity. The preschool child is selfish, self-centered, and demanding. The training for this child should be a compromise between too much expression and too much repression. Children who have learned to deny themselves and consider the wishes of others, yet who have not been repressed to a state of timidity and reticence, are likely to have the balanced emotional responsiveness of normal children entering school. Preschool children exhibit jealousies and tantrums, but the child who has obtained neither status nor attention through these expressions will find more acceptable means for obtaining self-gratification. Yet most children enter school life with a handicap because they are entering a life in which they share the stage with 30 others and are coming from a life in which they are the center of all activity and the world revolves about them. It is true that the home has the primary responsibility for guiding children in their emotional development, but the school gains little by pointing to the shortcomings of the home training.

EARLY ELEMENTARY SCHOOL YEARS

Social influences have modified children by the time they arrive at school; nevertheless they are still very much *individualists*. They will play with others for only brief periods. It is an ideal time to develop self-reliance and the ability to fullfill responsibilities—attributes of value throughout life.

Emotional expression. Primary school children are cheerful and happy. They are curious and will take a keen interest in new experiences. They enjoy play and can amuse themselves. They are friendly to others, but do not sustain an interest in other children.

They are not excessively timid or afraid and exhibit self-confidence.

At this period of life children may display contrasting and even conflicting emotional traits. They may be exuberant, eager, overactive, assertive, aggressive, adventuresome, and daring. They may be overly dramatic. They can be unduly sensitive and will exhibit pronounced negative emotions, such as anger and jealousy. However, the same children can be most sympathetic in their concern for the misfortunes and trials of others. Their emotions are usually of short duration, however pronounced they may appear to be.

Evidences of emotional maturation. During the primary years children should be learning to accept disappointments and disagreeable tasks. They should be learning to control anger, fear, and other negative emotions. They should forget anger and grudges. They learn to respect others and refrain from interrupting and quarreling. They learn to control or reduce possessiveness. They learn to obey rules and wait their turn, as a kindness to others. They learn to do their work promptly and show reasonable persistence.

Too often the teacher assumes that children will learn by observation which conduct is not accepted. However, explanation of accepted and unaccepted conduct and the reasons will usually hasten the maturation process.

LATER ELEMENTARY SCHOOL YEARS

During the fourth through sixth grades of school, children show the maturing effects of socialization. Emotionally they are actually much more stable and mature than is generally recognized.

Emotional patterns. Individualistic children in the 9- to 11-year age span are acquiring orderly habits of work and play. They assume increasing responsibility and self-reliance. They adjust quite well to frustration

and conflict, and, although they occasionally are upset emotionally, they recover quickly. They are not prone to brood or worry. They have a more lasting interest in friends and share their pleasures and possessions. They have learned to respect the rights and property of others and conform to the social and moral requirements of their group.

Although the children's interest span is increasing and their self-control is improving, they are sensitive to failure and are easily discouraged. In their intense desire to achieve and even excel, these youngsters may appear to be argumentative and antagonistic. However, a better interpretation would be that this merely expresses a combination of boundless vitality and extreme competitiveness, a product of the modern American culture.

Many children in this age group do considerable daydreaming. All normal people do some daydreaming, but this age level is the high point for daydreams. Not ridicule, criticism, or punishment, but tasks that interest and keep the child occupied in gratifying accomplishment will reduce daydreaming.

Some of these children are boisterous and noisy, not with asocial tendencies, but as a manifestation of physical vitality and self-expression. Timely counseling will help the child to acquire the insight essential to the necessary adjustment.

Some children in this age level are still very shy, and teachers frequently overlook them. After all, the boisterous child is more easily remembered. The shy child is usually a lonely child, perhaps with exaggerated feelings of inferiority because of insecurity, poor home environment, lack of specific skill, or other factors—real or imaginary.

JUNIOR HIGH SCHOOL YEARS

During the period when children are 12 to 14 years of age, their interest in self is transposed to interest in the group. The tendency of youngsters to gang together at this age is a common observation. No biological reason accounts for the phenomenon. It is a social attraction to the members of the same gender, and hence is called the homophilic period. It is not a homosexual phenomenon. The reason may be that girls tend to be almost 2 years in advance of boys in physiological and social development and to have interests both more advanced and more diverse.

Group loyalties. Attempts to break up a group are met with determined resistance and generally are unsuccessful. Directing the group into wholesome channels usually proves profitable. The intense loyalty of the individual self to the group identity can be the most potent force motivating children. To them it is more important that they have the approval of their peer group than that they get approval elsewhere. Teachers and parents find that when the standards of the group conflict with those of the school or home, the group will exert the greater influence. Guiding the group, rather than competing with it, can be effective.

Emotional patterns. The marked individualism of previous years is displaced by a cooperative approach. Self-gratification comes from the praise and approval of the group. Status within the group is the primary goal. New interests of the child do not tend to appear except as they are accepted and fostered by the group. Reliance on the support of the group doubtless avoids some personal frustrations and conflicts and can be of value unless the standards and mores of the group range outside of social norms. Leadership exerts itself in the groups, and, if it is directed into proper avenues, the training opportunities are valuable. Ability to lead asserts itself in many forms, from the very highest to the browbeating level.

Many youngsters at this stage of life may be inordinately self-conscious and painfully shy. This in itself can leave its mark on the personality, but the greatest scars occur when the shy, self-conscious youngster develops serious doubts that he or she is normal. Assurance that all normal people, especially those at this age, experience the discomforts of shyness and self-consciousness can relieve his or her concern and fears.

Children who can fit into no particular group find themselves persons who walk alone. From this may develop the beginning of a tendency to be a lone wolf. Patterns of emotional adjustment acquired at the junior high school level often determine the direction of emotional mold throughout life. In appraising the child's emotional behavior, the teacher might well ask, What will be the significance of this tendency 20 years hence?

PUBERTY

Precisely considered, puberty refers to the age at which the reproductive organs become functionally mature. It occurs at some time between the ages of 12 and 17 years. In the female, menstruation occurs and she takes on the typical secondary female characteristics of body contour, breast growth, and pelvic enlargement. In the male, seminal discharge and a change of voice are indices of the climacteric called puberty.

In its practical, broader sense, puberty is considered the complete change that occurs at the time of maturation of the reproductive organs. It is more than a physical change. It involves social, emotional, and mental change as well. From the standpoint of school practice this is an important concept because some children experience a *negativism* at this stage of life. Negativism is characterized by withdrawal, reticence, and marked timidity. These children are somewhat perplexed by the changes through which they are passing, and, as with all persons, something they do not understand is disturbing. They will recover from the negativism in about 6 months, even without counseling, but they can be helped measurably by being told that they are going through a transition that all normal persons experience.

SENIOR HIGH SCHOOL YEARS

Adolescence, the period of youth, is not a pathological state. It does involve special problems related to emotional development that result in frustrations and conflicts. Adolescents find themselves in a social environment considerably more complex than anything they have encountered previously. A combination of inexperience and immaturity may find them unequal to the situation, and thus they make improper or inadequate adjustments. Adolescence is not a sudden, overnight change. It runs a course of about 5 years and includes the ages from 15 to 20 years, when the adult level is attained.

Heterosexuality. Adolescence is characterized by an interest in the opposite sex. To the boy the girl becomes physically and socially attractive. The self obtains gratification from the attractiveness of the sexes; emotional responses rise to the highest level on the positive side, yet also may fall to the extreme on the negative side. Intense emotional responses of this phase of life may be of fleeting duration—an index of the level of emotional maturity.

Transition to adulthood. This is a period of transition from childhood to adulthood and is characterized by marked inconsistency. At times a youth may act as mature as a 30-year-old adult, but during the next hour may exhibit the emotional pattern of a 10-year-old child. It is a period of emancipation in which youths wish to be recognized as individuals in their own right. Parents who still think of them as children may insist on childish standards and requirements, a source of frequent parent-youth conflict. Youths resent restraints and orders. Although youth lack experience, they possess considerable ability.

Therefore both teachers and parents need to consider the viewpoint of the student and to provide whatever compromises and counsel the situation may merit. Suggestions, not orders, are the effective instruments.

In expressing their desire for emancipation, some youths, girls as well as boys, go to the extreme of revolt against their parents, teachers, school, community, and even society. They are students of high intelligence as well as of average mentality. These are the "youth in revolt" of our time. Defiance of the established patterns and order of things seems to give them a certain self-gratification. They appear to obtain a feeling of identity or individuality. With rare exceptions they pay dearly for their revolt for many years to come when they find they are not readily accepted by those who normally would accept them, and they find themselves going down the road of life alone.

Youths need guidance to avoid this tragic role. To express individuality, but within the range of social requirements and with respect for the rights of others, must be learned. As an attention-getting device, revolt can exact a high price in future years. This the teenager must be helped to understand.

Social conflict. Youths live in an adult world, made to adult order, and controlled by adults. They possess a high level of self-esteem. Yet failure and frustration are frequent, with both deep and superficial scars.

Emotional maturation consists of adapting demands of the self to the demands of the social world. Children mature as they learn that some problems of social conflict have no ready solution, but are something they have to live with; therefore they must not permit these problems to cause too great an emotional reaction. During maturation youths learn that problems that disturb them extremely today will become, with the mellowing of time, of little consequence. They should strive to develop social traits of sincerity, congeniality, courtesy, tact, fairness, industry, and thoughtfulness.

Emotional patterns. Adolescents are idealistic and sensitive. They are insecure and seek assurances from their own peer group. Yet they are eager to be approved and accepted by older people—hence the disturbance they suffer when they must choose between the conflicting demands of their peer group and those of older people. The cliquishness and group loyalty of youths doubtless serve to provide some degree of social security. Students of high school age are also concerned about their masculine and feminine roles. They may be demonstrative, even border on exhibitionism, to obtain the attention and recognition they seek. Yet, though they are anxious about their status, they are seeking a mature set of values. Perhaps the best single index of the emotional maturation of high school students is to be found in the maturity of the values they are acquiring.

An interesting phenomenon that is not new but is more pronounced than in past generations is the frequent conflict between high school girls and their mothers. This conflict arises partially from the girl's desire to be emancipated from the dependence of childhood to the independence of adulthood—to be recognized as an individual in her own right. The mother, on the other hand, still considers her daughter a child and tends to treat her accordingly. Overprotection, however well-intended, interferes with the daughter's style and is resented. Contradictory respect for and antagonism toward the parents also may be extended to teachers and other adults. Though this conflict dissolves, the dissolution can be hastened by honest adult attempts to understand the youth's position and to make reasonable compromises between the demands of the youth and the edicts of adults.

High school students should acquire a philosophy of life as well as day-to-day goals. They should develop confidence, courage, self-esteem, self-reliance, self-discipline, orderliness, humor, adaptability, and an interest in people. They should learn to accept monotonous tasks, gain satisfaction from doing things well, and accept criticism and facts about themselves. They should strive to obtain the maximum benefit from their various experiences to assure themselves of at least optimum social maturation.

UNREST OF HIGH SCHOOL YOUTHS

High school youths exhibit the same unrest that is found on the campuses of colleges and universities. Many of the same conflicts plague the high school students that plague the college students and equally seriously affect their mental well-being. In any phenomenon as complex as the unrest of youth, many factors in various combinations account for the disturbed behavior. In considering some of these causative factors, attention must be directed to just how they can affect impressionable youths at various levels of maturation. The mental health implications are readily apparent.

World tensions. The conflict between capitalism and communism is the background of life for all people in the world. This conflict has gone on for more than a quarter of a century and could well continue for another half century.

Conflict of ideologies is not new. Conflict between the Moslems and the Christians lasted for 3 centuries. There were frequent skirmishes but no major outbreaks, and the conflict finally became submerged in the Age of Discovery, the Renaissance, and the Industrial Revolution. For almost two centuries, the Chaldeans and the Greeks were rivals in the field of science. This rivalry became dissolved in the sea of problems that beset both nations. Today, an ideological conflict and a science rivalry are repeated. These, too, will pass in the wake of new discoveries, new interests, and new events.

If everyone in the United States pessimistically acted on the premise that another world war was inevitable, surely we would be reduced to ashes. We must choose to proceed on the premise that if we are resolute, and work on peace, we shall find peace. We must prefer to deal in terms of difficult problems to be solved, not in terms of civilization reduced to rubble. Youths must be helped to understand that not threats from without but decay from within our nation is the danger we face, and that youngsters, too, have a responsibility to build a stronger nation for themselves today and for future generations.

National tensions. Within a highly competitive free enterprise democratic nation where there exists a kaleidoscope of different economic, social, educational, political, and religious groups, each striving for status and even advantage, conflicts are inevitable. These conflicts and related tensions are accentuated in times of great national strains, and the United States is now passing through the most fantastic period in all its history, a period of fluid transition, seeking new values, new standards, and new directions. This nation has gone through many crises and upheavals but has always demonstrated a magnificent capacity to resolve its problems. Living in times that make history is interesting, although somewhat inconvenient. With further experience and subsequent maturation, the student develops an understanding of various social interactions and becomes more comfortable with these interactions.

Contempt for authority. All normal people have a certain degree of resentment of authority. We resent the authority of parents, teachers, principal, professor, dean, policeman on the beat, traffic officer, boss of the

gang, general manager, or anyone else who has authority over us. If the nation is to survive, its institutions must be effective, and to be effective, authority must be delegated and exercised. It is necessary to accept authority, to respect authority, and even to honor authority. It is the misuse or abuse of authority that should become the concern of youth and adult alike.

Antiestablishment. As an adjunct of the distaste for authority many youths express their disdain for the establishment. Partially this arises from the fact that they are not a part of the establishment and do not relish their position on the outside looking in. Of course, this is a distorted view. They do belong to the society that is the establishment but do not have a place on the top rung of the ladder nor a place in the sun. Like others, they will have to work patiently and earn a place on the ladder of life.

Competition. In the United States, competition has been a significant factor in the amazing advance of the nation in its economy, science, discovery, education, and other respects. Perhaps the United States has become so highly competitive that it is destroying itself. At least, many youngsters have become disturbed and discouraged by the intense competition for grades, the suicidal competition in athletics, and the effect of economic and social competition on their fathers and mothers. Youngsters want no part of such a "rat race." Maybe they are right in their desire for a life of peace, productivity, and creativity at their own pace. Perhaps they envision a much better life than the one now prevailing in the United States. On this issue they should be heard.

Depersonalization of society. We are a nation of more than 200 million people on the run, and we find little time and few opportunities for forming friendships. Mass participation gives a youth a feeling of nonentity, that there is no place for him or her as an individual; there is no feeling of identity, of worth, of status. It must be pointed out that a person need not get entirely bound up in the mob. There are opportunities for participation in small groups, with one or two persons or acting by oneself. Youth needs both to create opportunities and to take advantage of opportunities that are available. No citizen needs to feel that he or she does not belong to this nation and its people. Every high school student should have identity.

Hypocrisy of adults. In an imperfect world of imperfect people a certain degree of hypocrisy is inevitable and perhaps should be both expected and accepted. This is true of youth as well as of adults. Rank hypocrisy should be exposed and frowned on as rank dishonesty. Youths have a point in identifying a lack of integrity and honesty in the adult population. Having made this point, youngsters should now complete the picture by themselves, living up to their high standards, values, and honesty and demonstrating a laudable integrity.

Success-oriented society. Youngsters protest that today's mad scramble, 8-hour day is meaningless and leads nowhere. They feel that life should be made more meaningful. Youths should be encouraged in their quest for new values, for new purposes in life. Perhaps the present-day adult generation's standards and values need a reexamination and a thorough revision.

Permissiveness. Youths take advantage of today's permissive society but do not truly like what they see or do. They both resent and emulate adults and want proper guidelines laid down for them to live by. Not too much repression and not too much permissiveness is the formula youths want.

Guilt feelings over unearned affluence. Youths today know they are given too much and do not feel right about it. They derive much more satisfaction in doing things and earning things on their own.

Inability to achieve and fear of failure. Idealistic, imperfect youths are frustrated by their inability to reach many of the goals they set for themselves. Perhaps the goals are set too high and should be lowered. Often an inability to achieve reflects a lack of self-discipline. The many diversions and distractions make concentration on study and self-growth discouragingly difficult.

Television and movies. Television has become the most powerful and influential force in the United States. It brings human frailty and opulence into the living room. It gives the nation ringside seats in the slaughter of war, brutality in the streets, and the various violent phenomena of society. Television and movies depict the abnormal in American life, the blasé, and even the distorted. For no group is the television more of a desert wasteland than for youths. The school can help measurably to counter the influence of insulting commercials and the questionable culture of television programs.

In attempting to understand the "angry young men and young women," it is well to keep in mind that society is uncomfortable for them. They are a minority group having no influence and no voice. They have nothing meaningful to contribute to society. Yet they find themselves with an affluence they have not earned, and they accept it with uneasiness and reluctance. There is a crying need to help them understand that in attending school and applying themselves diligently they are preparing themselves for more meaningful roles in society. The future need of the nation is competent, well-educated citizens who can provide the expertise and leadership to lead the nation out of its present dilemma. High school faculties have a responsibility and an opportunity to help youth sift out and explore the many problems and conflicts that disturb them. This is education's number one priority.

Certain guidelines can be an aid to teachers at all levels. Perhaps the elementary school teacher strategically is in the key position.

Desirable *attributes* to develop in children are:

Kindness
Honesty
Neatness
Sharing
Fair play
Cooperation
Thoughtfulness
Consideration
Self-pride
Courteousness
Obedience
Respect for privacy
Desire to do what is right
Respect for persons, rights, property, parents, and
authority

Desirable *practices* for children are:

Saying thoughtful things
Good manners
Proper dress
Sportsmanship
Relation to strangers
Keeping clean
Showing appreciation
Doing for others

Justifiably, it could be asserted that many students develop these qualities on their own. However, with specific effort on the part of the teacher to develop these qualities, all students will better acquire these highly desirable attributes and practices. Schools have an obligation to teach something besides academic subject matter. Teaching that lasts is teaching that develops personal traits and attributes so necessary for adjustment to a highly competitive society. As yet, we have no devices or procedures to measure these qualities in children, but there is ample evidence that children can be beneficially modified through schools' efforts

to improve the ability of students to better themselves.

INDIVIDUAL DIFFERENCES

There is no convenient pattern of emotional maturation. Every person is unique—the product of an interaction of constitution and environment. Every student can be expected to have assets and liabilities of varying degrees. The teacher who can recognize each child's good qualities and give them proper recognition is truly a great teacher. A greater teacher is the one who can also recognize each child's deficiencies and help him or her set up a program of constructive readjustment. Every child needs security as well as faith, love, and acceptance. Every child needs direction and guidance. These are indispensable ingredients of mental health.

QUESTIONS AND EXERCISES

1. What factors can account for the differences in temperament, or emotional mold, in children?
2. Why is it important that the teacher never lose sight of the fact that every child is self-centered and wants attention?
3. What distinguishes negative emotions from positive emotions?
4. Why is it important to explain to a child why his or her conduct is not proper?
5. What is the responsibility of a teacher toward a youngster who has pronounced aggressions?
6. What could be the cause of excessive daydreaming by a 12-year-old?
7. What should be the role of parents, physicians, and schools in dealing with the hyperactive child?
8. Is there a contradiction in saying that in the school a youngster must learn to cooperate and learn to achieve independence?
9. "The youngster who is secure in his status in the home will accept the values of his peer group rather than those of his home." What is the significance of this statement?
10. What can parents do to guide the group, or gang, their children belong to?
11. What can be done for a junior high school youngster who is not accepted by any group?
12. What are the problems of the high school youngster who has a problem of delayed maturation?

13. What counseling should be provided for the youngster with delayed maturation?
14. What are some indications of the inconsistency of youth?
15. The 18-year-old male may be basically heterosexual, but also retains some of the earlier homophilic tendencies. Explain.
16. What causes some youths to be at war with the adult world?
17. What are some common faults of adults when dealing with youths?
18. What should be done about the domineering sixth grader?
19. Should a markedly obese elementary school teacher lead class discussions on nutrition? Support your contention.
20. How can a teacher help students to see themselves as others see them?

REFERENCES AND SELECTED READINGS

Amly, M. C.: Ways of studying children, New York, 1959, Teachers College, Columbia University.

Bach, M.: The power of total living, New York, 1977, Dodd, Mead & Co.

Blaine, G. B., and McArthur, C. C.: Emotional problems of the student, ed. 2, Seattle, 1971, Spectrum Books.

Braga, L., and Braga, J.: Learning and growing, a guide to child development, Chapel Hill, N.C., 1975, Preston-Hill, Inc.

Brunk, J. W.: Child and adolescent development, New York, 1975, John Wiley & Sons, Inc.

Chapman, A. H.: Management of emotional problems of children and adolescents, Philadelphia, 1965, J. B. Lippincott Co.

Chiang, H., and Maslow, A. H.: Healthy personality readings, Cincinnati, 1969, Van Nostrand Reinhold Co.

Collen, M. F.: Multiphasic health testing service, New York, 1978, John Wiley & Sons, Inc.

Dalton, R. H.: Personality and social interaction, Boston, 1961, D. C. Heath & Co.

Despert, J. L.: Emotionally disturbed child, Garden City, N.Y., 1970, Doubleday & Co., Inc.

English, O. S., and Pearson, G. H. J.: Emotional problems of living, ed. 3, New York, 1963, W. W. Norton & Co., Inc.

Faas, L.: Emotionally disturbed child, a book of readings, Springfield, Ill., 1975, Charles C Thomas, Publisher.

Gesell, A., et al.: The child from five t[...] New York, 1977, Harper & Row, Pub[...]

Hamburg, M., and Hamburg, M. V.: H[...] problems in the school, Philadelph[...] Febiger.

Hockbaum, G. M.: Health behavior, Basic Concepts in Health Science Service, Belmont, Calif., 1970, Wadsworth Publishing Co., Inc.

Illingworth, R. S.: The normal child, ed. 3, Atlanta, 1975, Churchill Livingston.

Jourard, S. M.: Healthy personality: an approach from the viewpoint of humanistic psychology, ed. 3, New York, 1974, The Macmillan Co.

Kahn, J. H.: Human growth and the development of personality, ed. 2, New York, 1972, Pergamon Press. Inc.

Lippman, H. S.: Treatment of the child in emotional conflict, ed. 2, New York, 1962, McGraw-Hill Book Co., Inc.

Long, N. J., Morse, W. C., and Newman, R. G.: Conflict in the classroom, Belmont, Calif., 1965, Wadsworth Publishing Co., Inc.

Mayer, G., and Hoover, M.: When children need special help with problems, New York, 1961, Child Study Association of America.

Mussen, P. H., Conger, J. J., and Kagan, J.: Child development and personality, ed. 4, New York, 1974, Harper & Row, Publishers.

Nixon, R. E.: Art of growing: a guide to psychological maturity, New York, 1962, Random House, Inc.

Ridenour, N.: The children we teach, New York, 1960, Mental Health Materials Center.

Rogers, C. R.: On becoming a person, Boston, 1961, Houghton Mifflin Co.

Samuels, H.: Mental health (contemporary topics in health science series), Dubuque, Iowa, 1975, William C. Brown Co., Publishers.

Saul, L. J.: The childhood emotional pattern: the key to personality, its disorders and treatment, New York, 1977, Van Nostrand Reinhold Co.

Sinecore, J. S.: Health, a quality of life, ed. 2, New York, 1974, The Macmillan Co.

Stevenson, A. C., et al.: Genetic counselling, ed. 2, Philadelphia, 1977, J. B. Lippincott Co.

Trapp, P. E.: Readings on the exceptional child, New York, 1962, Appleton-Century-Crofts.

Van Osdol, W. R., and Shane, D. G.: An introduction to exceptional children, ed. 2, Dubuque, Iowa, 1978, William C. Brown Co., Publishers.

Zachry, C. B.: Emotion and conduct in adolescence, for the commissions on secondary school curriculum, Westport, Conn., 1968, Greenwood Press, Inc.

When any calamity has been suffered
the first thing to be remembered is, how
much has been escaped.

Samuel Johnson

CHAPTER 5

Departures from normal health, growth, and development

Every school can expect to have children who deviate from the normal. Some deviations will be minor and affect the youngster little or not at all. In other instances the deviation may be of a nature that so markedly limits the child that special provisions must be made. Whatever the deviation, there are correct ways and incorrect ways to deal with the situation. There are ways to make it possible for children to make the most of whatever endowment they have and to make them feel they are accepted, regular members of the group. Handled incorrectly, children with deviations can be made to feel that they are outsiders, with resulting harm to mental health.

Generally speaking, normal children are eager to accept and assist the child who has some deficiency. It is essential that all children understand the various aspects of the total situation and what their proper role is in the best interest of their classmate with a deviation. Nothing in all of a teacher's experience will be more rewarding or more gratifying than to make a normal, or near-normal, school life possible for the child who has some departure from the normal. Sometimes the opportunity or even the demand of the

teacher may be great; at other times it may be small. Perhaps the need is that of aiding in having the child directed to a physician, perhaps in helping the child to help himself or herself to better health, or perhaps in assisting the child to do the best with what he or she has. Whatever the situation, the teacher's present contribution may well benefit the individual through all the years of his or her life.

Teachers are eager to do everything reasonable for children who deviate from the normal range of health, growth, and development, but are hesitant to act because of a lack of confidence in their knowledge of such conditions. No teacher, neither an elementary classroom teacher nor a secondary school health educator, should be considered an expert on any of these conditions, but the teacher can have a fundamental understanding of their essentials. Such knowledge gives the teacher the confidence to participate actively in a program for the betterment of the child.

RESPONSIBILITY OF THE SCHOOL

Schools do not have a recognized legal responsibility for the correction, or even the improvement, of health defects in any child. The responsibility is recognized as a professional obligation of the teaching profession to do everything reasonable for the health and well-being of every child in school. This professional obligation can be fulfilled in various ways:

1. It may simply be a matter of bringing a child's condition to the attention of the parents.
2. It may be a follow-up of such a referral.
3. It may require counseling with the parents on means for obtaining necessary professional services.
4. It may mean seeking outside financial or other aid to obtain the corrective services the child needs.
5. It may require that the teacher carry out certain instructions from the child's physician or other practitioner.
6. It may be a matter of adapting the school program to the needs of the specific child.
7. It may mean helping the child to help him- or herself in solving health problems that are not directly under the supervision of any practitioner.
8. Most important of all, it may simply mean that the teacher fully understands the child's condition and problems and is able to make the school life more enjoyable and effective because he or she understands the condition and its various implications.

A teacher need not have the technical background of a Sir William Osler. The province of a teacher is neither diagnosis nor therapy. What the role requires is an understanding of how and why various deviations affect the individual child in the pursuit of school life. The teacher needs to know what factors in the school can affect the child favorably as well as unfavorably. Above all, the teacher should have an appreciation of what can be done for the best interests of the child.

LOW VITALITY

A teacher's attention is quickly drawn to children who seem to lack the vitality of other children. These children seem to function at a low level. To move appears to be an effort. Other than their general sluggishness, no symptoms distinguish these children. They may be of normal height, weight, and general growth.

Although many of these children exhibit no pronounced disorders, a thorough examination by a physician usually will ferret out a combination of minor deficiencies that produce the low vitality. Low thyroxin output, anemia, chronic low-grade infection, malnutrition, and visual fatigue account for the sluggishness, and the physician will readily diagnose these conditions. He or she will undertake treatment of the child for these disorders and notify the school of its responsibilities in rejuvenation of the child.

Many times the causes of low vitality are not basically organic, but are primarily functional. Children with low vitality seldom are taken to a physician, and, unless the school makes concerted efforts to help them, they go through school dragging around, disinterested in everything about them, and destined to be social liabilities.

Inadequate rest is more frequently a cause of sluggishness in a child than is generally recognized. Some homes lack any semblance of a regular schedule, and the children get to bed at almost any hour of the night. In addition, sluggishness becomes a habit with some children. A child who has been permitted to loaf through childhood is a neglected child. It is more important that children acquire effective practices for applying their ability than it is that they acquire the usual classroom factual information. The school has both an opportunity and an obligation to develop the best possible work practices for children in keeping with their ability and vitality.

In practice, the school should have a true evaluation of the capacities of a child with low vitality. Further, the school should plan a definite program for improving the general vitality of the child. Such a program should include a regular routine of living, activity sufficient to stimulate muscle tone and circulation, no excessive tension, no excessive fatigue, adequate rest, balanced diet with midmorning and midafternoon lunches, and immediate medical care for illness, whether infectious or organic. Spectacular results are not the rule. Steady, gradual improvement should be the goal. The teacher's personal gratification in being of tangible value to such a child is one of the finest rewards of teaching.

MALNUTRITION

Severe or pronounced malnutrition is relatively uncommon among the children in the United States today, but moderate and mild malnutrition is far more prevalent than is commonly known. A teacher can easily recognize pronounced obesity and underweight, but children with the usual type of vitamin deficiency and lack of sufficient protective foods are not readily detectable. Although the general school health program should be planned to promote the nutrition of every schoolchild, certain children merit special attention because of recognized or suspected nutritional needs.

Obesity. Children more than 10% overweight for their height and age are considered obese. In some children overweight of more than 10% may not visibly affect health adversely during childhood, but the long-term effect may be to lower the level of health. Although no physical effect may be discernible, obesity will reduce both the effectiveness and enjoyment of living. A child who carries around an excess weight of 15 pounds is likely to fatigue easily. Although the added burden may not tax a normal heart, a slightly defective heart may be burdened seriously. Obese children are handicapped in play and in muscular reactions. They frequently are the object of taunts and ridicule and may be considered different by their associates. Being classed out of the normal category is not conducive to the best mental health for the developing child.

Obesity can result only from eating more calories than one uses. Even when a glandular disorder exists in which organic substances readily turn to fat, the organic compounds must come from what a person eats. The remedy for obesity is to eat less or expend more calories or both. Any child who is obese has been eating too much. He or she has established dietary practices that lead to caloric excess. Long-established family dietary customs, perhaps of foreign national origin, patterned to the needs of people who work in the fields or at other manual labor, may well produce obese children who become conditioned to excessive eating. Once this psychophysiological pattern is established, obese children find it progressively more difficult to reduce their intake. Their problem is both physiological and psychological.

Hunger is basically physiological and is governed essentially by the sugar level of the blood. When the blood sugar level is low, a person experiences sensations of hunger. Immediately after a meal, the blood sugar level is high. This high level affects the output of insulin from the pancreas. Insulin converts excess blood sugar to stable glycogen, which is stored in the liver. This results in a low blood sugar level and hunger. It is apparent that consuming carbohydrates (e.g., sugars) to relieve hunger may shortly cause a reaction of high insulin output—low blood sugar and increased hunger. For this reason reducing diets are high in proteins and low in carbohydrates. Proteins satisfy hunger without an appreciable increase in insulin output.

Children who can reduce their caloric intake by 600 calories a day should lose a pound a week. This is a wholesome weight-reduction rate. Cutting down on portions and using proteins to allay between-meal hunger are the two points that must be emphasized. If at all possible, dieting should be done under medical supervision. Encouragement from the teacher and cooperation from the home complete the picture.

An example of a low calorie and high protein diet is one that includes grapefruit, eggs, steak, lamb, chicken, fish, lettuce, tomatoes, combination salads, dry toast, and nonfat milk. Salt is ruled out of the diet and no fried foods (e.g., eggs) should be eaten. Children need not suffer from hunger so long as they use proteins to satisfy their hunger. Once they have reduced their weight to the desired level, the teacher should help them establish permanent dietary practices that will keep their weight within the normal range.

When there is a combination of underweight and illness or even a low level of health, it is the province of the medical profession to find the underlying causes. Yet the observant teacher can initiate the chain reaction that brings the child and physician together. Eliminating the obstacles to good health is more important than bringing the child's weight up to that of the group norm. Putting weight on some of these young bean poles is beyond the ability of the pediatrician. Some underweight children gain a few pounds on a high calorie diet, supplemented by emulsions and a routine of reduced activity and extended rest. Yet those who remain thin despite this special program may well be as healthy and live as long and vibrantly as any of the others.

In practice the school correlates its efforts with the home and family physician. As a minimum the teacher should confer with the parents when concerned about a child's weight. Usually the parents, too, are concerned and express the wish that something could be done. Proposing a health examination is in order. From the examination may come a recommended program to which the school may be asked to contribute. Or it may elicit this sage advice from the physician, "The child is healthy and normal in all respects, including weight for his particular constitutional type."

Specific nutritional deficiencies. It obviously is not the role of teachers to diagnose deficiency diseases. They may suspect that a specific condition is the result of a nutritional deficiency. Perhaps if, as a health project, each child records the family menus for a week, the suspicions of the teacher will receive further support. Yet in the absence of medical diagnosis and direction, the teacher's province is primarily that of education that results in desirable knowledge, attitudes, and practices. A teacher with ingenuity and a sincere interest in the child can utilize the school lunch, the home, and self-interest to achieve a gradual yet tangible improvement in his or her general condition. A well-thought-out plan to assure the child of the necessary quality foods is basic. "Drugstore vitamins" should not be taken without a physician's prescription.

Digestive system disturbances. Most digestive disturbances in school-age children are accompanied by symptoms and signs that serve as warnings that something is wrong in the digestive system. The symptoms might include a mild upset from which the child recovers in a relatively short period of time. It is not for the teacher to diagnose what the disorder is; rather, it is the teacher's responsibility to provide immediate care for the child. This may involve obtaining medical service, hospitalization, home care, or providing care in the school building.

Symptoms are descriptive of what the sensations are that the patient experiences. This may include such things as nausea, pain, elevated temperature, irritability, or headache.

Signs are descriptive of what can be seen by observing the patient. This could include flushed skin; restlessness; red, watery eyes; or facial grimaces. Mild symptoms and signs do not necessarily denote a mild illness.

It is not in the province of the teacher, nurse, or administrator to make a diagnosis when a child becomes ill while at school. It may be a difficult task for a physician to make the necessary diagnosis. This becomes apparent when one lists just a few disorders of the digestive system to illustrate what is involved:

Gastroenteritis

Upset stomach

Ulcers

Appendicitis

Injury

A teacher's responsibility begins the moment he or she receives word of the child's illness. The teacher then initiates action in the best interests of the child by following procedures such as those presented in Chapter 9. A child with abdominal pain merits the immediate services of a physician. Parents of the child should be contacted, and the school should aid the parents in deciding the best course of action.

ENDOCRINE DISTURBANCES

Neither the classroom teacher nor the director of the school health program is expected to be an expert on glandular disorders. Yet an understanding of some of the disorders that may likely be found in a school population can be of value to the teacher and to particular children. Parents and the teacher's school superiors hold in high regard the teacher who understands children with special problems.

Diabetes mellitus. Although it is generally considered a disease of later life, since the average age of the more than 1,500,000 diabetic persons in the United States is 55 years, diabetes mellitus does occur among school-age children and occasionally among preschool children. Medical authorities point out that for every four known cases, three unrecognized cases of diabetes exist.

Most persons who have diabetes can keep well and lead healthful and useful lives. Careful attention to the physician's instructions can safeguard the subject's health. In this respect the school can be of appreciable service to the diabetic student.

Diabetes mellitus is usually the result of a deficiency in the insulin output of the islands of Langerhans in the pancreas. It also may be caused by a deficiency of the glycogenic hormone of the anterior pituitary gland. A deficiency of these hormones results in a high level of blood sugar (hyperglycemia) and sugar in the urine (glycosuria). Lassitude and weariness result; there is a pronounced thirst after meals, and, with the subsequent consumption of water, there is frequent urination. Increased hunger, a drawn expression, and a loss of weight may occur. The mouth is dry, the tongue red and sore. Dry skin, itching, eczema, and boils occur. The eyes are affected, and neuritis, numbness, and tingling of the hands and feet occur. Marked weakness results from the inability of the muscles to use available fuel.

Some diabetic students may be on a restricted diet, which may be sufficient to control the condition. The physician or parents should inform the school of the prescribed diet and routine for physical activity. The teacher should guide the child in adherence to the prescription. In the absence of such information, the teacher will have to regard the child as any normal member of the group.

Children under insulin treatment will probably receive their injection at least an hour before coming to school. The peak of the effect may occur a short time after arrival at school. Or it may appear late in the afternoon, and a low blood sugar level (hypoglycemia) may result. The condition is commonly spoken of as insulin shock and is characterized by trembling, faintness, palpitation, unsteadiness, excessive perspiration, and hunger. Orange juice, which contains carbohydrates, produces recovery in a few minutes. Some children carry a supply of carbohydrates and begin to ingest them immediately on the appearance of symptoms. The other children soon accept the procedure, and it becomes part of the school life. It is indicative of a mentally hygienic school environment.

Hypoglycemia. Abnormal behavior in children can arise from an unusual body chemistry and, as a consequence, mask the true cause and nature of the illness. Hypoglycemia is one of these conditions. The dominant factor is a low level of sugar in the blood, responsible for periods of irritability, confusion, depressions, lethargy, complaints of weakness in the extremities, and inability to concentrate. As soon as a physician puts the patient on a selective diet, there will be an improvement in the patient's behavior.

Hyperthyroidism. Youngsters with a basal metabolic rate above plus 10 may be considered to have a hyperthyroid condition. During childhood the children are healthy, thin, but strikingly robust, active, energetic, high-strung, and perhaps nervous and highly excitable. They never seem to tire and seldom are ill. As adolescents they may be restless, energetic persons who are perpetual doers and workers. They may be impatient and impulsive. Life is at a maximum function for these persons from early in the morning until late at night. To be idle is their biggest trial.

The need for a routine or plan for everyday living is urgent with some of these children. In this, guidance from the teacher can be helpful. To harness this energy and direct it

into productive channels is the objective. Routinization of the day helps to slow down the dizzy pace.

Persons with excessive hyperthyroidism obviously need medical supervision.

Hypothyroidism. Children with extreme hypothyroidism (cretinism) do not attend school, but children with marked thyroxin deficiency are present in our classrooms. They are disinterested and slow, need constant coaxing and forcing, are chronically late, and do poorly in their schoolwork. They perspire very little, have a slow reaction time, fatigue easily, sleep heavily, and are often accused of being lazy loafers. Life is a real effort for these children. In practice, teachers should exercise patience and strive to understand the child's limitations. A duty-possessed teacher who lacks understanding could do infinite harm by harrassing such children every hour of the day.

Endocrine therapy can do much for these students. Frequently treatment transforms them into alert, energetic, active, and bright-eyed children who for the first time, as expressed by one of them, "really know what it is like to live." Sometimes at puberty, nature brings about this sudden reversal from a dull, lackadaisical child to a highly animated, vivacious adolescent.

RHEUMATIC FEVER

Rheumatic fever is an insidious disease that overtakes a child stealthily. Although it undoubtedly is infectious, the causative agent is not known. However, physicians generally agree that a certain type of infection is the forerunner of rheumatic fever. Group A *beta*-hemolytic streptococcus, producing a sore throat, is the recognized source of rheumatic fever. From this primary infection two additional phases can be delineated in the evolution of rheumatic fever:

1. Middle phase—dormant phase, which lasts 2 or 3 weeks after the sore throat

and during which no visible symptoms appear; child seems completely recovered from sore throat.

2. Final phase—acute rheumatic fever, which lasts from 2 or 3 weeks to several months.

Although most afflicted children have the services of a physician and the condition has been diagnosed, some children appear in the classroom without the benefit of medical advice. It is not the province of the teacher to diagnose rheumatic fever, but the teacher who recognizes certain danger signals can contribute immeasurably to the child's welfare by bringing the matter to the attention of the parents. Early detection may prevent the most serious complication—rheumatic heart disease.

Specific symptoms do not exist in every case of rheumatic fever, but enumeration of the various symptoms that have been observed will encompass the symptoms of any specific case. They include fever; irritability; undue fatigue; nosebleeds; pallor; pain in the joints, arms, and legs; jerky and twitching motions; poor appetite; loss of weight; and a lack of interest in school activities. The teacher will make no mistake in contacting the parents of a child with several of these symptoms because there obviously is something wrong with the child and he or she should not be in school.

Prevention of rheumatic fever. Rheumatic fever is not communicable; therefore prevention is directed toward the conditions that are forerunners of it. Prevention of the spread of throat infections in the school should have an indirect effect on reducing the incidence of rheumatic fever. Prompt medical treatment for any throat infection may prevent it from becoming the forerunner of rheumatic fever.

Since rheumatic fever tends to run in families, members of the patient's family should be informed of the need for a well-balanced diet, adequate rest, early treatment of respiratory infections, and regular medical supervision. A child with rheumatic fever will receive long-term medication from the physician to prevent repeated attacks.

Classroom adjustment. When children who have recovered from rheumatic fever return to the classroom, their activities will be guided by the instructions of the attending physician. If the disease has impaired the heart, a well-planned program will be proposed to the school, but, if no cardiac complications have occurred, the children should be made to feel that they are normal members of the group. Participation within their limits is imperative for the children. Overprotection produces feelings of dependence and anxiety. Confidence of children in their ability to live normally is worth cultivating.

CARDIOVASCULAR DISORDERS

Approximately 1% of schoolchildren in the United States have a diagnosed cardiac disorder. Together, rheumatic fever and its accessory, rheumatic heart disorder, cause more disability than any other disease of childhood. A second important cardiac disorder of childhood is congenital heart defect. In both congenital heart defect and rheumatic heart disorder, the everyday management or supervision of the child is all-important. A teacher who knows what should and can be done is in a position to make an invaluable contribution to the well-being of the child.

Congenital heart defects. A child may be born with a defective heart. Some defects are so severe that the child does not survive to school age. Other defects are of such a nature that the child can attend school. Some congenital heart conditions can benefit from surgery; others cannot be helped by methods now known. Some congenital heart disorders are so minor that they can almost be ignored. Others are not serious enough to prevent a child from attending school; yet the child is in need of everyday supervision and management. From this range in degree of defect it is apparent that some knowledge of these defects will enable the teacher to cooperate effectively with the child's physician and fully understand his or her instructions.

Many cardiac patients can participate in the regular classroom activites. Restriction or limitation should not be imposed except on instruction from the child's physician. Many of these children limit their own activity when necessary because of the distress of fatigue. A physician may rule out competitive sports for children because in the excitement of competition they may be oblivious of fatigue. Restrictions imposed by the physician are only those that must be imposed because, for children to be mentally healthy, it is desirable that they live as normal a life as possible. It is essential that children develop a wholesome, positive attitude toward their capacities and abilities. The teacher should emphasize what they can do and give less emphasis to what they cannot do if they are on a restrictive regimen.

Rheumatic heart disease. Two out of three rheumatic fever patients suffer damaged hearts. A single attack may cause minor damage, but recurrence of the disease will likely cause further damage to the heart. Rheumatic fever "licks the joints but bites the heart." With regular medical supervision, attacks can be prevented from recurring.

During the acute stage of the infection the heart muscle may be affected. This muscle inflammation (myocarditis) may weaken and enlarge the heart. At times the outer heart covering is inflamed (pericarditis). As the infection declines, the heart tends to return to normal size. Permanent injury usually is the result of inflammation of the valves of the left half of the heart. During the healing process scar tissue forms, which prevents the valves from opening or closing properly.

About a third of the children with rheumatic fever show no evidence of heart damage; about one third more show signs of cardiac injury, but can lead practically normal lives.

No limitations should be placed on the child except those advised by the physician. From the physician's advice the teacher makes such classroom adaptations as are indicated. Such adjustments may include permission for the child to be late to school, special transportation, restricted recess and physical education activity, a minimum of stair climbing, between-meal lunches, and rest periods. As much as possible children should be made to feel that they are not abnormal but can, with some exceptions, participate in the regular work of the classroom.

If children should experience a cardiac crisis, the teacher should allow them to assume a comfortable position. They may find it comfortable to lie flat, but, if they have difficulty in breathing, they should be permitted to sit up. Giving them plenty of air and loosening clothing may be of help. The poise of the teacher while waiting for the physician will be important in effecting composure in both the subjects and their classmates.

Hypertension. High blood pressure is not frequent among children of school age, but it does occasionally occur among boys of high school age. Among girls of this age the condition is extremely unusual. High blood pressure (hypertension) is not caused by a disorder of the walls of the arteries, but perhaps by overstimulation of the vasoconstrictor nerve fibers that govern the contraction of the arteries. This excessive contraction of the vessels indirectly produces an elevation in blood pressure. Certain renal, endocrine, vascular, and cerebral disorders may also account for hypertension.

Even in a normal person systolic blood pressure may vary considerably, but in hypertension the systolic pressure consistently will be above 160 mm Hg. Sometimes the condition is functional, being the result of mental and emotional tensions. If their tensions are relieved, these persons improve considerably. Sometimes the condition is organic, perhaps caused by a substance produced in the kidneys that affects the vasoconstrictor center of the brain. From this center originate the impulses that travel along the vasoconstrictor nerve fibers.

In practice the school should rely on the students' family physicians for guidance in making any necessary provisions for students with hypertension. Some physicians forbid participation in vigorous athletics, but otherwise approve the normal activities of a typical high school. With this prescription the student enjoys a normal existence. Often the vascular pressure returns to normal.

ANEMIA

Anemia literally means without blood (Gr. *An*, without; *haima*, blood), but in its practical sense anemia means a condition in which the red corpuscle count or the hemoglobin content of the blood is low or both deficiencies are present. Actually, anemia is not a specific disease, but a symptom that may arise from various causes.

Skin color is not an index to the condition of the blood. Pallor, of itself, does not denote anemia. Pale lips and fingernails may be somewhat indicative, and a pale inner lining (conjunctiva) of the eyelid may be associated with anemia. A better general indication is the lack of vitality and endurance of the child. Since oxygen available for the tissues depends on adequate red blood cells and hemoglobin content, the anemic child becomes breathless quickly and is unusually fatigued and uncomfortable. Surprisingly some anemic children will not be denied in physical contests and will exert themselves to the limit to keep up with the group. Ane-

mic children frequently are missed until a physician makes a count of the red blood cells and a hemoglobin determination.

Anemia occurs most frequently among girls. Perhaps biologically girls are more prone to anemia, but usually the condition is preventable.

Several classes of anemia are recognized, but two of them are most likely to be found in children of school age. Other types occur rather infrequently.

Chlorosis, which is the anemia of preteen-age children, occurs among girls and results in a sallow complexion. It occurs less frequently than formerly because of improved nutrition. In most girls with this type, the anemia is caused by poor nutrition, although sometimes it results from the inability of the red marow cells to produce sufficient red blood cells.

The most frequent type of anemia that occurs in school-age children is *nutritional anemia* caused by dietary deficiencies or the inability of the body to utilize the constituents of the diet. Iron, proteins, and copper are essential for the production of red blood cells. Yet the human male needs only about 0.006 to 0.010 g of iron daily, since the iron fraction of hemoglobin is used over and over again. A female needs four times as much iron as a male. Too much milk in the diet may displace such valued sources of iron and protein as egg yolk, liver, and other meats.

In the school, anemic children may be helped by supplementary feedings, reduced activity, and extra periods of rest. However, primary supervision of the child should be by the physician who likely will prescribe medication to stimulate the production of red blood cells and formation of hemoglobin. If children who lack normal vitality are not under medical supervision, the teacher performs a service by arranging for thorough health checkups for them.

DISORDERS OF POSTURE

In the typical school situation, posture is not regarded as an important factor in the promotion of student health. True, a deviation in posture usually does not produce a serious threat to health. Yet, like other physical disorders, postural defects in children should be the concern of all school personnel, not just the responsibility of the health teachers and school nurses.

A child does not stand in a straight line but in four counterbalancing curves—cervical, thoracic, lumbar, and sacral. These vertebral curves are not in perfect compensating alignment but must be supported by the skeletal muscles. Whether a child is standing, walking, or sitting, four criteria can be applied as the index of good posture: (1) head erect, neck back, and chin level; (2) no exaggeration of vertebral curvatures; (3) chest lifted slightly; and (4) shoulders held broad, without tension.

In standing, the body weight should be over the center of each foot, and the feet should be toeing straight forward. In walking, a rhythmical gait with a free and easy leg swing should be supplemented by a free and easy arm swing. The feet should be nearly parallel. In sitting, the hips, knee, and ankle should point straight ahead and be flat on the floor.

Most poor posture is functional, that is, it results from carelessness in habits, and a considerable amount results from poor muscle tone. Deformities of the skeleton and joints account for a very small percentage of poor posture.

Which is cause and which is effect, poor posture or poor health? In many youngsters poor health reflected in poor muscle tone leads to poor posture, which leads to further poor health in a downward spiral. In other youngsters, slovenly habits reflected in poor posture have a deleterious effect on health

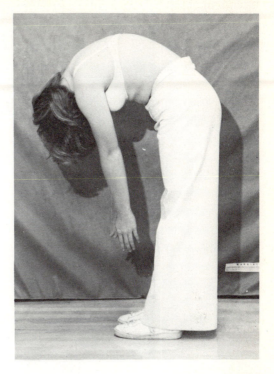

Fig. 5-1. Proper stance for scoliosis checkup. Marked arching of the back reveals any misalignment a student may have. (Courtesy Marion County Health Department, Salem, Ore.)

with a downward spiral of both posture and health.

In recent years school nurses and health instructors have been greatly concerned about *scoliosis* in junior high and senior high school students. The term scoliosis is applied to the condition in which there is a lateral curvature of the vertebral column. To identify a curvature the subject bends forward and arches the back. The person doing the testing runs his or her fingers along the spines of the vertebrae to identify a curvature. The condition often occurs first among junior high students and appears more frequently in girls.

The usual procedure is to line up a physical

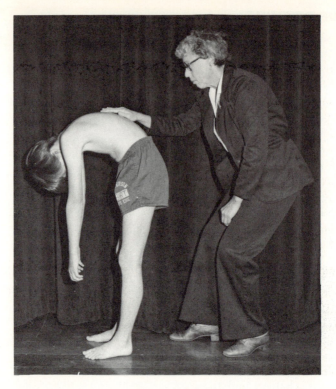

Fig. 5-2. Scoliosis detection program. School nurse examining vertebral column for possible deviation. (Courtesy Marion County Health Department, Salem, Ore.)

education class and, like a mass inoculation, the line passes along one after another (Fig. 5-1). Some schools obtain parental approval by having parents sign a printed permission card. Other schools carry out a publicity program and inform the parents to notify the school if they have objections to having their children tested (Fig. 5-2).

Round shoulders may be a concern of both the school health department and the physical education staff. Likewise, *visceroptosis* (often referred to as abdominal paunch) is a condition the health and physical education personnel are concerned about. Whether the corrective program is conducted on a group or individual basis, the need is to develop muscle tone.

Perhaps the greatest contribution of good posture is the mental health attributes of confidence, euphoria, and vitality that proper posture can provide. Good posture is essential to a vigorous state of health, and it provides the extra dividend of a striking personal appearance.

DEVIATIONS OF THE RESPIRATORY SYSTEM

Some noninfectious chronic conditions of the respiratory system are of minor consequence. Others are significant in terms of reducing the effectiveness and enjoyment of life. Occasionally, life itself may be threatened.

Nasal congestion. All persons experience

some congestion of the nasal passages, but usually it is a temporary condition resulting from an excessive production of mucus associated with coryza or other respiratory infection. Although it is temporarily distressing, the accumulation of mucus is not serious, being a natural response to irritation of the mucous tissue. A chronic or permanent congestion may be caused by mucus or can be a mechanical obstruction such as a stemmed growth (polyp) of mucous tissue. Except for the inconvenience, some of these congestions are not too serious, whereas others need constant medical care or correction by surgery.

Sinusitis. The sinuses of the skull are air cavities lined with the same type of mucous tissue that lines the nasal passages. Two frontal sinuses, one above each orbit, and two maxillary sinuses, one in each upper jawbone beneath the orbits, have narrow passageways, or ducts, that empty into the nasal passages. Exhaled and inhaled air passes into the ducts and sinuses. These structures are properly considered part of the respiratory tract. Even normally the mucous tissue lining the sinuses secretes a small to moderate amount of mucus. Mechanical or bacterial irritation can produce an excessive amount of mucus (ozena), with resulting congestion. Until the irritation is removed, the overproduction of mucus is likely to continue. Persons with constricted ducts may have sinus congestion, with devastating pain.

To use home or patented remedies to deal with excessive mucus is fraught with considerable danger. Nasal sprays that contain astringents may constrict blood vessels and, for a while, reduce mucus output. However, these sprays in time will be highly irritating to the sensitive tissue, and serious damage may result.

In practice the school should identify children with chronic sinusitis and set into action the chain of events that will bring the child into the office of a physician. If a cure is not possible, the physician at least will relieve the child of much distress.

Deviated septum. At least half the adults in the United States have some degree of deviation of the partition that separates the nares, but most deviations are of no particular significance. Deviation can occur without a nasal fracture.

In children, only when the deviation is so pronounced that one of the nasal passages is closed will surgery be advised by the physician. When the condition is so markedly pronounced, the teacher will observe that, although the youngster has no difficulty in breathing under ordinary conditions, slight exertion requires mouth breathing. Closing the open naris by pressure with the finger and asking the child to exhale forcibly will indicate the degree of obstruction in the other passage. Mouth breathing is not necessarily objectionable, but the chronic condition that produces it usually requires correction.

Enlarged turbinate bones. On the lateral surface of the nares, the scroll-shaped turbinate bones may be sufficiently enlarged to obstruct breathing. It is an infrequent condition in children, but, if present, is discovered in the typical health examination of schoolchildren. Excessive production of mucus as well as any obstruction in the nasal passage is a discomfort, if not a hazard to well-being.

Allergy. Hypersensitivity can affect the respiratory tract in a variety of ways. Hay fever, bronchial asthma, bronchitis, and croup are end products of allergies that affect the respiratory system. Although some of these conditions exist when the child enters school, others do not become evident until the child is in the teen years. Sometimes allergies do not appear until adulthood. Because of the factor of inheritance, children with a family history of allergy should be considered to have a possible respiratory allergy if they display chronic respiratory disturbances while in school. Unwittingly some teachers, suspecting an infectious condition, exclude children from school only to discover that they have an allergy. Had they studied the health record form of these students, they might have avoided this embarrassment.

Under medical supervision, children with respiratory allergies usually carry on the normal activities of school life. An asthmatic attack in school may appear dramatic, but should not be alarming. Generally the students themselves know what action to take. A sitting position is usually more comfortable than any other. For many children exhalation is the more difficult mechanism, and a siege may leave them near exhaustion. Poise and assurance on the part of the teacher may help the student to relax.

DISORDERS OF THE ORAL CAVITY

Disorders of the oral cavity are not an urgent life-and-death matter; yet they play an important role in the quality of health, the length of the prime of life, and life expectation. Early detection and correction are dictated if the child's present and future well-being are considered.

Caries and cavities. The process of dental decay is called caries; the end result of decay is the cavity. The process is initiated by the *Lactobacillus acidophilus* (LA) organism and can be expressed in the equation

$$LA \rightarrow Enzyme + Carbohydrate = Acid$$

Disintegration of the enamel occurs as the acid dissolves it.

Dental cavities occur more frequently than any other disorder that schoolchildren experience. Yet, of itself, a simple cavity may have no effect on health. However, it may progress to a point at which the tooth is de-stroyed or must be extracted. Loss of several teeth, without compensating dentures, can affect a person's dietary practices, and, what is more serious, the cavity can be an avenue of invasion for disease-producing organisms that can pass, via the pulp cavity, to the apex of the tooth root and produce an abscess.

It is not the province of teachers to examine children's mouths. To prevent the children from having caries, they can carry on a program to encourage effective practices of dental care, including a visit to the dentist at least twice a year. Whenever a child with a special dental health problem comes to their attention, counseling an immediate visit to the dentist is the minimum service they owe to the child.

Abscess. An infection in the gum or at the apex of a tooth root may be painful or virtually painless. Toxins produced at the abscess can travel about the body and cause serious impairment of vital tissues. Any gum involvement, including the familiar gum boil, which is an abscess, is a warning of the need for immediate professional attention. Prompt action may save the tooth and prevent injury to the general health.

Pyorrhea. Pyorrhea is an infectious or mechanical irritation of the periodontal membrane, which attaches the tooth to the gum and bone. A red margin of the gum around the neck of the tooth is indicative of this irritation. If permitted to continue, the irritation may seriously damage the membrane. Since the periodontal membrane does not have the capacity to rejuvenate itself, the tooth becomes permanently loosened and may have to be extracted.

Gingivitis. Any inflammation of the gum may be termed gingivitis, but in its general usage the term designates infection by two known pathogens, *Bacillus fusiformis* and *Borrelia vincentii*. Commonly called trench mouth, or Vincent's disease, the condition is characterized by inflammation and even ulceration of the gums and other parts of the mouth, bleeding, excess salivation, and considerable soreness.

Gingivitis does not often occur in the healthy child. Malnutrition, poor general health, inadequate rest, and poor mouth care predispose to gingivitis. The infection can be treated successfully by the dentist, but improvement in general health also should be sought.

Malocclusion. Marked overbite or underbite and poorly aligned teeth create mechanical problems that eventually destroy the supporting tissue. For children with these conditions, the services of an orthodontist are a necessity, not a luxury. Before their school days are over, by some means, these children should have the services of an orthodontist. Once the teeth are permanently set, as in adulthood, it may be too late. Correction of these conditions when a child is 15 years of age or younger means a possible 70 years of benefit. A conscientious teacher will do everything possible to see that the child receives the necessary service. The child is not the only one to benefit. Nothing in the teacher's professional experience is more gratifying than to watch the change in a child who has benefited from orthodontics.

DISORDERS OF VISION

With a function as complex as vision and a structure as remarkable as the human eye, the wonder is that the incidence of defective vision is not greater. Every school expects to have children whose vision is not normal. Standard screening tests usually detect children with more pronounced vision disability, and a professional practitioner's examination will locate even the slightest disability. Teachers who observe their students closely can be helpful in detecting children whose posturing, squinting, inattention, or poor progress may be due to their inability to see normally.

Myopia. Nearsightedness is a heritable tendency and is usually caused by elongated eyeballs. The image falls in front of the retina unless the object is close to the eye. Thus close objects can be seen quite clearly, but distant objects are blurred. Fortunately, concave lenses will compensate for the extra length of the eye bulb. Although nearsighted children may be able to read without glasses, they will become less distressed and fatigued with proper glasses. They also will see better at various ranges.

Hyperopia. Farsightedness is caused by an eyeball so short that the image literally falls behind the retina. With a great deal of effort, a farsighted child can see near objects by overworking the delicate muscles of accommodation. Visual fatigue sets in very quickly with such strain. A tendency to become cross-eyed is possible. Convex lenses can compensate for the farsightedness so that the child can read with a minimum of strain and fatigue.

Astigmatism. Irregularities in the curvature of the cornea and lens prevent a true focus of the eye, and a blurred image with discomfort results. Astigmatism requires carefully prescribed glasses and, in some instances, frequent renewal of the prescription. Contact lenses frequently prove highly satisfactory. For effective and enjoyable living, the child with astigmatism needs glasses of accurate prescription.

Amblyopia. Dimness of vision without known cause can occur in people of all ages. No discernible lesion in the eye structures is present. A disturbance in the optic nerve is a possible cause. It is known that certain metallic poisons, certain toxins, alcohol, tobacco, and uremic conditions can be responsible for the disturbance, but in children usually no specific cause can be identified.

Amblyopia may begin with a central or peripheral spot where there is little vision. The condition may enlarge slowly and will progressively interfere with vision. Visual disturbance will be more pronounced in bright light.

Fortunately, amblyopia in children usually clears up spontaneously, but every child with dimness of vision should be under the supervision of an ophthalmologist for periodic checkups.

Strabismus. *Cross-eye*, not cross-eyes, is descriptive of strabismus, since only one eye is crossed because of a shortened extrinsic muscle that turns the eye inward. Ophthalmologists can correct many conditions of strabismus by treatment or surgery or a combination of procedures. Early attention to the condition is essential. The accommodation or acuity of one or both eyes may be affected in some children if the condition is untreated. Such children exhibit posturing and other signs of difficult vision. The alert teacher will call this difficulty to the attention of the child's parents.

Ptosis. A drooping of one or both upper eyelids is usually an inherited condition in which the nerves that stimulate the elevating muscle do not conduct impulses. Paralysis of the muscle may come on gradually during the school life of the child. If the paralysis is bilateral, children will naturally tilt their heads back in order to see through the small apertures formed by the backward tilt of the head. Ptosis is a symptom of myasthenia gravis and can be corrected adequately with drugs. Occasionally surgery may be necessary.

HEARING DISABILITY

Most children who have some hearing loss acquire it gradually. The audiometric test will determine hearing disabilities, but the alert teacher can observe indications that a child has hearing difficulties. Children who cannot hear well will often posture, are inattentive, copy, and make poor progress. Faulty pronunciation and an unnatural voice are hints that the child does not hear well.

Conduction deafness. Almost all hearing loss in children is caused by disturbances of the outer and middle ear that interfere with the conduction of sound. Excessive wax (cerumen), ruptured or rigid tympanic membrane, rigidity of the ligaments of the bones (ossicles) of the middle ear, mucus congestion of the middle ear, and rigidity of the oval window of the spiral shell (cochlea)—all can interfere with sound conduction. Some of these conditions can be corrected, and most are amenable to treatment.

Perception deafness. Nerve deafness or perception deafness is relatively rare in children of school age. It may be caused by an injury or disease in the neuron or inner part of the ear. Infected gums or gallbladder can be the primary cause of perception deafness. It also can result from meningitis, influenza, and drugs such as quinine and salicylates. Extremely high body temperature can also result in perception deafness.

Some types of hearing loss cannot be prevented or corrected. However, hearing aids can compensate for much of the deficiency in persons with impaired hearing. Today prescriptions for hearing aids are written with the same precision as prescriptions for glasses. Some people are unable to hear the sounds of high frequencies, and the hearing aid is prescribed to compensate for this specific deficiency. Wearing a hearing aid is now just as acceptable as wearing spectacles.

In addition to letting the parents know that a child has a hearing defect, the teacher can be of further service by helping children to understand that wearing a hearing aid is a sensible thing and not a stigma. How fortunate the child is to have a disability for which science has a relatively simple solution, rather than to have some disability for which nothing can be done!

NEUROLOGICAL DISORDERS

Two neurological disorders, epilepsy and chorea, from which some students suffer and which cause the uninformed teacher considerable concern, are worthy of discussion. An understanding of the two conditions and the proper care of the afflicted children gives a teacher the assurance necessary for dealing with any episode involving these children.

Epilepsy. From its Greek derivation, the word *epilepsy* literally means a seizure. Being merely descriptive of clinical symptoms, the term is not satisfactory, but it usually is employed to designate recurrent fits and periods of unconsciousness.

Grand mal is the more serious type of epileptic seizure. Essentially it is a convulsive seizure with the following characteristics:

1. Aura, or sensory disturbances (e.g., light or taste) sometimes preceding and giving warning of the attack
2. Sometimes a shrill and startling cry
3. Sudden loss of consciousness and falling backward
4. Pupils dilated; eyes open at beginning of seizure
5. Tonic spasm—drawing up limbs in rigid, flexed position
6. Clonic spasm—intermittent contraction and relaxation with thrashing about of arms and legs
7. Spasm of respiratory muscles—no breathing and blueness of the face
8. Spasm of jaw muscles—biting the tongue results in bloody foam
9. Relaxation, prolonged stupor, and profound sleep

The active convulsion lasts less than a minute and terminates in exhaustion. During the seizure an attempt should be made to protect the child from injury. It is sometimes possible to catch the individual and prevent a fall. Moving the child out into a clear space away from hot and sharp objects may prevent injury. The seizure should not be resisted. Children who have only two or three grand mal seizures during the school year usually continue school attendance. When seizures becomes so frequent as to disrupt the class, the child should remain at home until medication can control the seizures somewhat. The cause of epilepsy is unknown, but sedatives can reduce the severity of seizures and increase the length of time between seizures.

Typical minor attacks (petit mal) are characterized by a transitory (3- or 4-second) loss of consciousness without falling and only minor, if any, muscular twitching. These children attend school without any particular incidents.

Chorea. Commonly called St. Vitus' dance, chorea is characterized by convulsive twitchings, especially of the facial muscles. Grimaces and arm and body jerking occur, with some remission from time to time. The disorder usually follows a siege of rheumatic fever or other infection, which sometimes has gone undiscovered. Toxins appear to affect one of the motor control centers of the brain, and the incoordination results. Most of these children can be treated very effectively.

Because of the effectiveness of modern treatment, children with chorea are not encountered as frequently in school as in former years. Yet they are encountered. After ascertaining that children are under medical care, the teacher should try to treat them as normal members of the class. It may be helpful for the child to avoid undue excitement and fatigue. If a child with chorea is not under treatment, the school should take steps necessary to make medical care available to him or her.

DELAYED MATURATION AND GROWTH

A typical school population will have children who are retarded in either or both maturation and growth. Most of these children show little concern over their delayed growing up, and there is no reason why the teacher should be concerned and thereby intensify their concern. So long as these children possess a good level of health, they should be accepted as normal members of the group. In all likelihood the child's physician will have nothing to offer that might hasten growth and maturity and will not deem any action on his or her part necessary. Eventually the child will mature into adulthood. Although the student may never attain average adult height and weight, growth will take place. To assure a disturbed child that his or her final level of growth and development will be within the normal range is a service that the teacher can contribute.

ACCELERATED MATURATION AND GROWTH

Whereas boys show most concern about delayed growth and development, girls are more likely to be disturbed by acceleration of maturation and growth. Yet girls can be assured that there are many illustrious women who have traveled the same road. To adapt to her situation is the girl's goal. To despair is to take an emotional approach. If the precocity is the result of an overactive adrenal cortex or other physical causes, usually little or nothing can be done. Sometimes the accelerated maturation and growth occurs while the girl is relatively young, causing her to attain adult physiological maturity at an early age. A girl who understands her assets and places primary emphasis on these will usually make a wholesome adjustment. Indeed, many make these assets the springboard to outstanding achievement.

DEVIATIONS IN MENTAL HEALTH

Major and minor mental disorders are the province of the medical profession, but the teaching profession is in a most strategic position to give wholesome, positive assistance to the child who exhibits personality deviations. Most of these deviations are not serious, but they do detract from the child's effectiveness and enjoyment of life and may become serious if nothing constructive is done to correct the deviation.

In undertaking to aid children with a personality deviation, the teacher must obtain as complete an understanding of the children and their background as is practical. Then the teacher must strive to answer the cardinal question, What motivates this conduct? Any constructive program of readjustment is certain to yield the child some benefit and in many cases will produce the optimum of readjustment.

Undue shyness. A shy child is a lonesome child. The shyness may be an expression of too marked a feeling of inferiority. It may be a fear of failure or embarrassment. It can be mere habit. It may be a lack of preschool opportunities to associate with children of the same age. It can be a reaction to imaginary guilt.

A teacher with ingenuity will contrive situations in which the child will associate closely with one, two, and then several of the group. If the shyness is to be overcome, it is essential that a child be brought gradually into the activities of the group. It is most helpful for the teacher to express high regard for the child and to point out that the other children in the class feel the same way. The solution is gradual readjustment, not medical treatment.

Tendency to be a "loner." Children who seek to be alone, to do everything on their own, may never have learned to play or work with others. They may not feel equal to the group, or they may feel that the group does not accept them. Perhaps home background or an imaginary deficiency is the genesis of the tendency.

Constructive readjustment would require opportunities for group participation, perhaps indirectly at first. Self-esteem must be bolstered, particularly in terms of contributions to the class and school.

Restlessness and easy distraction. A thyroid disorder, malnutrition, or inadequate rest may be the cause of restlessness. Uneasiness may be caused by a feeling of inadequacy. Lack of success and its subsequent gratification may lead to disinterest.

If physical disturbances have been ruled out, a child should be motivated to take an interest in school activities by assistance in attaining success and by learning to enjoy success. If the child has a short attention span, a reshuffling of the daily schedule may be helpful.

Excessive daydreaming. Physical health may be of significance in accounting for daydreaming. Inadequate rest, visual fatigue, and a low level of vitality may be present. A lack of success, with a resulting escape into fantasy, may be the primary factor. Children who obtain self-gratification entirely in a dream world must be brought out into the world of reality through assigned tasks that require that they focus their attention away from themselves.

Anxiety states. An overanxious, tense, apprehensive child shows an inability to relax. Fear of censorship, fear of punishment, or fear of failure may underlie the anxiety state. Identification with an older person who is tense and unrelaxed can be the source of the child's tenseness.

Helping children to assess their own abilities and success can yield tangible results. These children need to be assured of the importance of their role in the home, in

school, and with their associates. That they are held in high esteem by those about them can be helpful. Readjustment usually is a slow process.

Sitting on sidelines. Frequently from mere habit some children have been conditioned to be spectators, not participants. The busy elementary schoolteacher unintentionally permits children to slide into this mode of life. In other children, fear of failure or embarrassment can be primary factors. The child who likes to be coaxed is usually seeking attention in a manner society does not approve.

Devising situations in which the child is naturally a participant is not difficult. If the new practice is associated with success, it will likely become habitual.

Hysteria. Occasionally a child of school age will display hysteria. This type of person usually is highly unstable and has a tendency toward explosive conduct. Adjustment generally is inadequate. In true hysteria a person may become unconscious or semiconscious, with an absence of sensation. A form of functional paralysis may result. Such an episode is an unwholesome escape from reality. Paralysis is imaginary and can be removed merely by the suggestion that the paralysis is gone. The great need of this person is insight into his or her real motives, with guidance in learning to adjust wholesomely to frustration and conflict.

In pseudohysteria persons may go into a tantrum or a violent display of temper. Helping them to see themselves as others see them is essential. The first step in readjustment is for others to disregard the tantrum or display. Rebuilding these persons' ability to adjust to the trials of life may be a long process.

Some pseudohysteria is passive. As an attention-getting device children may pretend that they have fainted. The less attention given to them, the sooner recovery will occur. They will abandon this form of behavior as soon as it becomes apparent that others know why they do it.

Chip on the shoulder. The belligerent, pugnacious, quarrelsome youngster is the defensive youngster. Perhaps an exaggerated feeling of inferiority, a feeling of rejection, or a defensiveness because of a lack of status can account for this personality mold. Perhaps the youngster cannot find success in school life and other activities and resorts to the one superior attribute he or she has—physical force. Some of these youngsters are diagnosed as "brain damage" cases. Oddly, physicians control some of these children with tranquilizers and others with stimulants. The youngster becomes obedient, cooperative, and socially adjusted.

Suspiciousness. Occasionally a child may be overly suspicious, exhibiting a marked distrust of others, even to the point of suspecting everyone of taking advantage of him or her. This defensiveness may express a feeling of extreme insecurity and perhaps inadequacy. The home situation may be reflected in the attitudes and general conduct of the child.

Selfishness. A youngster who lacks consideration for others and is possessive, particularly in relation to material things and even to the extent of being greedy, may merely have acquired a distorted set of values. Insecurity can account for the egomania expressed in extreme selfishness. Such youngsters can acquire new values under a regime that emphasizes respect and consideration for others and the importance of other than material things.

Excessive moodiness. The depressed or moody youngster usually lacks incentive or purpose in life. A child coming from a home in which life is a very gloomy affair may reflect this at school. Perhaps a physiological basis does exist, but, whatever the youngster's physiological endowment, he or she

can be challenged through worthwhile purposes. Desirable self-gratification can be attained and received from accomplishment.

Exaggerated emotionalism. An overly responsive child—even the overly dramatic child—expresses a pattern outside of the normal. The child who is ecstatic one moment and in the depths of sadness or depression the next moment exhibits an unhealthy emotional instability. Whether this expresses an attention-getting attempt or other motive, the child can be benefited by helping him or her to understand that such extreme emotionalism is neither usual nor acceptable.

Hypochondria. The child who finds he or she can get attention by having a pain or other physical complaint may resort to this ruse whenever an uncomfortable or trying situation is encountered. Expression of an imaginary pain can be an escape mechanism or an attention-getting device. Perhaps the school has failed to give the child the recognition he or she should have from normal acceptable accomplishment or performance. However, distinguishing true pain from pseudo pain is not always a simple task. To make too big an issue of the matter, whether in error or in truth, can compound the problem. When there is little doubt that the pain is imaginary, then obtaining a statement from a physician that no physical disorder exists is a desirable first step. A matter-of-fact approach suggesting that the pain is leaving can produce a surprisingly effective acceptance by the youngster. On the impressionable child the effect of suggestion may not be spectacular, but suggestion can help to produce the desired wholesome outlook of the normal child.

Hyperkinetic child. "Hyperactive child," "brain injury child," and other designations identify the overactive child syndrome characterized by combinations of signs and symptoms portraying a youngster who is frequently labeled a renegade or outlaw but who, in effect, is a youngster with a serious problem that cries out for recognition and understanding. Perhaps 4% of children in grade school are in this category, and boys outnumber girls six to one. The syndrome is not confined to children, but the incidence in the adult population is much lower than that in children because many recover spontaneously with the aging process.

A whole gamut of characteristics occurs in these youngsters, but not all of them in any one child. Yet, the different combinations are readily identifiable as the condition with which we are concerned. The child may be fidgety, easily upset, easily distracted, restless, noisy, disobedient, talkative, continually in motion, irritable, impatient, cantankerous, defiant, and impulsive. The child cannot concentrate for more than a minute, rarely finishes tasks, talks out of turn, does not respond to discipline, does not follow directions, acts or speaks on impulse, cannot sit still, gets into things, has temper tantrums, and usually is regarded as antisocial. Generally, the child displays these symptoms and signs only when in a familiar place or situation. Perhaps there is a possible explanation if we could understand why the child acts differently in an unfamiliar setting. Another unique phenomenon is that many of these youngsters have a history of accidental poisoning in preschool days.

Teachers are inclined to dismiss these children as "spoiled brats," victims of permissiveness in the home, attention seekers, bullies, and otherwise undesirable; yet these are not normal children and actually are ill. Their abnormality appears to be based in an inborn error of metabolism. This diagnosis of the biological basis for the condition is strengthened by the dramatic change produced by stimulants. Physicians report that stimulants such as amphetamines (pep pills) tend to calm the hyperactive child. The duration of the effectiveness of the medication is short. In addition, there is the ever-present danger of an overdose. Some physicians report success with tranquilizers.

If brain damage exists in any of these children, it is not of a physical or anatomical nature. Brain malfunctioning is more likely the result of a biochemical aberration not completely understood as yet. There is some evidence, although decidedly limited, that a genetic factor exists. The possibility of a developmental anomaly also exists.

A teacher with a pupil who fits this category can take several steps in the best interests of the child. Consultation with the school's personnel counselor, if one is available, should be a first step. Through the administration, a conference with the child's parents is in order. One outcome of this consultation should be the decision to refer the child to a physician best able to deal with this particular type of child. The physician may start the child on drugs to stabilize behavior. During this time the teacher and the parents will be instructed to make special efforts to get the child into more normal patterns of behavior. Particular emphasis will be placed on a routine schedule with activities and tasks that the child is able to succeed in and in which gratification can be found. Episodes of overactivity can be handled by guiding the child into more sedentary activities and providing the child with an associate or associates who can share the interests and calm the behavior of the disturbed child. How long the physician will keep the child on drugs will depend on many developments, particularly the child's adjustment to the school environment.

MENTAL HEALTH PROMOTION

Education accepts as both a professional obligation and a privilege the opportunity to promote the mental, emotional, and social growth as well as the physical growth of the child. All children can be helped in their total growth. The normal child can attain an even higher level of mental, emotional, and social growth with effective supervision. Those children with minor mental and emotional disabilities can overcome their difficulties when understanding and dedicated teachers give them the necessary insight and guidance. Many of the lesser behavior problems can be managed in the classroom. Even the children with marked or gross emotional difficulties can be helped by direct and indirect action from the school.

Mental health programming in the classroom usually is not formally structured. Yet a recognizable program usually is in operation in schools in which there is an awareness of the opportunity to make the greatest possible contribution to the overall development of each youngster. Such a program logically has four basic aspects.

First is a mentally hygienic environment in which each child feels he or she has status, is accepted by classmates and teacher, is challenged to develop his or her abilities, and succeeds to a gratifying degree. A teacher cannot create a perfect environment, but can create one that, although not perfect, can provide for a high level of emotional, mental, and social development for most, if not all, students. This situation is not attained by chance. It results from planning and application.

Group social interaction can be used to the benefit of all youngsters in the classroom. It means tailoring the school life to the patterns of living that provide opportunities for varieties of human interaction.

There are certain things that rightfully can be expected of the teacher in the role of an educator:

1. Understand his or her own behavior
2. Separate personal problems from the classroom and school life
3. Respect each youngster
4. Understand individual differences
5. Understand the cause-and-effect relationship of deviant behavior
6. Maintain an atmosphere neither too rigid or severe, nor too permissive
7. Strengthen desirable behavior through recognition and even praise
8. Deal with behavior problems not serious enough for professional care
9. Substitute acceptable behavior for deviant behavior

Second is the individual guidance the teacher gives individual youngsters. An able, discerning, understanding, conscientious teacher who seeks to know each child—his or her strengths, weaknesses, and particularly needs—can guide into the proper channels those youngsters who have special problems in emotional and social adjustment. This implies a person-to-person, or a one-to-one, approach. It requires some degree of ability in counseling, in understanding children, and in assisting children to understand themselves. Mutual deliberation enables children to develop their abilities to deal with their own problems.

Third is the organized, cooperative, total guidance program of the school or the school system, which is designed to deal with gross emotional or mental health difficulties. It begins with the general observation of the classroom teacher and his or her recognition of the problem. Staff conferences, discussions with the nurse, physician, principal, school counselor, and parents may lead to the necessary action to deal with the problem of the child under consideration. Fortunately, more people are being prepared to aid the classroom teacher in working with problems of deviant behavior in students.

Fourth is the use of consulting services other than those in the school. Referral is through the parents to the professional services a particular youngster may need. Public schools generally have not accepted the use of outside professional mental health services, preferring to leave entirely to the parents any decision in this sphere that should be made. Schools must reconsider their reluctance to recommend that the services of a professional mental hygienist be obtained for a grossly maladjusted child. The stigma of mental and emotional deviation has dimmed in recent years, and the school should not be reluctant to recommend the employment of available community professional services when the school has exhausted its own resources or recognizes its own inability to be of value to the child. A youngster with 60 or more years of life ahead is entitled to the best possible start on this long journey.

APPRAISAL

The age-old aphorism, "Know the child," should be extended to, "and know what might befall the child." A teacher has no acknowledged final legal responsibility for a child's health, but educators recognize a professional responsibility for the welfare of each schoolchild. This obligation is most fully discharged when the teacher understands deviations as well as the normal. This basic understanding translated into action through continual alertness cannot but resound to the benefit of every student under the supervision of a teacher with this competence. Translated into numbers represented by an entire staff of teachers, it is easy to visualize the possible impact on human health that can be exerted by teachers well prepared to fulfill their school health obligations. Here is opportunity for those who will prepare themselves for this role.

We have seen in this chapter that we are not dealing with something mystical, bewildering, or totally obscure. We deal with those things we can understand, with some conditions in which the teacher can be of primary assistance, and with other conditions in which the knowledgeable teacher can play a secondary contributing role. From a mod-

est beginning of basic knowledge the t can continue to extend and expan knowledge through a combined prog..... ... study and practical experience.

Perhaps special emphasis should be given to the likelihood that today children are in regular attendance in school who but a few years ago would have been invalids at home. This is a result of the phenomenal advances of recent years in the medical field. Physicians may prescribe school attendance for pupils with what appear to be extreme deviations from normal. Yet, as the teacher becomes familiar with the capabilities of these pupils, he or she soon accepts the child as one of the group and easily makes whatever adjustments are indicated. Most important, this growth or maturation in the teacher reflects itself in increased confidence and in a more meaningful service to pupils.

A teacher who feels inadequate to deal with a particular problem in mental health should seek assistance. To disregard the problem or to take a fatalistic point of view is to neglect his or her professional obligation to help each child attain the highest possible level of effective and enjoyable living.

QUESTIONS AND EXERCISES

1. Indicate some deviations from the normal in children that should be disregarded or even ignored in the school.
2. What are some of the indications that a teacher is maturing in the conduct of the school health program?
3. What is the legal responsibility of the school for the correction of defects in a pupil?
4. What is the professional responsibility of the teacher for the correction of defects in a pupil?
5. What role can a teacher play in aiding the excessively obese child to lose weight?
6. What should be the course of action of the school in dealing with a student who is listless, slow, inactive, disinterested, and chronically late?
7. After a child has had an epileptic seizure while in school, what should the teacher say to the other children in the class?

8. The teacher can do nothing directly about accelerated or delayed growth and maturation, so why should the teacher be concerned?

9. A teacher can be so overly concerned about a pupil with a heart disorder that he or she may be the cause of the child developing into a "cardiac neurotic." Explain.

10. Why can it justifiably be said there is as great a danger of a child with a defect or disorder underparticipating as there is of overparticipation?

11. What does it mean and what should the teacher do if a child's physician reports, "The child has a functional heart murmur, but it should be disregarded, and she should be treated like any other child"?

12. Under what circumstances should a teacher be concerned about medication for a schoolchild?

13. Explain the statement, "For the growing child with a malocclusion the services of an orthodontist are not a luxury."

14. What agencies or organizations in your community are interested in helping children with vision and hearing disorders?

15. A schoolchild needs a hearing aid, but the parents do not buy one. What should the school do?

16. What can be done by a teacher for the youngster who does not enter into group activities but always tends to be alone?

17. What is meant by this expression: a mentally hygienic environment?

18. What is meant by the expression "mutual deliberation?"

19. In terms of its influence on the mental health of the students, what is the most important factor in a classroom?

20. What are some resources a teacher can call upon for consultations relating to students with health problems?

SELECTED READINGS

Bonvechio, R. L., and Dukelow, D. A.: Responsibilities of school physicians, J. School Health 31:21, Jan. 1961.

Eisner, V., and Oglesby, A.: Health assessment of school children, VIII, the unexpected health defect, J. School Health 42:348, June, 1972.

Ellis, R. W. B., and Mitchell, R. G.: Diseases in infancy and childhood, ed. 7, Atlanta, 1973, Churchill Livingston.

Facts on the major killing and crippling diseases in the United States today, New York, 1965, National Health Education Committee, Inc.

Feingold, D. A., and Bank, C. L.: Developmental disabilities of early childhood, Springfield, Ill., 1977, Charles C Thomas, Publisher.

Holloway, P. J.: Child dental health, ed. 2, Chicago, 1975, Year Book Medical Publishers, Inc.

Jolly, H.: Diseases of children, ed. 3, Philadelphia, 1976, J. B. Lippincott Co.

Keith, J. D., Rowe, R. D., and Vlad, P.: Heart disease in infancy and childhood, ed. 2, New York, 1967, The Macmillan Co.

Kendig, E. J., and Chernick, V., editors: Disorders of the respiratory tract in children, ed. 3, Philadelphia, 1977, W. B. Saunders Co.

Krugman, S., and Ward, R.: Infectious diseases of children, ed. 5, St. Louis, 1973, The C. V. Mosby Co.

Licht, S. H., editor: Therapeutic exercise, ed. 2, New Haven, Conn., 1961, Physical Medicine Library, vol. 3, The Williams & Wilkins Co.

Lum, M. C.: Current concepts in the rise of nonprofessional assistants in school health services—a selected review, J. School Health 43:6, June, 1973.

National Office of Vital Statistics, Public Health Service, U.S. Department of Health, Education, and Welfare: Health statistics, Washington, D.C., 1965, United States Government Printing Office.

Pelton, W. J., et al.: Epidemiology of dental health, American Public Health Association Monographs, Cambridge, Mass., 1969, Harvard University Press.

Silverthorne, N. H., Anglin, C. S., and Schusterman, M.: Principal infectious diseases of childhood, ed. 2, Springfield, Ill., 1966, Charles C Thomas, Publisher.

Turner, C. E., Sellery, C. M., and Smith, S. L.: School health and health education, ed. 7, St. Louis, 1976, The C. V. Mosby Co.

Wallace, H. M., and Goldstein, H.: Child health in the United States, Pediatrics 55:176-181, Feb. 1975.

PART TWO

Organization of the school health program

All are born to observe order, but few
are born to establish it.

Joubert

CHAPTER 6

Basic plan of the health program

A basic plan or blueprint is essential to any important undertaking, particularly one such as the school health program, which is expected to deal with the diversity of factors and situations related to human well-being. Although the plan for school health must have a basic pattern or framework, it should be sufficiently flexible to adapt to any situation or need. To be functional it must be practical. It should be adjusted to the needs of the students and must be in harmony with the background of both the school and the community.

There is no such thing as the only school health program. Many plans have their merits. However, it is important to recognize that school health programs in the United States are legal responsibilities of both public education and public health. School health laws in the state of Illinois reveal the shared legal relationship of the two community governmental agencies of education and health. The school code pertaining to physical examination states in part, "physical examinations as prescribed by the Department of Public Health including vision screening tests, shall be required. . . ." The Critical Health Problems and Comprehensive Health Education Act for Illinois Schools states that the Office of the Superintendent of Public Instruction (Illinois Office of Education)

"shall establish the minimum amount of instruction time to be devoted to comprehensive health education at all elementary and secondary grade levels."

Because of this mutual concern, several different administrative patterns of school health programs are often employed. The school health service aspect of the program may be placed under the jurisdiction of the local health department. Some schools operate under a joint administration of school health shared by the board of education and the health department. The most common pattern places the school health services under an associate superintendent for special services or associate superintendent for pupil personnel services.

How the program is administered is not of great importance so long as agreement on program objectives and a very real and cooperative working relationship exists between the school personnel and the health professionals. Serious difficulties have arisen in schools that have not had the benefit of leadership from professionally trained school health nurses and school health educators. Without such leadership, misunderstandings may arise over program priorities, based on a failure to understand the difference between the educators' objective to teach and the health professionals' goal to treat or to cor-

103

rect. Although the objectives are different, they are not mutually exclusive but instead serve to complement and strengthen each other. The student's full effectiveness in the teaching and learning situation cannot be achieved if he or she is not at optimum health nor can optimum health be achieved or maintained without benefit of education.

AUTHORIZATION OF SCHOOL HEALTH PROGRAMS

Inherent in the American system of schools is the principle that the local board of education is responsible for the schools of its district. This principle acknowledges that the closer a governmental agency is to the people, the more likely it is to be in tune with the situation in which it functions. Accordingly, extensive authority and responsibility have been delegated to the local school board. However, as illustrated in the Illinois situation, state laws make certain requirements of the school districts. In addition, state departments of education, through regulation, have set standards that local school districts must meet. Such legislative and regulative requirements have applied to school health programs.

State legislation. States pass two forms of legislation that affect the school health program: permissive and mandatory laws. In practical terms, permissive legislation simply recommends or encourages the local board of education to institute certain procedures that are beneficial to the health and well-being of schoolchildren. Permissive laws are couched in such language as "school districts should provide" or are "encouraged to provide." The conditions or procedures outlined in the law are recommended but not required. Therefore the school board has the option to accept or not accept the recommendation set forth in the law.

However, in the case of mandatory legislation, laws are authoritatively ordered. The state requires the local districts to carry out

the provisions of the law. This requirement is obligatory, meaning that no exceptions to the law are permitted. Ideally, such legislation is drafted in broad outlines so that the state department of education can interpret the legislation and write guidelines to schools for implementing the requirements. Such guidelines are usually developed by persons who have had extensive school experience and who are recognized for sound administrative judgment and knowledge of successful school practices. The terminology of mandatory legislation contains such phrases as "the school district shall provide" or "must include." Statutes may further indicate the areas of health instruction and charge the state superintendent of instruction with responsibility for providing materials and advisory services for the schools throughout the state. The state department of education in cooperation with the state department of health may also be required to prescribe a program of health examinations of students in the elementary and secondary schools. The state superintendent of public instruction is charged with the implementation and enforcement of these statutes. Enforcement is exercised through school standardization requirements.

Among other requirements, in order to qualify as standard, the school district must meet the state standards for health services, health instruction, and school sanitation. Failure to meet these requirements may place the district in a probationary status for a specified period of time. Failure to meet requirements within this time period may disqualify the district from participation in certain state school aid funds.

Advocates of legislation to assure health protection and promotion for *every* schoolchild in the state assert that many school boards have very little understanding of school health work. The thinking of board members and administrators is conditioned by the old classical education they received.

The practical value of health in the school may not be fully appreciated. State recognition of the importance of health in the school will assure *every* schoolchild of at least a minimum of health promotion and health understanding.

State education department initiative. Some states seek to achieve the same goal through prescription by the state board of education. The state board sets up standards for school health services, health instruction, and a healthful school environment. Again, those districts failing to meet requirements may be declared substandard and ineligible for certain state financial aid.

In practice, these provision are not carried out ruthlessly and dictatorially. Great leniency is granted by giving ample time for the development of health programs. Only in those districts in which the school board or administration actually resists the development of an adequate school health program will the ultimate in enforcement be exercised. The important thing is the health of the students, not the state aid or the prerogative of school boards and administrators.

Responsibilities of the local board of education. Sovereignty or ultimate authority rests with the people. Except such authority as the states have granted to the federal government through the federal constitution, the people have vested their authority in the 50 states to be exercised within their own borders. Local governmental units have only such authority as has been granted to them by the state legislature through specific legislation and accepted practice. Unless otherwise specified or prohibited, local school boards have broad authority to make such provisions for their schools as they deem necessary to discharge their responsibilities to the school-age children of their district. From common practice, certain authority and responsibility of the school for health promotion have become generally accepted.

1. School health promotion is vested in the board of education. In practice, although the superintendent and his or her professional staff propose the program, such proposal is merely a recommendation to the board. Only as the board approves the plan can the program have official status. The board can make the program as extensive as it sees fit. It can appropriate such funds as it deems necessary for the health program.

2. All phases of the school health program must comply with state laws and their implementing regulations. In practice, the state provisions serve as minimum standards. A board of education properly may set standards or requirements higher than the state provisions, but not lower. If a state statute provides that all students participating in interscholastic athletics must have a health examination before the season in which they are to compete, the local board on its own initiative may also require such an examination of all who participate in intramural sports. What a prudent and farsighted board that would be!

3. A board of education has the authority to require every child to have a health examination before entering school and at such other times as it deems reasonable. Some boards have made provisions for exceptions on religious grounds. Other boards have made no exceptions, contending that a health examination does not constitute medication. The Washington State Supreme Court has upheld this point of view.

4. A school board can require immunization against a particular disease as a condition for admission to school. Here religious rights definitely do enter in, and provisions for exceptions should be made. In the event of an epidemic or threatened epidemic, the board may exclude those children from school whose parents refuse permission for immunization on religious grounds.

5. The school can pass rules governing school attendance. It can extend this authority to include provisions for exclusion

and readmission in control of communicable diseases. Although legal isolation and quarantine are functions of the health department, the school can assert control of communicable diseases insofar as this control is part of the school program.

6. A board may require daily inspections for indications of communicable disease.

7. A child may be excused from sex education if the parents of that child object to the instruction on the basis of religious belief.

8. School boards may specify the areas of health instruction, going beyond any requirements of the state, but including the state requirements in the program.

BASIC DIVISIONS OF THE HEALTH PROGRAM

In a world that gets progressively more complicated, it is refreshing to find a group,

especially an education group, that is striving to simplify its program. Two decades ago the school health program in general use consisted of seven phases or divisions. Repeated reassessment and realignment have sifted to the following three basic divisions: (1) school health services, (2) health instruction, and (3) healthful school living (Fig. 6-1).

In a well-integrated school health program no pronounced demarcation of the divisions exists. They are interdependent and support and supplement each other. In actual operation the divisions do not exist; they are essentially creations for organizational and administrative convenience. There is *one* school health program with three different aspects. Whether a particular activity belongs under one aspect or division is primarily academic. How effectively it functions is the significant consideration.

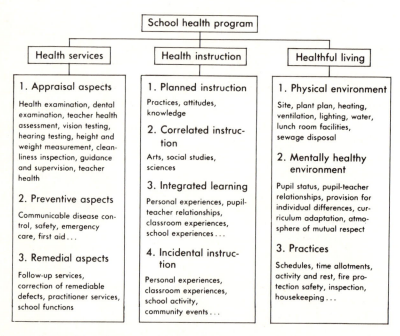

Fig. 6-1. Organization of the school health program. For purposes of planning and administration, three distinct phases of the program are recognized, but in actual function the three phases constitute a cohesive integrated contribution to the total school program.

SCHOOL HEALTH SERVICES

School health services constitute those school activities directly concerned with the present health status of the schoolchild. It is only natural that the school should concern itself with the health condition of the children because the health of the students and the type of education program in which they participate are interdependent. The children can do their best work only if their health condition will permit them to participate to the extent that the school program requires. A child with low vitality will have little interest in any school program. A school program in turn must be adapted to the physiological and emotional health levels as well as the intellectual level of the child. More than this, the program should be designed to develop the highest possible level of physical and emotional health in the child.

School health services can reinforce the efforts of the parents and the family physician in promoting the health and well-being of children. The school setting provides an unusually good vantage point from which to observe and assess the health of children. Teachers and nurses, because of their experience of observing many children, have a ready-made standard against which to compare and evaluate a child's health status and behavior. Those children who deviate from the expected normal range of health status or behavior are readily apparent to teachers and nurses. As Eisner and Callan have stated:

The classroom teacher should become the focus of case finding and the child's behavior and functioning should become the primary indicators of his or her health. If this were done, school physicians could devote their time and attention to those children who have been identified as having problems. . . .*

School health services of this type can have a profound effect on children's health and

*Eisner, V., and Callan, L. B.: Dimensions of school health, Springfield, Ill., Charles C Thomas, Publisher, p. 51.

their eventual development as healthy and mature adults. The healthy adult whose preadult years were marked by proper supervision of health, growth, and development enjoys a high level of well-being built on a solid foundation of two decades of planned health promotion. An accumulation of 12 years of organized school health services will have a beneficial effect on a person's health for the remaining years of his life. The healthy, well-educated student in school becomes the effective and happy adult citizen of the community, freely giving of his services and influence to his neighbors and his nation.

Scope. The school has a fundamental concern for all aspects of the child's health and well-being. No child should suffer the burdens of illness or defects resulting from conditions that are preventable or correctable. Although the parents have primary responsibility for the health care and supervision of their children, the school cannot ignore the needs of children who are neglected or abused. In fact, when parents fail in these responsibilities, the school must be the child's advocate as well as defender.

Traditionally, school health services have been considered a part of preventive medicine. Emphasis is given to health appraisal activities that identify those conditions or problems interfering with the child's educational progress, and the results of that appraisal are used to inform the parents about their children's health needs. Such programs have operated on the assumption that any treatment needed by the child should be provided by the family physician. Unfortunately, large numbers of children today come from families and homes that do not have or cannot afford the cost of private medical care. Nevertheless, the emphasis on prevention is still the proper role for school health programs in the total health care scheme.

School officials have had a tendency to view

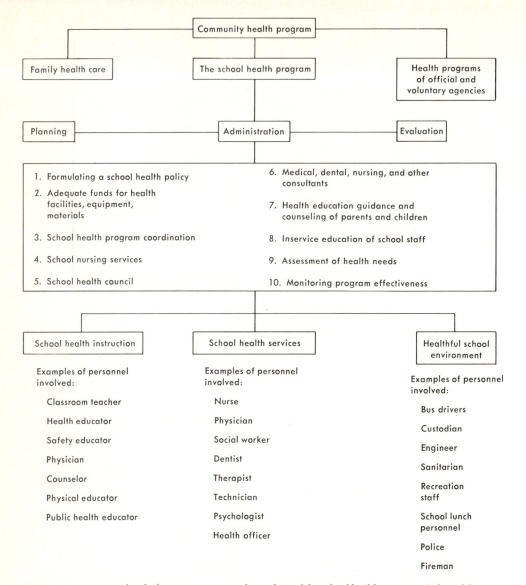

Fig. 6-2. Organizational and administrative interrelationships of the school health program. (Adapted from Illinois Comprehensive State Health Planning Agency [191 6/30].)

their child health responsibilities too narrowly. As a consequence, school health services have, in too many instances, become isolated and unrelated to the community health program. Even though the focus of such services is on preventive activities, it is essential that they be related to and coordinated with other agencies in the community so that comprehensive and continuous health care may be available for children and families.

Recently, new patterns of health care have

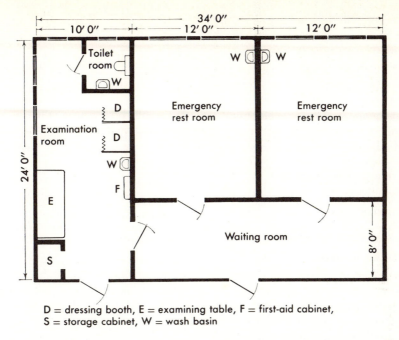

Fig. 6-3. Health services facilities. A simple yet efficient plan for complete health services needs, which permits a variety of arrangements.

been developing. Title 19 of the Social Security Act is intended to make comprehensive medical services available for those families who are unable to pay for them. This program is popularly known as Medicaid. For services to be effectively used, the interrelationship of school and community health programs must be fully understood, so that the necessary cooperation as well as coordination can be achieved (Fig. 6-2).

Appraisal. Complete evaluation of each child's health includes health examinations by a physician, dental examinations, health assessments and observations by the teachers and nurses, screening of vision and hearing by the teachers, weighing and measuring, and inspection of cleanliness.

Health guidance and supervision. In a well-conducted school health program provision is made for aiding students in directing their own health. This includes all processes necessary to acquaint students with their health status and the sources and channels for developing their health assets. It aims to help the students in their health self-direction. The school supervises the children's caring for their own health. An important part of the health education program includes individual and small group counseling of both students and parents. Such supervision must be planned, be well-organized, and have recognized spheres of responsibility.

Prevention. Control of communicable diseases, safety promotion, first aid, and emergency care are not only opportunities for school service, but are also responsibilities for doing everything reasonable to prevent disasters of all proportions.

Remedial measures. Although the school is not expected to treat or to correct defects, it does have a responsibility to assist the child and his or her family in securing the necessary health care. Whether such services are provided by the private physician or through some community agency will depend on the circumstances of individual students and their families. Effective follow-up depends on school personnel. Health education can play a fundamental role in developing an understanding as to why health care is needed and where the needed service may be located.

Facilities for health services. From both necessity and recognition of the importance of health services, well-planned adequate health facilities should be provided. Various plans have proved satisfactory. Existing rooms can be remodeled satisfactorily. Necessarily, plans must be adapted to needs and available space.

A suite of four rooms can be arranged to provide the necessary quarters. Such a plan provides a waiting room, examination room, and two emergency rest rooms, as illustrated in Fig. 6-3. The examination room can be used for a variety of purposes—health examinations, dental examinations, x-ray examinations, hearing and vision testing, first aid, and conferences. Equipment will be determined by the requirements of the physician, the dentist, and the nurse. One emergency lounge for girls and one for boys can prove invaluable (Fig. 6-3). Space devoted to facilities for health service is well invested. The director of the health program, the nurse, or other suitable person should be in charge of the health rooms.

HEALTH INSTRUCTION

Formal planned classroom health teaching is designed to prepare students to make the proper decisions throughout their lives on matters affecting their health. The very nature of health allows for a great variety of approaches in instruction. Diverse methods, techniques, and combinations have been effective in health instruction. In the final analysis any program of health instruction must be appraised in terms of the extent to which it modifies persons in their understanding and practice of health principles. Instruction that promotes the development of favorable attitudes and understanding and that results in a pattern of living enabling the individual to attain the highest possible level of health meets the true goal of all health teaching.

Elementary school. During the early years of school life health instruction is directed primarily to the establishment of recognized health practices and the inculcation of desirable health attitudes. Health knowledge may be used as a vehicle for promoting health practices and health attitudes. Elementary school children will acquire valuable health knowledge that may be associated with pleasant experiences, but health knowledge should always be considered a means to an end—better health. As such, health knowledge should be regarded as secondary to health attitudes and practices in promoting an effective elementary school health instruction program.

Junior high school. The idealism and group tendencies of junior high school students make an ideal setting for the promotion of community health interests and ideals. Interwoven with the concept of respect for the welfare of one's neighbors are the interrelationships that exist between personal and community health. Practices and attitudes are fortified with further knowledge.

Senior high school. Health attitudes and practices developed in the previous years are fortified by knowledge gained in the high school from a sound scientific basis. Since for many students this will be their last opportunity for formal health instruction, high school health teaching should endeavor to prepare young people to accept responsibility for their personal health as well as that of their future families. Students should be encouraged to sustain their interest through self-directed study of health problems. Sources of health information, health services, and health products are of particular importance in high school health instruction.

HEALTHFUL SCHOOL LIVING

From the beginning of public school education in the United States, communities have shown a special pride in their new up-to-date school buildings. The school building denoted a monument to the culture of the community and the people's concern for their children. With this concept was the connotation that the school environment consisted of the physical plant, and a costly building per se constituted an ideal environment for learning. It was a static concept.

The present-day dynamic concept of the environmental factors in the school is well expressed in the designation *healthful school living*. It denotes a social situation in which children develop their potentialities in effective and enjoyable living. Children's educational, emotional, and physical development will have the stimulation and motivation essential to their fullest attainment. It is expressed in the atmosphere of the classroom, the corridors, the gymnasium, the playground, and every other place about the school. It incorporates factors that affect the physical, mental, and social health of the child. In so doing, it includes the physical plant, its equipment, the personnel, and the practices within the school.

If an atmosphere of wholesome living is to be created, all plans and activities must be focused on the child's need for wholesome development. The physical, esthetic, cultural, moral, emotional, social, and all other aspects of the experiences and needs of the child must be met by the school. It properly should create in every child a pride in being a part of the school, an elation in the level of living in which to participate.

The physical plant with its site, proper living conditions, ideal sanitary equipment, and general attractiveness represents a first essential in healthful school living (Fig. 6-4). How the teaching staff utilizes and incorporates these assets into the life of the student will determine whether the school is truly a place of healthful living. To have a lunchroom with adequate space and sanitary equipment is not enough. The practices in the lunchroom and the general atmosphere are equally important. Children need guidance in learning to appreciate and live fully in even the most ideal physical environment. Out of this appreciation should evolve the social values so important to the present and future citizen.

When the physical plant is not of an acceptable standard, the intrepid teacher can instill in the children a desire to better the conditions under which they are learning. Even to appreciate what is and what is not commendable in the school is an achievement in personal growth. Out of these experiences can come improvements in school, home, and community.

After all, people are the most important elements in the school environment. The quality of these people can be noted in their values, attitudes, activities, and attainment. Healthful school living is an important aspect of the quality of life.

Responsibility for environmental health. Parents, school board members, architects, administrators, teachers, custodians, lunchroom personnel, and students are responsible for the environment of the school. United responsibility combined with collective effort produces the environmental conditions conducive to the atmosphere necessary for healthful school living.

Factors influencing environmental health. The attitude of the school community constitutes the all-important background for environmental health. First, those concepts

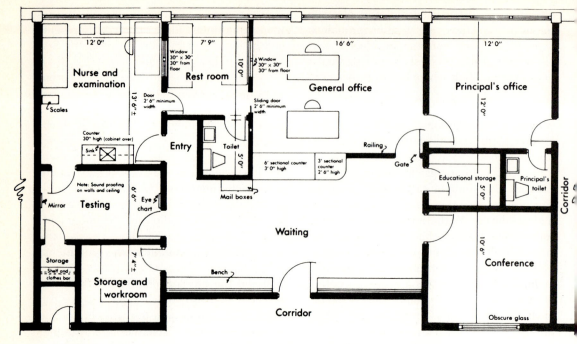

Fig. 6-4. Administrative area in an elementary school. Functional planning includes health services facilities in the administration center. (Courtesy Denver Public Schools, Denver, Colo.)

which the parents hold as standards and put into effect by their own contribution and interest establish the pattern or mold for a healthful school environment. Through the board of education, this attitude will project itself into attractive, functional school buildings, which are safe, efficient, sanitary, and commodious. It will lay the groundwork for an effective school program that will assure the children of an opportunity to develop their potentialities. This community support makes it possible for the school staff to create an atmosphere in which children can live effectively and enjoyably.

A second factor is a well-planned, well-constructed sanitary school plant. This implies a suitable site; functional architecture; adequate heating, ventilation, and lighting; safe water supply; approved disposal facilities; and essential accessory school equipment.

A third factor is the practices of the school. From custodial housekeeping, to lunchroom decorum, to group courtesy, to opportunities for self-status, many practices contribute vitally to healthful school living. Capable teachers can utilize fully the available facilities and opportunities to create a mentally and physically healthy environment.

Healthful school living can be reduced to a rather simple equation:

$$\frac{\text{Functional}}{\text{school plant}} + \frac{\text{Wholesome}}{\text{practices}} = \frac{\text{Healthful}}{\text{school living}}$$

SCHOOL HEALTH PERSONNEL

In the organization of the school health program an essential consideration is the role of the various members of the school staff. The health responsibility of each staff member and the correlated functions of the staff as a whole should be well defined and understood. Some overlapping and duplication is inevitable and frequently desirable. However, duplication should be avoided. If each member of the school staff conscientiously and competently discharges his or her health responsibilities, the ingredients of a balanced, effective school health program are provided.

Administrator. There can be no greater obstacle to a first-class school health program than an administrator who knows little or nothing about school health and cares less. Conversely, there can be no greater asset to a school health program than an administrator who has a thorough understanding of the school health program and appreciation of the contribution of the school to child health.

Some school administrators fail to appreciate the integral relationships between child health and the educative process. As a result, health instruction may be viewed as less important or peripheral to the school's central mission. Such administrators may resist vigorously any attempt to develop a health program, or may exert a passive resistance, which may discourage even the most enthusiastic health educator.

Every state expresses a need for the education of school administrators in the fundamentals of school health. Some states require work in health education as a qualification for an administrator's certificate. Confidence engendered by knowledge expresses itself in a positive leadership in matters of school health.

Both the superintendent and the principal have responsibilities in the health program. However, in practice it is the principal who deals directly with the program. The following list of an administrator's health responsibilities cites those of the principal, although the superintendent may be concerned in a sanctioning role:

1. Provide the organizational structure and administrative leadership necessary for a total school health program:
   a. Emphasize health promotion as a basic objective of the schools
   b. Provide an adequate budget for the program
   c. Provide adequate supervision of the program
   d. Employ qualified staff to implement program activities
2. Establish a complete school health services program including:
   a. The health appraisal and screening activities necessary for assessing children's needs
   b. Teacher observation as an important part of health appraisal
   c. A functional system of health record keeping in order to help provide follow-up health care
   d. An organized plan for medical emergencies
   e. Regular school nurse–teacher conferences
3. Establish effective school-community relationships that are characterized by:
   a. Regular communications between the school, the home, and community health agencies
   b. Health education counseling of parents regarding the health needs of their children
   c. Cooperation with health agencies and parents in securing health and medical care
4. Establish an effective program of health instruction, which would include:
   a. A plan of health instruction that is comprehensive and articulated from one educational level to another, beginning in the primary grades and continuing through senior high school
   b. A curriculum guide made available for teacher use at all educational levels
   c. Allocation of sufficient time to the program
   d. Health education materials made available to ensure effective instruction
   e. Regular in-service health education preparation provided for school staff
   f. Coordination of health services and health instruction
5. Provide the conditions needed for a healthful school environment, including:
   a. A physical environment conducive to the health of students and staff
   b. The facilities and equipment for effective teaching and service
   c. Appropriate standards of food handling
   d. A program to promote school safety
   e. Policies and procedures that promote the social and emotional well-being of students and staff

School physician. During the past 20 years school administrators have experienced increasing difficulty in obtaining medical services for schools. Physicians in private practice have had less and less time and inclination to serve the school, except to examine athletes or others for activity programs. Most physicians feel that their offices in clinics are more conducive to good medical practice than the school setting. The small and medium-sized school systems have been forced to operate without the services of a school physician or have been obliged to provide makeshift arrangements for the occasional service of whatever physician could spare a morning for a clinic or some special health problem. Only a few metropolitan school districts with large enrollments have full-time physicians. Even among large school districts, such a position is decidedly the exception rather than the rule.

First, there is a limited supply of physicians interested in the position. A school physician should have training beyond that of the general practitioner, including special preparation in the normal growth and development of children. He or she must be interested in mental health, immunization, and special problems in child health. An interest in and knowledge of public health, public relations, and factors in the community and home that affect child health are basic.

Another factor accounting for the small number of full-time school physicians is a lack of interest on the part of school boards and school administrators. Perhaps this reflects a lack of general public acceptance of the proposal that schools should retain a full-time physician. Doubtless the element of cost enters in.

In some instances, providing medical services at the school may be the most effective procedure. Under such conditions the board of education arranges with a practicing physician or physicians for specified medical services in the school. The physician may be scheduled to appear at certain school buildings at a given time for work in programs to control communicable diseases. Examina-

tions or immunization clinics may be conducted. A set pay schedule is prearranged.

Some schools arrange for physicians' services through the local medical society. If properly administered, this type of modified, part-time medical service can be satisfactory.

Whatever the administrative arrangement, there are certain recognized functions of the physician who serves the school:

1. Participate in the planning of the school health services program
2. Conduct health examinations
3. Provide medical consultant service in the school
4. Advise the administration on problems of school health
5. Advise parents of children with defects or disorders
6. Assist in exclusion and readmission in the program for control of communicable diseases
7. Provide necessary health services for in-service training of school personnel
8. Provide emergency care
9. Coordinate health services with the health instruction program
10. Coordinate the school health program with the public health program
11. Assist in informing the public of the operation of the school health services
12. Serve as adviser on medical aspects of the school environment

It must be emphasized that the school physician does not correct defects or provide treatment for children except in an extreme emergency. His or her role is primarily one of appraisal and prevention. In a consulting capacity the school physician functions in the corrections program by advising parents of the need for professional services for children with disorders. The school physician is a guardian of the schoolchild's health.

Director of the school health program. Terms such as director, supervisor, and coordinator are used to designate the same general assignment, depending on the section of the country, legal designation, adoption by state education departments, terminology of particular schools, or just convenience. The term *director* indicates the person who has immediate responsibility for the direction of the school health program, whether serving as the director for the elementary school, the secondary school, or the entire school health program. Whatever the responsibility, the school health director first and foremost should be an educator.

In addition to educational background, the school health director should have a special interest and preparation in school health work. Because of the necessity of working with children, teachers, custodians, and other school personnel, the school health director should be a well-adjusted person who is able to get along with people.

Large school systems employ full-time health directors with full-time and part-time assistants. One has a full-time director with a full-time assistant who directs the elementary school program and a part-time assistant director in each high school building. The part-time directors teach health classes as part of their duties. The elementary school assistant health director serves the elementary teachers in promoting their health programs. Modifications of this plan are in vogue and usually are adapted to the particular needs of the system.

Medium and small school systems may engage a full-time school health director who administers the entire health program and has no other duties. Other school systems may divide the director's time between health and physical education or health and some administrative assignment. Often the school health directors devote about half of their time to classroom health instruction in either the junior or senior high school. Time spent beyond teaching can be devoted to integrating health instruction with the rest of the health program in the high school. Also, it may be possible to give assistance to the elementary schools in planning, organizing, promoting, and implementing their health programs. The following plan, with some

modification, should be considered a minimum for any school system, regardless of how small it may be.

To have one person in charge of school health is sound educationally and administratively. If that person has a deep interest in the health program and is prepared professionally, he or she may be a principal, a home economics teacher, a science teacher, a physical educator, any other staff member, or a nurse with a background in education. The important thing is that the person be qualified. This was superbly expressed by a school superintendent who said:

> I am looking for someone to take charge of health work in our high school. I want someone who has more than just a superficial knowledge of health. If the extent of a health director's knowledge is to urge a student to go to a dentist twice a year, or take a bath, or have his eyes tested if he has visual difficulties, I will not need him. The run of classroom teachers knows that much.
>
> When I engage a person to direct instrumental music, I expect him to know far more in that field than any other member of the faculty. I do not expect him to be an Arturo Toscanini. Neither do I expect a health director to be a Sir William Osler, but I do expect him to be trained so that he has more than a superficial knowledge of health.

Certainly a person with a teaching major in health education, or with a school nursing background could be qualified to direct a school health program. Ideally, such a person would have had school experience and additional graduate study leading to the master's degree in health education. Again, it is important to emphasize that the purpose of the school health program is educational: better health through education. The school health director should supervise the following program:

Health administration

1. Develop an overall school health policy and program for the consideration of the administration
2. Exercise direct supervision over the health program
3. Assume the role of the coordinator between the school, the home, and the individuals and agencies

in the community that can contribute to the health of the child

4. Keep all school personnel thoroughly informed on all aspects of the school health program, particularly the role of each person
5. Issue health notices and announcements
6. Provide special programs for exceptional children
7. Accept responsibility for special health programs that may arise in the school
8. Set up a program for the promotion of teacher health
9. Provide for evaluation of the school health program

Health services

1. Arrange for necessary facilities for health services, including emergency rooms
2. Make arrangements for health examinations, dental examinations, and special clinics
3. Arrange for screening of hearing, vision, and posture of the students early in the school year
4. Interpret health records and health data
5. Promote immunization programs and follow through on the number of students protected through immunization
6. Establish a functional health record keeping system
7. Establish a program of systematic teacher observation for deviations from normal health
8. Provide channels through which referrals may be made easily and effectively
9. Confer with teachers, nurses, attendance coordinator, and others regarding students absent excessively
10. Assume the overall direction of the follow-up program in securing correction of the defects
11. Serve as a health resource person for teachers when special occasion requires
12. Serve as health counselor for students with health problems or health needs
13. Assume responsibility for control of communicable diseases, including exclusions and readmissions
14. Assume responsibility for developing and for providing first aid and emergency care
15. Accept responsibility for the promotion of teacher health

Health instruction

1. Using all available resources, set up a complete health education program
2. Coordinate health instruction from grade to grade
3. Obtain instructional materials for the teaching staff
4. Serve as a health resource person for all teachers needing assistance in their health instruction programs
5. Arrange necessary in-service health preparation of the teaching staff

6. Provide for periodic review of the health instruction program
7. Provide health instruction evaluation instruments
8. Serve as adviser or resource person for student groups or committees participating in health activities or health programs
9. Teach regularly scheduled health classes or conduct special sessions for other health educators

Healthful school living

1. Assume responsibility for all factors related to safety and sanitation in the school
2. Provide for regular inspections for safety and sanitation
3. Assume responsibility for the correction of all hazards existing in the school
4. Plan and supervise a program of safety promotion
5. Provide a program for fire prevention and building evacuation
6. Provide a system of accident reporting and follow-up procedures
7. Make regular appraisals of the mental and social environment of the school
8. Provide means for building up a better relationship among students and faculty

Not enough school systems have recognized the role of the school health director. Those that have a competent health director are strong advocates of the principle of having a definite person responsible for the school health program. Administrators, especially, value the services of a school health director. The cost is relatively low and actually is an investment in better health for the children of the school.

School nurse. Perhaps the ideal is a school health nurse, prepared in education and public health as well as nursing, who works full time on school health work and is on the school payroll. These nurses are properly called teacher-nurses. Many schools have nurses who meet these specifications. Other schools have the services of nurses on the staff of the county or city health department. In the latter case the nurses divide their time between the school and their public health duties. The two responsibilities do not necessarily conflict. Budgeting the nurse's time is frequently difficult, but whatever time is made available to the school will yield a valuable contribution to the school health program. Some phases of school health services are distinctly the nurse's province. In other areas they assist or supplement what is being done by others. To list their duties will suggest the possibilities of their services:

1. Administrative and supervisory responsibilities
   a. Assist with formulation of the school health program and its policies
   b. Establish a health record keeping system and implement its use
   c. Assist with the development of the school's communicable disease control program
   d. Assist with the development of an accident prevention and emergency care program
   e. Assist with the in-service education of school staff regarding school health practices
   f. Promote a healthful school environment
2. Health appraisal responsibilities
   a. Assist physicians and dentists with examinations given at the school
   b. Evaluate health needs of children who are referred by teachers
   c. Retest children with questionable vision and hearing defects
3. School health program coordination responsibilities
   a. Conduct follow-up and counseling of parents regarding child health needs
   b. Conduct regular nurse-teacher conferences
   c. Coordinate the school health program activities with those of the community and state health agencies
4. Health instruction responsibilities
   a. Participate in the care and education of handicapped children
   b. Conduct health counseling of students
   c. Conduct classes and give demonstrations on care of the sick, control of communicable diseases, and first aid
   d. Serve as a resource person to the teacher for health instruction

Some school districts financially unable to employ a school nurse have relied on the school health director to assume many of the tasks usually performed by the nurse. Moderate-sized systems have found that a double team of health director and school nurse has been the formula for a dynamic, effective school health program.

Public health nurse. Many school districts do not employ a school nurse but utilize the services of the public health nurse. In many instances the school district pays nothing for the service of the public health nurse, who is paid by the county or city health department. In other cases the school district contributes a certain amount of funds to the county or city health department as payment for service.

The public health nurse who divides his or her time between public health and school nursing services usually has a prearranged schedule for working at certain schools at certain times of the day. This permits the school administration and staff to plan in advance for the nurse's visit. Some of the duties of the nurse include establishing communicable disease control measures and serving as consultant on many child health questions. The nurse is also available on special call from the school. He or she can, in fact, carry on the usual functions of the school nurse.

Because public health nurses are family health oriented, they are in an ideal position to coordinate the health work of the school with what is done and can be done in the home. Nurses can also use their knowledge of the home background of children to make necessary adjustments in the school health programs. The public health nurse who serves the school is an invaluable member of the school health team.

School health coordinator. The school health coordinator—more generally for the elementary school, but also in the junior high school and senior high school—provides leadership in coordinating all school activities in the area of health. A coordinator in the building facilitates effective use of all health resources and facilities in the school, the home, and the community.

A health coordinator is appointed by the principal or other administrative head of the school. In a large school the coordinator may have no other major responsibility. Or the coordinator may have regular classroom responsibilities, perhaps dividing the time between teaching and coordinating duties.

A health coordinator serves directly under an administrator (usually the principal) and frequently works with a health council or committee that assists in formulating general policies and aids in the solution of problems requiring group consideration. Certain functions usually are the direct responsibility of the health coordinator:

1. General program coordination responsibilities
   a. Assure effective functioning of school health activities
   b. Inform school staff about the total school health program
   c. Establish effective communication between the school, the home, and community health agencies
   d. Provide leadership in promoting a safe and healthful school environment
   e. Plan the periodic evaluation of the total school health program
2. Health service coordination responsibilities
   a. Develop the school's health service activities
   b. Establish teacher observation and child referral and follow-up procedures
   c. Assist teachers to assess student health needs
   d. Establish the school's plan for health counseling of students
   e. Interpret the school's emergency care policies and procedures to teachers and staff
3. Health instruction coordination responsibilities
   a. Develop a systematic and articulated health instruction program from level to level
   b. Plan the in-service preparation of teachers in health education
   c. Plan the effective use and sharing of health education materials and equipment
   d. Involve parents and others in developing the health education curriculum
   e. Secure and distribute new health education materials to teachers

A health coordinator should have academic preparation in personal, school, and community health, experience in health education, and, above all, a sincere interest in health promotion. On-the-job experience fanned by enthusiasm can flare into a highly effective health coordinator with a complete school health program that meets the present and future needs of the pupils.

In several states the use of health coordinators has become a well-established practice. It is of interest and significance that the State Board of Education in Oregon has passed a regulation that all schools shall appoint a health coordinator.

Dentist. In the United States between the years 1925 and 1935 a considerable number of schools and local health departments had full-time dentists on their staffs. Duties of the dentist consisted essentially of dental examinations of elementary school pupils, although some health department dentists did corrective work for children whose parents were unable to pay for the services of a dentist. Today few schools employ a dentist, even on a part-time basis.

In some communities dental treatment programs have been located in schools. In other communities school-administered programs may pay for dental care that is provided in public clinics or through contracts with private dentists.* When dental examinations are conducted at school, it is essential that careful planning between representatives of the school and the dental society be carried out. The schedule for examinations can then be set, and the necessary communication with and cooperation of parents can be secured. Through various media the parents are informed of the program. A dental record card for each child is supplied by the school, but the dentist supplies his or her own instruments for the examinations. All examinations are done at the school, and the dentist makes out a record card for each child. After making a duplicate for the

---

*American Academy of Pediatrics: School health: a guide for physicians, Evanston, Ill., 1972, American Academy of Pediatrics, pp. 132-133.

school, the original is sent to the parents, who thus are informed of their child's dental health status.

Even when the dentists are paid on a clinical fee basis by the school board, this type of program serves only as the first step in assuring every youngster the benefit of a thorough dental examination. Yet it is an important first step.

Dental caries is now recognized to be a preventable disease. Therefore dental health education becomes one of the most important aspects of any school dental health program. Because some parents fail to appreciate the importance of good dental care, it is necessary to make a special effort to secure their cooperation in helping their children develop the desired oral health practice being taught in the school. Thus a significant outcome of the school dental program is its carry-over benefits to the parents and entire family.

A recent innovation in the school dental program has been fluoridation in the classroom. Following an explanation of the program, parents are asked to designate whether they wish to have their children participate in the program, which takes about 10 minutes 1 day a week.

To fully expose the surface of teeth so that the fluoride will be most effective, a dry run of brushing and flossing with nonwax floss and a medium stiff brush precedes the flushing. Each child in the program receives a paper cup half filled with water containing 2 ppm fluoride (Fig. 6-5). This is "swished" around in the mouth for 60 seconds before the cup and water are discarded in a metal container. This experiment is of too recent vintage to answer the question of how effective it is. The fact that teachers willingly participate in the program is in itself important.

Elementary classroom teacher. An elementary school with teachers well prepared in health has the foundation for an effective school health program. Elementary classroom teachers have both an opportunity and an obligation to aid youngsters in building up and maintaining a high level of health. Nothing teachers do will be more gratifying than what they do in behalf of the health of the children under their supervision. Most of the health duties of elementary teachers are integrated with the normal routine of classroom life:

1. School health service responsibilities
   a. Perform health appraisals of all children in class
   b. Maintain continuous observation and alertness to pupil health needs
   c. Participate in screening of vision, hearing, and the physical growth and development of children in class
   d. Isolate and refer children suspected of having a communicable disease
   e. Make referrals to appropriate persons as well as follow through to assure that children receive needed care
   f. Provide first aid and emergency care when no other designated person is available
   g. Utilize health appraisal information to promote the health interests of children in class
2. School health instruction responsibilities
   a. Observe health practices of children
   b. Encourage children to evaluate and to improve their own health behavior
   c. Motivate children to establish good health practices
   d. Prepare children for medical and dental examinations so that this experience becomes a part of the health instruction
   e. Provide direct health instruction of children
3. Healthful school environment responsibilities
   a. Be informed about basic health principles
   b. Maintain his or her own health as an example
   c. Maintain a continued alertness for potential hazards in the classroom and school environment
   d. Establish classroom routines that are conducive to positive interpersonal relationships and good mental health
   e. Encourage children to accept responsibilities for an orderly and sanitary environment

Secondary school health educator. Fortunately for the students, the schools, and the health education profession, the time is fast

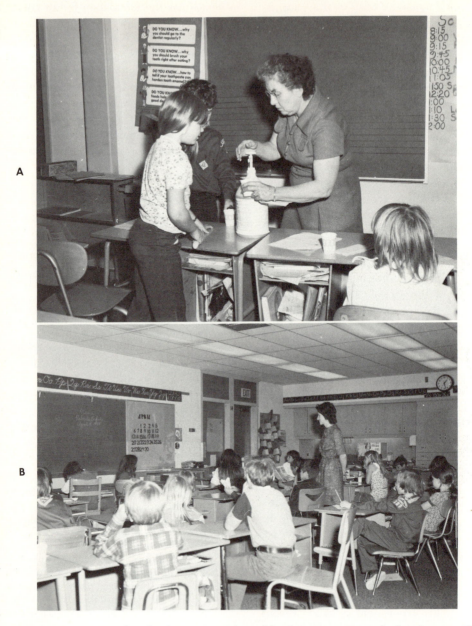

Fig. 6-5. A, Passing out fluoridated water to members of the class participating in the dental project. The teacher fills the cups with water containing 2 parts per million of fluoride. **B,** Fluoride "swishing" for about 60 seconds. It is recognized that no one has demonstrated that fluorides can penetrate dental enamel, but this program is based on the assumption that fluorides penetrate the softer tissues of the oral cavity. (Courtesy Corvallis Public Schools, Corvallis, Ore.)

passing when anyone available is assigned to teach health in the junior and senior high school. Certainly a minimum requirement should be a minor in health with supporting courses in biology and the social sciences. Health educators in the high school are in a strategic position to affect beneficially the lives of all students with whom they have contact in their health classes. Here is an opportunity for public service that can be totally gratifying. The duties and responsibilities of health educators include most of those already identified for classroom teachers. However, the following represent special or unique functions of the health educator:

1. Serve as a health counselor for students
2. Serve as a resource person in health education for other faculty members
3. Accept the leadership in developing a functional and effective health education curriculum
4. Be able to correlate and to integrate health education experiences with other areas of the curriculum
5. Accept the responsibility for providing first aid instruction to others as well as provide first aid in emergencies
6. Provide the leadership for the school's efforts in promoting the physical and mental well-being of the total school health environment
7. Accept leadership in conducting school health program evaluation

Physical educator. A physical educator is in a strategic position to offer much to the health of the schoolchild. The responsibility of the physical educator is definitely to promote physical and mental health in children in addition to helping them develop physical strength and skills. The physical educator contributes to the child's health and well-being in many ways:

1. Constantly observe the health status of children and detect deviations from normal
2. Recommend exclusion of students from classes when an apparent indication of communicable disease exists
3. Motivate and assist students in establishing good health practices

4. Develop understandings and practices relating to cleanliness and the prevention of infection
5. Develop an appreciation of the role of community health services in safeguarding health
6. Develop an appreciation of the relationship of diet to health
7. Create an interest in health skills as an attribute for more effective and enjoyable living
8. Promote safety practices
9. Provide first-aid and emergency services
10. Develop an appreciation of the nature of fatigue and the need for rest
11. Adapt student activities to the capacities of the students
12. Promote wholesome boy-girl relationships through coeducational classes and recreation
13. Promote mental health as expressed through emotional control
14. Cooperate with physicians and parents in providing special activities
15. Rehabilitate students who have recovered from illness or defects
16. Assume responsibility for good posture
17. Assume responsibility for excellent grooming
18. Maintain a healthful school environment in cooperation with the students

Secondary school classroom teacher. All secondary school classroom teachers have a contribution to make to the school health program. Certainly opportunities for health discussions arise in every class. Home economics classes especially provide repeated opportunities for health instruction. Nutrition, family life, and homemaking encompass health aspects. More than just imparting health instruction, all secondary school teachers have an opportunity to observe students daily and thus be concerned directly with the health of the students. The health responsibilities of the high school teacher are not many, but they are important:

1. Observe students continually to note any deviations from the normal
2. Report to proper administrators when a student appears to be in need of health counseling
3. Cooperate with the administration in preventing the spread of communicable diseases
4. Maintain sanitary, safe, and congenial environmental conditions in the classroom

5. Note the kind of questions students ask regarding health and assume some responsibility for helping them to find accurate answers
6. Recognize requirements and activities that may jeopardize health
7. Assume responsibility for first aid and emergency care
8. Analyze particular area or areas of subject matter for the purpose of making the content more functional in terms of the health needs and problems of the students

Custodian. The custodian is concerned with a healthful physical environment—cleanliness, ventilation, lighting, heating, water supply, sewage disposal, safety factors, floors, exits, walks, and fire equipment. He or she also has a direct responsibility for pupil health and should be regarded as a member of the school health team. A qualified custodian is one with the proper training to meet the present requirements. Health protection and promotion are two of his or her most important functions.

Other personnel. Lunchroom workers, clerks, bus drivers, and other school employees can make contributions to the health program. A first essential is that they understand that they are part of the program to promote health. Second, they should be made to feel that their role is an important one. Third, they should have specific instruction in the performance of their tasks in the light of health protection and promotion. It is the composite contribution of everyone in the school community that builds the complete school health program.

QUESTIONS AND EXERCISES

1. Interpret the aphorism, "All are born to observe order, but few are born to establish it."
2. What are the merits and demerits in the American system that places responsibility for public school education in a local board of education?
3. Compare the practice of having the state legislature set up standards for school health programs with that of having the state education department prescribe what the school health programs shall be.
4. Courts have held that, when a school requires a child be immunized, the child's parents can object on religious grounds, but requiring a health examination is not an infringement on the child's religious rights. How do you explain the possible paradox?
5. Why should the school be concerned with the present health status of a child?
6. What activities in the school health program are preventive measures?
7. A school and its teachers have no legal responsibility to remedy defects and disorders in a child; why do they do so?
8. What is the true goal of health instruction?
9. What besides an ample sanitary school plant is necessary for healthful school living?
10. What can be done to correct the situation where an inadequate health program exists because the superintendent or principal is lacking in knowledge of school health or is not interested?
11. Which is the better arrangement: to have a full-time school physician or to have the school patrons take their children to their family physician?
12. Evaluate the statement, "To employ a competent school health director is to invest in the present and future health of the children of the community."
13. What qualities and preparation do you want in a school health director?
14. Compare the relative merits of having a public health nurse serve the school and having a school nurse hired by the school district.
15. Appraise the statement, "No one in the entire public school system is expected to wear as many hats as the elementary school teacher."
16. Of all the valuable services the elementary teacher gives to pupils, what rank order do you give to health, and why?
17. Explain why the physical educator's relationship to students gives the teacher a unique opportunity to contribute to the health of the students.
18. Why is it important to promote coeducational classes in the schools?
19. What activities and requirements in a high school may jeopardize the health of the students?
20. Why is the school custodian regarded as a member of the school health team?

REFERENCES AND SELECTED READINGS

American Academy of Pediatrics: School health: a guide for health professionals, Evanston, Ill., 1977, American Academy of Pediatrics.

Byrd, O. E.: School health administration, Philadelphia, 1964, W. B. Saunders Co.

Cromwell, G. E.: Nursing in the school health program, Philadelphia, 1963, W. B. Saunders Co.

Eisner, V., and Callan, L. B.: Dimensions of school

health, Springfield, Ill., 1974, Charles C Thomas, Publisher.

ESPDT: does it spell health care for poor children? A report by the Children's Defense Fund of the Washington Research Project, Inc., 1977.

Foord, A.: Health services for children of school age. In Sartwell, P. E., editor: Maxcy and Rosenau's preventive medicine and public health, ed. 9, New York, 1965, Appleton-Century-Crofts.

Grout, R. E.: Health teaching in schools, ed. 5, Philadelphia, 1968, W. B. Saunders Co.

Haag, J. H.: School health program, New York, 1965, Holt, Rinehart & Winston.

Jenne, F. H., and Greene, W. H.: Turner's school health and health education, ed. 7, St. Louis, 1976, The C. V. Mosby Co.

Joint Committee on Health Problems in Education of the National Education Association and the American Medical Association: School health services, ed. 2, Washington, D.C., 1964, National Education Association Publications.

Joint Committee on Health Problems in Education of the National Education Association and the American Medical Association: Suggested school health policies, ed. 5, Chicago, 1966, American Medical Association.

Kilander, H. F.: School health education, ed. 2, New York, 1968, The Macmillan Co.

Mayshark, C., Shaw, D. D., and Best, W. H.: Administration of school health programs: its theory and practice, ed. 2, St. Louis, 1977, The C. V. Mosby Co.

Miller, D. F.: School health programs: their basis in law, New York, 1972, A. S. Barnes and Co., Inc.

Nemir, A., and Schaller, W. E.: The school health program, ed. 4, Philadelphia, 1975, W. B. Saunders Co.

Oberteuffer, D., Harrelson, O. A., and Pollock, M. B.: School health education, ed. 5, New York, 1972, Harper & Row, Publishers, Inc.

Teamwork in school health, Washington, D.C., 1962, American Association for Health, Physical Education, and Recreation.

Wallace, H. M., Gold, E. M., and Lis, E. F., editors: Maternal and child health practices, Springfield, Ill., 1973, Charles C Thomas, Publisher.

PART THREE

School health services

CHAPTER 7

Appraisal aspect of health services

Whether traveling into outer space or to a nearby vacation spot, it is essential to establish a takeoff point in order to measure the length of the journey. During the course of the trip, readings or measures must be taken periodically to determine the traveler's exact location at a given time, as well as how much progress has been made. This analogy applies to the health history of the individual and to those activities designed to improve health status.

Health appraisal is essential to a student's welfare. It can give assurance to the child, the parents, and teachers that his or her present health is at a satisfactory level, or it can give a warning that the health status is not satisfactory, thus providing a forewarning of possible danger ahead. It can indicate where strengths and weaknesses exist and where special attention might profitably be applied. It can give an accounting of progress or lack of progress in the health program of each child. It can serve as an experience that motivates a child to take pride in his or her health. It can motivate children to maintain and as much as possible to improve their quality of health.

An appraisal of health is an evaluation or assessment of the present health status of the individual. It is more than a static inventory, since it deals with the relationship of a person's health attainment to his or her basic endowment and with the consequent adjustment to life needs. Appraisal of health denotes a positive approach in which major emphasis is placed on the health assets of a person, and deviations and deficiencies are appraised in terms of the degree to which they obstruct or interfere with effective and enjoyable living.

Health appraisal is a continuing process. From the entrance health examination, to the observations by the classroom teacher, to the last health examination or other health evaluation in the final year of high school, the appraisal of health traces the course of each child's health status throughout his or her school career. However, in the final analysis the appraisal of health is not an end in itself. It is a means to an end—a means to better health for the student. Its value comes from its use, and the appraisal of health will thus contribute to the general well-being of the youngster.

FUNDAMENTAL OBJECTIVES

The ultimate objective of the health appraisal program is the improvement and maintenance of the student's health. Several more immediate objectives, including the following, are the avenues through which the final goal can best be reached.

1. Develop in the student an understanding and interest in his or her health status
2. Establish a lifelong practice of having one's health status evaluated at regular intervals
3. Establish the basis on which to construct a life program of health promotion
4. Help the parents to understand the health status and needs of their children
5. Enable the school to understand the health endowment of each pupil so that the child and the school program will be adapted to the best interests of the student
6. Establish a wholesome physician-child relationship
7. Establish a wholesome dentist-child relationship
8. Develop in each child an appreciation of the value of professional services, methods, and techniques
9. Discover deviations from normal
10. Assess changes in individual health status

HEALTH EXAMINATION

A health examination is a means to an end, and potentially it is perhaps the most effective single instrument mankind possesses for elevating the general standard of health. In keeping with the present-day positive approach, the physician's examination of the child is designated a *health examination*, not a medical examination or physical examination. The physician looks for evidences of health. Any defects found are considered to be obstructions to the true goal of health. The first consideration of the physician is evaluation of the health status of the child. Determination of specific conditions that interfere with the best possible health of the child is the second consideration.

Purpose. The importance of the health examination is reflected in the multiple purposes it serves:

1. Make a comprehensive, meticulous appraisal of the child's status
2. Be sufficiently informative to be of value to parents and to school personnel
3. Discover defects
4. Provide professional counsel for any existing deviation
5. Indicate the extent to which the school program should be modified to benefit the child
6. Secure medical supervision and corrections as indicated

7. Provide a valuable health experience for the child
8. Determine the fitness of the child to participate in the school program

Legal requirements. In some states the legislature specifically has provided that the state board of education shall prescribe a program of health examinations for pupils. Under this provision the state board of education sets examination requirements to which local education districts must conform.

In some states the local education boards specifically are granted legislative authority to provide a program of health examinations for pupils. However, in the absence of any such specific legislative authorization, courts have held that a board of education has the authority to specify that a health examination is a requirement for admission to school. This authority can be extended to include health examinations for other purposes, such as participation in athletics. However, courts stipulate that the exercise of this authority shall be *reasonable*.

Usually exceptions are made on religious grounds, although a question arises as to whether a health examination constitutes medication. The Washington State Supreme Court ruled that the University of Washington Board of Regents was within its authority in requiring that all students matriculating at the university have x-ray films of the chest. The court further ruled that the board acted properly in denying exceptions for religious reasons because an x-ray examination is not a form of medication.

In practice the state board of education establishes a pattern for a health examination program, which guides the local education board in the exercise of its legal responsibility and authority.

Examination schedule. An annual health examination for every schoolchild might be ideal, but in practice is hardly attainable. Cost, scheduling problems, time consumed, and parental objections to apparently unnecessary repetitions have combined to make the annual school health examination an academic question. Actually, from the standpoint of practical health protection and promotion, modifications can be made that will yield approximately the same end result as the annual examination.

One modification is to give children a health examination when they enter school, another in the fourth grade, and a third in the eighth grade. Supplemental examinations are made as indicated by screening by the teacher or nurse and for participation in athletics. Even this relatively modest program did not gain wide acceptance. As a result, a further modification has been practical and effective and each year appears to be gaining wider acceptance. This program is outlined here.

Pupils entering school for the first time. Children who are to begin school in the fall should be examined sufficiently early to permit an adequate follow-up on recommendations of the examining physician. June has been found to be the most satisfactory month for the preschool examination.

Pupils referred through screening by the teacher or nurse. Alert teachers and nurses frequently are the first to detect that a child is not up to his or her normal health status. Both minor and serious deviations are recognized by the informed and observant teacher, who has an excellent opportunity to observe the child during the many hours of close association each day. The teacher or nurse informs the parents or guardian of the child of the observation. Parents refer the child to a physician. When the school has a nurse available for consultation, parents or guardian should be contacted by a teacher-nurse referral channeled through the principal, although the teacher may make the actual contact with the parent. Even though the teacher may be unsure of the necessity for having a pupil examined, it is prudent in this

case to err on the side of caution and to speak to the parents about the advisability of having the child checked by the physician.

Students participating in vigorous athletics. Any student participating in interscholastic athletics should be examined just before the beginning of the sports program in which he or she is to participate. The physician's certification of the student's fitness to participate in athletics will indicate any limitations or restrictions. A physician's certification of fitness for every participating athlete should be on file in the school before the students are even permitted to practice for an interscholastic sport. Following an injury, illness, or other incapacity, the student should be permitted further participation only on the recommendation and under the supervision of a physician. Students participating in vigorous intramural sports should also be examined before the season of participation.

Pupils new to the system. If an acceptable health record is received from the school the pupil previously attended, an examination may be deemed unnecessary. If there is no health record or a doubtful health condition exists, a health examination is in the best interests of the child.

Pupils entering seventh, eighth, or ninth grades. In schools organized on the 6-3-3 basis, examination as a requirement for admission to junior high school is both sound and easy to administer. Middle schools would have the examination in the eighth grade. In schools on the 8-4 plan, this requirement will apply for admission to high school.

• • •

A few school districts have inaugurated the plan of giving all graduating seniors a health examination 4 to 8 weeks before graduation. Thus, in addition to an evaluation of the academic status of the student at the time of graduation, the school also provides a record of the health status of the graduate. In some communities, service clubs have made the health examination a gift to the graduating seniors.

Preparing the students. A health examination should be considered a valuable opportunity and the physician a valued friend. This positive attitude can be developed only by planned effective health instruction, fortified by an exchange of individual experiences among the students and the utilization of events and incidents that provide opportunities for learning about the importance of the health examination. A positive attitude, supported by knowledge and wholesome personal experiences, is the equation for proper preparation for the health examination for child and adult.

Methods for obtaining examinations. A variety of methods and combinations of methods are used by various school districts in obtaining health examinations of school-children (Fig. 7-1). The particular method best suited to conditions in the community should be used. This particular method or plan should be worked out jointly by the school and representatives of the parents, the health department, and the medical society. The final plan may include parts of several methods or may be limited to one of the recognized methods.

Examination in the family physician's office. Since the family physician frequently knows the background of the child and family, he or she is in an excellent position to make a comprehensive appraisal of the child's health. A commendable physician-patient relationship exists. Ideal conditions for examination usually prevail, and labora-

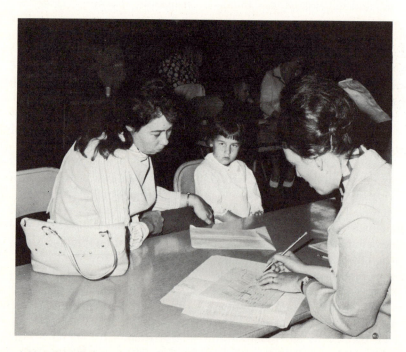

Fig. 7-1. Child and family history taken by a qualified volunteer. Using competent people from the community can be a highly effective vehicle for promoting public support. (Courtesy Tillamook County Health Department, Tillamook, Ore.)

tory facilities are available for tests indicated by the clinical examination. Parents frequently accompany the child to an examination by the family physician, and a highly profitable physician-parent-child conference can be held. An additional benefit is the likelihood that families without a recognized family physician will select a physician who serves subsequently in that capacity. A concept of parental responsibility for health services is always worth cultivating.

Three disadvantages are possible in conducting the examination in the family physician's office. First, a lack of uniformity both in the examination and the reporting may result. This can be reduced by using a standard examination form. Second, the physician may fail to use the opportunity for effective health instruction. Third, possibly only a small percentage of schoolchildren will actually have an examination.

A growing concern to educators and physicians alike is the large number of children who come to school from homes where the parents either cannot afford or do not accept responsibility for the needed health and medical care of their children. An added complication is the lack of medical services available to the disadvantaged and to children of the lower socioeconomic levels. This problem is particularly acute in many of the major cities in the United States today. Special federal legislation has been enacted, such as the amendments to the Social Security Act and Titles V and XIX (popularly known as Medicaid), which are designed to provide comprehensive health services for child and youth. The intent of this legislation is to provide medical care for all those who are unable to pay for it. Although providing direct health care for children is not considered to be a responsibility of the school, nevertheless school personnel should not overlook the health care needs of children. School officials should inform themselves of state and federal legislative provisions for child health ser-

vices. Indeed, school administrators, teachers, and school nurses are advocates for the health of school-age children and youths. It is they who must communicate the health needs to the family and to the appropriate community health officials.

While supporting the principle that students should have regular medical examinations in the office of their own family or personal physician, this ideal is not likely to be achieved in the near future. Because of these circumstances, periodic school health examinations are likely to be conducted in a variety of patterns depending on the needs, the attitudes, and medical resources available in the community.

Examination by health department physician. In some districts the health department staff conducts all, most, or a few selected health examinations. Clinics for preschool examinations, pre-junior high school examinations, and athletic examinations may be held in the health department office or in a school building (Fig. 7-2). This method has special value for small or isolated school districts.

Examination clinics held in the school building. These clinics are conducted by practicing physicians selected through arrangement with the local medical society. Most of the advantages of the examination in the private office are retained, and the convenience appeals to many parents and some physicians. Parents of elementary school-age children are usually invited to be present at the time of their child's examination. Parents are an important source of information regarding the child's health history. Having the parent available facilitates interpretation of any significant medical evaluation as well as clarification of any recommendations for follow-up care or treatment. When parents are not present, the school nurse later visits the home to explain the examination findings to the parents. In unusual cases the physician may have a conference with the parents to

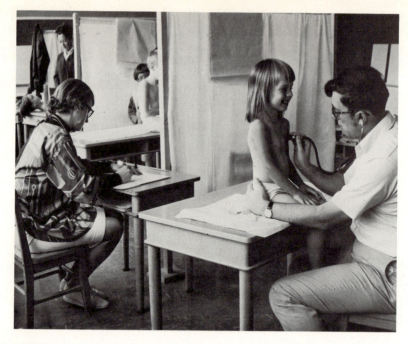

Fig. 7-2. Clinical examination by a physician, one stop on the journey through the multiphase entrance examination. A nurse recorder conserves the physician's time and energy. Other stations just ahead await the pupil. (Courtesy Tillamook County Health Department, Tillamook, Ore.)

explain certain aspects of the child's health status.

Examination by the regularly appointed school physician. These examinations constitute a principal function of the school physician.

Multiphasic entrance health examination. A recent innovation has been the development of a multiphasic health examination to provide a free examination for every entering child through a team approach using medical, dental, paramedical, and other personnel in a methodical, standardized procedure on something of an assembly line operation. The plan is fostered jointly by the county health department and the school administration. The procedure follows a pattern such as this:

1. Completion in advance of medical history questionnaire by the parents

2. Review of medical history by a trained health person such as a nurse

3. Test of child's hearing by audiometrist with audiometer; referrals are rechecked by a senior audiometrist

4. Amblyopia team member examines the child's vision; a private practitioner ophthalmologist examines children referred for eye problems; this is an on-the-spot examination

5. A speech therapist evaluates the child's speech (Fig. 7-3)

6. A private practitioner dentist makes a record of the child's dentition

7. A technician with a phonocardioscan screens each child for significant heart abnormalities; the phonocardioscan record is appraised by the physician who conducts the final examination (Fig. 7-4)

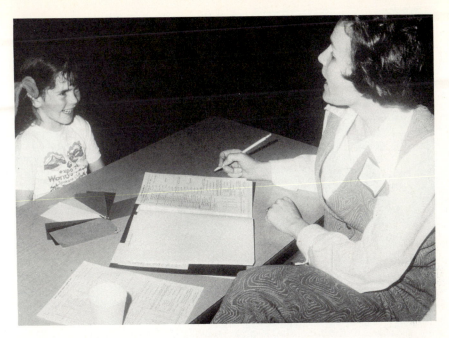

Fig. 7-3. Speech therapist screening for speech difficulties. Far more pupils have speech problems, a neglected disability, than is generally recognized by classroom teachers. Testing for speech difficulties is a part of the multiphasic entrance examination and should always be conducted by a competent speech therapist. (Courtesy Tillamook County Health Department, Tillamook, Ore.)

8. Each child is given a clinical examination by a physician who also reviews the previous findings of other personnel; a pediatrician is available for consultation; the team of physicians is composed of private practitioners as well as health department medical physicians

9. Laboratory tests as recommended include (Fig. 7-5):
   a. Hematocrit
   b. Serum albumin
   c. Plasma vitamin A
   d. Urinalysis

10. Vaccines, particularly rubella, are administered as indicated by medical history and approved by parents

11. Evaluation for the benefit of the parent either by a nurse or a physician as circumstances provide

This in-depth program assures a thorough methodical appraisal of a child's health status. Health department personnel serve without cost to the school or the parents. Private practitioners may donate their services or may be paid a fee by the school board. Thus every child whose parents approve is assured of an all-important thorough entrance examination. Parents still have the option of taking their children to their family physician.

Time and place of the multiphasic entrance examination are optional, depending primarily on local circumstances. The examination may be conducted in June or the first week of school in September. If adequate facilities are available in school buildings, examinations could be scheduled in all of the buildings where children enter school, or one school building could be designated for all examinations. Under some circumstances

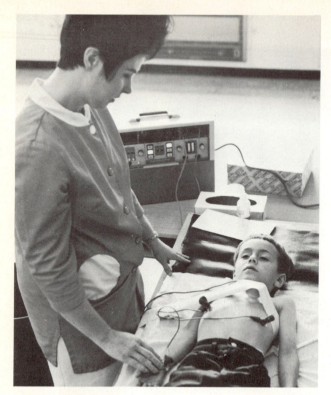

Fig. 7-4. Phonocardioscan test. Conducted by a technician furnished by the state heart association, the test identifies cardiac disorders. Questionable heart patterns are interpreted by a cardiologist whose recommendations may include electrocardiograms and other tests. Using newly developed procedures is in the true tradition of school health programs in doing everything possible in behalf of each child. (Courtesy Tillamook County Health Department, Tillamook, Ore.)

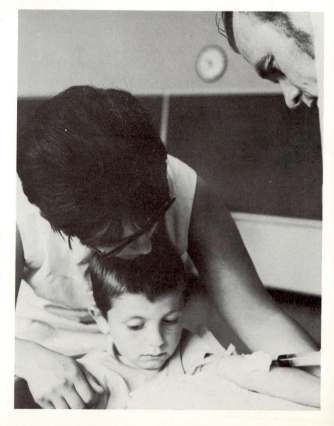

Fig. 7-5. Drawing blood sample. Test to include hematocrit, serum albumin, and plasma vitamin A. A urinalysis is also included in this particular multiphasic examination. Few school districts will have entrance examinations as extensive as shown here, but this pioneering may well be a forerunner of things to come. (Courtesy Tillamook County Health Department, Tillamook, Ore.)

the decision may be made to have the examinations conducted in the quarters of the county or city health department.

The 1967 amendments to Title XIX of the Social Security Act added a requirement to Medicaid that directs attention to preventive services and to early detection and treatment of diseases in children eligible for medical assistance. For example, in the state of Illinois, those children who receive Aid to Dependent Children (ADC) or medical assistance are eligible for services under this program for the period from birth to age 20 years. This extension to Title XIX of the Medicaid program is commonly known as Early Periodic Screening Diagnosis and Treatment (EPSDT). In Illinois it is called Medichek and it is conducted jointly by the Department of Public Aid and the Department of Public Health.

The extended services provided under the Medicaid (Title XIX) program include:

1. Periodic health appraisals (Fig. 7-6), including health history and physical examination, with emphasis on growth, development, and nutritional status. (The schedule includes four medical checkups during the first year, annual checkups to age 6 years,

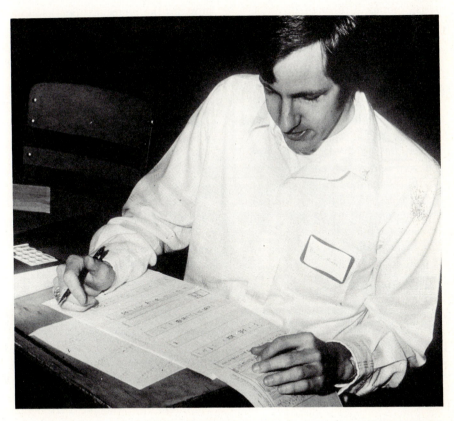

Fig. 7-6. Electronics in modern school health programs. Food intake questionnaires are picked up at the history station and taken to a side room to be calculated. After calculations are completed the results are taken to the nutrition education station, which the child and mother will eventually reach. (Courtesy Tillamook County Health Department, Tillamook, Ore.)

and then at ages 10, 14, 17, and 20 years.)

2. A comprehensive immunization program and updating of previous immunization; including measles, polio, diphtheria, pertussis, and tetanus.

3. The periodic screening for urine sugar and protein, hemoglobin, or hematocrit determinations and tuberculosis testing. (Vision and hearing screening are provided annually from ages 3 to 8 years and thereafter at ages 10, 12, 14, and 16 years.)

4. Screening when indicated to detect specific conditions including lead poisoning, sickle cell abnormality, and venereal disease.

5. Dental examinations as provided on an annual basis from age 3 through 20 years.

Emphasis is given to follow-up care and treatment of the health problems discovered through these screening activities.

School officials and especially health educators are urged to inform themselves about the aforementioned federal and state services, which are provided through Medicaid, that are available to the children of their respective communities. With the development of new programs of health services, school health education must accept the leadership and responsibility for informing children and parents about these important community services and resources.

Payment. The method by which physicians are paid for their examining services is determined by local practices, by the method used to obtain examinations, and by individual circumstances. Any one or all of the following four common methods of payment may be in use:

1. The parents pay the family physician on a private basis.

2. Under the provisions of the extended Medicaid program (EPSDT), physicians and dentists are paid for conducting examinations and for any further diagnostic work or treatment that may be required as a result of their medical appraisals.

3. In some instances, the board of education pays practicing physicians for conducting health examinations of schoolchildren. A board of education legally can pay a physician for an examination of a schoolchild whether the examination is conducted in the physician's office or elsewhere.

4. Because of the frequency of medical examinations and the need to reevaluate the fitness of an athlete for competition, special arrangements are usually made for students participating in the interscholastic athletic program. One such approach is for the school to employ a team physician who gives the preseason medical examinations and who also provides the medical supervision of the athletic program.

5. Occasionally community service clubs pay for the health examination of schoolchildren, but usually on a selective basis—hardship cases, athletes, seniors—rarely on a school-wide basis.

The examination. Techniques for conducting an examination are the province of the medical profession, but various factors relating to the examination are of interest and importance to all school personnel.

Whether the preschool examination is conducted in the physician's office or elsewhere, the family history and child history portions of the examination form should be filled out by the parents in advance of the examination time. It should be logical for the parents to be present at the preschool and referral examination, although there may be some question of the necessity for the parent to be present at junior high school or athletic participation examinations. At the preschool examination the physician will include tests for vision and hearing.

For children who are in school and are scheduled to be examined, the school may test vision and hearing and record height and weight on the examination form. In addition, the school can assume responsibility for having the parents complete the history portion of the form if such information is not on record.

Optimum time for an examination is 15 minutes, and 10 minutes should be regarded as minimum. Every phase of the examination should be thorough. A superficial examination may be worse than none at all if it gives a false feeling of security. It is recognized that in 7 minutes one physician may conduct the actual medical aspects of the examination just as thoroughly as another physician who takes 15 minutes for the entire examination. The difference comes in the amount of health counseling that is included. An examination is a magnificent opportunity to impress youngsters with the importance of *their* health. To get a person to appreciate the value of his or her own health is the most difficult single task in health education, and here is the best possible teaching situation for that purpose. Informing students of their health assets and complimenting them on favorable points can create a wholesome *health esteem,* an essential to a high level of lifelong health promotion.

In addition to the history of health behavior and experiences, a standard health examination usually includes an evaluation of the following:

1. General appearance
2. Height and weight
3. Head and neck, nose and throat
4. Vision and hearing
5. Thorax, heart, and lungs
6. Abdomen and genitalia
7. Skin
8. Muscular and skeletal systems
9. Posture, gait, and feet
10. Neurological system

When examinations are held at the health department or school, a nurse may serve as recorder for the physician, which conserves time and energy for the physician. If there is no nurse, some physicians appoint a teacher to record their findings as they call them off.

The enactment of the Family Education Rights and Privacy Act of 1974 has brought about a new sensitivity among school officials concerning students' records. This law requires that all educational records be open to students and their parents or guardians. The confidential nature of records, including health records, and the recognition of the individual student's rights places a heavy responsibility on school officials. This concerns both the appropriateness of health information that is recorded and also the necessity for proper interpretation of this information.

Examination record form. Medical societies, public health societies, and public health departments have developed model health examination forms. The particular form adopted by any school district should be one approved by the local medical society. Usually, in practice the state department of education, state department of health, and state medical society jointly develop a form for use by schools throughout the state. In the absence of such a form the local school board should ask the local health department and local medical society to recommend a form for use by physicians examining schoolchildren.

One such concise, practical health examination form is reproduced in Appendix B. This is not to be looked on as *the* model form, for while it satisfies most requirements for such a recording, modifications of this form have been found to be highly satisfactory. Forms that are too long or too short have obvious disadvantages.

If the form is to be used for day-to-day reference, a lightweight cardboard (index Bristol) should be used rather than sheet paper. However, if data from this form are to be transferred to a school record card for everyday use by the teacher, sheet paper (20-pound bond) is adequate.

When the health department cooperates

in the school health program, the school health administrator should furnish the department with a duplicate report for each child examined within the district served by the health department. The original copy should be kept by the school the child attends. A separate form is used for each health examination the child has during his or her school career. Examination records should be available for use, not filed in an inaccessible cabinet.

The point is that health record information must be made available to both the family and to the school. It is the parents who will, in most cases, initiate the action needed to follow up health care. For teachers, especially at the elementary school level, it means using the student's records in ways that will help the child to achieve his or her optimum growth and development.

An effective and appropriate use of health records can best be achieved by placing them on file in the principal's office or in the school health office if a full-time nursing service is available. Here the student's cumulative health records can be kept on file and be regularly augmented with reports of the periodic physical examinations that the student receives during the years of elementary and secondary schooling.

Health record card. The health record card brings together in one record essential health information supplied by the parent, physician, nurse, and teacher. It may be a light cardboard (index Bristol) card 8×10 inches. One side records personal and family histories; height; weight; results of vision, hearing, and susceptibility tests; annual health summary; immunizations; and physician's recommendations. The reverse side can record the child's illnesses as well as the regular observations by the teacher. The health record form presented in Appendix B illustrates one type of form that has proved to be highly satisfactory.

A card is provided for each pupil when he or she enters school for the first time. The card goes with the student from grade to grade, precisely as does the academic record, and at the close of the student's senior year in high school is filed with the academic record. If the student transfers to another school system, the original health record form should accompany the scholastic record. A duplicate health record card is retained by the original school.

A health record card is a means to an end, not an end in itself. It is there to be used. It can be used in conferences with the nurse, the parent, and the physician or in a conference of the teacher with all three. It is a means of sharing information and can quickly point up the health status of each child in the school. It can indicate desirable or attained health advances. It can tell the teacher what is happening in relation to the health of the child.

Report to parents. When parents are present at the health examination, it is logical that the attending physician verbally inform the parents of findings of special significance. When parents are not present at the examination, a routine report can be sent to them on a formal report form if nothing of special importance has been discovered. This form can be mailed by the health department. In the absence of a health department school nurse, the director of school health, the principal, or the teacher can mail the report or send it home by the child. When some condition that merits immediate attention has been discovered, an early home visit by the nurse, the health director, or the teacher is in order. Even when the examination reveals no special problem or a very minor health problem, a person-to-person conference with parents has many possible values (Fig. 7-7). The follow-up to any examination program is an index of the vitality of the whole school health program. As a

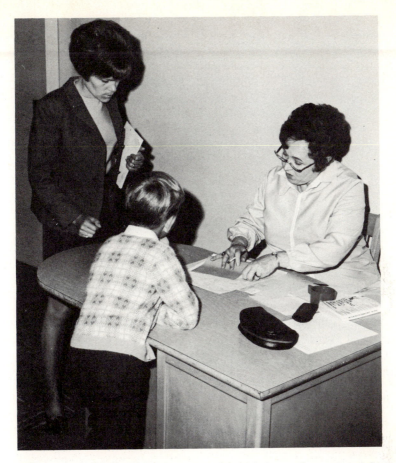

Fig. 7-7. Explanation of examination results to parent. A qualified nurse having the confidence of the parent makes the results of the examination highly meaningful in terms of the child's health status. (Courtesy Tillamook County Health Department, Tillamook, Ore.)

phase of the remedial aspects of health services, the follow-up is given special consideration in Chapter 10.

DENTAL EXAMINATION

Although both the physician's and dentist's examinations are designed to evaluate, protect, and promote the student's health, the two examinations have basic differences that have led to different administrative practices. Some schools provide for a record of the dental examination on the health exam-

ination form. This section of the form is thus filled out by the dentist, since the physician is not qualified to make the dental examination. Most schools use separate record forms for the dental examination and keep the dental examination program distinct from, yet correlated with, the general health examination program. Dental examinations are far more frequent than the general health examinations, which further justifies a special dental examination program.

Purpose. Dental cavities are the most

prevalent of all defects in America's school population. A simple dental cavity may have no demonstrable effect on health. Yet, if permitted to progress, a simple cavity could result in a loss of the tooth, with possible indirect effects on health. Most important, an apical abscess may develop as a consequence of the cavity, and vital structures of the body may be affected by the toxins formed at the abscess.

Because dental disease is so widespread, the urgent need is to reach children who must have treatment if they are to avoid the effects of permanent dental disorders and handicaps. This is a serious problem that interferes with the child's educational progress and poses a direct threat to his or her general health. Schools must take the initiative in helping to identify those children who are in need of immediate dental treatment. This is of particular concern for those children coming from families of lower socioeconomic status. Public health authorities have estimated that half of all the children in the United States under 15 years of age have never seen a dentist. The percentage is even higher among those children who come from homes of extreme poverty.

The dental profession is vigorously pursuing a program of preventive dentistry. The American Dental Association through its Bureau of Dental Health Education is giving significant leadership in promoting dental health education and in actively supporting schools in their efforts to develop more effective programs of health education. Dentists recognize the importance of an effective teamwork relationship among dentists, public health agencies, and the schools if the goal of positive dental health is to be achieved.

A minimum dental health appraisal program is an annual examination, supplemented by observations and referrals from teachers, nurses, dental hygienists, and parents. The traditional role of the school in conducting dental screening programs is to identify those children who are in need of special care. However, the participation of dentists in such programs is now being questioned. Dentists correctly point out that examining children in schools is not the most effective use of their skills. Moreover, given the fact that most children will need treatment, it is not a wise use of the dentists' time nor the public's money to confirm what is already known. Thus it is more efficient to make maximum use of the dentists' time in correcting and treating children's problems and to rely on the teacher, nurse, dental hygienist, and parents for screening and referral.

Methods for obtaining examinations. Whenever possible, the ideal is to have the child's dental examination performed by his or her own personal dentist. Toward this end, it is recommended that schools establish policies that children may be excused in order to secure examinations from their own family or personal dentist during school hours. In some instances dental inspections, as opposed to dental examinations, have been given by a dentist or dental hygienist in special clinics held at the schools (Fig. 7-8). Although dentists prefer to use their offices to conduct examinations, dental inspections can be given with the aid of mouth mirrors, explorers, and flashlights. Such a program can serve a useful purpose if it is an integral part of the school health program and emphasis is placed on the educational value of the activity. Teachers can take this opportunity to integrate the inspections with the unit on dental health education, to acquaint children with the role of the dentist or dental hygienist, and also to stimulate the interest of children and their parents in good dental care.

As previously pointed out, regular dental screening is included as a part of the ex-

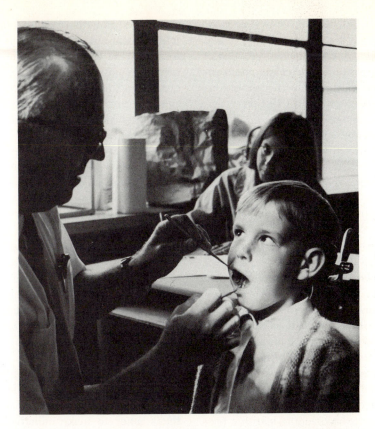

Fig. 7-8. Dental examination. Proper lighting and headrest provide the dentist with the necessary "props" for a clinical examination. (Courtesy Tillamook County Health Department, Tillamook, Ore.)

tended Medicaid program. Because of the magnitude of the dental health problem and because of the need to reach children early enough to initiate a program of preventive dentistry, Medicaid provides for an annual dental screening examination beginning at age 3 years.

The emphasis here is placed on early diagnosis and treatment. The form for dental screening should include recommendations for treatment. Payment is provided to dentists for both their diagnostic and treatment services.

A school health instruction plan properly includes dental health, provides knowledge, and establishes attitudes and ideals for the pupils that should motivate them to want good dental health. Education of the parents in dental health can be promoted through school bulletins, pamphlets, conferences, newspaper articles, radio and television programs, and addresses by dentists, dental hygienists, nurses, or other qualified speakers.

Examination record form. When all examinations are done by the family dentist, the dentist will maintain his or her own examination record form. Medichek provides a dental examination and follow-up treatment form. Other variations may be necessary in special circumstances.

Follow-up. Since the dental examination is

merely a means to an end, it is important that emphasis be placed on having dental treatment done. Establishing the practice of having dentists give schoolchildren a certificate indicating that all dental corrections have been made serves both the child and the school. It is a motivational factor for the child, and it promotes pride in his or her attainment. It also provides the school with a record of the child's dental status and an indication of the effectiveness of its dental health program.

HEALTH ASSESSMENT BY THE TEACHER

Typically, an elementary school level teacher has a class for most of the school day throughout the school year. This extended period of association with children provides the teacher with an unusual vantage point from which to develop special understanding and insight into the personality of each student. Experienced teachers come to appreciate that an understanding of a child's total personality including his or her health status is essential to the teaching-learning process.

Over the course of a school year, the teacher is able to form a general concept of each child's physical, emotional, and social characteristics as well as behavior patterns. Although teachers may not be able to diagnose specific health problems as could the physician or dentist, they can nevertheless develop an acute sensitivity to any variations from an individual child's behavior. Teachers who have had the benefit of formal preparation concerning the characteristics of healthy children and in specific methods of evaluating the health status of children are a vital source of health information. Experience has shown that teachers are usually aware of those children in their classrooms who have health problems. Conversely, it is very seldom that an independent examination will

reveal a child with a serious health problem who has not already been identified and referred by the teacher. Although the old concept of a classroom morning inspection has generally given way to the principle of continuous observation of children, there are ways by which the teacher's observational and referral abilities can be improved through practice. One such procedure is to utilize the school nurse to conduct an annual review of the students in class. Another opportunity is the review of each student's progress during the regular parent-teacher conference. These reviews provide the teacher with an excellent opportunity to check his or her observations and evaluations with those of the nurse and the parents. In addition, it serves to develop the understanding and trust among teachers, parents, and school health personnel that is so important to the effective follow-up of children's health problems.

The school nurse can conduct special inservice conferences on child health and school health procedures that will enable the teacher to make effective child health evaluations. In such conferences, the nurse can acquaint teachers with those readily observable signs of health problems as well as those that reflect healthy growth.

Evaluation record form. A school health record card such as the one illustrated in Appendix B contains points that the teacher can observe and serves as an evaluation record form for the teacher. If these points are used, the teacher can get a practical evaluation of a child's health. This record card might be supplemented with a general classification of the child's health as A, B, C, D, or E for the teacher's own guidance.

When no such health record form is available to the teacher, one can be devised to suit the purpose. It can be simple and easily scored and understood. A form should be completed for each child.

HEALTH EVALUATION

Name _____ Date _____ Health rating: A B C D E

Parent _____ Family physician _____

_____

Muscle tone _____ Posture _____ Coordination _____

Vitality _____ Endurance _____ Nutrition _____ Skin _____

Eyes

Inflammation _____ Styes or crusted lids _____ Squinting _____

Ears

Inflammation _____ Discharge _____ Wax _____ Earache _____

Nose and throat

Nasal discharge _____ Nose bleed _____ Mouth breathing _____

Sore throat_____

Oral cavity

Lips _____ Gums _____ Oral hygiene _____

Behavior

Restlessness _____ Drowsiness _____ Aggressiveness _____

Tenseness _____ Instability _____ Timidity _____

Cooperation _____ Industriousness _____ Orderliness _____

_____

Height _____ Weight _____ Hearing: R _____ L _____

	Both eyes	Right	Left
Vision:	W 20/	W 20/	W 20/
Vision:	WO 20/	WO 20/	WO 20/

Health assets _____

Deficiencies _____

Attention needed _____

Comments:

In scoring the evaluation form, the teacher uses the most meaningful designations. Words, symbols (o, x), and check marks can be used. Blue pencil marks to designate meritorious points and red marks to designate deficiencies help to point up health assets and liabilities. Although this evaluation is an assessment of the present level of a child's health, it could have further value if a follow-up plan for day-to-day health improvement is initiated with the child. Occasionally the evaluation brings to the teacher's attention a condition that should be referred to the parents.

Daily observation. In addition to the more comprehensive evaluation, the health-minded teacher will observe both positive and negative indications of the child's health at any given moment on any given day. Outward indices of changes in health are not generally pronounced, but the teacher becomes so well acquainted with the pupils that minor changes in a child's condition will be observed. Most gratifying to the teacher is the gradual improvement in health that many of the pupils will display.

Report to parents. Normally the evaluation is for the teacher's own use. When a child has no particular health deficiency and appears to be in normal health, the teacher makes no special report to the parents as a consequence of the health evaluation. Occasionally a child will show a pronounced deficiency that should be reported to the parents. At times a child may show a sudden pronounced decline in health. Referral to the family is in order because any acute change in health can be serious. Likewise any chronic condition that appears to lower a child's effectiveness and enjoyment in living should be discussed with the parents. All referrals should be followed up, because for the best interests of the child it is important to know what has been done and what is being done.

CONSERVATION OF VISION

Vision is a priceless heritage, and the school is responsible for doing everything reasonable to conserve and protect that heritage for every schoolchild. A child with normal vision for school purposes is fortunate. Perhaps equally fortunate is the child with a slight visual defect that is detected early in its course and the necessary correction made. Not only is the efficiency of the child's sight involved, but also the personality of the child, if the required treatment is not given.

A child who is farsighted (hyperopic) may sit and stare out of the window, relaxed and contented, and perhaps watch every detail of a bird building a nest. To look in the distance is both relaxing and restful for the child with this condition. The child who is nearsighted (myopic) does not stare at the bird building a nest. Perhaps he or she does not even see the tree. Instead, the myopic child may be buried in a book, no bother to the teacher or anyone else, whereas the hyperopic child may be a worry to the teacher because of his or her apparent inattention. The farsighted child may develop into an active, outdoor, extroverted person, interested in athletics and vigorous activities. A nearsighted child, on the other hand, is more apt to be withdrawn and interested in reading and related interests.

From 2% to 5% of schoolchildren will have amblyopia, a dimness of vision. These youngsters will have difficulty in the standard Snellen vision test. In screening these children, the school does not diagnose the condition as amblyopia. Diagnosis or identification of the condition is the province of the certified professional eye specialist.

A school's vision conservation program logically can be divided into four phases: (1) vision screening tests, (2) observation, (3) health record, and (4) follow-up.

Vision screening tests. A vision screening test is not a selective diagnostic test, but a

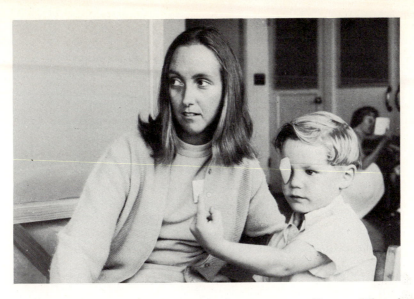

Fig. 7-9. Vision examination by a specially trained volunteer Jayceette. (Courtesy Tillamook County Health Department, Tillamook, Ore.)

method of identifying those children who are most likely to need a more thorough diagnostic examination (Fig. 7-9). Some children who need further examination may be missed, and some who do not need further care will be selected. Indeed, whether the deficiency revealed by the screening is serious or even significant is for the professionally trained practitioner to determine. Thus the teacher is not a vision-testing expert. Rather, he or she shares in the screening process to identify those children who may have visual problems. Defects in visual acuity are the result of hyperopia, myopia, astigmatism, and muscle imbalance. Children in the first and second grades tend to be farsighted. Nearsightedness in children develops at about the level of the fourth grade. Most children who need glasses will show the need by the time they are in the seventh grade.

Schools should give at least one test of color discrimination during the child's school experience.

Test schedule. It is now recognized that

vision screening should begin before the child enters school or as early as age 3 or 4 years. This preschool screening is important for the early identification of the condition amblyopia, so that early corrective procedures may be initiated. Beginning in preschool, children should be tested on an annual basis through the early grades to age 8 or 9 years. Thereafter, the screening can be reduced to a schedule of once every 2 or 3 years and on a referral basis.

At the high school level, vision screening of all students in health classes as a learning experience can be helpful in identifying children who need a thorough eye examination. An observant staff of teachers who note those students exhibiting visual fatigue or other visual difficulty will refer them to the health director or nurse. Actual screening is done by the health director or the nurse. Few high schools give a vision screening test to all their students. Yet the time would be well invested.

Test procedures. The best known and

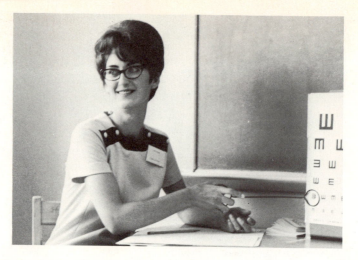

Fig. 7-10. Vision examination by a specially trained volunteer Jayceette. (Courtesy Tillamook County Health Department, Tillamook, Ore.)

most widely used test for vision screening is the *Snellen test.* Although apparently simple, this test has been found through experience to be extremely reliable and valid in identifying loss of visual acuity. Experience indicates that the "tumbling" E chart is as effective as the multiple letter chart, whether readers or nonreaders are being tested (Fig. 7-10). The test is a valuable educational experience. Procedures can be enumerated in a series of steps:

1. Explain the purpose of the test to the children in the classroom
2. Show the chart to the children as a group and conduct group practice trials until they understand the test thoroughly
3. Demonstrate how to cover the eye not being tested by holding a 3 × 5 inch card by the corner in front of the eye so that the eye is open and is not disturbed
4. Do testing in a room where there are no distractions; the classroom is usually unsatisfactory for obvious reasons
5. Hang a clean chart vertically in an uncluttered space so that all possible glare is eliminated
6. Place the child being tested so that the light comes from the side, rear, or overhead; do not face the light
7. Focus an intensity of light of 8 to 12 footcandles, whatever the source, on the chart
8. Be sure that the 20-foot reading line on the chart is at the child's eye level when standing
9. Draw a chalk line or make a tack line on the floor 20 feet from the chart so that the child may toe this mark as he or she stands and reads the chart
10. Test each child individually
11. Have each child toe the 20-foot mark and keep both eyes open. Place a fresh 3 × 5 inch card over each eye in sequence
12. Begin with the 50-foot line on the chart and let the testing proceed from left to right; using a card with a 1-inch hole, expose only the letter you wish the child to see; proceed from line to line downward to include the 20-foot line; reading three out of four symbols successfully at a particular level is evidence of satisfactory vision
13. Check for possible farsightedness by using a pair of convex or "plus" lenses (framed glasses containing a pair of 2.25 diopter convex lenses); if the child can read the 20/20 line with the glasses on, it is an indication of farsightedness
14. If the child wears glasses, first test with glasses, then without glasses; test both eyes first, then the right and left eyes separately; record in the same order
15. Note any unusual actions such as tilting of the head, blinking, scowling, or squinting
16. The numerator that denotes the distance from the chart is always 20

17. The denominator is the lowest line the child can read successfully
18. If the child correctly reads the 20-foot line with the right eye, the score is right 20 over 20 (normal)
19. If he or she can read only the 50-foot line at a distance of 20 feet, the record is 20 over 50
20. After the tests are completed, keep the chart out of sight until the next time for testing

These instructions should be followed very closely. Some practice is necessary to gain skill.

Interpretation of the test is not difficult in most cases. For school purposes, 20/20 is normal. Occasionally a child with 20/20 vision may have a vision defect, but the teacher is not expected to ferret out every conceivable irregularity of the eyes. A child with 20/30 vision is probably nearsighted, although the teacher determines merely that the child has difficulty in seeing, not that the child is nearsighted. A child with 20/10 or 20/15 vision is probably farsighted. For jet pilots 20/10 vision is normal; good hitters in baseball find 20/15 vision to be an advantage, but for the school 20/20 is normal.

It must be pointed out that any vision testing done by the teacher or nurse in the school is a screening test. If the Snellen test or just observation indicates the child's vision may not be normal, through the parent the child should be referred to an eye specialist. It is of some interest that a combined survey and experiment in Oregon public schools indicated that the plus sphere test screened out very few cases of vision difficulty not identified by the Snellen test. This study indicated that discerning observations, competent screening with the Snellen test, and an effective referral and follow-up program will fulfill the obligation of the school in vision conservation.

Observation. An observant teacher who knows what to look for can identify children who have vision trouble before the Snellen test is ever conducted. The signs of eye trouble in children listed by the National Society for the Prevention of Blindness, Inc.* are the best guide for the teacher to use.

Behavior

Rubs eyes excessively
Shuts or covers one eye, tilts head or thrusts head forward
Has difficulty in reading or in other work requiring close use of the eyes
Blinks more than usual or is irritable when doing close work
Stumbles over small objects
Holds books close to eyes
Is unable to participate in games requiring distance vision
Squints eyelids together or frowns

Appearance

Cross-eyed
Red-rimmed, encrusted, or swollen eyelids
Inflamed or watery eyes

Complaints

Cannot see well
Dizziness
Headaches } after close eye work
Nausea
Blurred or double vision

Any suspicion of vision trouble should be followed up to protect the valuable heritage of sight.

Follow-up. After conducting the Snellen test, the teacher should follow definite steps:
1. List pupils needing further vision examination
2. List pupils to be checked by the school nurse
3. Arrange conference with the nurse
4. Record results of the conference
5. Refer to parents, using a special form
6. Schedule follow-up visits by nurse or teacher if parents take no action following original referral
7. Record results of Snellen test made with new glasses child is wearing

---

*From Signs of eye trouble in children, New York, 1959, National Society for the Prevention of Blindness, Inc.

REPORT ON EYE CONDITION

Date _____

Pupil _____

Address _____

_____
Parent or Guardian

Symptoms that may indicate vision difficulty have been observed in your child _____

_____

The school urges you to consult a doctor at once for professional advice.

_____ Signed _____
School   Teacher

EXAMINING DOCTOR'S REPORT TO THE SCHOOL

Visual acuity

Without glasses   **With glasses**

Right _____ Left _____   Right _____ Left _____

Explanation of condition _____

Time of next examination _____

Restrictions on eye work _____

Other recommendations _____

Date _____ Signed _____
                   Examiner

Actually this program is relatively simple; yet the dividends are considerable in terms of sight-saving and effective and enjoyable living. Here are both an obligation and an opportunity for service to the schoolchild, which the truly professional teacher will fulfill.

CONSERVATION OF HEARING

The first obligation of the school in the conservation of the hearing of children is the prevention of hearing loss. In this role the school can serve in several spheres. It can educate children on proper action to prevent injury to hearing. It can inform parents on measures to avoid possible hearing loss in their children. Equally important, the school can follow established practices to prevent hearing loss in children enrolled in the school.

Prevention of hearing loss. Most hearing defects are preventable, and the school, through understanding and an effective approach, can contribute directly to the prevention of hearing loss. Several factors can be involved in hearing loss, and various measures can be taken to protect the hearing of children. The school and the home, with full understanding, working together in a common purpose, can best serve the interests of any child whose hearing may be threatened. Several factors can be involved and should be given necessary consideration:

1. Any foreign object in a child's ear canal may cause hearing loss and even lead to infection. Usually it is wise to have a physician remove the object.
2. Hard packed wax in the ear canal can be softened by warm oil and then removed, but when the wax is soundly embedded it should be removed by a physician.
3. A discharging ear should have the immediate attention of a physician.
4. Some of the common infectious respiratory diseases such as measles, scarlet fever, and diphtheria can develop into a complication of middle ear infection and result in damage to the hearing apparatus.
5. Frequent colds can affect hearing, and, when there is a possibility of this happening, the services of a physician should be enlisted.
6. Blowing the nose hard, particularly through one nostril, can force infectious material into the eustachian tube and middle ear, resulting in hearing loss.
7. A child with a history of ruptured eardrum should have a physician's approval before swimming.
8. No child outgrows a hearing loss. He may adjust to the condition, but medical service is necessary to assure improvement or complete recovery in hearing.

Nowhere does a "stitch in time" apply more aptly or with more certainty than in measures directed toward alleviating a condition threatening hearing. *Action Now* should be the school motto in matters of hearing conservation.

Discovery of hearing impairment. Loss in hearing acuity is frequently so gradual that it is imperceptible to the person concerned. Unconsciously a person adapts to a gradual loss of hearing. People with normal hearing do a certain amount of lip reading, and the person whose hearing is declining relies more and more on lip reading. Often the teacher will observe behavior symptoms of hearing difficulty such as posturing, inattention, faulty pronunciation, unnatural voice, poor academic progress, and copying.

However, many children with a hearing defect do not show behavior changes, and a hearing screening test is a more reliable device for the discovery of hearing defects than is the child's outward behavior.

Hearing screening tests. Many adults with markedly defective hearing could have normal or nearly normal hearing if the defect had been discovered when it first began to develop. Youngsters with a small hearing loss, by ingenuity, can compensate for the deficiency, and neither the child, the teacher, nor the parents may be aware of the deficiency in the early stages. A hearing screening test will identify the child who has a hearing loss. In addition to being the first stage in the prevention of further hearing loss, the test may be a step to more effective hearing in the immediate future.

It must be recognized that the hearing screening test is but the first of six steps:

1. Screening test
2. Evaluation of school progress
3. Preliminary medical screening
4. Parent interview
5. Examination and care by family physician
6. Adjustments based on recommendations

Test schedule. Recognizing the importance of early detection and early treatment, public health officials are recommending that the screening of hearing be conducted on a schedule similar to that of vision screening, which commences during the preschool period. Since hearing losses are often related to middle ear infections that occur frequently among children in the lower grades, screening at this level should be done on a yearly basis and every 2 years in secondary school.

Test procedures. An accurate and reliable hearing screening program requires the use of a pure tone audiometer and a trained audi-

ometrician to do the testing. Although school districts may have their own audiometer available, increasingly state departments of public health are providing the equipment and the trained personnel to conduct the hearing tests. This not only is an excellent service to schools but also helps to assure more accurate and reliable test results, which reduce the problem of both overreferrals and underreferrals (Fig. 7-11).

The conventional auditory screening program involves a two-step process including (1) a sweep check method and (2) a threshold

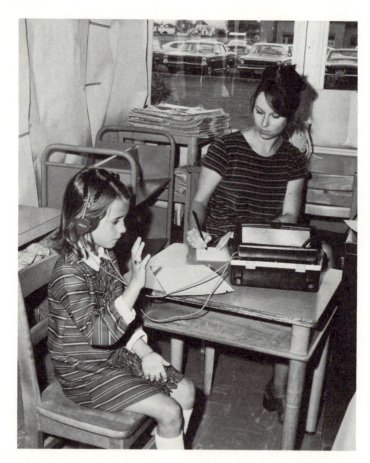

Fig. 7-11. Hearing test conducted by a professional audiometrician. Today's refined audiometers have replaced the unreliable whisper test of past vintage. (Courtesy Tillamook County Health Department, Tillamook, Ore.)

level test. Testing should be carried out individually in a quiet room at the school that the child attends. In the sweep check screening, the tone is presented at a consistent 25-decibel level of intensity, starting with the frequency of 6,000 hertz (Hz) or cycles per second and then sweeping through the several different frequencies as follows: 4,000, 2,000, 1,000, 500, and 250 Hz. Those children who are able to hear each of these tones are considered to have normal hearing and to have passed the screening test. However, those children who fail on two or more of

these frequencies are given a retest as a check against false referrals. The second step, or threshold level testing, in effect determines the profile of an individual child's hearing, revealing the exact decibel level at which the tone can be heard for various frequencies included in the testing range as shown on the audiogram (Fig. 7-12). The tone is presented at a loud level that the child can hear and then is reduced by 5-decibel decrements until the child can no longer hear the tone. The procedure is then reversed, increasing the intensity by 5-decibel

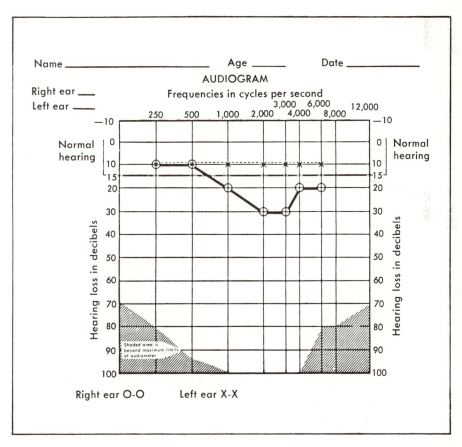

Fig. 7-12. Audiogram. The diagram indicates normal hearing in the left ear, but in the right ear a loss of 20 decibels at frequencies of 1,000, 4,000, and 6,000 cycles per second and a loss of 30 decibels at frequencies of 2,000 and 3,000 cycles per second.

increments until the exact level at which the child can hear the tone or frequency is established.

The threshold testing proceeds from 250 Hz and continues to 500, 1,000, 2,000, 4,000, and 5,000 Hz. Those children who have a hearing loss of 30 decibels at two or more frequencies or a loss of 35 or more decibels at a single frequency are referred for a diagnostic evaluation of their hearing.

Follow-up. The next step is to review the child's progress in school and look for a possible relationship to hearing acuity. Following this review of school history, the child may profitably be given an examination of the ears, nose, and throat by the health officer or school physician if one is available. The next step is an interview with the parents. After explaining the findings, the nurse or other school representative obtains a history of ear trouble and related disorders. The parents are then urged to refer the child to a physician. All information obtained up to this point is made available to the physician. A physician's examination and recommendation for care are the logical outcome of the previous attention given to the child. It now is a problem for the medical profession, but the school may be called on to contribute to the final step—adjustment.

Many persons and even organizations may work together to help a child with defective hearing make the necessary adjustment. The program may include special classroom seating, tutoring in academic subjects, instruction in lip reading, guidance, speech therapy, and auditory training.

HEIGHT AND WEIGHT MEASURES

Perhaps the practice of weighing and measuring has been the most firmly established aspect of the school health program. At one time teachers literally worshipped at the shrine of the height-weight-age tables, but fortunately that delusion has vanished.

Purpose of the measures. The primary purpose of recording the height and weight of children is to interest them in their own growth and well-being. As a health education project, it is invaluable. Emphasis should be placed on interesting children in their own condition, not in comparing them with a standard table or with other children. Each child is an individual, and no two are alike. One may be tall and heavily built; another may be short and slender. An effort should be made to interest each child in his or her own condition and in those procedures that are best for each individual.

Procedures. A group discussion and an analysis of the significance of height and weight should precede the weighing and measuring. Other aspects of health can be incorporated into such a discussion to develop a desirable interest in each of the children.

Formal records should be made three times a year—the first week of school, the first week of the second semester, and the final week of the school year.

Because of the natural interest in one's growth, this activity of weighing and measuring height can be effectively correlated with classroom health instruction. The opportunity to observe growth firsthand by recording their own height and weight not only stimulates the students' interest but also develops their appreciation of the wide range of variation in growth and the individual differences that characterize the growth patterns of normal, healthy children. It is also through this activity that students develop a basic understanding of the relationship that exists between such health-related activities as diet, exercise, and rest and growth. The scales and height standards should not be confined to the nurse's office but should be made available for regular student and classroom use, since they are an effective aid for the instructional program.

Evaluation. Weighing and measuring are not without merit. Ingenious teachers make weighing and measuring a stimulating group and individual experience. Even the location of the scales can be significant. To complete the picture, an extensive group discussion should grow out of the experience. Individual teacher-pupil conferences may be indicated. No child should lose status as a result of the weighing and measuring. Every child should "gain." If a child is in good health, the fact that he or she is shorter and less heavy than others is of minor significance. The child may have a father who is barely 5 feet tall and a mother even less than 5 feet tall. Height and weight, as a part of a total picture, may have significance. In this light, weighing and measuring is an aspect of health appraisal. Extreme underweight or extreme overweight may present opportunities for the teacher to be of service to the child.

HEALTH GUIDANCE AND SUPERVISION

A student's health status is important, and the school traditionally has accepted the role of supervising the health of the child during school hours. In practice, such supervision at school corresponds to the type of immediate supervision the conscientious parent would exercise in the home. However, more than just the protection and maintenance of the child's health are inherent in the school's supervision.

Any school health program must be appraised in terms of its effect on the health of the individual student. No phase of the program has a more direct effect on the immediate health of the student than does the guidance and supervision phase. The effect will be reflected in the future well-being of the student if the guidance and supervision have been effective in developing the student's ability to accept responsibility for his or her own health. This phase must be a carefully planned, integrated program that is centered on the student's needs.

School administrators have experienced increasing difficulty in obtaining medical service for the school. Physicians in private practice have had less and less time and inclination to serve the school, except for special purposes. Small- and medium-sized school systems have been forced to proceed without the services of a school physician or have been obliged to provide makeshift arrangements for occasional service of a physician who can spare a morning for a clinic on some special health problem. With the exception of several large metropolitan school districts, there are very few physicians available for school health guidance and supervision.

Absence of a school physician does not eliminate an effective program of health guidance and supervision, but makes it even more necessary. Indeed, proper use of available private medical services depends on an effective school guidance program. Such a program not only should guide the health of the student but should also develop the student's ability to guide his or her own health.

Basic concepts. The Education Policies Commission stated, "Guidance is a way of helping boys and girls to plan their own actions wisely, in full light of all the facts that can be mustered about themselves and about the world in which they live and work."

Health guidance is concerned with the process of acquainting individuals with various ways in which they may discover and use their natural endowments in order to live to the best advantage of themselves and society. Guidance means accepting each pupil as an independent personality. Effective guidance means developing the student's ability in self-guidance. If the student continues to lean heavily on the counselor, the guidance has not been effective. As revealed

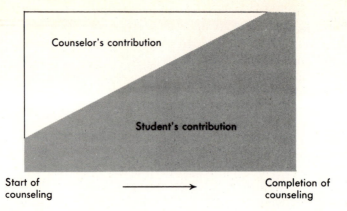

Fig. 7-13. Counselor and student contributions in health counseling. At the outset the counselor makes a considerable contribution, but reduces his or her role as students increase their contributions. The final objective is to develop students' abilities to rely on their own resources.

diagrammatically in Fig. 7-13, the guidance person should play a diminishing role and the student an increasing role in the guidance.

Responsibility. The school health program and the school general guidance program experienced a parallel growth in the United States, since both health and guidance grew out of the transition to functional education. Both are concerned primarily with students as individuals and with their overall well-being. Because of the direction in which education is now developing, guidance is no longer incidental, but an integral part of the total education process. Leaders in education support the view that all teachers have a role in guidance. These leaders also recognize that school health personnel are in a strategic position to make a unique contribution to the school guidance program and consequently to the fullest development of each student.

Although health guidance has long been accepted as an essential school service, the questions of how the school guidance program should be organized, how it should be administered, what it should encompass, who should participate, and what profes-

sional training for health guidance is necessary have never been clearly answered. Some school districts in the nation have established health guidance programs in response to existing local situations. This pragmatic pioneer approach is commendable, and the experiences of these independent and widely dispersed districts have served as pilot studies. A synthesis of the positive findings of these experiences into a practical, workable, well-defined program of health guidance is needed.

In a study conducted by H. E. Petersen,* a group composed of 75 nationally recognized guidance specialists, 75 health education specialists, and 100 secondary school health educators agreed on the guidance functions of health educators in the public school programs. As do other members of the school staff, the health educator has incidental responsibilities in other areas. However, the major guidance responsibilities of the health educator were given as follows:

1. Home and family problems
   a. Parent-student relationship

---

*Study conducted at Chico State University, Chico, Calif.

2. Boy-girl relationships
   a. Adjustments to other sex
   b. Dating
   c. Going steady
   d. Marriage
   e. Sex problems
3. Personal-social problems
   a. Appearance
4. Mental health problems
   a. Conflicts
   b. Frustrations
   c. Fears
   d. Depressions
   e. Insecurity
   f. Marked inferiority feelings
   g. Personality clashes
   h. Oversensitivity
   i. Daydreaming
   j. Overcompensation
5. Physical health problems
   a. Vision
   b. Hearing
   c. Speech
   d. Orthopedic disorders
   e. Skin
   f. Posture
   g. Feet
   h. Nutrition
   i. Overweight
   j. Underweight
   k. Fatigue
   l. Diabetes
   m. Epilepsy
   n. Cardiac disorders
   o. General health
6. Vocational and placement problems
   a. Health requirements
   b. Health assets and liabilities

Perhaps the most significant finding of Dr. Petersen's study was that guidance specialists almost unanimously agreed that secondary school health educators have an extremely important role to play in the guidance program that they thus far have failed to fulfill. It was felt that school health personnel should participate actively as members of the school guidance team, since they see secondary school students every day of the school week and are in a position to acquire an understanding of each youth's capabilities, interests, needs, and liabilities. Health personnel

develop a desirable rapport with these young people, which can be of enormous value in the general guidance program. This rapport, plus the professional knowledge of the health education staff, affords the opportunity for health personnel to make a distinct contribution to the overall school guidance program. Although some independent health counseling will be both necessary and justified, school health personnel should think of their contribution as part of the total guidance program.

In this context, health education should not be thought of exclusively as an academic subject. Health instruction is a means to an end, and the overall goal is the fullest possible development of a student's endowment. The quality of well-being the student maintains and his or her ability to make the necessary decisions relating to personal health reveal the application of health knowledge.

Counseling is a procedure of guidance and a form of mutual deliberation that consists of examination of the items that will aid a child in comprehending his or her problem and understanding its solution. The school counselor does not make the final decision, but may aid the student or the parent in arriving at a solution. The final decision does not rest with the counselor. Counseling may help a child to see his or her health needs and to find the medical or other service required. It may be a matter of working out a pattern of living to attain a maximum level of health. Counseling also can be instrumental in helping each child develop a full appreciation of the valuable asset good health is, and to inculcate a determination to promote and protect that asset. Counseling may be an avenue through which a student visualizes future needs and accomplishments.

Primary responsibility for the health of the child must always rest with the parents, but the school is in a strategic position to complement and supplement the efforts of the parents by dealing with the expressed and observed health problems of the individual students. After all, the best and fullest development of each child is the cardinal objective of the school. Subject matter is important, but serves as a means to an end—the development of the student. It is incongruous to teach children about health and then disregard their existing health problems. The extent to which individuals can succeed and the heights to which they can rise are conditioned by the quality of their health. It is incumbent on everyone in the school health profession to do everything possible to assure children the fullest possible development of their native endowment as a vehicle for effective and enjoyable living today and in the unpredictable years ahead.

The guidance role of the elementary school teacher and the secondary school health educator is to help students understand their problems, to see possible solutions, and to know which professionals and agencies may be of service in helping them solve their problems.

Organized health guidance makes health instruction more effective by focusing the students' interest on the appraisal of their own health status, thus making health knowledge personally identifiable and more meaningful.

Student appraisal of personal health. If students are to develop the ability to guide their own health actions, they must have an interest and an understanding of their health. In the final analysis, the student's own health is the concern and object of the whole program and is the logical vehicle by which the program is promoted and the way in which self-guidance is developed.

Whether health education is a required or elective course, an effective course sequence is one in which all students take a semester of health instruction during their first year in high school. In the 8-4 plan it would be in the ninth grade, and in the 6-3-3 plan it would fall in the tenth grade. A second semester course would be taken during the senior year.

The emphasis of the first course might be on an appraisal of personal health and the development of a health inventory. Although it is recognized that a thorough technical health examination is necessary for a precise evaluation of an individual's health, nevertheless various outward indices that the student can appraise do exist.

Emphasis should be on the positive aspect of health with interest in health evaluation, not diagnosis of disease. Wise use of medical service is an obvious corollary. Following this rather extended discussion of appraisal of personal health, each child, using a health inventory approach, makes an evaluation of his or her own health status. The health teacher-counselor then schedules individual conferences with each member of the group. At the beginning of these teacher-student conferences, the teacher often takes more initiative in making suggestions for guidance. However, the aim is to reduce the extent of the teacher's contribution and to allow students to guide themselves. An individual's growth in self-guidance is an important index of the teacher's effectiveness.

As an outgrowth of the student's interest in personal health, the alert teacher will ensure that all materials used in the health education class are of practical value in promoting health. The student-centered concept should be projected to all student experiences that might have personal health implications. The senior high school health education course can provide a culminating as well as an integrating experience for the student. Ideally, it will serve as a basis for the student's understanding and attitudes toward health, which will make for life-long practices that are both healthful and productive.

Guidance that follows this pattern will

Teaching	Counseling
1. The teacher needs to know pupils so that educational objectives are attained and normal growth processes encouraged.	1. The counselor needs to know pupils in terms of specific problems, frustrations, and plans for the future.
2. The subject matter outcomes (or objectives) to be attained are known to the teacher.	2. The subject matter of the interview is unknown to the counselor and sometimes unknown to the counselee.
3. The teacher is responsible for encouraging growth toward objectives partially determined by the social order (citizenship, honesty). The teacher has a responsibility for the welfare of the culture.	3. The counselor is responsible for helping the counselee resolve his own personal problems. The counselor has a responsibility for the welfare of the counselee.
4. Teaching starts with a group relationship and individual contacts grow out of and return to group activities.	4. Counseling starts with an individual relationship and moves to group situations for greater efficiency or to supplement the individual process.
5. The teacher is responsible for the welfare of many children at one time.	5. The counselor is responsible for only one person at any one time.
6. The teacher carries on most of her work directly with children.	6. The counselor works with and through many people. Referral resources and techniques are of considerable importance.
7. The teacher uses skill in group techniques with great frequency—whereas interviewing skills are used less often.	7. The counselor uses interviewing skills as a basic technique.
8. The teacher uses tests, records, and inventories to assist the instructional (educational) process.	8. The counselor uses tests, records, and inventories to discover factors relating to a problem. The results are used for problem-solving (therapeutic) purposes.
9. The teacher has many tools (curriculum outlines, books, workbooks, and visual and auditory aids) to increase her effectiveness.	9. The counselor has no tools that are used with all the counselees. She must first help the counselee discover problems and their causes and then the individually appropriate sources of assistance.
10. The teacher needs to increase her information relating to instructional activities.	10. The counselor needs information not frequently used by teachers; information about occupations, training institutions, colleges, apprenticeship programs, community occupational opportunities, placement, referral resources, social service agencies, and diagnostic and clinical instruments.
11. The teacher has a "compelled" relationship. Children are required to be there.	11. The most effective counseling comes from a voluntary association. The counselee must want help and must feel that the counselor can be helpful.
12. The teacher deals with children, the majority of whose adjustments are happy and satisfying.	12. The counselor's clients are disturbed by frustrations. They are often characterized by emotional tensions, previous disappointments, and lack of confidence.
13. The teacher is much concerned with the day-to-day growth of pupils and with their general development.	13. The counselor is concerned with the counselee's immediate problems and choices, but she is also interested in helping the counselee develop workable long-term plans.
14. The skillful teacher tries to develop many abilities that increase her instructional effectiveness.	14. The skillful counselor tries to develop many of the abilities used by a wide variety of highly technical specialists, psychiatrist, clinical psychologist, test technicians, occupational information specialists, social workers, visiting teachers, juvenile delinquency workers, placement officers, etc.

logically encompass preventive and remedial aspects of health. Need for immunization or the correction of defects, by its very nature, suggests the value of guidance.

Teaching and counseling. In many respects teaching and counseling are similar. Many of their objectives are the same. Teaching attempts to obtain these objectives through classroom situations. Counseling seeks these objectives through counseling relationships. Very few treatises in the field of education have as much to offer the teacher as these concise statements. Teachers who study the following principles will enhance their knowledge and effectiveness as teachers. Here is an opportunity for providing professional self-growth. This distinction is admirably made by the Michigan State University Institute of Counseling, Testing and Guidance in the outline on p. 157.

HEALTH AND THE TEACHER

A teacher can be the source of communicable diseases, and appropriate measures should be taken to prevent any spread of disease from teachers to students. School boards, school administrators, and parents should concern themselves with those factors that can affect the health of teachers as well as the students. Responsibility for the teacher's health does not rest entirely with the teacher.

Health examination of the teacher. Some school districts require a health examination certificate of every teacher employed by the district for the first time. The examination usually includes a test for tuberculosis. Other districts require an annual x-ray examination of the chest, but no general examination. A third approach requires an examination every third year and an annual test for tuberculosis, supplemented by additional examinations following illness or as otherwise indicated. From a practical standpoint this plan has merit. It is a standard any school district can attain, and it will assure a good appraisal of each teacher's health. A few schools achieve the ideal of an annual health examination, including a test for tuberculosis, which is supplemented by additional examinations as indicated.

There is no legal question of the board's authority to require that all teachers have health examinations. Usually the state department of education and the state health department, with the cooperation of the state medical society, develop a standard examination form. Local school districts may have their own health certificate forms or may accept the report used by any practicing physician. Logically the board of education that requires a health examination of its teachers should pay for the examination. This has been the practice of private industry and should be followed by school districts. A test for tuberculosis is usually obtained without cost, and some physicians perform the health examinations without charge to the teacher. Yet the school, which benefits by the examination, should assume all or at least part of the costs involved.

Promotion of teachers' health. Many conditions and factors in the school can contribute wholesomely to the promotion of the health of the teaching staff. None of these factors is novel or unique; some or all of them exist in many schools today. Further, they place no great burden on the school administration or the school patrons. An investment in these factors is an investment in a better school, with an end result of students who are better prepared.

Teaching loads not to exceed 40 hours a week with midmorning and midafternoon breaks yield a better quality of work in school as in industry.

Lounges for teachers provide the opportunity for necessary relaxation away from the pressing tasks of the classroom.

Lunch hour should have a minimum of responsibility. If the responsibility for supervision of the lunchroom and noon-hour activities is divided among the teachers, all will have some lunch hours that are free for relaxation.

A healthy emotional environment in the school is one in which tensions are resolved as soon as possible and in which teachers know their status, feel they are appreciated, are reasonably secure, succeed, and know they can rely on the support of their administrators in solving special problems.

Sick leave of 10 days a year with pay and an accumulation of sick leave up to 60 days help to assure the district that only well teachers are in the school. The implications are clear, although some school boards fail to appreciate the economy of the plan.

Medical and hospital insurance is always available, and teachers should expect to pay the premium. However, group programs often offer a better policy and should be encouraged by the school administration.

Tenure may prevent the discharge of a teacher merely on the whim of one administrator. Terms of tenure should be stated in the teacher's notice of appointment. No person is totally secure, but tenure does make a teacher somewhat more secure professionally. However, tenure is not a license to neglect professional duties and do slipshod work. It is a reciprocal agreement.

Retirement provisions have health implications, especially when teachers may retire voluntarily before 65 years of age because they feel that they no longer can do an adequate job. All measures designed to aid the teacher carry with them obligations on the part of the teacher to give the students the best possible education. Students, teachers, and parents benefit from the school's efforts to promote the highest possible level of health for the teaching staff.

QUESTIONS AND EXERCISES

1. Explain the contention that health appraisal is a continuing process.

2. What is the primary objective of the health examination?
3. What are the disadvantages of conducting a physical examination at the school?
4. Who should decide how frequently a normal elementary school child should have a health examination?
5. How does the legislation known as Medicaid benefit the school health services?
6. If certain parents do not arrange to have their children checked by a dentist, what can the school do?
7. Who should have access to the child's health record form?
8. What is meant by a unified concept of a child's health?
9. Referral of a child by the school is to the parents, not to the physician. What is the significance of this procedure?
10. Why is it important to start the screening for vision and hearing in preschool?
11. Propose a program to have all elementary school children have at least one dental examination per year.
12. What measures should the school take when a child has been found to have a hearing defect?
13. Why is it unnecessary for all schoolchildren to have a threshold test of their hearing?
14. What is the purpose of a screening examination as opposed to a diagnostic examination?
15. What are some of the benefits that can come to students from effective health guidance?
16. Why have health educators failed to fulfill their responsibilities in health guidance?
17. What are some common objectives of teaching and counseling?
18. Why should the school administration concern itself with the health of all teachers in the school district?
19. Why is the health of the teacher a significant factor in the school health program?
20. What is the responsibility of the local board of education for the health of the teachers?

REFERENCES AND SELECTED READINGS

American Academy of Pediatrics: School health: a guide for physicians, Evanston, Ill., 1972, American Academy of Pediatrics.

Alderman, M. H.: White House Conference on Health, Nov. 3-4, 1965, Public Health Reports 81:111, Feb. 1966.

Cornacchia, H. J., and Staton, W. M.: Health in elementary schools, ed. 4, St. Louis, 1974, The C. V. Mosby Co.

Collen, M. F.: Multiphasic health testing service, Atlanta, 1975, Churchill Livingston.

Eisner, V., and Callan, L. B.: Dimensions of school health, Springfield, Ill., 1974, Charles C Thomas, Publisher.

Gabrielson, I. W., et al.: Factors affecting school health follow-up, A. J. Public Health 57:48, Jan. 1967.

A guide for vision screening of school children in the public schools of California, Sacramento, Calif., 1957, Department of Education.

Haag, J. H.: School health program, ed. 3, Philadelphia, 1972, Lea & Febiger.

Haag, J. H.: Consumer health: products and services, 1976, Philadelphia, Lea & Febiger.

Hall, G. S.: Aspects of child life and education, New York, 1975, Arno Press, Inc.

Hanlon, J. J., and McHose, E.: Design for health: the teacher, the school, and the community, Philadelphia, 1963, Lea & Febiger.

Hart, C.: Screening in general practice, Atlanta, 1975, Churchill Livingston.

Harvard child study project: Developing a better health care system for children, vol. 3, Philadelphia, 1977, Ballinger Publishing Co.

Joint Committee on Health Problems in Education of the National Education Association and the American Medical Association (Moss, B. R., Southworth, W. H., and Reichart, J. L., editors): Health education, Washington, D.C., 1961, National Education Association.

Joint Committee on Health Problems in Education of the National Education Association and the American Medical Association: Suggested school health policies, ed. 5, Chicago, 1966, American Medical Association.

Jones, A. J.: Principles of guidance, ed. 6, New York, 1970, McGraw-Hill Book Co.

Miller D. F.: School health programs: their basis in law, New York, 1972, A. S. Barnes Co., Inc.

Nemir, A., and Schaller, W. E.: The school health program, ed. 4, Philadelphia, 1975, W. B. Saunders Co.

Oberteuffer, D. O., Harrelson, A., and Pollock, M. B.: School health education, ed. 5, New York, 1972, Harper & Row, Publishers.

Pollock, M. B., and Oberteuffer, D.: Health science and the young child, New York, 1974, Harper & Row, Publishers.

Smolensky, J., and Bonvechio, L. R.: Principles of school health, Boston, 1966, D. C. Heath & Co.

The Snellen eye chart, New York, National Society for the Prevention of Blindness.

Suggested school policies, ed. 4, Washington, D.C., 1966, American Association for Health, Physical Education, and Recreation.

Wallace, H. M., Gold, E. M., and Lis, E. F., editors: Maternal and child health practices, Springfield, Ill., 1973, Charles C Thomas, Publisher.

Wheatley, G. M., and Hallock, G. T.: Health observation of school children, ed. 3, New York, 1965, McGraw-Hill Book Co.

Illness is one of those things which a man
should resist on principle at the outset.
Bulwer-Lytton

CHAPTER 8

Preventive aspects of health services—control of communicable diseases

The school today is concerned with the prevention of all possible diseases and defects. Yet in day-to-day practice its primary attention is directed to the prevention of communicable diseases, even though the incidence of infectious diseases in the school population continues to decline. Perhaps this very decline is but a reflection of the school's attention to the problem.

COMMUNICABLE DISEASE

Disease is a harmful departure from the normal state of health. A communicable disease is one that can be transmitted from one person to another or from other animals to man. It involves parasites that are pathogenic to humans. Most of the organisms involved are microscopic, although some of the worms and even mites that affect man are visible to the unaided human eye. Of the microscopic pathogens, bacteria cause the greatest number of communicable diseases. However, true fungi and protozoa are serious offenders also.

INFECTION AND DISINFECTION

Infection is the successful invasion of the body by pathogenic organisms under condi-

tions that permit them to multiply and harm the body. The mere presence of organisms in the body does not comprise infection. At a given moment a high percentage of persons harbor pneumococcus bacteria in the lungs without having pneumonia, and all of us have billions of *Streptococcus albus* on the skin without having acne. Harm to the body usually is caused by the toxin (biological poison) produced by the organism, although some organisms invade and damage tissues directly. To multiply and thrive, human pathogens require a temperature of about 98.6° F (37° C), moisture, alkalinity, darkness, and nutrients. The human body provides these optimum conditions.

The body reacts to infection by increased production of white cells of the blood, elevation in body temperature, inflammation caused by blood gorged in the localized area, and pain. These body defenses may be sufficient to overcome the infection.

Disinfection is killing or removing the pathogens of infection or arresting their activity so that the defense mechanisms of the body can overcome the invader. Disinfection mechanisms are as follows:

1. Oxidation of the organism

161

Table 8-1. Incidence of acute and chronic illness by sex per 100,000 persons 5 to 14 years of age, 1957, State of California*

Diagnosis	Boys	Girls
Common cold, sore throat, cough, nasopharyngitis	1776	1774
Accidents	1010	848
Bronchitis and chest cold	254	175
Asthma and hay fever	223	133
Intestinal influenza	209	270
Indigestion	205	213
Common childhood diseases	240	190
Allergies (other than asthma and hay fever)	169	118
Diseases of ear and mastoid, including deafness	120	100
Migraine and headache	98	128
Chronic tonsillitis or sore throat	93	152

*Courtesy California State Department of Public Health, Sacramento, Calif., Health Survey, 1957.

2. Dehydration (desiccation) of the organism
3. Hydrolysis (hydration)
4. Coagulation of cell proteins
5. Destruction of enzymes

Chemical disinfectants are generally used for infections. Tincture of iodine, Argyrol, gentian violet, Mercresin, Metaphen, Merthiolate, Zephiran, and alcohol dilutions are examples. A disinfectant must be effective without causing damage to living tissues.

CONTAMINATION AND DECONTAMINATION

Contamination is the presence of human pathogens or nonpathogenic organisms (*Escherichia coli*) of the alimentary canal on inanimate objects, which cannot react. Thus one speaks of a contaminated handkerchief, glass, water supply, or quart of milk, but one speaks of an infected finger, tonsil, or intestine. Water is said to be contaminated if it contains *Escherichia coli* because it is assumed that discharges from human beings are infesting the water, since these nonpathogens inhabit the human colon. Milk is a good medium for human pathogens, but other inanimate objects are poor media because pathogens live but a matter of seconds in light, dryness, and low temperature. Inanimate articles, other than milk, water, and solid foods, that harbor pathogenic organisms are called fomites.

Decontamination is killing or removing the pathogens and *Escherichia coli* in or on inanimate objects. Several methods can be used, such as burning, heat, drying, ultraviolet rays, and highly concentrated chemicals such as Lysol.

As shown in Table 8-1, not all acute or chronic illnesses are caused by pathogenic organisms, but have other causative factors, such as those for migraine and allergies.

CAUSATIVE AGENTS

Knowledge of the classification and nature of organisms causing diseases in humans is essential to a working understanding of the nature of infectious diseases. Most human pathogens belong to the plant kingdom, as shown in Table 8-2 on p. 163.

CLASSIFICATION OF COMMUNICABLE DISEASES

Many different systems have been devised for classifying communicable diseases. Each system has a particular basis for classification. Some systems combine several factors. A simple yet comprehensive classification accepted by many people in the health field is

Table 8-2. Classification of pathogens of man

Plants		Animals	
Bacteria (split fungi)		**Protozoa (one cell)**	
Bacillus (rod-shaped)	Bacillary dysentery	Ameba	Dysentery
	Brucellosis	Spirochete (spiral)	Syphilis
	Diphtheria	Plasmodium	Malaria
	Tuberculosis		
	Typhoid fever	**Metazoa**	
	Whooping cough (pertussis)	Roundworm	
Coccus (spnerical)	Furunculosis (boils)	Tapeworm	
	Gonorrhea	Trichinella	Trichinosis
	Scarlet fever		
	Streptococcal throat infection		
Spirillum (spiral-shaped)	Cholera		
	Rat-bite fever		
Rickettsia (small bacteria)	Rocky Mountain spotted fever		
	Typhoid fever		
Virus (ultramicroscopic)	Chickenpox		
	Coryza (head cold)		
	Influenza		
	Measles (rubeola)		
	Mumps (parotitis)		
	Poliomyelitis (infantile paralysis)		
	Rabies		
	Smallpox (variola)		
True fungi			
Mold	Mycosis		
	Tinea (ringworm)		
Yeast	Blastomycosis		
	Dermatophytosis		

one that recognizes four different classes of communicable diseases. Each class title is descriptive of the diseases in the group and incorporates a suggestion of the mode of transmission.

The four classes and some of the more common diseases in each class indicate the nature of this classification:

1. Respiratory diseases
   a. Chickenpox
   b. Coryza (head cold)
   c. Diphtheria
   d. German measles (rubella)
   e. Influenza
   f. Measles (rubeola)
   g. Meningococcus meningitis
   h. Mumps (parotitis)
   i. Poliomyelitis (infantile paralysis)
   j. Rheumatic fever
   k. Scarlet fever
   l. Smallpox (variola)
   m. Streptococcal throat infection
   n. Tuberculosis
   o. Whooping cough (pertussis)
2. Alvine (intestine) discharge diseases
   a. Amebic dysentery
   b. Bacillary dysentery
   c. Salmonellosis
   d. Typhoid fever
   e. Serum hepatitis
   f. Viral hepatitis

3. Open-lesion diseases
   a. Furunculosis (boils)
   b. Gonorrhea
   c. Impetigo contagiosa (gym itch)
   d. Rabies
   e. Syphilis
4. Insect-borne diseases
   a. Malaria
   b. Rocky Mountain spotted fever
   c. Tularemia
   d. Yellow fever

In the normal school situation the respiratory diseases constitute by far the greatest problem in disease control. A teacher rarely will encounter the other diseases.

TRANSMISSION OF INFECTIOUS DISEASE

Humans are the great reservoir of organisms that cause disease. Although other reservoirs exist, the great problem in the control of communicable disease is the prevention of the transmission of organisms from one person to another. The increase in population, the increase in travel, and the congregation of the populace in large cities have made the problem of control increasingly difficult. Yet technical advances in disease control have kept ahead of the difficulties that have been created.

Pathogens are transmitted by direct or indirect contact or by an intermediate host.

Direct contact is the most common means of transfer of infection. Three conditions are necessary for transfer of disease by direct contact—the infectious material must be fresh, the distance traveled must be short, and the elapsed time must be brief. Material may be transferred through handshaking, kissing, coughing, or sneezing. Normal air does not contain enough virile pathogens to cause infection by inhalation, but sneezes and coughs containing water droplets or sprays may provide a means of transfer. Respiratory diseases are transferred by direct contact. Most of the respiratory diseases are acquired by carrying the organisms to the mouth via the person's own hands. Open-lesion diseases also are transmitted by direct contact.

Indirect contact involves an intermediate vehicle between the reservoir and the prospective new host. The infectious material may be old, the time interval long, and the distance great. Alvine discharge diseases are usually transmitted indirectly via water, milk, or foods. Respiratory diseases may be spread by indirect contact via handkerchiefs, towels, and eating utensils, although the usual method of spread of respiratory disease is by direct contact.

An *intermediate host*, the third method of transmission, accounts for the transfer of insect-borne diseases. A specific insect or other intermediate host acquires the organism from an infected person or lower animal and transfers the organism to another person. In some instances the organism spends part of its life cycle in the intermediate host, but in other cases the transmission is a mechanical transfer.

BLOCKING ROUTES OF TRANSMISSION

If one visualizes a person as the original reservoir of infection and another person as a prospective new host, then the organisms must travel by one of several routes from the reservoir of the new host. If these routes can be blocked, the new host will be protected from contracting the disease. First, the organisms must escape from the reservoir. Their ability to travel is practically zero; therefore they must rely on vehicles of transmission. Conditions outside of the human body are decidedly unfavorable to pathogens; hence the organisms must enter the new host shortly after leaving the reservoir. Several means are available for blocking the routes of transmission of disease.

Early diagnosis is essential to all methods for blocking the routes of transmission. Since diseases vary in their mode of transmission, identification of the disease makes it possible to concentrate on blocking the specific routes over which the organisms of that disease may travel.

Control of the social contact route is the most difficult to handle effectively. In a democratic society the citizens enjoy a personal freedom that makes both voluntary and compulsory restriction difficult to establish. An informed citizenry, willing to undergo some personal inconvenience for the protection of others, is a primary necessity in control of disease. In addition, citizens who practice sound principles of personal and community health may aid measurably in controlling disease spread by social contact.

Isolation of persons with diagnosed cases can be an effective means of controlling the social contact route. Also helpful is quarantine of exposed susceptible persons during the period in which they might transmit the disease if they are infected. These are legally enforced measures, but persons who are ill can go into voluntary isolation and, by thus avoiding social contact, prevent the spread of disease. This is citizenship of the highest order.

Control of the air route is based on an understanding of the three principal ways by which infection may be spread via aerial contamination—droplets, droplet nuclei, and dust. *Droplets* are the fine drops of moisture composing the spray of coughs and sneezes. Moisture sustains the bacteria for several seconds so that inhalation could carry virile organisms into the respiratory tract of a susceptible host. However, the droplets settle to the ground rather quickly. *Droplet nuclei* are minute particles from the evaporation of droplets and, being small and light, may float in the air for minutes. *Dust* can become contaminated from droplets and droplet nuclei and thus be a vehicle for the transmission of disease.

Control measures of airborne infection are in need of further analysis. Evidence does not warrant the general use of ultraviolet irradiation and glycol vapors. Ventilation and oiling of floors and other objects may be helpful in the control of transmission, but the evidence is inconclusive. The old admonition, "Cover that cough and sneeze," is still the very best measure. Bacteria exhaled during normal breathing are not a danger.

Control of the water route is highly effective through community water treatment plants, sewage treatment, and the prevention of stream pollution. The same procedures apply to private and semipublic water supplies.

Control of the milk route is possible through testing of herds for tuberculosis and brucellosis, pasteurization of milk, inspection of dairies, and examination of dairy employees.

Control of solid food route is focused on sustained inspections and sanitary safeguards for the cultivation, production, distribution, and preparation of food. Special attention is given to those foods that are consumed raw, such as products from truck farms. Supervision of sanitation in restaurants and establishments for the production or preparation of foods, such as canneries and bake shops, has been fruitful.

Control of the insect route depends on a knowledge of the pathogen, the insect, and the disease itself. Control measures are directed toward the destruction of the intermediate host. Elimination of breeding places and the use of insecticides and larvacides are direct means that are highly effective. Theoretically, insect-borne diseases can be controlled completely.

RESISTANCE AND IMMUNITY

Resistance is the general ability of the body to ward off pathogens. Several factors in the body act as barriers or defenses against all organisms pathogenic to the human being. These mechanisms are nonspecific in their action, attacking all foreign organisms with varying degrees of effectiveness.

Human skin serves as a mechanical barrier, and its moderate acidity provides an unfavorable medium for pathogens. Mucous secretions of the respiratory tract interfere with pathogens, which the hairlike cilia of the mucous cells propel outward. The acid of the stomach and high alkalinity of the intestines are defenses against pathogens. Salinity of the tears protects the eyes and eyelids against infection. Fever is the body's response to disturbance by the invading parasites. Since most pathogens are inactivated at temperatures above 100° F, a fever makes easier the body's task of destroying organisms.

Perhaps the most important defense mechanism is *phagocytosis*, the process of enveloping, dissolving, and absorbing microorganisms. White cells of the blood (leukocytes) and fixed (endothelial) cells of the liver, spleen, and lymph nodes are phagocytes, capable of destroying pathogens.

Immunity is complete resistance to a disease and is specific for a particular disease. Immunity to one disease does not ensure immunity to any other disease because immunity is the result of specific chemical substances (antibodies) that neutralize a particular toxin or cause bacteria to stick together or to precipitate.

Active immunity exists when a person's own body has produced the antibodies either through an attack of a disease or by inoculation with an antigenic substance that stimulates the body's lymphoid cells to produce antibodies. The length of time active immunity lasts varies with different diseases. Second attacks are common in coryza, influenza, and pneumonia and are rare in chickenpox, measles, mumps, poliomyelitis, and scarlet fever. Inoculation during infancy against diphtheria, pertussis, and tetanus may produce lifelong immunity. Artificial active immunization is available for diphtheria, measles, mumps, poliomyelitis, rabies, Rocky Mountain spotted fever, scarlet fever, smallpox, tetanus, typhoid fever, and whooping cough.

Passive immunity is attained when antibodies formed in lower animals or human beings are injected into another person. Passive immunity is of short duration; the borrowed antibodies tend to exhaust their cycle and disappear as the blood is renewed. An example of passive immunity is the *infantile immunity* of the first 6 months of life. Antibodies from the mother diffuse through the placenta into the bloodstream of the fetus. The injection of serum (convalescent serum) from a person who has had measles into a susceptible child who has been exposed to measles is another use of passive immunization. Convalescent serum should be injected within 3 days after exposure to the disease if the serum is to be effective. Passive immunization is used but little today because of effective active immunization and treatment.

CYCLE OF RESPIRATORY INFECTIOUS DISEASES

Respiratory infectious diseases follow a characteristic cycle of six stages or periods—incubation, prodrome, fastigium, defervescence, convalescence, and defection (Fig. 8-1).

Incubation is initiated by the invasion of pathogens. During the incubation period organisms are multiplying, but the infected person displays no symptoms. The incubation period varies from one disease to another and from one person to another with the same disease. Usually the disease is not communicable during the incubation period, although measles and chickenpox can be transmitted during the last 3 days of the incubation period.

Prodrome is initiated by the first symptoms of illness. Symptoms of the prodromal period

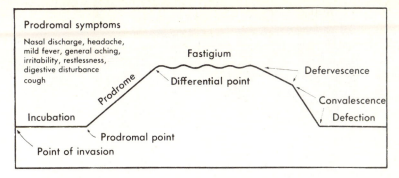

Fig. 8-1. Course of an infectious respiratory disease. All respiratory infections follow the course indicated on this graph. In the school the prodrome and convalescence periods pose the greatest problems in disease control because the infected person may be well enough to be up and around and thus will expose others.

are the same for all respiratory infections and are those of the common cold—nasal discharge, watery eyes, mild fever, headache, general ache, irritability, restlessness and perhaps a cough, and digestive disturbances. This period lasts about a day, and a definite diagnosis cannot be made. Since the person often thinks he or she has just a cold, he or she may continue a usual mode of life and expose many people during the highly communicable stage. Teachers should be alert to observe prodromal symptoms in children as the signal of impending danger.

Fastigium represents the height of the disease. It is initiated by the differential point at which characteristic signs of the specific disease make diagnosis possible. Since the person is now home or in a hospital, not many people are exposed, although this period is a highly communicable one.

Defervescence is a decline in the severity of the disease. A new disease may produce a *relapse*, but usually the case proceeds to convalescence.

Convalescence or recuperation represents a difficult problem in control of the spread of disease. The disease may still be transmissible, and, if the patient mingles with other persons, he or she may communicate the disease.

Defection is a casting off of organisms and may coincide with convalescence. Recovery from a disease does not imply the end of communicability. Isolation time is based on the termination of defection, which is when the person has cast off all organisms.

INFECTIOUS RESPIRATORY DISEASES

Although the list of known infectious respiratory diseases is extensive, certain of them affect the school population and are of particular interest to the teacher. An understanding of the characteristics, mode of transmission, and control measures for these diseases can be of value to the teacher in his or her efforts to prevent the spread of disease. Although the teacher at no time attempts to diagnose a particular ailment, knowledge of the various diseases enables him or her to have the necessary confidence to take effective action.

Chickenpox. A fairly prevalent, although not serious, disease among schoolchildren, chickenpox can become widespread.
1. *Infectious agent:* unidentified virus
2. *Source of infection:* respiratory discharges; lesions of the skin of infected persons
3. *Mode of transmission:* directly from person to per-

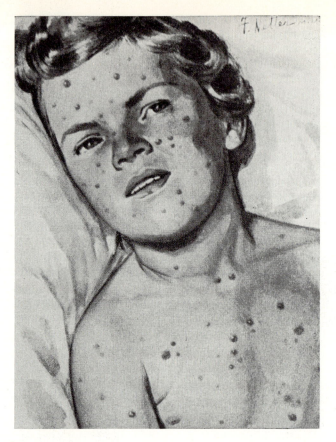

Fig. 8-2. Chickenpox. Fully developed eruptions with lesions at various stages of development are shown. (Courtesy Merck, Sharp & Dohme.)

son; indirectly through objects with fresh respiratory discharges from the mucous membranes and skin of infected persons

4. *Incubation period:* 14 to 16 days
5. *Description:* mild constitutional symptoms; slight fever; few eruptions and mostly on covered surfaces; eruption at various stages of development in the same area (Fig. 8-2)
6. *Control measures for the school:* exclusion for minimum of 7 days.

Coryza (head cold). Typical coryza merits more attention than usually is given. It can be a forerunner of other diseases.

1. *Infectious agent:* unidentified viruses
2. *Source of infection:* nose and mouth secretions of infected person
3. *Mode of transmission:* directly by sneezing and

coughing; indirectly from objects with fresh respiratory discharges of infected person

4. *Incubation period:* 1 to 3 days
5. *Description:* nasal discharge; watery eyes; mild fever; headache; general aches; irritability; cough
6. *Control measures for the school:* exclusion for 3 days

Diphtheria. An entirely preventable disease, diphtheria still appears in school populations.

1. *Infectious agent:* Klebs-Loeffler bacillus
2. *Source of infection:* secretions from throat and nose of carrier or active case; also skin lesions
3. *Mode of transmission:* person to person or objects (including milk) contaminated with discharges from throat and nose of carrier or infected person
4. *Incubation period:* 3 to 5 days
5. *Description:* early symptoms not striking; onset

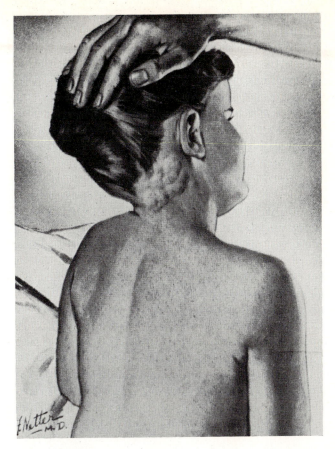

Fig. 8-3. German measles. The fine macular eruptions are rose pink in color. Note the marked enlargement of the lymph nodes, characteristic of German measles. (Courtesy Merck, Sharp & Dohme.)

insidious; temperature not high; illness greater than symptoms indicate; throat sore and has gray membranes; blood-tinged nasal discharge

6. *Control measures for the school:* exclusion of suspected case until released by health authorities following successive negative nose and throat cultures. *Preventive measures:* reimmunization of all students entering school for the first time

German measles (rubella). Often referred to as 3-day measles, rubella is a distinctive disease in its own right and appears among primary school pupils.

1. *Infectious agent:* unidentified virus
2. *Source of infection:* nose and mouth secretions of infected persons
3. *Mode of transmission:* directly from person to person; indirectly from objects contaminated with fresh discharges from nose and mouth of infected person

4. *Incubation period:* 16 to 18 days
5. *Description:* mild symptoms; slight fever; eruptions varied but often rose pink and small; lymph nodes on neck behind the ear swollen and sensitive (Fig. 8-3)
6. *Control measures for the school:* exclusion merely for sake of infected child; isolation of no practical value

Hepatitis, infectious. Infectious hepatitis is an acute involvement of the liver that occurs sporadically or epidemically. It occurs most frequently in autumn. Poor sanitation and overcrowded living conditions appear to increase its spread. An uneventful recovery after 7 or 8 weeks of illness is usual. Mild symptoms and malfunction of the liver may persist for more than a year. About 12% of the patients suffer a relapse, usually because of overactivity or other indiscretions.

1. *Infectious agent:* heat-resistant virus
2. *Source of infection:* usually milk or other food contaminated by fecal discharges of an infected person; feces and blood may be infectious before, during, or after the occurrence of hepatitis
3. *Mode of transmission:* both sporadic and epidemic types usually transmitted from feces of infected person by way of the hands, which come in contact with milk, food, water, etc.; infection from direct contact or fomites and direct fecal contamination of water possible; transmission via blood from transfusions, medical instruments, or biologicals possible
4. *Incubation period:* 15 to 35 days
5. *Description:* prodromal signs include fever, headache, lassitude, nausea, anorexia, fatigue, and marked tenderness and pain in the liver; jaundice appears about the fifth day and then fever subsides; not all patients develop jaundice
6. *Control measures for the school:* recognition of disease; exclusion from school until readmitted by attending physician or health department; improved sanitary and hygienic practices in food handling, handwashing, and disposal of sewage; food handlers in school cafeteria should be checked for possible latent infectious hepatitis

Hepatitis, serum (inoculation hepatitis, transfusion jaundice). This form of hepatitis occurs following such procedures as blood transfusion, plasma therapy, and inoculations in which the virus is present but not known to be present in the blood of a donor. Inoculation into the blood of a recipient means a transfer of organisms into a new host.

The inoculation period of serum jaundice usually is about 2 to 4 months. Onset is rather gradual. Clinical manifestations and treatment are very much the same as in infectious hepatitis.

It is apparent that serum jaundice can be prevented by laboratory tests of the blood of prospective donors. A history of the donor's health problems can be helpful as a preventive measure, but an accurate assay of the blood is most reliable.

Measles (rubeola). A highly communicable disease, measles occurs in 3-year cycles.

1. *Infectious agent:* unidentified virus
2. *Source of infection:* secretions from nose and mouth of infected person
3. *Mode of transmission:* directly by sneezing and coughing from person to person; indirectly from objects contaminated with fresh respiratory discharges of infected person
4. *Incubation period:* 10 to 12 days
5. *Description:* nasal discharge; eyes red and sensitive to light; eyelids swollen; irritability; moderate

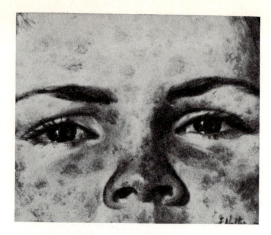

Fig. 8-4. Measles. Characteristic appearance of the eyes in measles showing puffy eyelids, lacrimation, and swelling of caruncula and mucous lining of eyelid. (Courtesy Merck, Sharp & Dohme.)

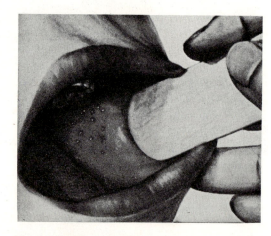

Fig. 8-5. Koplik spots. These red and white pinpoint eruptions on the buccal mucosa are one of the most important signs of measles. (Courtesy Merck, Sharp & Dohme.)

fever; hacking cough; Koplik spots on buccal surface of mouth; dusky red skin eruptions that tend to coalesce (Figs. 8-4 and 8-5)
6. *Control measures for the school:* exclusion for not less than 5 days after appearance of rash; exclusion of contacts only if symptoms appear; immunization recommended

Meningococcus meningitis. One of the most feared of the respiratory diseases, meningococcus meningitis can now be treated successfully if it is discovered early.

1. *Infectious agent:* meningococcus (spherical bacterium)
2. *Source of infection:* nose and throat discharges of carrier or person with active case
3. *Mode of transmission:* directly from person to person; indirectly from objects contaminated with fresh discharges from nose and throat of carrier or person with active case
4. *Incubation period:* 6 to 8 days
5. *Description:* acute onset; intense headache; fever; nausea; stiff neck; irritability
6. *Control measures for the school:* exclusion until recovery, usually minimum of 14 days, or until released by health department following negative laboratory tests; exclusion of contacts in same household for 7 days from last exposure

Mononucleosis. This disease is an acute infection that occurs in epidemic form among children and youth, but more often is sporadic. It usually lasts from 1 to 3 weeks, but involvement of the lymph system and general fatigue and weakness may last for months. Recurrences are frequent, but usually are short lived.

1. *Infectious agent:* unidentified virus
2. *Source of infection:* probably discharges from nose and throat of infected person
3. *Mode of transmission:* probably by direct contact with infected person
4. *Incubation period:* 5 to 15 days
5. *Description:* fever; sore throat; headache; fatigue; chilliness; malaise; general involvement of lymph system, hence use of name glandular fever; white cell count of the blood varies between 10,000 and 20,000; excessive agglutinins present in the blood
6. *Control measures for the school:* recognition of disease; no legal isolation, but patient should not return to school until so advised by attending physician

Mumps (parotitis). Involving the salivary glands primarily, mumps nevertheless is properly classified as a respiratory disease.

1. *Infectious agent:* unidentified virus
2. *Source of infection:* saliva of infected person
3. *Mode of transmission:* droplet spread by direct contact; indirectly from objects contaminated with fresh saliva of infected person
4. *Incubation period:* 18 days
5. *Description:* slight fever; tenderness and swelling over the jaw and in front of the ear, one side or both sides; involvement of ovaries and testes may occur in persons with mature reproductive system

6. *Control measures for the school:* exclusion until the disappearance of swelling and tenderness; immunization of 12- to 18-year-old boys recommended

Poliomyelitis (infantile paralysis). Long a greatly feared disease, poliomyelitis can now be considered one of the highly preventable diseases.

1. *Infectious agent:* Brunhilde, Lansing, and Leon or types 1, 2, and 3 viruses
2. *Source of infection:* discharges from nose, throat, or bowel of person with active case or of carrier
3. *Mode of transmission:* directly from person to person, although history of association with other patients is infrequent
4. *Incubation period:* 7 to 14 days
5. *Description: abortive* form presents characteristics of severe coryza—fever, headache, sore throat, nasal discharge, watery eyes, general ache, irritability; *neurological* form includes stiff neck and back and muscle tenderness and weakness; *paralytic* phase involves motoneurons and produces paralysis of one muscle or a muscle group of one extremity of muscles used to breathe or swallow
6. *Control measures for the school:* exclusion of suspected case until released by health authorities, usually 7 days or for duration of fever; home contacts excluded at discretion of health authorities. *Preventive measures:* immunization of all pupils and students

Rheumatic fever: Insidious disease.

1. *Infectious agent:* group A beta-hemolytic streptococcus, producing sore throat
2. *Description:* primary phase—identified as severe sore throat; middle (dormant) phase—no particular symptoms or signs, may last for 4 weeks with apparently complete recovery; final phase—acute rheumatic fever lasting for 2 to 3 weeks; without treatment recurrence of primary phase possible; damage to heart or other organs may occur
3. *Control measures for the school:* effective prevention by use of antibiotics at early stage of recognized infection

Scarlet fever and streptococcal throat infection. These diseases are commonly classed together.

1. *Infectious agent:* hemolytic streptococci
2. *Source of infection:* nose and throat discharges of person with active case or a carrier; articles soiled with these discharges
3. *Mode of transmission:* directly by coughing and sneezing from person to person; indirectly via handkerchiefs, clothing, and other objects that reach the mouth; from contaminated milk
4. *Incubation period:* 3 to 5 days

5. *Description:* sore throat; fever; nausea; vomiting; flushing of cheeks; pallor about mouth; if rash occurs, it is on the neck and chest and is a fine scarlet goose-pimple type that blanches when pressure is applied
6. *Control measures for the school:* exclusion for at least 7 days or until all abnormal discharges have disappeared; a sore throat is always a signal for exclusion

Smallpox (variola). Entirely preventable.

1. *Infectious agent:* unidentified virus
2. *Source of infection:* lesions of mucous membrane and skin of infected person
3. *Mode of transmission:* directly by person-to-person contact; indirectly through objects contaminated by discharges from lesions of infected person
4. *Incubation period:* 12 days
5. *Description:* 2 or 3 days of severe illness with headache, backache, and fever that subside when rash appears; eruptions first occur on exposed surfaces; small elevations (papules) develop into pustules all at the same time
6. *Control measures for the school:* exclusion of suspected case until released by health authorities, usually until scars have healed. *Preventive measures:* revaccination of children on entering school

Tuberculosis. In the high school population, tuberculosis still remains a serious problem.

1. *Infectious agent:* tubercle bacillus (Koch)
2. *Source of infection:* open lesions of persons with pulmonary tuberculosis
3. *Mode of transmission:* direct contact by kissing, from hands, and from droplets from sneezes and coughs; indirectly from contaminated drinking and eating utensils, perhaps contaminated dust; repeated, not casual, exposure is necessary
4. *Incubation period:* minimum 1 month, usually considerably longer
5. *Description:* primary or first infection type involves infection of the lymph nodes along the windpipe (trachea) and bronchi; usually no discernible general symptoms and therefore frequently missed; recovery spontaneous, with infected lymph nodes becoming fibrous and calcified, as revealed by subsequent x-ray plates. Primary form always precedes secondary form. Secondary or reinfection type has gradual onset; chest x-ray plates reveal the condition long before constitutional symptoms appear. General symptoms may be fatigue, fever, cough, loss of weight, dullness, and finally expectoration of blood. The condition is now far advanced and should have been detected earlier. Few patients contract secondary type before 15 years of age, but occurs in high school population, particularly among girls
6. *Control measures for the school.* Preventive measures: routine examination of all students exposed to active case; periodic chest x-ray examination of students 15 years of age and older; referral of all students observed to be lacking in usual vitality

COMMON SKIN INFECTIONS AND INFESTATIONS

Skin conditions that are communicable in themselves are not a life-or-death matter, but they can be a trying problem to the secondary school as well as the elementary school. Much of the nuisance effect can be eliminated by an understanding of the common communicable skin diseases.

A skin infection is a condition in which the pathogen penetrates the skin and causes harm. A skin infestation is a condition in which the parasite remains *on* the skin and causes harm.

Impetigo contagiosa (gym itch). In elementary schools impetigo may spread quite widely from a single unrecognized case. Early recognition is important.

1. *Infectious agent:* streptococci and staphylococci
2. *Source of infection:* skin lesions of infected persons
3. *Mode of transmission:* directly by contact with discharge of skin lesions; indirectly from objects contaminated with such discharges
4. *Incubation period:* 2 to 4 days
5. *Description:* systemic manifestations usually are absent except in infants; lesions first appear as pin-red stains that are fluid-filled and wet, then fill with pus, and finally form a crust that appears as though it were pasted on; the face (particularly the butterfly area about the mouth) and hands are commonly involved, but other parts of the body may be affected, particularly the scalp; pressure generally causes pus to escape from beneath the oval-shaped crusts
6. *Control measures for the school:* exclusion from school until the pustules have healed. *Preventive measures:* encourage prompt treatment, which consists of soaking crust until it can be removed and applying 5% ammoniated mercury ointment or sulfa ointment to the infected area; some schools have ointments available for the student's own use, and in some instances at the request of the parent or student, teachers have assisted

the student; a physician's services should be obtained if possible; emphasis on general personal health promotion helps to avoid any wide spread of impetigo

Pediculosis (lousiness). This condition is a classical example of infestation.

1. *Infesting agent:* head or body louse
2. *Source of infestation:* infested person or his or her personal belongings
3. *Mode of transmission:* directly from infested person; indirectly by contact with clothing of infested person
4. *Incubation period:* ova hatch in 1 week and mature in 2 weeks
5. *Description:* the louse egg (nit), larva, or adult louse on the scalp or other parts of the body or in the clothing; nits attached to the hair shaft; occasionally a severe secondary infection
6. *Control measures for the school:* exclusion not necessary if proper insecticide has been applied to scalp, skin, and clothing; inspection of possible contacts and use of effective insecticide for infested pupils. *Preventive measure:* emphasis on bodily cleanliness

Ringworm (tinea). The term *athlete's foot* applies only to ringworm of the feet. Ringworm can affect all parts of the body. Common dermatophytes are often present on healthy skin and cause disease only when favorable conditions prevail.

1. *Infectious agent:* several types of fungi
2. *Source of infection:* lesions on body of infected persons; objects contaminated by the fungi or their spores
3. *Mode of transmission:* directly by person-to-person contact with lesions; indirectly from objects contaminated by the fungi or their spores
4. *Incubation period:* unknown
5. *Description:* lesions often circular, clear in the center, with vesicular (fluid) borders; not widely distributed; crusting not present; itching common; foot ringworm (athlete's foot) more common in adults; the body, face, and head forms are more common among children, especially in warm weather.
6. *Control measures for the school:* exclusion when lesions of exposed parts of the body are present until treatment has been effective; in foot ringworm, exclusion from privileges of swimming pool and gymnasium. *Preventive measures:* personal cleanliness; thorough drying of feet after bathing; use of sandals; gymnasium and shower room cleanliness; regular inspections and treatment; keep feet dry by sprinkling with talcum powder to deny moisture to the fungi

Scabies (the itch). The common term *7-year itch* is often used to designate scabies. Both male and female mites live on human skin, but the female burrows into the superficial layer of the skin to deposit eggs. The female can be seen with the unaided eye, but the male, being half her size, is not readily detected. The parasites are short-lived, the male dying after mating and the female after she has laid her eggs. Larvae are hatched in 4 to 8 days.

1. *Infectious agent: Sarcoptes scabiei* (itch mite)
2. *Source of infection:* person infected with the mite
3. *Mode of transmission:* directly by contact with infected person; indirectly from underclothing, bedding, towels, and other objects of the infected person
4. *Incubation period:* 1 to 2 days
5. *Description:* itching of the skin often unbearable; frequent locations—the waist, armpit, and crotch; at times, lesions on the face, scalp, and arms; when infection is mild, systemic symptoms are negligible, but severe infections may result in fever, headache, and discomfort
6. *Control measures for the school:* exclusion from school until successfully treated with an effective miticide (e.g., 5% sulfur ointment). *Preventive measures:* personal cleanliness

In the consideration of the control of infectious disease the teacher need not be limited to specific detailed symptoms. Any time a child has a sore throat, fever, or watery eyes, the teacher should prudently assume that he or she has the beginning of an infectious respiratory disease. Skin eruptions that exhibit inflammation are likely to be infectious as contrasted with noninflamed skin areas such as occur in eczema.

Although the usual incubation period for each disease has been stated, atypical cases may have an incubation slightly shorter or considerably longer. These deviations from the usual incubation patterns do not alter the general prodrome characteristics of the disorder. A teacher who watches for typical prodrome symptoms quickly identifies the child in the early stages of any of the usual infectious respiratory diseases. Skin disorders will also be recognized early in their development.

RESPONSIBILITY FOR CONTROL OF COMMUNICABLE DISEASES

In the control of communicable diseases both legal and professional responsibilities must be considered. Responsibilities as written into law or into sanitary codes represent the minimum desirable control essentially in terms of restrictions. Over and beyond these legal responsibilities are the moral or professional responsibilities assumed by individuals and groups. These professional responsibilities add measurably to the effectiveness of the control of disease.

Public health personnel. Health is recognized as a prime essential of the people. Primary authority for the protection and promotion of the people's health rests with each state. The state has taken such measures as have been necessary to protect and preserve the health of those subject to its authority.

Health authority is vested in the police power of the state. Police power is the authority of the people, vested in the government, to enact and enforce laws to protect the health and general welfare of society. It is the power to promote public welfare by regulating and restraining the use of property and liberty. It is based on the concept of the greatest good for the greatest number and may operate to the inconvenience of one individual or family in the interests of the common good. Yet it allows for personal freedom insofar as such freedom does not work to the detriment of others.

State legislatures delegate authority to a state board of health to set up rules and regulations governing the health of the people. Accordingly the health board passes regulations that govern the control of communicable diseases. This includes the imposition of isolation and quarantine, milk control, water treatment, and all other measures necessary to the control of disease. Thus a state board of health has legislative authority to set up a sanitary code to govern health, which includes control of communicable diseases in the state. The state code specifies the time and terms of isolation, quarantine, and other control measures.

State health boards set up a division of communicable disease control to deal specifically with the immediate problems of the prevention of the spread of disease. Personnel of the division are specialists in specific phases of the control program. These professional workers may deal with any problem of disease control anywhere in the state. Or they may leave the control to local health personnel and will be available for consultation or special services if requested by local health officials.

The state delegates many of its powers to subdivisions of local governments to exercise within their own borders. Through enactment of law the state legislature delegates to counties the power to control diseases. The state also grants charters to cities giving them absolute self-rule (home rule) to exercise within their own borders and within specific limits or fields. Police power thus delegated to the municipalities enables them to control communicable diseases within their own geographical borders.

In terms of direct effect on the individual citizen, it is the county or city health department that is charged with legal responsibility for the control of communicable diseases. A city or county board of health passes regulations that govern the activities concerning the control of communicable disease. Standards may not be lower than those of the state code, but may be higher. Thus if the state code sets the isolation period for a particular disease as 7 days, the local code may require 9 days, but not 6 days. In practice the local code usually coincides with the state code.

Local health personnel are charged with legal enforcement of isolation and quarantine and such other provisions as pertain to disease control. However, a health official is a public servant and accepts the professional responsibility of giving every service possible that may aid persons or families with communicable diseases. Professional service is extended to others in the community as well. A particular recipient of public health service is the school, and properly so, since in the school population a considerable number of cases of communicable disease will occur in any given year. The school is free to call on the public health personnel for advice and other control services. A cooperative working agreement between the health department and the school benefits both agencies, but more especially serves the children and community.

At the outset of each year a conference between the health department staff and the school administrators fosters a better understanding of the function of both groups and a better program of control. If possible, the public health nurse should be scheduled for regular visits to the school and be available for special calls from the school. The nurse can thus assist the school in problems of exclusion and readmission as well as advise it on other health problems.

The director of the public health department should be available to assist the school with especially difficult problems that occur in its program for control of communicable diseases. In addition, the director has the legal authority and responsibility to make final decisions relating to isolation and quarantine. Termination of isolation by the health department automatically clears a child for readmission to school.

Health departments sponsor immunization programs. When the prevailing local practice is that each family physician performs all immunizations, the health department carries on extensive public health education programs. In addition, health department personnel contact homes with children in need of immunization.

Private physician. Practicing physicians have always been the key figures in the control of communicable diseases. It is they who diagnose and supervise each case. They are in the best position to advise as to the best interests of the patient. Modern health codes require that they report cases of certain diseases to the local health departments. For their convenience special forms and franked envelopes are available. They can quickly fill out the forms and mail them to the health department, which then assumes responsibility for enforcement of isolation and quarantine without interfering with the physician's medical supervision of the case. Physicians properly accept responsibility for the health of the public as well as for the welfare of their private patients.

Today's practicing physicians advise clients to have their children artificially immunized, and they do the immunization as a routine part of their medical service to the family. Through this practice the physicians of the nation are largely responsible for the high percentage of children who enter school immune to diseases for which artificial immunization is recommended.

Parents. An obvious health responsibility of parents is to carry out such recognized health measures as will protect their own children and all other children. Parents assume this duty by observing their children for symptoms of disease during the morning of each school day, keeping them home when symptoms of communicable disease are present, and following the practices recommended by the school and required by the health department. Parents have legal responsibilities when isolation has been imposed officially. More than this, parents have a moral obligation to go beyond legal requirements and do everything reasonable to prevent the spread of disease. The formula for effective control of communicable disease consists of civic-minded parents who work cooperatively with an alert school staff and a competent health department (Fig. 8-6).

School personnel. Promotion of immuni-

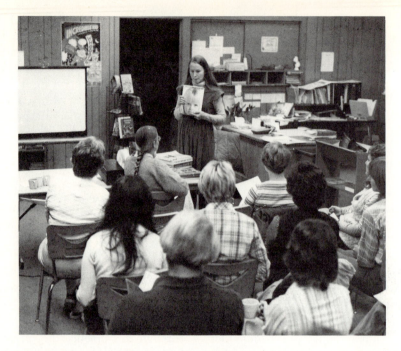

Fig. 8-6. Prevention of communicable disease. Evening classes conducted by the school or public health nurse for parents of elementary school children means an effective first line of defense against communicable disease spread. (Courtesy Benton County Health Department, Corvallis, Ore.)

zation, early recognition of symptoms of disease, and effective control of exclusions and readmissions are the means by which the school staff carries out its responsibilities in communicable disease control.

Smallpox immunization that was once required by law for school entrance is no longer required for children in the United States. Massachusetts has required diphtheria immunization for entrance to school. In some states the state department of education sets the requirement. However, in general, immunization as a prerequisite for entrance to school has been left to local school boards. Courts have held that a board of education has the authority to require such immunization as a condition for entrance to school. However, provisions of the requirement must be reasonable. Exceptions must be made on religious grounds, and a board could not require immunization for some uncom-

mon disease. In practice, boards usually require immunization against diphtheria only.

It is recognized that compulsory immunization is instituted in the interests of the child, and in many school districts it may still be desirable. Where effective public and school health education programs have been operating for several years, voluntary immunization can displace the compulsory program.

Teachers who are prepared to recognize early symptoms of communicable disease and who make proper inspections, reviews, and observations of children, perform a highly valuable service in the control of communicable diseases. Early detection of disease can mean early exclusion, with benefit to the individual affected as well as to the child's classmates. It is relatively simple to exclude children and to refuse readmission until all communicability has passed, and it is highly effective.

Teachers as well as the school nurse can advise children and parents on matters relating to disease control and thus assist children and families to follow the desirable course of action. Knowledge leads to understanding and harmony that will operate to the best advantage of all concerned.

IMMUNIZATION PROGRAM

In the best democratic tradition an immunization program should be based on voluntary participation. Basic to an effective voluntary immunization program is an informed public that understands the importance of preventive measures and the effectiveness of present-day immunization practices. A voluntary immunization program in which more than 85% of entering school pupils have been immunized against diphtheria and poliomyelitis would be successful in preventing all outbreaks of epidemic proportions. Yet all children should be protected, and all parents should understand the importance of immunization. The most effective instrument for health education is an epidemic, but it is also the most costly; neither health officials nor schools want epidemics in any form. Although the public health agencies assume primary responsibility for public health education, the school has both an opportunity and an obligation to educate parents in the importance of immunization for all children. To be effective, adult health education must be continued over a long period. In the absence of such a long-term program and until such a program can be developed, compulsory immunization may be necessary to assure every child the protection to which he or she has a right.

Compulsory immunization against diphtheria, measles, rubella, and poliomyelitis as a requirement for entrance to school is an accepted concept. When thus required, immunization should be available to all children through the services of the family physician or of a clinic. The school board may legally pay the cost of such immunization on whatever basis the program is organized. Such an appropriation is an investment in lives saved, health preserved, family and community stability maintained, and education continued without needless interruption.

In the event of an epidemic, health authorities may deem it advisable to require immunization as a requisite for school attendance. A conference of school officials and health authorities can formulate a program of emergency immunization. Students who refuse immunization on religious grounds may be placed under quarantine by the public health department until the danger is past. Courts have held this to be a reasonable exercise of the authority of the health department to control communicable diseases.

Because there have been no cases of smallpox reported in the United States during the past decade and none in the world since 1977 excepting a laboratory accident, public health officials and physicians have concluded that smallpox immunization of schoolchildren is no longer necessary.

Diphtheria-tetanus-pertussis. Combined immunization for diphtheria, tetanus, and pertussis is highly effective and practical. The effectiveness of each immunization seems to be increased by the activity from the others.

Diphtheria toxoid is produced by propagation of the diphtheria bacillus in a broth medium at 37.5° C. Under these conditions the bacillus produces toxin. The bacteria are then killed with phenol, and the toxin is filtered out. This toxin is treated with formaldehyde and alum so that it is no longer a dangerous poison. It now is designated alum-precipitated toxoid. Tetanus alum-precipitated toxoid is produced in much the same way. However, pertussis-immunizing material is produced by killing phase I strains of the pertussis organism and injecting the dead organisms into the person to be immunized.

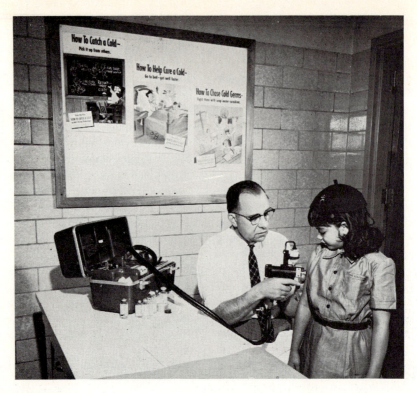

Fig. 8-7. Hypospray (jet gun) for diphtheria-tetanus-pertussis shot. No needle or syringe is used and there is no chance for the pupil to get infectious hepatitis when the physician uses this method of immunization. (Courtesy Denver Public Schools, Denver, Colo.)

The first inoculation of multiple (trivalent) antigens is an intramuscular injection into the arm (Fig. 8-7). It usually is given between the third and sixth months of infancy, plus a reinforcement inoculation within 3 to 12 months. All children entering school for the first time should be reinoculated. This should be a minimum requirement. Reinoculation of the entire school population will be recommended by the health officials if any cases of diphtheria are reported in the community.

The *Schick test* for susceptibility to diphtheria is seldom used today. An injection of 0.1 ml of toxoid is necessary. Physicians agree that, if an injection must be given, it should be an immunizing dose, and thus the child is spared a second shot.

Poliomyelitis (infantile paralysis). The Salk procedure of immunizing against poliomyelitis is successful in about 75% of the persons who receive the inoculation. Active immunity against poliomyelitis is attained from inoculation with a nonliving form of the poliomyelitis viruses. Not all human bodies appear to be capable of producing antibodies when the antigen of poliomyelitis is introduced into the body.

The immunizing material for poliomyelitis is produced by a fairly elaborate process. The trivalent poliomyelitis vaccine contains types 1, 2, and 3 strains of poliomyelitis virus. Each virus is grown separately in tissue culture on living kidney tissue of rhesus monkeys. Long periods of time are required for the viruses to multiply in adequate numbers. Tissue cultures containing each type of virus are clarified to remove extraneous matter. To stimulate multiplication of the organisms, tissue culture fluid containing high concentrations of the virus is then incubated at 37.5° C. The live viruses are later killed by the addition of formaldehyde. This material of dead viruses is then refrigerated and checked to ascertain that it is sterile and the viruses are dead. The three vaccines are then pooled in equal amounts to make the final trivalent vaccine.

Various schedules are used, but immunization procedure usually consists of an initial intramuscular injection of 1 ml, the second injection of 1 ml 2 to 4 weeks later, and the third 1 ml injection after 6 or 7 months. Since July, August, September, and October are the months of high incidence of paralytic poliomyelitis, immunization should be done considerably in advance of this season, although any time of the year apparently is acceptable.

Sabin vaccine consists of attenuated live viruses in a medium such as a liquid or a lump of sugar. Type 1 vaccine can be given to a child as young as 3 months old. Six weeks later type 3 vaccine is given, and 4 weeks later type 2 vaccine is given. For the child in the early months of infancy, vaccine in liquid form is most practical. As soon as the child can take a lump of sugar, the vaccine in sugar lump form can be used.

A newly developed oral trivalent live poliovirus vaccine has an advantage of conferring simultaneous immunization against all three types of poliomyelitis viruses. A dose may be given in a teaspoon or in a paper cup. If a cup is used, a small amount of chlorine-free water is added. This type of vaccine may also be given absorbed in bread, cake, or a cube of sugar. Two doses are given within a period of 8 weeks, and the age to begin administration is between 6 weeks and 6 months.

Schedule for immunizations. Various immunization schedules have been recommended, all with merit. No standard sched-

Table 8-3. Recommended schedule for active immunization of normal infants and children*

2 mo	DTP†	TOPV‡
4 mo	DTP	TOPV
6 mo	DTP	§
1 yr		Tuberculin test‖
15 mo	Measles,¶ rubella¶	Mumps¶
1½ yr	DTP	TOPV
4-6 yr	DTP	TOPV
14-16 yr	Td#—continue every 10 years	

*From: Report of the Committee on Infectious Diseases, ed. 18, Evanston, Ill., 1977, American Academy of Pediatrics.
†DTP diphtheria and tetanus toxoids combined with pertussis vaccine.
‡TOPV trivalent oral poliovirus vaccine. This recommendation is suitable for breast-fed as well as bottle-fed infants.
§A third dose of TOPV is optional but may be given in areas of high endemicity of poliomyelitis.
‖Frequency of repeated tuberculin tests depends on risk of exposure of the child and on the prevalence of tuberculosis in the population group. For the pediatrician's office or outpatient clinic, an annual or biennial tuberculin test, unless local circumstances clearly indicate otherwise, is appropriate. The initial test should be done at the time of, or preceding, the measles immunization.
¶May be given at 15 months as measles-rubella or measles-mumps-rubella combined vaccines.
#Td—combined tetanus and diphtheria toxoids (adult type) for those more than 6 years of age, in contrast to diphtheria and tetanus (DT) toxoids, which contain a larger amount of diphtheria antigen. *Tetanus toxoid at time of injury:* For clean, minor wounds, no booster dose is needed by a fully immunized child unless more than 10 years have elapsed since the last dose. For contaminated wounds, a booster dose should be given if more than 5 years have elapsed since the last dose.

Concentration and storage of vaccines: Because the concentration of antigen varies in different products, the manufacturer's package insert should be consulted regarding the volume of individual doses of immunizing agents. Because biologics are of varying stability, the manufacturers' recommendations for optimal storage conditions (e.g., temperature, light) should be carefully followed. Failure to observe these precautions may significantly reduce the potency and effectiveness of the vaccines.

Table 8-4. Primary immunization for children not immunized in early infancy* †

Under 6 years of age

First visit	DTP, TOPV, tuberculin test
Interval after first visit	
1 mo	Measles,‡ mumps, rubella
2 mo	DTP, TOPV
4 mo	DTP
10 to 16 mo or pre-school	DTP, TOPV
Age 14-16 yr	Td—repeat every 10 years

6 years of age and over

First visit	Td, TOPV, tuberculin test
Interval after first visit	
1 mo	Measles, rubella, mumps
2 mo	Td, TOPV
8 to 14 mo	Td, TOPV
Age 14-16 yr	Td—repeat every 10 years

*From American Academy of Pediatrics: *School health: a guide for health professionals*, Evanston, Ill., 1977, American Academy of Pediatrics.
†Physicians may choose to alter the sequence of these schedules if specific infections are prevalent at the time. For example, measles vaccine might be given on the first visit if an epidemic is underway in the community.
‡Measles vaccine is not routinely given before 15 months of age (Table 8-3).

ule exists, but most will approximate the ones in Tables 8-3 and 8-4. Individual physicians may deviate considerably from them. Combination polyvalent vaccines are now available for immunization against several diseases in one injection, and the advantage is obvious.

Special immunization practices. In practice, immunization against certain diseases is not advocated, except under special circumstances. When a disease is peculiar to a special area (endemic), health authorities may recommend immunization of all persons in that area, particularly those who are likely to be exposed. Thus in the Bitter Root area of Montana, endemic for Rocky Mountain spotted fever, health authorities have recommended that persons living in the area be immunized against that disease.

Normally mass immunization against typhoid fever is not advocated, but, if an outbreak occurs in a community, health authorities and physicians may advise all susceptible people to be immunized. The program is on a voluntary basis, not a compulsory one.

For mumps, prepuberty immunization will protect the body through the critical transition years to adulthood. As a possible preventive for exposed men who lack prior immunity, it is better to use special gamma globulin that gives temporary immunity and thus prevents possible sterility. High school boys exposed to mumps and lacking prior immunity should have a physician's counsel on the advisability of gamma globulin administration.

Because German measles in a mother during the first 3 months of pregnancy can cause the birth of defective infants, there has been an urgency to develop an effective vaccine. Now such a vaccine exists, and all girls should be immunized before the age of 12.

No proposed preventive for tuberculosis has been generally accepted in America. However, a tuberculin testing program is being urged by health departments and practicing physicians. The tine test of the Mantoux skin test can be given at school age with a retest as recommended by the administering physician or the department of health. The tine test uses no needle but a disposable gadget with four tiny prongs. The tines are coated with protein from dead tubercle bacilli. If the punctured area becomes inflamed within 2 or 3 days, it is then a positive reaction, indicating there has been tuberculous infection. A chest x-ray is then taken to determine whether the infection is active or whether it is a past involvement now contained. The same procedure is used with the Mantoux skin test.

When susceptible preschool children are known to have been exposed to measles, diphtheria, or whooping cough, the family physician may advise passive immunization.

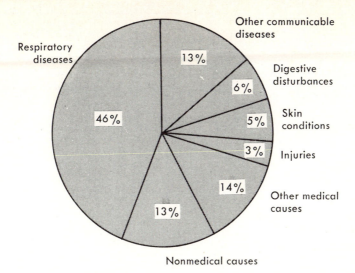

Fig. 8-8. Chart showing causes of absence from school. All causes of absence must be considered, but respiratory diseases always command major attention. (Courtesy Metropolitan Life Insurance Co.)

However, this procedure normally does not involve the school population.

SCHOOL–PARENT–HEALTH DEPARTMENT PRACTICES

Any effective program requires teamwork based on complete understanding. Well-informed parents who understand the role of both the school and the health department are essential to effective control of communicable disease (Fig. 8-8). A health department carries on a continuing program of health education, keeping the public informed of the activities of disease control. Logically the health department and school develop a program of joint action in disease control and work hand in hand in administering the program. After all, both are public agencies created to serve the public. Too frequently the school is remiss in making clear to parents just what it seeks to do to control communicable disease and how it proposes to carry out its program.

School bulletin on control practices. To prevent misunderstanding and possibly avoid ill feeling, the school should compose a state-

ment of its policy and program for control of communicable disease. Issuing the bulletin on attractive bond paper or cardboard will encourage the parents to keep the bulletin in a convenient place. It should be sent to the home during the first week of the school year. The bulletin should be clear and concise.

DETECTION OF COMMUNICABLE DISEASES

In an orderly plan for detecting the early symptoms of communicable disease, the teacher utilizes three procedures—inspection, review, and observation.

Inspection for communicable disease on one or two mornings during the first week of school is a means of enabling the teacher to become familiar with the distinctive physical characteristics of each child as well as to identify any existing infectious disease. Thereafter the inspection is conducted only during an epidemic or threatened epidemic.

A daily morning *review* for detection of communicable disease is followed when no epidemic exists or threatens.

Observation for communicable disease is

HEALTH BULLETIN

Everyday living brings with it exposure to infection and other dangers to the health of children. Recognizing this, the teachers and principals of your schools have organized an intensive program to protect the health of your children during the coming year. The success of the program will depend greatly upon the cooperation of the parents. Knowing that parents are eager to protect the health of their children, teachers propose to parents:

1. If your child appears to be ill before he is ready for school, for his own good keep him home. Any of the following symptoms may indicate illness:

Flushing	Fever
Repeated sneezing	Sick feeling in the stomach
Sniffles	Diarrhea
Red or watery eyes	Skin eruption
Eyes sensitive to light	Rash
Nasal discharge	Skin peeling
Sore throat	Pain
Sluggishness	Cough
Irritability	Dizziness
Paleness	Headache

2. If after coming to school your child becomes ill, for his own good the child will be either brought home immediately or given proper care at school until it is advisable to take him home.

This action on the part of the home and the school will protect the health of your child and every other child in school.

Let us remember:

(a) Serious illness appears to be but a trifle at the outset.

(b) A cold is in itself serious enough and often develops into something more serious.

(c) Your child's health is more important than a perfect attendance record.

_____

Principal

(Save this bulletin for use throughout the year.)

---

the continual survey of the children during the school day for any indications of illness.

Inspection for communicable disease. Whenever an epidemic threatens or is present, a complete inspection (Table 8-5) of each child should be made each school day at 9:00 and 11:40 A.M. Experience has proved that if the inspection is made just before lunch, rather than at 1:00 o'clock, the teacher can avoid the awkward situation of returning a child who has just come from home if symptoms of illness are found (Figs. 8-9 and 8-10). Three plans for the inspection are used. In the first method the teacher stands at the door and inspects each child who enters the room. In the second method all the children enter the room and take their seats, the teacher sits or stands in a convenient place, and the children pass by for inspection. In the third and most satisfactory method the pupils remain in their seats as the teacher passes up the aisle and inspects to the right and to the left. This plan is recommended highly because it allows economy of time and a more natural, relaxed situation.

With practice, teachers develop their own

Table 8-5. Communicable disease inspection

Inspection	Directions to child	Stigmata
For respiratory disease		
1. General condition	How do you feel?	Facial expression, listlessness, irritability, sneezing
2. Eyes	Move your eyes about.	Watery eyes, inflammation, puffiness, redness
3. Nose	Tilt your head back.	Discharge, inflammation, odor
4. Skin	Do you feel hot?	Flushing, hot, cold, clammy
5. Forehead	Raise the hair from your forehead.	Eruptions along hair line
For skin infection		
6. Chest	Open your shirt (or dress).	Eruptions, redness, irritation
7. Hands and wrists	Pull up your sleeves and spread your fingers.	Eruptions, redness, irritation

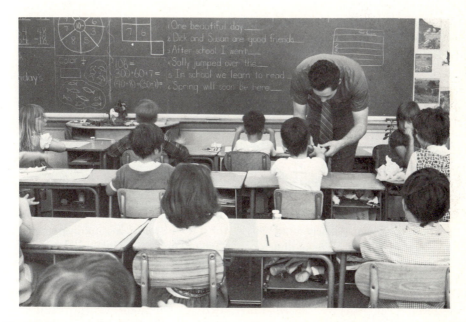

Fig. 8-9. Communicable disease inspection by the teacher. Primary grade pupils fortunate to have a highly competent teacher who is well versed in school health practice. (Courtesy Corvallis Public Schools, Corvallis, Ore.)

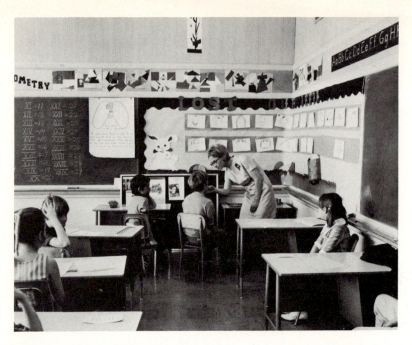

Fig. 8-10. Referral examination by the nurse. A combination of a teacher having basic health knowledge and a nurse available for consultation assures the schoolchild of continuous health protection. (Courtesy Corvallis Public Schools, Corvallis, Ore.)

procedures and techniques. They are looking for deviations from the normal and are not making a diagnosis. As they get to know the normal characteristics of each child, they will quickly recognize any deviations from normal conditions. In making an inspection for communicable disease, teachers are "suspecticians," not diagnosticians.

Daily morning review. Under normal conditions when no epidemic threatens or is present, it is not necessary to make a close inspection of the children. A fairly rapid daily morning review will detect signs of illness or other deviations from the normal. At the opening of the morning session, while the pupils are seated and before classwork begins, the teacher can observe each child as he or she stands at the front of the room. The teacher looks up one row and down the next, viewing the appearance of each child and noting any deviations from normal. The following points should be noted: facial expression, flushing of skin, pallor of skin, catarrhal discharge, watery or red eyes, restlessness, lassitude, coughing, and sneezing.

If it is indicated by the review, a close inspection of a particular child should be made.

Continual observation. A child may be well at the opening of school in the morning and become ill before the noon hour. Teachers with an appreciation of the importance of the control of communicable disease will detect any symptoms of disease children exhibit because they will continually observe children for deviations from the normal. They will be looking particularly for prodromal symptoms of respiratory disease. Children themselves are helpful because they inform the teacher when they do not feel well.

ISOLATION OF A CHILD AT SCHOOL

A child with the symptoms of a communicable disease should be segregated immediately. An emergency lounge is ideal for a child who appears to be but slightly ill and may recover in a short time or who possibly may not have a communicable disease. This child should lie comfortably on a cot in a moderately darkened room and should be kept warm with blankets. Someone should be in attendance or responsible for visiting the child at intervals. This attending person should be an adult, but if this is not possible a responsible sixth-grade child or an older one can serve. The attending child should be sufficiently removed from the ill child to eliminate transmission of disease.

If the isolated child does not seem to improve in a reasonable time, the parents should be contacted and arrangements made to take the child home. At times it is not possible to get in touch with the parents; in that case it is probably best to keep him or her in the emergency lounge. If the child should become seriously ill and no contact with the parents can be made, the family physician should be called and his or her advice followed. Failure to reach the family physician within an hour would justify calling some other physician. Since the call is in the best interest of the child, the parents will be responsible for the cost of the physician's services.

EXCLUSIONS

A question of considerable concern to classroom teachers is their responsibility for the exclusion of children who appear to have a communicable disease. Teachers readily recognize their professional responsibility to do everything reasonable in behalf of the child's health, but knowledge of legal aspects and administrative procedures gives teachers the necessary confidence to deal competently with exclusions caused by communicable diseases.

Legal aspects. Do teachers themselves have the right to exclude a child for suspected communicable disease? If it develops that the child's condition was not communicable, can teachers be held legally liable for their act? These two vital questions have been answered definitely by the courts. The classical decision was laid down by the court in the case of *Stone* v. *Probst,* in which parents instituted a civil suit against a public school educator for excluding their child from school because of suspected communicable disease. The key sentence of that decision is this:

Pupils who are suffering, or appear to be suffering, from a communicable disease may menace the well-being of all pupils and therefore should be denied the privilege of school attendance.*

It is significant that the court emphasized the mere *appearance* of the symptoms of communicable disease is sufficient basis for exclusion. The court did not require proof that the well-being of other pupils was being menaced, but merely that their well-being *may* be menaced. The court did not assert that the school may exclude the child, but that it *should* exclude the child. This decision means that, if teachers have reason to believe a child has a communicable disease, they should exclude the child. When they exercise this responsibility, the teachers' action should be reasonable and reflect what a person of ordinary prudence would do. If it is subsequently found that the child did not have a communicable disease, all concerned should be pleased. It is inconceivable that any jury would ever hold the teacher liable for such reasonable actions. Courts recognize that at times the individual must be incon-

---

*Supreme Court of the State of Minnesota, 165 Minn., 1925, 361, 206 NW 642; appeal from the District Court, Hennepin County.

venienced in the interests of the general good.

Administrative procedures. Various situations require different methods, and typical examples illustrate standard procedures:

1. If the child is not well, but some doubt exists as to whether the condition is communicable, he or she may be isolated in the emergency lounge.

2. If no doubt exists that the child is quite ill and very likely has a communicable disease, the child should be taken home. First, the parents should be called to make certain that someone is home. If someone is at home, an adult, preferably, should drive the child home. One of the child's parents may come after him or her. If neither of these alternatives is possible and no adult is available, a responsible student may walk home with the ill child. A sixth-grade student can carry out this assignment. Under no circumstances should the ill child walk home alone. All decisions to exclude a child should be channeled through the principal's office.

3. In a doubtful case the teacher should rely on the school physician for a decision and, if no physician is available, rely on the school nurse. If neither is available, the collective judgment of three or four teachers is in order. If the group of teachers agree that exclusion is advisable, the principal should be notified and steps taken to transport the child home.

4. When circumstances are such that the ill child rides home in a bus, he or she should sit with the bus driver, away from other children.

READMISSIONS

The problem of readmission of children with questionable symptoms after they have had a communicable disease does not occur so frequently as does that of exclusion of children with questionable symptoms. However, some of the school's knottiest problems are questions relating to readmission. Yet, by following established authority and procedures, the school can find acceptable solutions to the various questions of readmission.

Legal aspects. In general, courts have held that it is the responsibility of the parent to demonstrate that the child is not in a communicable state and thus should be permitted to attend school. This interpretation is best expressed in the case of *Martin* v. *Craig:*

> It is the responsibility of the parents to prove otherwise if the child is not to be denied the privilege of school attendance.*

When doubt exists as to communicability, the parents must resolve the doubt by obtaining a written clearance from the health department or a practicing physician.

Administrative procedures. The school properly should be reasonable in readmitting a child who has been ill with a communicable disease, but it also has an obligation to susceptible children who are in school. Usually action in the interests of the many is also in the best interests of a child who has been ill. Certain cases and situations are easy to administer, whereas others are difficult, as examples illustrate:

1. If the child has been under official isolation or quarantine, an official statement of release by the health department is the certificate of readmission to school.

2. If no official isolation has been in force but the child has been under the supervision of a private physician, the school can properly request the physician's written statement that the child is in a noncommunicable state. A standard form makes the physician's reporting task easier.

3. If there has been no supervision by either the health department or a physician, the school has its most difficult readmission

---

*Supreme Court of North Dakota, April 22, 1919, 42ND213, 173 NW 787, Mand. 81. Schools 157.

problem. In some states the state department of education requires that any child absent from school for illness for 5 or more consecutive school days must present a statement from a physician that the child does not harbor a communicable disease. A better approach is for each local school board to establish an official policy on readmission. Details of the policy and procedures should be developed cooperatively by the school administration, the local physicians, and the health department. Thus a form that includes space for the physician to include the nature of the illness and instructions for the school can be developed.

Normally the requirement of a statement from the physician after a child has been absent 5 consecutive school days is practical and effective. However, parents may be tempted to send the child to school on the fifth day to avoid calling a physician. If the child appears to be somewhat ill on his or her return on the fifth day, or fourth day, or any other day, it should be the policy of the school to require a physician's certificate of clearance. This should apply to every child who has returned after illness if there is any doubt about his or her being in a noncommunicable state.

In practice when a child has been absent for a day or two, the teacher should attempt to judge whether or not symptoms such as nasal discharge indicate that the child should remain home for another few days. In this case the school calls the parent and diplomatically suggests that for the best interests of the child it might be wise to keep him or her home for another day or two. With the judgment of the nurse and other staff members, the teacher can make the necessary decisions in the more difficult situations.

Repeated controversy on readmission is an indication of an inadequate program for educating parents on policies and procedures of disease control. Where parents are well-informed and cooperative, children will be kept out of school until there is no doubt that the child should be readmitted. Tact and diplomacy from school personnel are needed, not high-handed police methods, when misunderstanding or controversy develops. After all, the school as well as the parent is concerned with the same thing—the best interests of the child who has been ill and of every other child in the school.

EPIDEMICS AND SCHOOL POLICIES

Experience has demonstrated that during an epidemic it is better to keep the schools in session unless the epidemic is extreme and all public gatherings are prohibited. This is a decision for the health department. When children remain in school during an epidemic, regular inspections and observations result in early detection and segregation of children with a communicable disease. This opportunity for control is important and should not be lost by default.

If the health department recommends that schools be closed, prohibiting groups of children in theatres, recreation centers, churches, and other places is properly in order. School personnel can assist by appealing to parents and students to follow health department regulations and remain away from public places.

Occasionally an outbreak of influenza or other respiratory disease in a school population may be so widespread that school officials, for academic and economic reasons, close the school. When more than half of the student body of a high school is absent because of influenza, it may be wise to close the school for the remainder of the week. Most of the schoolwork for that week would have to be repeated for the benefit of those who were absent. Although it is not done in the interest of controlling communicable diseases, it might be profitable academically and economically.

QUESTIONS AND EXERCISES

1. Explain the possible paradox that all cases of communicable disease are infectious diseases, but not all cases of infectious diseases are communicable.
2. What is each citizen's responsibility for the health of his or her neighbor?
3. "Infectious disease is but the reaction of the host to a parasite." Explain the statement.
4. What are the sources of disease that threaten a schoolchild?
5. What class of communicable diseases pose the greatest problem for the school, and why are these diseases so difficult to control?
6. An outbreak of 26 cases of infectious hepatitis occurred in a junior high school. Why was the school cafeteria suspected as the route over which the disease was transmitted?
7. What forms of isolation can a school use to prevent communicable disease spread?
8. What has led to the decision to eliminate smallpox vaccinations?
9. Explain the statement, "Skin infestation is found where cleanliness is not."
10. The fungus causing ringworm must have moisture and darkness in order to survive. Why should not constant application of talcum powder to the affected areas of the feet along with bright light clear up any case of "athlete's foot?"
11. What are the responsibilities of the county health department in controlling communicable diseases in the schools of a community?
12. Why do health officials contend that teachers are the first line of defense against the spread of communicable disease?
13. Why do epidemiologists maintain that, if 85% of children entering school have been immunized against diphtheria, smallpox, and poliomyelitis, there will be no major epidemic?
14. Salk versus Sabin poliomyelitis immunization—what are the relative merits?
15. What is the significance of sending an opening week bulletin to school parents making clear what the school plans to do in communicable disease control and what the parents might do?
16. Explain why in communicable disease control in the school problems of readmission can be more difficult than those of exclusion.
17. How would parents establish that their child is no longer in a communicable state and should be readmitted to school?
18. In communicable disease control in the school why should authority or power be the last resort?
19. Under what circumstances should a school be closed because of an epidemic?
20. List those communicable diseases that a teacher may have and that he or she may transmit to students.

REFERENCES AND SELECTED READINGS

American Academy of Pediatrics: School health: a guide for health professionals, Evanston, Ill., 1977, American Academy of Pediatrics.

Anderson, G. W., and Arnstein, M. G.: Communicable disease control, ed. 4, New York, 1962, The Macmillan Co.

Bach, M.: The power of total living, New York, 1977, Dodd, Mead & Co.

Bower, A. G., and Pilant, E. B.: Communicable diseases for nurses, ed. 8, Philadelphia, 1962, W. B. Saunders Co.

Burnet, F. M., and White, D. C.: Natural history of infectious disease, ed. 4, London, 1972, Cambridge University Press.

Christie, A. B.: Infectious diseases: epidemiology and clinical practice, ed. 2, Edinburgh, 1974, E & S Livingston.

Christie, A. B., and Christie, M. C.: Hygiene and food hazards, ed. 2, London, 1977, Faber and Faber.

Clark, R. L., and Cumley, R. W.: The book of health, ed. 3, New York, 1977, Harcourt Brace Jovanovich, Inc.

Cockburn, A., editor: Infectious diseases: their evolution and eradication, Springfield, Ill., 1967, Charles C Thomas, Publisher.

Dauer, C. C., et al.: Infectious diseases (American Public Health Association Vital and Health Statistics Monographs), Cambridge, 1968, Harvard University Press.

Gallagher, R.: Diseases that plague modern man, Dobbs Ferry, N.Y., 1969, Oceana Publications, Inc.

Grissom, D. K. (Kaplan, R., editor): Communicable diseases (Contemporary Topics in Health Sciences), Dubuque, Iowa, 1971, William C. Brown Co., Publishers.

Harvard child study project: Developing a better health care system for children, vol. 3, Philadelphia, 1977, Ballinger Publishing Co.

Herzlich, C., and Graham, D.: Health and illness: a social, psychological analysis, New York, 1974, Academic Press, Inc.

Holloway, W. J., editor: Infectious disease reviews, Mount Kisco, N.Y., 1974-1975, Futura Publishing Co., Inc.

Jenne, F. H., and Greene, W. H.: Turner's school health and health education, ed. 7, St. Louis, 1976, The C. V. Mosby Co.

Johnson, W.: Health in action, New York, 1977, Harper & Row, Publishers.

Jolly, H.: Diseases of children, ed. 3, Philadelphia, 1976, J. B. Lippincott Co.

Kendig, E. J., and Chernich, V., editors: Disorders of the respiratory tract in children, ed. 3, Philadelphia, 1977, W. B. Saunders Co.

Krugman, S., Ward, R., and Katz, S. L.: Infectious diseases of children, ed. 6, St. Louis, 1977, The C. V. Mosby Co.

Landon, J. F., and Sider, H. T.: Communicable diseases, ed. 8, Philadelphia, 1964, F. A. Davis Co.

National Center for Vital Statistics, Public Health Service, United States Department of Health, Education and Welfare: Health statistics, Washington, D.C., 1969, United States Government Printing Office.

National Lung Association, formerly National Tubercu-losis and Respiratory Disease Associati tion to respiratory diseases, New Yor Association.

Parry, W. H., editor: Communicable diseases. an demiological approach, ed. 2, (Modern Nursing Series), New York, 1973, Academic Press, Inc.

Report of the Committee on Infectious Diseases, ed. 18, Evanston, Ill., 1977, American Academy of Pediatrics.

Sartwell, P. E., editor: Maxcy and Rosenau's preventive medicine and public health, ed. 10, New York, 1973, Appleton-Century-Crofts.

Top, F. H., and Wehrle, P. F., editors: Communicable and infectious diseases, ed. 8, St. Louis, 1976, The C. V. Mosby Co.

Waldbott, G. L.: Health effects of environmental pollutants, ed. 2, St. Louis, 1978, The C. V. Mosby Co.

In life, as in chess, forethought wins.

Charles Buxton

CHAPTER 9

Preventive aspects of health services—safety, emergency care, and first aid

In modern school life the prevention of accidents has become as important as the prevention of communicable diseases. In terms of their effect on the school-age population, accidents loom as a greater threat to health and life than do the infectious diseases. Whether one thinks of accident prevention or safety promotion, there is ample justification for considering this activity a phase of the preventive aspects of school health services.

Just as the most effective prevention of communicable diseases is the positive approach of immunization, the most effective prevention of accidents is also the positive approach—safety promotion for effective living. Safety does not mean the elimination of all risk. Some risks are inevitable, even necessary, but needless risks can be eliminated. Safety extends the scope of human experience by anticipating and preventing conditions that would otherwise be injurious and even fatal. If it thus becomes possible for children to extend their adventures without mishap, the end result will be more effective and enjoyable living.

The child's environment is one of dynamic action and change. It cannot be a totally safe environment, but physical hazards can be reduced if they are recognized and modified. Children's behavior is normally fast moving and vigorous, which in itself may invite injury. Yet in the interest of safety no one would advocate that children just sit and do nothing. Behavior necessary for life's demands also may have to be modified to reduce or even eliminate unnecessary risk.

SCHOOL SAFETY PROGRAM

It is apparent that safety in the school does not imply the physical environment be converted into an accident-proof situation or that children's actions be completely restrained so that an accident cannot possibly happen. Rather, it means pursuit of the normal demands of life in an environment in which hazards are reduced to a practical minimum and the behavior of the pupils is adapted to safe and effective living.

Because of the high accident rate among children of school age, the promotion of safety is both a challenge and an opportunity for all school personnel. Not all accidents involving school-age children occur on school

Table 9-1. Leading causes of death of children by age groups, United States, 1975*†

Rank	Cause	No. of deaths	Rank	Cause	No. of deaths
5 to 9 years of age			7	Influenza and pneumonia	185
			8	Suicide	170
1	Accidents	3,033	9	Bronchitis, emphysema,	39
2	Malignant neoplasms	929		and asthma	
3	Congenital malformations	424	10	Nephritis	34
4	Cardiovascular diseases	232	11	Diabetes mellitus	30
5	Influenza and pneumonia	177	12	Cerebral hemorrhage	27
6	Homicide	136			
7	Diseases of the heart	134	**15 to 19 years of age**		
8	Bronchitis, emphysema,	29	1	Accidents	12,035
	and asthma		2	Homicide	2,008
9	Nephritis	25	3	Suicide	1,594
10	Cerebral hemorrhage	22	4	Malignant neoplasms	1,259
11	Diabetes mellitus	16	5	Cardiovascular diseases	716
12	Suicide	—	6	Diseases of the heart	426
			7	Congenital malformations	345
10 to 14 years of age			8	Influenza and pneumonia	323
1	Accidents	3,785	9	Cerebral hemorrhage	60
2	Malignant neoplasms	787	10	Bronchitis, emphysema,	55
3	Cardiovascular diseases	344		and asthma	
4	Congenital malformations	318	11	Diabetes mellitus	43
5	Homicide	249	12	Nephritis	38
6	Diseases of the heart	205			

*Based on data from the United States National Center for Health Statistics: Vital statistics of the United States, 1975, vol. 2. Mortality, part A.
†Rather than deal in death rates, the authors' experience is that the actual number of deaths is more meaningful for the student. The impact of actual numbers of deaths seems to be of more value to the student than ratios expressed in rates.

premises; yet a high number do occur at school. Although the immediate task is to prevent accidents today, the school safety program has the further value of turning out safety-conscious citizens better adapted to the hazards of modern life.

School population deaths

To get a perspective of the importance of accidents as a cause of death in the school-age population, it is desirable to review the causes of school-age deaths for a representative year. Complete and final data are available for 1975 and are representative of the year-to-year occurrence in the United States. Table 9-1 gives the official numbers of deaths

in each category of causes for various age groups.

These data reveal that in a year over 18,000 children of school age lose their lives in accidents. In the 5- to 9-year age group accidental deaths are more than twice as high as the combined total of the next two causes of death, cancer and congenital malformations. In the age group from 10 to 14 years the number of deaths caused by accidents is more than three times as high as the combined total of the next two causes of death, cancer and cardiovascular disease. In the 15- to 19-year age group the accidental deaths are more than three times as high as the combined total of the next three diseases causing death, cancer, diseases of the circulatory system, and diseases of the heart. Viewed in another light, accidents caused 42% of all deaths in the 5- to 9-year group, 45% in the 10- to 14-year group, and 57% in the 15- to 19-year group.

The 1975 records of the National Center for Health Statistics indicate that accidental deaths were much greater for boys than for girls of school age. From a difference of two boys to one girl in the 5- to 9-year age group, the gap widens to three to one in the 10- to 14-year group and four to one in the 15- to 19-year group.

More than 18,000 school-age youngsters 5 to 19 years of age lose their lives in accidents each year. The distribution is significant:

Motor vehicle	58%
Drowning	15%
Fires, burns	7%
Firearms	5%
Railroad	1%
Other	14%

These data point up the overall hazard to life encountered by the school-age youngster. The school should extract from these general figures information concerning what the relation of the school is to this accidental death picture and what this means to the school in terms of its obligation and opportunities.

School accidents

Studies and surveys reveal that about 43% of accidental deaths among school-age children are connected with school life. Of these accidents about 20% occur in school buildings, about 17% on school grounds, and about 6% on the way to and from school. In school buildings the gymnasium is the most frequent location of accidents, and about one third of the fatal accidents occur within the building. Another 20% of the fatal indoor accidents occur in halls and on stairs. Shops and laboratories account for about 18%, and

Table 9-2. Injuries to school-age children by location

Location	%
School buildings	24
School grounds	28
On way to and from school	5
Home	20
Other	23

other classrooms account for 14%. The remaining indoor accidents occur in various other locations. On the school grounds, 41% of fatal accidents occur during organized activities—football, 20%; baseball, 12%; playground apparatus, 9%; and other organized activities, 18%.

The 6% of fatal accidents among school-age children that occur while the pupil is going to or from school are mostly pedestrian–motor vehicle and bicycle–motor vehicle accidents.

Student injuries by location and grade level are reported by the National Safety Council (Table 9-2). Reports of accidents to schoolchildren that occurred in the school environment and elsewhere and caused injuries requiring a physician or causing at least a half day's absence were available from schools having a total enrollment of more than 1,900,000 students. In school buildings most accidents occurred in the gymnasium, with classrooms second. On school grounds football and unorganized activities in which running was involved caused most injuries. This report of the National Safety Council also indicated injury by grade levels (Fig. 9-1).

All grades have unjustifiably high accident rates. Fourth- to ninth-grade children tend to engage in vigorous activity, often with an abandon that leads to a high accident rate. The problem is to control and to modify vigorous activity, not to abolish it.

Through an orderly process of supervision

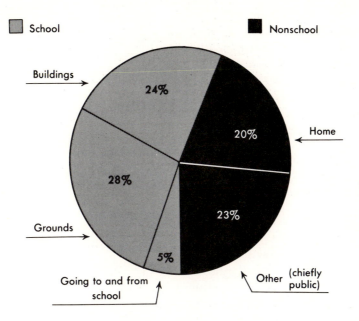

Source: reports to the national safety council from school systems with enrollment of about 1,940,000 students. Injuries requiring the attention of a doctor, or causing absence from school of one-half day or more.

Fig. 9-1. Chart shows injuries to students; the breakdown is by location at which the injuries occurred. In buildings about one third of the injuries occurred in gymnasiums and about one fifth in classrooms. On school grounds injuries occurred more during organized activities than during unorganized activities. (Courtesy National Safety Council.)

Table 9-3. Injury rates by location and grade level (per 100,000 students)

Grade	All injury rate	School building	School grounds	Going to or from school	Home	Other
Kingergarten to 3	11.2	1.4	3.4	0.8	3.5	2.1
4 to 6	16.3	2.4	5.4	1.0	3.6	3.9
7 to 9	23.7	7.8	5.5	1.0	3.5	5.9
10 to 12	24.1	9.0	7.1	0.6	2.2	5.2
All grades	16.6	4.0	4.7	0.8	3.3	3.8

and guidance, children can acquire less hazardous modes of activity.

A tabular presentation of injury rates can be revealing (Table 9-3).

Legal aspects

Teachers and other school employees run the risk of a lawsuit from injured students because of alleged negligence that causes injury.

In general, negligence is any conduct below the legally established standard for the protection of others against unreasonable risk of harm. Two basic types follow:

1. An act that a person of ordinary prudence or judgment would realize involves unreasonable risk to others
2. Failure to act for the protection of another

Thus negligence can be acts of commission or omission. The specific details of each case determine whether there has been negligent behavior. Harper has outlined the types of negligent behavior very well. According to him, an act may be negligent in any of the following circumstances:

1. It is not properly done; appropriate care is not employed by the actor
2. The circumstances under which it is done create risks, although it is done with due care and precaution
3. The actor is indulging in acts which involve an unreasonable risk of direct and immediate harm to others
4. The actor sets in motion a force, the continuous operation of which may be unreasonably hazardous to others
5. He creates a situation which is unreasonably dangerous to others because of the likelihood of the action of third persons or inanimate forces
6. He entrusts dangerous devices or instruments to persons incompetent to use or care for them properly
7. He neglects a duty of control over third persons who, by reason of some incapacity or abnormality, he knows to be likely to inflict intended harm upon others
8. He fails to employ due care to give adequate warning
9. He fails to exercise the proper care in looking out for persons whom he has reason to believe may be in the danger zone
10. He fails to employ appropriate skill to perform acts undertaken
11. He fails to make adequate preparation to avoid harm to others before entering on certain conduct where such preparation is reasonably necessary
12. He fails to inspect and repair instrumentalities or mechanical devices used by others
13. His conduct prevents a third person from assisting persons imperiled through no fault of his own*

Liability for negligent conduct is affected by the nature of both the act and its results. Carelessness is a relative term. In general, a person is considered to be careless or negligent when actions are not those of a person of ordinary prudence. If a pupil is injured because a teacher's actions were not those of a prudent person or the teacher failed to act, a lawsuit may be instituted by the parents and the teacher held liable. Each teacher is responsible for his or her negligence that results in physical harm to others. A teacher's administrative superior will be held liable when he or she directs the teacher to do some dangerous act resulting in injury to a pupil or fails to correct a hazardous situation that has been reported by a teacher. The teacher must have tangible evidence that the administrator was notified of the hazard.

A school board is usually not liable for its own negligent acts, since it is a government entity and thus is immune to lawsuit unless the board consents to a suit. Washington has a permissive law that is effective in permitting suits against school boards. California, New York, New Jersey, and Connecticut have annulled this common law immunity, but these annulments are exceptions to the basic philosophy. However, at present there is a slight trend toward abolishing the theory of nonliability for school boards. Many legal authorities question the justice of common

---

*From Harper, F. V.: A treatise on the law of torts, Indianapolis, Ind., 1938, Bobbs-Merrill Co., pp. 171-176.

law nonliability, contending the theory survives entirely by virtue of its antiquity. They further contend that it is harsh and unjust to require the teacher alone to suffer. However, so long as nonliability for school boards exists, the teacher must proceed with the knowledge that he or she alone may be held liable for any pupil injury. In Connecticut, New Jersey, and New York judgments against teachers may be paid out of the school funds.

However, courts are in the process of altering the whole legal structure relating to responsibility of public servants and agencies. On the very day, June 6, 1978, that the voters of California approved Proposition 13, limiting property taxes, the United States Supreme Court handed down a decision that stripped away a layer of immunity local governments previously enjoyed, that is, protection from damages in civil rights suits. A previous decree held that counties and cities can be sued for antitrust violations.

These rulings will prompt many local governments to give second thoughts to the services they provide. This especially applies to proprietary services such as health services, water and sewer systems, garbage disposal, and regulatory activities. Teachers and school administrators recognize that the direction being taken by the United States Supreme Court affects the operation of schools as well as other governmental agencies.

Teachers are not often defendants in lawsuits that allege negligence has resulted in injury to a pupil. Teachers tend to be conservative, and their conduct usually is prudent. Courts recognize the problem of close supervision of 35 or 40 children at a given moment, and only when the teacher has displayed deplorably poor judgment does the court tend to hold him or her liable. The low premiums for liability insurance for teachers attest to the small likelihood that a teacher will be a defendant in a lawsuit resulting from injury to a pupil.

The best safeguard against such a lawsuit is a well-planned functioning program for the prevention of accidents to pupils. Such a program will also be assurance to the parents that the school has taken definite steps to reduce student injuries to a minimum. The safety of the students is the first consideration, but here, as usual, student and faculty interests are one.

Prevention of accidents in school

Not all accidents can be anticipated and one cannot foresee all situations that cause accidents. Yet most hazardous conditions can be recognized and unsafe practices detected if the school has a well-organized safety program. Safety programs, financially speaking, are not costly. What they demand is vision, organization, leadership, and cooperation. They should be programs that are put into action, not just programs on paper. A well-planned program evaluates the conditions and practices in the school in terms of safety and then undertakes to modify those that are not adequate.

A necessary first step in the prevention of school accidents is to make a survey to detect all potentially hazardous conditions. It should be a *positive* survey in which all *Yes* answers denote acceptance and all *No* answers denote need for correction. The following survey form is one that from experience has proved highly satisfactory and that any school can adapt to its use.

SURVEY OF CONDITIONS AND PRACTICES AFFECTING SAFETY IN THE SCHOOL ENVIRONMENT
Reporting of accidents

1. Are accident report cards or forms available?
2. Is a complete written report on file for every accident that results in an injury?
3. Is a special study made of the causes of each accident?

4. Is an adequate constructive follow-up made after each accident analysis to prevent recurrence of the accident?
5. Is a rapid inspection made of the building each morning and a thorough inspection once each month?
6. Are adequate first-aid equipment and personnel available?

Fire protection

1. Are vacant rooms, basements, and attics free from inflammable material?
2. Is there proper insulation between heating equipment and inflammable material?
3. Are there two or more exits from every floor with doors swinging outward?
4. Are there adequate fire escapes on buildings of two or more stories?
5. Are fire extinguishers of an approved type provided for every 2,000 square feet of floor space?
6. Do the older pupils know how to use the fire extinguishers?
7. Are fire alarms centrally located?
8. Are fire drills so proficient that the building can be emptied in an orderly manner in less than 3 minutes?
9. Are student organization and lines of exit well established?

Gymnasium, pool, and locker rooms

1. Is equipment in good condition?
2. Are all exposed projections covered?
3. Is the floor treated to prevent its being too slippery?
4. Are doors of a safe type?
5. Are fountains in a safe location?
6. Are definite rules for the use of the gymnasium and pool posted and practiced?
7. Are students properly dressed for gymnasium activities?
8. Is horseplay prohibited?
9. Is unsupervised use of the gymnasium and pool prohibited?
10. Are pool users classified according to skill?

Halls and stairs

1. Are all obstructions removed?
2. Are the floors and stairs treated to prevent them from being slippery?
3. Are worn or broken stairs replaced?
4. Are railings provided so that every person using the stairs can hold a railing?
5. Is undue congestion of hall traffic prevented by changing routes, practices, and schedules?
6. Are horseplay and running in the halls prohibited?
7. Are stairs taken one step at a time?

Shops, laboratories, and home economics rooms

1. Is all equipment in good repair and inspected daily?
2. Are all possible safety devices and attachments available and used?
3. Are good housekeeping practices followed?
4. Are lighting and space adequate?
5. Are machines stopped for oiling and adjustment?
6. Are safety rules posted and practiced?
7. Are students properly instructed in the use of equipment?
8. Are horseplay and running prohibited?
9. Is the unsupervised use of the shop, laboratory, or home economics rooms prohibited?
10. Are first-aid supplies immediately available?

Classrooms and auditoriums

1. Are all obstructions removed?
2. Are exposed projections covered?
3. Are sharp objects placed in protected places?
4. Are radiators and electrical fixtures properly protected?
5. Are dropped objects picked up immediately?
6. Is an orderly routine followed, with running and pushing prohibited?

Playground

1. Is the playground space allocated in terms of safety?
2. Is apparatus in safe condition and checked regularly?
3. Are children taught the proper use of each piece of apparatus?
4. Is supervision always provided when the playground is used?
5. Do beginners receive special instructions and supervision?
6. Are horseplay and stunting prohibited?
7. Are caution and courtesy stressed at all times?
8. Do the children assume cooperative responsibility for playground safety?

Athletics

1. Is the playing area constructed in terms of safety?
2. Are all hazardous obstructions removed?
3. Is approved equipment used?
4. Has every participant received medical approval?
5. Is competent supervision always provided?
6. Are the participants properly trained and sufficiently skilled?
7. Is parental approval required for participation in vigorous athletic events?
8. Is parental approval required if students are to be transported for athletic contests?
9. Are adequate first-aid and medical services available?

Going to and from school

1. Are intensive studies made of hazards children may encounter going to or from school?
2. Are specific routes outlined for students?
3. Are the routes direct, requiring a minimum use of roadways and busy intersections?
4. Are stop and go signals, stop signs, school signs, police supervision, and one-way streets used to the greatest advantage?
5. Are ice, glass, and other hazardous obstructions removed from walks?
6. Do children stay on the walks and in crosswalk lanes, and do they obey rules, signs and traffic directors?
7. If school traffic patrols are organized, are the patrols under proper adult supervision?
8. Is maximum use made of traffic enforcement officers and facilities?
9. Are bus riders given instruction on entering and leaving the bus as well as conduct in the bus?
10. Are bicycle riders given special instruction and supervision?
11. Are student motor vehicle drivers given special instruction and supervision?
12. Are the parents enlisted in the safety program to and from home?

School safety organizations

School life becomes increasingly organized as school functions expand, but organization is necessary for effective action. Various plans for the promotion of safety are in operation, but three plans are in most general use. The first has a general *School Patrol* unit with subdivisions such as traffic patrol, fire patrol, and building and grounds patrol. The second plan recognizes three independent but correlated patrols—traffic, fire, and building and grounds. The third plan provides merely for a school safety patrol that directs and controls student pedestrian traffic near the school.

A *school safety patrol* is perhaps most valuable as a safety education measure, but its value in accident prevention should not be minimized. Careful planning and supervision are necessary. Standard rules governing the operation of safety patrols have been adopted by states and on a national level by representatives of the National Safety Council, National Congress of Parents and Teachers, National Education Association, American Automobile Association, National Association of Chiefs of Police, and the United States Office of Education. Standard rules have been published by the National Safety Council. Any school planning to have a safety patrol should obtain a copy of the complete rules from the National Safety Council. If standard rules for safety patrols have been developed on a state level, these should guide the schools within that state. A condensation of the rules will indicate the essential requirements of a safety patrol.

Standard rules for operation of school safety patrols. Experience has led to the development of standards and procedures that provide an optimum basis for the operation of a school safety patrol. These proposed rules are universally applicable and provide for the full effectiveness of the safety patrol.

Function. The functions of the school safety patrol are (1) to instruct, direct, and control the members of the student body in crossing the streets and highways at or near schools and (2) to assist teachers and parents in the instruction of schoolchildren in safe practices in the use of streets and highways at all times and places.

Patrols should not be charged with the responsibility of directing vehicular traffic, and they should not be allowed to direct it. They should not function as police.

Administrative support. The approval, support, and encouragement of all school authorities are essential if the safety patrol is to function effectively.

Selection. Patrol members, either boys or girls, ordinarily should be appointed by the principal or faculty sponsor. They should be selected from the upper grade levels. Patrol service should be voluntary and allowed only when the student has written approval of the parent or guardian.

Size and officers. The number of members on a school patrol should be determined by local factors such as street and highway conditions, number of intersections, volume of vehicular traffic, school enrollment, and number of school dismissal times.

Every patrol should have a captain and one or more lieutenants. Other officers may be appointed as required. Officers should serve for at least one school term; other members may be changed periodically.

Instruction, training, and supervision. Safety patrols are a means to extend traffic safety education beyond the classroom. Therefore careful and thorough instruction, training, and supervision of patrol members are essential if the patrol is to be efficient and continuous. School officials are responsible for the operation of school safety patrols.

Insignia. The standard insignia for patrol members is the white Sam Browne belt made of 2-inch wide material. It must be worn in plain view at all times while the patrol member is on duty. If the visibility of patrol belts must be increased when worn over white or very light clothing, either a narrow dark stripe at or close to each edge of the belt or a Federal yellow–colored belt may be used. Some schools outfit the members of their traffic patrol with bright yellow raincoats. Others use vests or coats with fluorescent orange stripes.

Increased visibility of patrol members if needed. If the patrol member cannot be seen as far away as the safe stopping distance for legal speed at that location, one of these procedures should be followed:

1. Select another location for the patrol-protected crossing.
2. If the selection of another crossing is not practical, station an auxiliary patrol at the approach to the crossing so that

he or she can be seen in time for a driver to make a safe stop or other driving adjustment.

3. If it is not practical to select another crossing or to use an auxiliary patrol member, place an effective flashing or other signal or sign to warn of a school crossing ahead.

Warning flags. Warning flags are used only as auxiliary equipment and *only* where necessary to increase the distance at which patrol members may be seen.

All warning flags should be approximately 24 inches square, made of colorfast, Federal yellow–colored material, and fastened along one edge to a rod approximately 4 feet long. The flag may bear the word *School* or the words *School Crossing.* The flagstick should be held upward and outward at an angle of about 45°.

Position and procedure. The patrol member must stand on the curb, not in the street, and restrain the children until there is a gap in traffic. When a gap occurs, he or she steps aside and motions for the children to cross the street in a group.

Relation to traffic signals and police officers. At intersections without any traffic control, the traffic may be sufficiently heavy to require the assignment of a police officer at those times when children are going to and from school.

At intersections where traffic is controlled by a police officer or a traffic signal or both, the safety patrol member will assist by directing children across the street in conformance with the directions of the signal or the police officer.

Hours on duty. It is essential that patrol members be on duty at all times when children are crossing streets or highways in going to and from school. The patrol members should reach their posts at least 10 to 15 minutes before the opening of school in the morning and at noon and should remain on duty until the tardy bell. At dismissals they should leave their classes 2 or 3 minutes before the dismissal bell and should remain on duty until all pupils who are not stragglers have passed their posts.

Bus duty. If pupils are transported to and from school by bus, patrol members should be assigned to bus duty. The function of the bus patrol is purely that of assisting the bus driver. School authorities should instruct children to obey both the bus driver and any patrol member assigned to bus duty.

Fire patrol. A fire patrol inspects buildings for fire hazards, periodically checks emergency exits and fire escapes, is familiar with the use of school fire fighting equipment, and directs regular fire drills. Officers of the fire patrol are elected by the pupils, and their duties include the following:

FIRE CHIEF

1. To consult with the principal about planning drills, mapping exits, and assigning duties to the fire squad
2. To assist the principal in calling, supervising, and reporting drills
3. To promote education on fire drills and fire prevention in the school through such means as assembly programs, personal appearances in rooms, organizing committees, and contacting the local fire department
4. To instruct fire squad members in their duties and to check on the performance at the time of each drill
5. To plan the meetings of the fire squad and act as presiding officer

ASSISTANT FIRE CHIEF

1. To assist the chief as directed and to take his or her place when absent

CAPTAINS

1. To supervise drills in different parts of the buildings
2. To check the completion of drills and notify the chief as soon as the section is free of occupants
3. To instruct and supervise room marshals and inspectors in performance of duties

ROOM MARSHALS (TWO FOR EACH ROOM)
No. 1 marshal

1. To lead the class in formation to point of safety outside of the building
2. To set the pace for the class along the route of exit

3. To assist No. 2 marshal and the teacher in taking roll and accounting for all pupils
4. To report to the captain on the completion of the drill

No. 2 marshal

1. To close windows, turn off lights, see that everyone is out of the room, and close the door
2. To follow the class, keep the formation compact, and prevent anyone from going back
3. To become the leader of the drill in case an exit is blocked and necessitates a reverse in direction (Marshals must be familiar with all alternate exits.)
4. To assist the teacher in supervising the pupils in the maintenance of strict fire drill discipline

INSPECTORS

1. To inspect all special rooms (close windows, turn off lights, see that room is clear of occupants, and close the door)
2. To report to the captain on completion of duties (Every conceivable place in the building where there might be persons not under direction of a teacher should be inspected. These stations would include offices, nurse's room, lavatories, gymnasium, and dressing rooms. Not more than two or three simple inspections should be assigned to one inspector.)
3. To leave the building promptly and report to their proper groups

Pupils who are members of the fire squad should be selected and trained in their duties so that a drill can be held during the first week of school. The first drill should be announced to the teachers in advance and should be staged as a slow-motion rehearsal. Special training should be given to pupils of the kindergarten and the beginning first grade. A meeting of the fire squad should follow each of the first drills so that imperfections can be corrected. Numerous suggestions for the improvement of future drills will be forthcoming from the pupils.

Building and grounds patrol. A building and grounds patrol is appointed to prevent disorders and accidents on the school premises. Patrol members assist teachers in preventing dangerous play practices on the playground and in preventing horseplay in the building. In addition, the patrol helps to keep the grounds in order by inspections for broken glass, refuse, uneven surfaces, holes, defective playground equipment, loose boards and railings, slippery floors and stairs, and other hazards. Patrol members also help handicapped pupils and greet and guide visitors.

School safety council. A school safety council is organized in some buildings and, under effective faculty supervision, can be valuable in both accident prevention and social experience. However, to avoid over-organization in the school, many administrators prefer to have patrols operate as self-contained units or under the general surveillance of the student council.

Evaluation

A school safety program can be evaluated entirely in terms of student safety knowledge, practices, and attitudes since the program encompasses safety education. Yet a school safety program must also be appraised in terms of the degree to which it reduces the incidence and severity of injuries to pupils. Repeated surveys must be made to determine the extent to which the program actually deals with the particular safety needs of the students. Records on accidents to students must be studied by month, time of day, place, age of pupil, nature of accident, nature of injury, and all other pertinent factors. In some schools an analysis of the activities of the pupils is the principal instrument used in evaluating the school safety program. That student practices in terms of established safety measures have improved is laudable, but practices are but a means to an end—accident prevention.

A new program may not yield immediate tangible results, nor will the most effective program yield spectacular changes, but an effective school safety program will produce a measurable reduction in the number and severity of injuries.

BLOCK HOME PROGRAM

With the deplorable rise in child molestation, abduction, abuse, and even homicide, concerned parents and educators have developed programs to protect their children when going to or from school. In some instances action is initiated by parents, and in other situations teachers propose that a program be put into action. In all events the program must be a cooperative enterprise with the parents, the neighborhoods, and the teachers working in harmony. Most block home programs are in elementary schools, but this program also exists in middle schools, junior high schools, and senior high schools.

The primary goal of the block homes program is to provide a haven for a child in distress. Although the program is school-based, it operates during the school vacation period as well as during school. Parents, as well as other adults, are asked to volunteer as participants. All volunteers fill out an application form. These applications are screened by the police, who indicate to the school any events in the applicant's file that would indicate the volunteer may not be acceptable for the program. In such a situation the school can merely notify the volunteer that a sufficient number of people have offered their service and thank the person for offering to help the program.

Guidelines for volunteers. The following guidelines are sent to the accepted volunteers.

We do not expect unfortunate incidents to occur as our students go to and from school, but we want to be prepared for any event.

You will not always be home when the students go by, but other nearby block home parents will be home.

Please display your block home sign in a prominent spot in a front window where it can be seen easily from the sidewalk or street.

Block home signs should be left up during summer as

well as winter. However, take the sign down if you plan to be gone for an extended period of time.

If a child comes to your home, do not give the child medication of any kind. If the child is slightly injured, call his or her parents or the school. If he or she is seriously injured, call the police department or the fire station. First aid should be given only to stop excessive bleeding or to restore breathing.

Do not offer a child food or beverages.

Do not call an ambulance, but call the police department and let the police decide if it is a matter for an ambulance.

Do not transport children in your own car. If a parent cannot be reached, call the school or the police department.

If a child has been bitten by a dog, call the dog control center and the police department.

Record all incidents that require your help as a block home parent and notify the school of any incident involving a child from the school.

Emergency telephone numbers:

Police department

Emergency _____

Other police business _____

Fire department

Fire calls _____

Other fire department business _____

Dog control

County _____   City _____

Instruction to children. In the explanation to the students, it must be emphasized that this program is to provide a home as a temporary refuge for children who are hurt, frightened, lost, bullied, threatened, molested, or badgered. Whenever a child feels that he or she is facing danger, he or she should seek a house posting the sign *Block Home*. Occupants of the house will recognize that the child needs adult help and will immediately admit the child to the house. While in the block house the child should obey the directions of the adult occupant. It will be a friendly home where the student can feel secure (Fig. 9-2).

Block homes should be used only when a child feels he or she needs the help of an adult. The mere fact these safety stations are available should produce a certain feeling of security. But there also can be additional

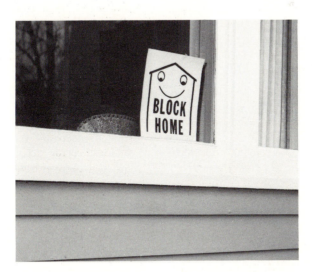

Fig. 9-2. Block home. A haven for a child in distress, homes with the identifying placard actually are inviting the child to enter. Informed children and a neighborhood of concerned citizens are the key to child protection.

security in numbers—in walking or cycling in groups of two or more. Knowing the location of block homes is an added safeguard.

EMERGENCY CARE

In any situation in which relatively large numbers of children are assembled, emergencies occur despite the best laid plans and thoughtful precautions. Wisdom dictates preparation for such emergencies. Experience indicates that such preparation need not be elaborate, but that it must be organized.

Planned program

One cannot possibly foresee every emergency that may occur in the school, nor is such foresight necessary. Emergency situations fall into patterns, and a school plan to take care of major illness, minor illness, and emergencies following accidents will take care of a school's needs. The program can be planned so that modifications will rarely be required and, if necessary, can be made readily.

Facilities for emergency care

1. Emergency lounges (one for girls and one for boys) each with at least two cots, adequate blankets, washbasin, soap, towels, chairs, and table
2. Splints, slings, gauze, rubber tubing
3. Emetic (e.g., mustard to produce vomiting)
4. Phone numbers posted at all phones
   a. Physicians   d. Clinic
   b. Ambulance   e. Fire department
   c. Hospital
5. Phone numbers filed
   a. Home of each child
   b. Child's family physician

Personnel assignments for emergency care

1. Person first in command and duties
2. Person second in command
3. Person third in command
4. Person to phone
   a. Physician   d. Home
   b. Ambulance   e. Fire department
   c. Hospital

With an organized program such as this the school is well prepared to meets its re-

sponsibility during emergencies. If the school emergency program is part of the community civilian defense program, the school should rehearse its procedures as part of the community rehearsal. Otherwise, on its own initiative the school should go through simulated emergencies.

Major illness

Occasionally a child in school may become seriously ill with high fever, severe pain, general distress, gastrointestinal upset, and even some indication of prostration. The condition should be considered serious, but not critical. It is not likely to be a matter of seconds; yet the teacher should handle the situation as if it were extremely important. A systematic procedure will apply to any situation:

1. Have the child rest on a cot in a moderately darkened room
2. Keep the child warm
3. Contact the child's home by telephone or other means
4. Carry out the parents' instructions
5. If the parents cannot be contacted within an hour, call the child's family physician
6. If the child's family physician is not available, call some other physician
7. State the condition of the child
8. Carry out the physician's instructions

It is apparent that in most occurrences of major illness the school will have met its obligation when it has carried out the parents' instructions.

Minor illness

A child in school may become mildly upset or ill. Perhaps a mild headache, slight distress, the aftereffects of overexertion, or a general malaise has developed. At least at the onset it may not be necessary to contact the home, since there is a good probability that after rest the child will be able to return to class and resume work:

1. Have the child rest on a cot in a moderately darkened room
2. Keep the child warm
3. Have someone in attendance or responsible for visiting the child at intervals
4. Use no drugs
5. If the illness appears to become more severe, follow the procedures for major illness

Emergency following accident

Specific first steps are necessary in virtually all accident emergencies, although not every measure applies to all cases. The order in which measures are carried out is determined by the particular situation:

1. Note whether the subject is breathing
2. Note whether air passages are obstructed, and remove any foreign bodies in the mouth
3. Note any profuse hemorrhaging
4. Note whether the subject is in a state of shock
5. Have him or her lie on the back with the head raised if his or her face is flushed, or lower him or her if the face is pale
6. If the student is vomiting, turn his or her head to the side
7. Loosen clothing, particularly if breathing is hindered
8. Place blankets or wraps under and over the student and keep him or her warm; injury usually produces a drop in body temperature
9. Do not move the subject unless absolutely necessary until a physician or an ambulance arrives
10. If it is necessary to move the child, apply a splint to the injured parts and handle the injured parts with extreme care
11. Give no liquids or solid foods
12. Confort and reassure the child; perhaps it is advisable not to allow the child to see the injury
13. Remain with the victim until a physician or ambulance has arrived

In case of really serious injury, as soon as the nature of the child's condition has been determined, the family physician should be called. The call should report the general condition of the child, including the pulse rate, whether the breathing is faint or heavy, the child warm and perspiring or cold and clammy, conscious or unconscious, and in pain. The physician also should be told of the nature and extent of injury, the nature of any bleeding, and possible fractures or dislocations.

Transporting the injured child by ambulance is the most satisfactory means of conveyance, but, if an ambulance cannot be obtained, care should be exercised in selecting a vehicle. A vehicle that will be most comfortable for the patient, not the vehicle easiest to recruit, should be selected.

When the injury does not appear to be serious, one may notify the home first. Whenever the parents are informed of an accident to their child, calmness and assurance are in order. Perhaps going to the home, rather than phoning, might be advisable. Report the kind of accident, the nature of the injury, and the condition of the child. If the child is being taken directly to a hospital or a physician's office, report the name of the hospital or physician. If the school and parents agree that the child should be taken home, suggest that immediate preparations be made for the arrival of the child.

FIRST AID AT SCHOOL

As the term implies, first aid is the assistance first given to the injured person and is aimed at the prevention of further harm. It is the temporary treatment given at the site of the emergency. It is the aid given by a skilled lay person before the subject is in the charge of a physician. At this point the first aid phase terminates and the lay person's first aid duty is done, unless he or she is directed by the physician to perform additional tasks. The correct first aid measures can reduce suffering, be instrumental in speeding up subsequent recovery, prevent permanent disability, and even save life (Fig. 9-3).

Basic philosophy

Every accident is tragic because it might have been prevented. Yet in an imperfect world of imperfect people accidents will oc-

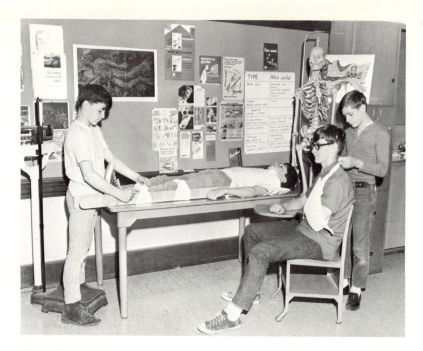

Fig. 9-3. First-aid practice. A junior high school unit on first aid properly includes a demonstration of knowledge and skill. (Courtesy Salem Public Schools, Salem, Ore.)

cur and emergencies that require people skilled in first aid will arise. There is nothing mystical about first aid. It simply involves recognized procedures for giving immediate help to an individual who has been injured. Yet simple though it may be, first aid can be of greater importance than the subsequent aid of a physician. Whether a major or a minor emergency exists, know-how is the important ingredient for resolving the situation, and every teacher should be trained in first aid.

Also, it should now be the policy of every school administrator to make sure that at least one person on the school staff or faculty is trained and skilled in the cardiopulmonary resuscitation (CPR) technique. This technique is now saving countless lives in emergencies involving cardiac arrest and the stoppage of breathing such as that caused by choking accidents.

Most first aid situations in the school are minor and subsequently are not brought to the attention of a physician. Even the most incidental injury should command the teacher's attention and care. Dealing with human health and life is a challenge to the teacher's best efforts. Parents should be informed of the first aid measures that were taken when their child has been injured or otherwise incapacitated.

Even in the best administered schools with well-organized and well-functioning safety programs, serious accidents occur. The poise and skill that enable school personnel to face the most serious situation, sufficient for whatever may be required, are usually the result of following recognized procedures and of assuming adequate self-reliance in many specific, although minor, emergencies over the span of time. All teachers should be prepared in first aid procedures so that, when the emergency arises, they will be equal to the occasion and confident in their ability to deal with the situation. First aid procedures are definite and specific, but not involved. Time given to a standard first aid course is well invested. In the absence of an opportunity to take a standard course, a study of first aid measures for typical emergencies of school life can be highly profitable to teachers who apply themselves conscientiously.

Guiding principles

A few basic principles or rules can guide the teacher in any first aid situation:

1. Be sure there is need for haste before you hurry. Many people needlessly rush blindly in emergency situations. Few emergencies require haste. If breathing is obstructed or profuse bleeding occurs or poison has been taken, haste is necessary, but it is difficult to envision any other emergency in a school that would require extreme haste.

2. Do the commonsense thing that is indicated. Often the correct thing may appear to be ridiculously simple; most first aid procedures are simple and obvious.

3. If in doubt, assume that the worst possible condition exists. If a child has a head injury of unknown extent and the teacher proceeds on the assumption that intracranial hemorrhage is present, the procedures will be more than adequate if the injury is of a lesser nature.

4. Even though your first aid procedure may not be beneficial, at least make sure that it is not injurious. Many well-meaning individuals, in their efforts to do something for an injured person, actually harm the victim. There are many things worse for the victim than to lie quietly on the ground while waiting for a physician and an ambulance.

If the victim is moved improperly, it may cause greater damage than the original injury.

Whenever a question of liability arises in the administration of first aid, the whole issue is based on the question of whether what was done was reasonable. Subsequent events may indicate that what was done was not the best that could have been done; yet in view of the circumstances it was sensible and perhaps what a person of ordinary prudence would have done.

GENERAL CONDITIONS AND INJURIES

Certain conditions and injuries involve the entire body. Aid in these conditions involves procedures different from those in which the injury is localized. In the school, five types of emergencies involving the entire body may occur—asphyxiation, shock, epileptic convulsions, fainting, and possible poisoning.

Asphyxiation

Any interference with aeration of the blood can be termed asphyxiation. There may be only a mild interference with aeration, such as a small obstruction to breathing or mild carbon monoxide poisoning. Or the interference may be so great as to stop the breathing completely. When the oxygen concentration of the blood drops appreciably, the vital respiratory and cardiac centers in the brain are affected and may not carry on their normal functions.

In the school, asphyxiation by the inhalation of gas is a rare occurrence. Asphyxiation usually occurs as a result of mechanical obstruction of breathing. This includes foreign bodies in the throat, larynx, or trachea, submersion in water, and strangulation.

First aid treatment for asphyxia consists first of removing the cause and second, providing air to the subject (Fig. 9-4). If the subject does not breathe, artificial respiration

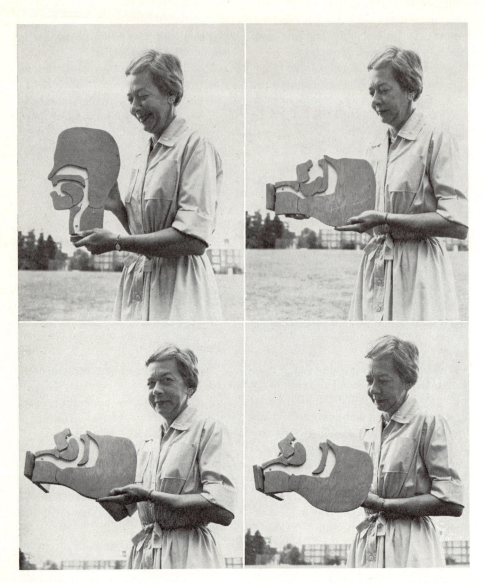

Fig. 9-4. Opening and breathing passages for mouth-to-mouth artificial respiration. **A,** Model showing normal respiratory passages in relation to associated structures. **B,** Model showing obstruction of the breathing passages when the tongue is retracted while the subject is in a supine position. **C,** Thrusting the jaw forward helps to widen the breathing passageway. **D,** Tilting the head far back and stretching the neck aids further in assuring a wide air passageway.

must be performed. Delay may cost the subject his or her life. Few persons can go without breathing for more than 5 minutes; therefore action to restore breathing should begin at once. Whether or not artificial respiration is necessary, certain other measures are helpful in producing recovery:

1. Loosen all clothing that interferes with breathing or circulation.
2. Keep the subject warm. Shock usually is present.
3. Provide ample fresh air.
4. Keep the subject quiet and at rest.
5. Summon a physician immediately, *even though the subject appears to be recovering fully*. The recovery may only be temporary.

Resuscitation is the revival of a person who is almost dead. In artificial respiration, breathing is produced by some agency outside of the subject's own body. If a pulmonary ventilator (pulmotor) and a competent operator are available, these should be used. In the absence of these mechanical means, manual artificial respiration should be used. At least one teacher in every school building should be trained in artificial respiration. Such training should be obtained from a skilled operator, which will provide ample opportunity for supervised practice. It is a skill that is mastered by explanation, demonstration, and supervised practice.

Mouth-to-mouth or mouth-to-nose artificial respiration, properly done, is the most effective method of rescue breathing other than the use of mechanical devices. It is not a difficult procedure and can be mastered effectively by any normal adult who can follow the prescribed directions:

1. Place the subject on his or her back at once right where he or she is; no need to loosen clothing or drain water from the subject.
2. Clear the mouth and throat of all obstruction.

3. Tilt the head far back in a "chin-up" position and the neck stretched.
4. Draw the lower jaw far forward, being careful not to depress the tongue. It is important that the jaw be held far forward to open the passageway of the throat.
5. Pinch the nose with the thumb and forefinger of the other hand.
6. Take a deep breath and, with your mouth wide and over the subject's open mouth, blow forcefully into the subjects breathing passageway until you see the chest rise.
7. Quickly remove your mouth when the chest rises and listen for exhalation. If the subject makes gurgling or snoring sounds, lift the jaw higher.
8. Repeat the process at the rate of 16 to 20 per minute for a school-age youngster until the subject begins to breathe normally.

While artificial resuscitation is being administered, a physician should be called. Once the physician arrives, he or she is in complete charge of the situation.

Shock

Shock is a depressed level of body function. It results from emotional upsets and from injuries of various kinds that involve a general blow to the body or localized injuries. Some degree of shock follows most injuries. Shock may occur at once or its onset may be delayed, even for 2 or 3 hours.

Symptoms of shock vary in degree, but the pattern is standard; usually the subject is conscious:

1. Cold clammy pale skin
2. Anxiety and fear in facial expression
3. Bluish lips and fingernails
4. Irregular breathing
5. Rapid weak pulse
6. Often chills
7. Limp relaxed muscles

A knowledge of the physiology of shock is helpful in providing the proper emergency care for a person in a shock condition. If death results from shock, it is caused by circulatory failure. Normally the heart pumps against a moderate amount of arterial pressure, which is necessary for normal contraction and output of the heart. Blood pressure is the result of constriction of the arteries and the viscosity of the blood proteins. These proteins cannot normally pass through capillary membranes. The injury or blow that causes shock produces dilation of the arteries and also makes the capillaries permeable to blood proteins; the proteins diffuse out of the capillaries. This relaxation of the arteries and loss of proteins by the blood causes a decline in blood pressure, which in turn causes poorer heart action, which produces a further drop in blood pressure. The downward spiral of blood pressure continues unless something reverses the course. Transfusion of blood plasma to the subject adds blood proteins, which will increase the blood pressure and thus start the recovery process. However, this is a procedure for a physician and hospital personnel. Teachers must concern themselves with first-aid measures.

First aid treatment for shock is simple, but highly important:

1. Keep the patient warm. Blankets, coats, and similar materials underneath and covering the subject help to prevent loss of body heat. Massage is not recommended.
2. Lay the subject on his or her back with the head low. A pillow should not be used, and he or she should not sit up.
3. Do not give the subject a stimulant or water unless instructed to do so by a physician.
4. If the subject must be moved, a stretcher should be used. An ambulance is best suited to convey a person in shock.

Epileptic convulsions

The United States has about 990,000 persons with epilepsy, which means about one in every 220 persons. Although the incidence is lower in the school population than in the general population, a teacher may be confronted with the problem of emergency care of an epileptic child during a seizure. With understanding the teacher can approach the task confident in the ability to handle the situation. For the prepared teacher a child in an epileptic seizure is not a frightening sight, but a signal for action that will be helpful to the child.

Minor (petit mal) seizures are characterized by a transitory loss of consciousness, with or without muscle tremors, and no other symptoms. If the child is standing, he or she remains in that position. The child may recognize that he or she has lost consciousness for 3 or 4 seconds, but will experience no particular ill effects. These children are not a problem in the school unless they develop the major form.

Major (grand mal) seizures are characterized by extreme convulsive thrashing about, followed by prolonged stupor.

First aid care of epileptic persons is rather simple:

1. Do not resist the seizure. Resistance neither shortens the time of the seizure nor reduces its intensity.
2. Get the person in the clear so that he or she will not be injured by striking something hot, sharp, or hard. If the child has a seizure while sitting at a desk, the first procedure indicated is to carry him or her to the free area in front of the room.
3. Open his or her collar if it is tight.
4. If the subject is swallowing the tongue, there will be an audible gurgling in the throat. The tongue has retracted and needs to be drawn forward. To do this, place a stick between the subject's

molars. With the fingers, draw the tongue forward. It may be necessary to hold the tongue forward for several minutes. If a wooden stick is not available, something else, such as rubber, may be used to hold the mouth open. Hard materials that may chip the teeth should not be used, but under no circumstances should the operator put his fingers in the victim's mouth without some such guard.

5. After the convulsion, place the subject on a cot and let him sleep.
6. Call the parents; usually parents indicate at the opening of the school year that their child is subject to convulsions and will instruct the school on what procedure they wish to have followed.

Children will accept a child who has an occasional seizure, but, if a child has seizures so often that the routine of the room is disrupted frequently, he or she should not attend school. The family physician should make the decision regarding whether the child's condition warrants discontinuance of school.

Fainting

The technical term for fainting is syncope. It may be induced by a psychological experience such as fright or by a physiological factor such as fatigue. During fainting the physiological change that takes place is dilatation of the large arteries in the abdominal cavity. This results in a shifting of the blood mass so that a disproportionately large share is in these vessels and a diminished amount is in the brain and surface areas. The reduced blood supply in the brain area is inadequate for consciousness. Paleness, or blanching of the skin, occurs and is the distinguishing symptom.

First aid care is based on the recognition that the blood supply to the brain must be increased:

1. Place the person in a horizontal position or with the head slightly lowered. Raise the legs to help hasten blood flow to the brain. Do not throw water on the person.
2. Following recovery of consciousness, the person should not return to a standing position too soon. After lying flat for perhaps 5 minutes, he or she should sit up for another 5 minutes before standing again.
3. If the child is sitting when he or she faints or appears likely to faint, the teacher, with his or her hand on the back of the child's neck, should lower the child's head between the knees.
4. After the child regains consciousness, a cold wet cloth placed over the forehead will produce a feeling of comfort and freshness.
5. If fainting is prolonged or recurrent, treat for shock and call a physician.

Possible poisoning

Occasionally a child at school may ingest poison such as toadstools, wild berries, roots, and some types of leaves (Fig. 9-5). Symptoms of ingested poisoning include discomfort in the upper abdominal region, cramps, pain, nausea, and vomiting. Some degree of prostration quickly sets in.

First aid care should start by making certain that the child actually has swallowed the substance suspected of being poison:

1. Administer the antidote recommended on the poison container.
2. Call a physician or poison control center, state the available information, and follow the instructions given.
3. If no medical service is available and the poison or its antidote is not known, give the subject two or three glassfuls of water or milk to dilute the poison.
4. Do not induce vomiting if a strong acid or alkali is taken because vomiting will

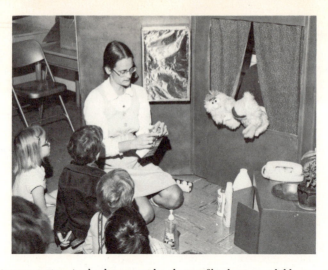

Fig. 9-5. Poisoning prevention. A school nurse, with a cluster of kindergarten children around her, puts on a puppet show on the dangers of poisons. With rapt attention the children enter into the experiences of the puppets. (Courtesy Benton County Health Department, Corvallis, Ore.)

further burn the mouth, throat, and esophagus. An acid can be diluted and neutralized by using two tablespoons of baking soda in a glass of water. An alkali can be neutralized with vinegar or lemon juice in water. A glass of the fluid usually is sufficient for a school-age child; too much fluid may produce vomiting. A glass of milk or the white of two or three eggs can act as stabilizers. Activated charcoal is accepted as a universal antidote.

5. Take the child directly to a physician or hospital.
6. Keep the child warm.

LOCALIZED CONDITIONS AND INJURIES

Perhaps it is an oversimplification to classify conditions as purely localized; an injury in one location of the body can affect the person's entire constitution. Yet most of those conditions and injuries listed as localized are more important in terms of their localized effect and affect the general body but slightly.

Wounds

An injury to soft tissues caused by violence is called a wound. Many classifications of wounds are possible, but purely descriptive terms are most meaningful and are applied here.

Abrasions occur when the superficial layers of the skin are scraped off, such as a brush burn or rope burn.

Contusions are bruises in which some of the tissues are ruptured, but surface continuity remains.

Incised wounds are those made by a sharp cutting edge.

Lacerated wounds are those with uneven or torn edges.

Penetrating wounds are those that penetrate internal organs.

Puncture wounds are deep and narrow, such as a pointed tool would cause.

First aid care should be concerned with

two factors—to stop bleeding and to prevent foreign materials from getting into the wound. Procedures must be adapted to the severity and nature of the wound, but certain steps apply to all wounds:

1. Elevate the part to stop bleeding. Over 90% of all wounds will stop bleeding simply if the affected part is raised, for example, when the person lies on the floor with the injured foot on a chair. By reducing pressure, this simple device provides a situation favorable for a clot to form.

2. If clotting does not occur, pack gauze into the wound.

3. As a third resort, put pressure on the severed vessel. If the wound is not deep and blood oozes out somewhat, a vein has been cut. Since veins carry blood *toward* the heart, the pressure point should be farther from the heart than is the wound. In deep wounds with gushing hemorrhage, an artery carrying blood *away* from the heart likely is involved. Then the pressure point should be between the heart and the wound.

4. A tourniquet of soft rubber can be used in place of manual pressure, but one must be certain a tourniquet is needed and properly applied. In more than half of the instances in which a tourniquet is used it is unnecessary and is frequently applied improperly.

5. If the wound is clean, small, and rather inconsequential, place a sterile gauze pad (e.g., Band-Aid) over the wound, and notify the parents of what has been done. Make the dressing snug, but not tight. Do not put a disinfectant on the wound. It is recognized that in school the teacher acts in the place of the parent (*in loco parentis*) in the control of health, and doubtless the parent would apply a disinfectant to the wound. Yet practice indicates that the teacher's role here is limited to first aid, and medication is not a first aid measure.

6. If the wound is serious or contains foreign materials, call the home. After stopping the hemorrhage, carry out the instructions of the parents. If the parents cannot be reached, contact the family physician.

Whenever indicated, place the injured part at rest by elevating it, splinting it, or placing it in a sling.

Nosebleed

Most nosebleeds are caused by a blow, but a sudden rise in blood pressure, violent activity, atmospheric change, and some local disorders may also cause the nose to bleed. Usually bleeding is confined to one nostril in what is known as Little's area. Along the nasal septum about 1¼ inches up from the opening, the mucous tissue is exceedingly thin and delicate. In this area the blood vessels are near the surface and can be ruptured easily.

First aid treatment is not always necessary because the bleeding often subsides spontaneously. If bleeding is profuse or persists, a series of measures should be followed until the first aid is effective in checking the flow:

1. Have the child sit erect with the head tilted back slightly, but not so much that the flow will be back into the throat.

2. Apply pressure to the sides of the nose by grasping it with the thumb and forefinger.

3. Place cold packs on the nose.

4. Irrigate the nose with spray, drops, or inhalant, using salt water or vinegar water (half water, half vinegar).

5. Pack the nostril with a long (2 inches or more) gauze roll about ¼ inch in diam-

eter. Be sure that sufficient length protrudes for grasping when the pack is removed. Be careful there is no blood flow back into the throat. Let a physician remove the gauze roll.

6. Call a physician immediately or take the child to a physician if the flow appears to be profuse.

Ear injuries

Bleeding or watery discharge from the ear indicates the possibility of a skull fracture and requires the same treatment as a head injury.

Bleeding from the ear canal may be caused by scratching and by probing the canal with a pointed article as well as by a direct blow. In itself, the bleeding may not be serious, but serious complications may develop. To arrest bleeding, have the child sit erect and still and apply a cold pack to the ear. Some bleeding may be desirable.

Foreign bodies in the ear usually can be removed quite easily. It may be sufficient simply to tilt the head. If the object will not swell in water, a syringe of moderately warm water may flush it out. If neither of these methods is successful, a physician should be consulted.

Eye injuries

Bleeding from an injury in the region of the eyes rarely is profuse. However, the bleeding should be checked by having the child sit erect and by placing a cold pack and light bandage over the area. There should be a minimum of pressure on the eyeball itself.

If any object penetrates the eyeball, no attempt should be made to remove the object. A cold pack to close the lids will serve until the child gets to a physician.

Most objects that get into the eye lodge in the mucous lining of the lid or on the eyeball. Embedded objects such as metal chips should be removed by a physician. Small objects such as dust particles can be washed out with warm water gently applied with a dropper. Other objects can be removed by everting the lid and cautiously wiping them off with a bit of moistened, sterile gauze or absorbent cotton. A most effective procedure is to approach the child from the rear and rest the fingers on the face and forehead, which prevents one from jabbing the child. With this technique, if the child should move, the operator's fingers and the applicator will move with the child's head.

Chemicals in the eye should be flushed out immediately with water. The eyelids should then be covered with a wet gauze pad while the child is en route to a physician.

Burns

A *burn* is an injury caused by dry heat; a *scald* is caused by moist heat, including that of hot fats. Burns are classified according to intensity:

1. First degree—redness of the skin
2. Second degree—blistered skin
3. Third degree—destruction of the outer layer of the skin
4. Fourth degree—destruction of all of the layers of the skin

A child reacts physiologically more violently to a burn than does an adult, and shock is always a threat when a child suffers a burn.

First aid measures depend on the extent of the burn. If the area is extensive or the burn is penetrating, the child should be referred to a physician as soon as possible. Until the physician takes charge, all measures should be directed toward the prevention and treatment of shock. Put nothing on the burned area. However, some physicians recommend cold water to relieve pain. If the burn is very minor, leave the area exposed to the air. Neither medication nor a bandage should be placed over the burn. The child could remain in school for the full day, and a note or phone call to the parents can explain the nature of the injury. If the burn is moderate, parents should be called and their instructions followed. The teacher should put nothing on the burn.

Sprains

A sprain is an injury to the soft tissues about a joint in which the ligaments, tendons, and even muscles are stretched or torn.

First aid care must be directed toward the prevention of swelling and further damage. Since it is the most common, care of an ankle sprain will illustrate the procedures:

1. Elevate the injured joint immediately. If the child is lying on the floor, he or she can put the foot up on a chair.
2. Wrap a gauze pressure bandage about the joint. The bandage should be very snug, but, if it appears to be too tight, a few clips with a scissors will allow adequate circulation.
3. Apply cold packs such as wet towels or ice bags.
4. Do not allow the child to bear weight on the joint.
5. Call the child's parents and carry out their instructions. Advise medical service because many sprains also involve fractures. In addition, proper care will assure complete recovery. Proper first aid adds measurably to an early and complete recovery.

Dislocations

A dislocation is a displacement of a bone from its normal position at a joint. In a dislocation soft tissues are under extreme tension, and improper handling of the injury may cause *further permanent damage*. A dislocated finger joint gives the finger a marked crooked appearance. A dislocated shoulder produces a drooped appearance, and the head of the humerus produces a prominence in the armpit.

First aid care must be directed to the prevention of further damage. If a finger joint is dislocated, it can be replaced by grasping the part of the finger beyond the dislocation and pulling steadily and strongly. Do not jerk. When the muscles fatigue as a result of the pull, they relax and the joint slips easily back into place. Wrap a splint (e.g., a tongue blade) along the finger, which is extended at rest.

A shoulder dislocation should be reduced by a physician. The principal first-aid measure is to support the arm comfortably in a sling until a physician is available. Older boys and girls may prefer to hold the injured arm in their other arm. This practice can be acceptable, though the sling has advantages during vehicular travel. Other dislocations (e.g., the elbow), should be given this same type of first aid care until a physician takes charge.

Fractures

Any break in a bone is called a fracture. Some fractures are readily recognized from the resulting deformity, but many fractures involve no visible anatomical change. Marked pain is sufficient for suspicion of possible fracture.

First aid measures should be based on the assumption that the fracture is serious and soft tissues are in danger. Further, the likelihood of shock is considerable. Several procedures should be followed:

1. Prevent further damage by gentle handling in order not to damage soft tissue.
2. Keep the patient comfortable.
3. Place full support under and completely across the possible fracture. The subject should not be transported unless an adequate splint supports the injured limb.
4. Keep the child warm to prevent shock or to counteract shock if it does develop.

5. Do not attempt to set the bone. If a bone fragment projects through the skin (compound fracture), do not attempt to put the bone back. Check any profuse bleeding by packing the wound with sterile gauze pads.

Head injuries

A blow to the head is often more serious than the teacher realizes. Children may receive a hard blow to the head and still not fall to the ground. Or if they do fall, they may get up immediately. Yet in either case the child may have suffered serious injury. All blows to the head should be regarded as serious.

A skull fracture with or without intracranial hemorrhage may result from a blow. The child does not have to be unconscious for the condition to be serious. If it is assumed that there is a possible skull fracture and first-aid is administered accordingly, proper care will also have been given should the condition be a lesser one, such as concussion. When brain concussion occurs, dizziness, nausea, slow respiration, weak pulse, and even unconsciousness indicate that it, too, is a serious condition.

First aid measures should emphasize a minimum of handling:

1. Place the child on his or her back with the head raised slightly if the face is of normal color. If the face is pale, keep the head level.
2. If no abrasions are present, apply cold towels or ice bags to the head.
3. Do not move the subject any more than necessary, and while en route to medical aid use a stretcher.
4. Keep the child warm.

Neck and back injuries

Pain in the neck or back caused by a violent accident is sufficient indication of a fracture of the vertebral column. Such fractures are more frequent than is commonly realized. The injury may be a slight chip, a complete fracture, or a displaced vertebra—all are serious. *Incorrect handling can cause permanent injury and even death.* In all such cases, it is wise to assume the worst and proceed accordingly.

First aid care emphasizes a minimum of handling:

1. Call for an ambulance. If the subject is comfortable, do not move him or her until the ambulance attendants arrive.
2. Do not let the child sit up or even raise the head.
3. If no ambulance is available and the subject must be moved, obtain a door, a wide board, or other flat wide surface.
4. Place the door beside the child so that it extends beyond the head and feet. Raise the child's near arm above the head. Three people should kneel alongside the board, reach over the subject, grasp his or her clothing on the far side, and gently roll the child slowly toward themselves so that he or she will be lying face down on the board. Another person at the head and one at the feet guide the head and feet as the child is rolled.
5. Keep the child warm. Shock usually accompanies fractures of the vertebral column.

FIRST AID SUPPLIES

Every school building should have at least one fully stocked, conveniently located first aid cabinet. In the elementary school the cabinet should be placed in the health services room if there is one. Otherwise the emergency rest room or principal's office are acceptable locations. In addition to at least one complete cabinet in the building, each classroom may have a first aid kit. This kit should be regarded primarily as a health education aid and secondarily as a device for first aid.

INVENTORY FOR FIRST AID CABINET

Suggested supplies	Purpose
Glass jars (2)	For applicators and blades
Blades, wood (500)	Splints, depressors
Wooden applicators (1,000)	Swabs, remove particles
Toothpicks (750)	Remove particles
Tincture of green soap	Wash injured parts
Absorbent cotton roll	Large pads or dressings
Sterile gauze, 4 in roll	Dressings
Sterile gauze, 3 × 3 in squares (100)	Protect injuries
Sterile gauze, 2 × 2 in squares (100)	Protect injuries
Compress on adhesive band, 1 in (100)	Protect injuries
Roller bandage, 1 in (12 rolls)	Dressings
Roller bandage, 2 in (12 rolls)	Dressings
Roller bandage, 4 in (12 rolls)	Dressings
Triangular bandage (4)	Sling, area coverings
Safety pins (24)	For triangular bandage
Adhesive tape, roll (widths ½ to 2 in)	Fasten splints and dressings
Scissors (blunt or bandage)	Cut dressings
Forceps (3 in pincer or tweezer type)	Grasp small objects
Eyedroppers (6)	Apply oil
Tourniquet (3 ft ¼ in rubber tube)	Check excessive bleeding
Splints (metal or yucca) (10)	Support
Ice bag (2)	Relief of swelling
Hot-water bottle (with cover) (2)	Local relief of pain
Mineral oil or petroleum jelly (nonmedicated)	Relieve irritation
Aromatic spirits of ammonia	Stimulant
Paper cups (100)	Receptacle

INVENTORY FOR FIRST AID KIT

Suggested supplies

Compress on adhesive band, 1 in (20)	Adhesive tape, roll ½ and 1 in
Sterile gauze, 2 × 2 in squares (10)	Scissors
Roller bandage, 1 in (1 roll)	Forceps
Roller bandage, 2 in (1 roll)	Paper cups (10)

A junior high school may profitably have a cabinet convenient to the physical education staff as well as an additional cabinet in the health services room or principal's office. If the school has a director of school health who assumes primary responsibility in emergency situations, one of the cabinets should be convenient for his or her use.

A senior high school will need a cabinet in the physical education offices as well as one in the health services room or principal's office. Two or three cabinets should be adequate for the typical high school, and one first aid cabinet may be sufficient. Note that no antiseptics are included in the accompanying list.

A responsible person should be in charge of first aid cabinets, kits, and supplies, and adequate supplies should be on hand at all times.

QUESTIONS AND EXERCISES

1. Should a school board and the faculty of a school district be legally responsible for preventing all risks involving its students?
2. Analyze the statement, "In the United States today accidents are a greater threat to the life of school-children than are the infectious diseases."
3. To reduce injuries among schoolchildren, why not eliminate physical education and recess?
4. In elementary schools, who is responsible for the promotion of safety?
5. While a high school physical education teacher was answering a phone call, one of the students in his class was badly injured on the trampoline. Would you regard the teacher as negligent or not negligent? Present your reasoning.
6. Should the common law immunity that exempts a school board from lawsuits be repealed in all states? What is your line of reasoning?
7. What is the value of a safety survey, who should conduct the survey, and what should the survey include?
8. Which usually is the more difficult to correct—unsafe conditions or unsafe practices, and what is the support for your decision?
9. What are the merits of advance emergency plans in the way of personnel, organization, and procedures?
10. Why do authorities on school health advise schools not to give medicine to pupils?
11. When a child is severely injured in school and the parents cannot be reached, who is liable for the ambulance and hospital costs if the teacher decides the proper action is to take the child to the hospital via ambulance?
12. Why is it correct to say that, to deal with shock properly, it is necessary to reverse the downward cycle of cardiovascular function?
13. If youngsters report to an elementary schoolteacher that three pupils have eaten toadstools, what should be her action?
14. Putting a disinfectant on a cut is not first aid and is not the province of the school in emergency care. Explain.
15. A fourth-grade youngster came into the school with a nosebleed of unknown cause. What procedures should be followed?
16. Indicate various emergency situations in which the best interests of the person will be served by having the person sit erect.
17. Ask a physician or other qualified person if a severely burned leg or arm should be put into cold water as an immediate first-aid measure.
18. What first-aid measures should be followed in the case of a junior high school student who has a painful injury of the ankle?
19. At noon hour a sixth-grade boy bumped his head against the school wall without falling, but later complained of feeling ill. What possible injuries could he have sustained, and what first-aid measures should be given?
20. Why is it highly desirable that every school building in this nation have at least one teacher with a Standard Red Cross First Aid Certificate?

REFERENCES AND SELECTED READINGS

Aaron, J. E.: Are you a safety educator? Safety Education **39:** March, 1960.

Accident facts, Chicago, published yearly, National Safety Council.

American Association for Health, Physical Education, and Recreation: Suggested school safety policies, Washington, D.C., 1964, The Association.

American Automobile Association: Teaching driver and traffic safety education, New York, 1965, McGraw-Hill Book Co.

American National Red Cross: Advanced first aid and emergency care, Garden City, N.Y., 1973, Doubleday & Co., Inc.

American National Red Cross: First aid textbook, rev., Garden City, N.Y., 1969, Doubleday & Co., Inc.

American National Red Cross: Standard first aid and personal safety, Garden City, N.Y., 1973, Doubleday & Co., Inc.

American National Red Cross: Home nursing textbook, Garden City, N.Y., Doubleday & Co., Inc.

Arens, J.: Dangers to children and youth, Durham, N.C., 1970, Moore Publishing Co.

Diehl, H. S., et al.: Health and safety for you, ed. 4, New York, 1969, McGraw-Hill Book Co.

Diehl, H. S., and Dalrymple, W.: Healthful living: A textbook of personal and community health, ed. 9, New York, 1973, McGraw-Hill Book Co.

Dzenowagis, J. G.: What they believe, Safety Education **41:** Dec., 1961.

Elder, A., and Farndale, W.: Environmental health technology, Elmsford, N.Y., 1978, Pergamon Press, Inc.

Florio, A. E., and Stafford, G. T.: Safety education, ed. 3, New York, 1969, McGraw-Hill Book Co.

Hanlon, J. J., and McHose, E.: Design for health: the school and community, ed. 2, Philadelphia, 1971, Lea & Febiger.

Henderson, J.: Emergency medical guide, ed. 2, New York, 1969, McGraw-Hill Book Co.

Home health emergencies, New York, 1963, Equitable Life Assurance Society of the United States.

Jones, K. L., et al.: Safety and first aid, San Francisco,

1971, Canfield Press, Division of Harper & Row, Publishers.

Marshall, R. L., and Abercrombie, S. A.: College centers, Safety Education **62:**26-28, Jan., 1963.

McCann, W.: New road barriers for safety, Science Newsletter **88:**38, 46, July 17, 1965.

Neuhas, P.: A hazard-free home, Today's Health **42:**54, Sept., 1964.

Reider, F.: Medical self-help training program, Public Health Report **80:**283, 1965.

Stack, H. J., and Elkow, J. D.: Education for safe living, ed. 4, Englewood Cliffs, N.J., 1966, Prentice-Hall, Inc.

Strasser, M. K., et al.: Fundamentals of safety education, ed. 2, New York, 1973, The Macmillan Co.

United States Public Health Service and United States Department of Defense: Emergency health care, Washington, D.C., 1963, United States Government Printing Office.

Weeden, V.: Beware the ides of April, Safety Education **40:**entire issue, April, 1961.

Healing is a matter of time, but it also is a matter of opportunity.

Hippocrates

CHAPTER 10

Remedial aspects of health services

Often a neglected area of school health services, the remedial aspects of the program are an index of the vision, completeness, and thoroughness of the health services of a school. Further, they reflect the concern of the professional staff for the long-range effect of the school's health program on the health of the children who have defects or disabilities. To give special attention to children with defects does not conflict with the basic philosophy that the school health program is concerned primarily with the normal child. This philosophy also acknowledges that each child should be served in terms of his or her needs in order to attain the highest level of health possible with his or her basic endowment.

IMPORTANCE OF FOLLOW-UP PROGRAMS

An essential first step in health service is to identify defects, but this becomes valuable only if action to remedy or correct the situation results. The school deals in futures; however small may be the defect, it can be important when considered in terms of the 60 or 70 years of life the child faces. Because of many unrecognized health obstacles, none of us attains 100% of our potential in effective

and enjoyable living. Thus it is imperative that any recognized defect, harmful to health, be corrected as soon as possible. It may not be a defect that threatens life. Yet, if it reduces the child's effectiveness and enjoyment in living, it merits correction. In some instances complete recovery of function may not be possible, but the child has the right to the recovery of whatever function can be attained.

In the correction of physical disorders the mental health component is often overlooked. Frequently a child with a disability develops an unwholesome self-identification. He or she considers himself or herself different and perhaps even senses an aura of stigma about his or her identity in the school situation. Each child wants to be distinctive, but not different.

An organic defect may lead to feelings of inadequacy and even to extremely deep-seated feelings of inferiority. This occurs even in children with a minor defect. The child may develop aggressive, even belligerent, attitudes as compensation for feelings of inadequacy. Sympathy is resented and leads only to further belligerence.

Fear of ridicule may cause the child to conceal the defect or even deny its existence.

Equally unfortunate is the tendency of some physically handicapped children to segregate themselves from their normal group. They may seek companionship with someone outside of the normal age or peer group. Children of their own age group are willing to accept a handicapped child, but find their efforts frustrated by lack of response on the part of the child with the defect.

A physical disability such as a defect of vision may hinder immediate educational progress, which aggravates the total problem. A combination of defective physical health, emotional maladjustment, and educational retardation more than triples the problem of correction and adaptation. Yet in the social evaluation of child defects these factors may exist in varying degrees. Even partial correction of a physical disorder may be sufficient to reverse the downward trend of maladjustment. To understand that some corrective devices are accepted may aid children in their adjustment. They can be helped to regard themselves as regular accepted members of their peer group. Correction of a defect may be only a starting point that sets off a chain reaction of total readjustment, but the direction of the reaction requires guidance.

Role of the school. A school has no recognized legal responsibility in the correction of children's defects; however, school personnel universally recognize a professional obligation to do everything reasonable to assure that every child with a remediable defect receives the necessary medical treatment. Inherent in teacher ethics is the acceptance of a personal obligation to supplement the medical service with other supporting services the school is in a position to give. The following four objectives will enable the school to fulfill its role in the follow-up program:

1. Promote corrective measures
2. Perform corrective functions
3. Assist in adaptation to noncorrectable defects
4. Rehabilitate after corrective work is done

Promote corrective measures. The most important and frequent function of the school in the follow-up program is the promotion of corrective measures. Although most parents take immediate steps to have their children's defects corrected, some parents will delay action. Lack of concern, lack of finances, lack of appreciation of the necessity for prompt action, wishful hope that some miracle may happen, and even gross neglect are typical causes of delay. None of these is a justifiable reason. In this day of medical insurance there should be no instances of total inability to pay for medical services, but such cases do occur. Yet even with the greatest financial hardship a solution to the problem can be worked out. All children in need of medical care are entitled to that medical care, and means should be devised to give it to them.

When parents have knowledge of their child's disability and the need for correction but neglect to arrange for the necessary medical care, the school can be the catalyst. Diplomacy and persistence may be required, but the goal is worth the effort. A considered methodical plan should be worked out.

The first step in such a plan is to learn whether the family has a definite plan. This information can probably be obtained from the child, an older sibling, the parents, or the family physician or pastor. If the parents have no plan, the school should consider what it may do in the child's behalf. To start with, there should be a conference of interested school personnel who may have something to contribute. Together this group could plan a course of action. Perhaps they will decide to have the school nurse visit and confer with the parents. In the absence of a nurse perhaps the school health director, the principal, or the child's classroom teacher will be designated to make the visit. On these assignments the teacher may have to be a combined salesman-promotor-middleman because the problem is to ensure medical treatment for the child.

When the school representative is not able to convince the parents of the necessity for corrective work, an indirect approach may then be tried by enlisting the assistance of others. Ministers have been successful in these missions. Employers of fathers may be influential. Union officials, lodge members, club members, even relatives of the parents in certain instances have been successful in this role. If the family has a family physician, the logical approach is through him or her. Unfortunately, children who need a physician often have the kind of parents who lack the foresight to see the need for a family physician.

When the basic problem is financial, the school can be helpful. However, the school representative should confer with the parents, who should designate the physician of their choice. They may ask for advice as to which physician to engage. Neither the teacher nor the nurse should designate a particular physician. It is proper, however, to suggest the names of various qualified physicians. If the parents cannot make a decision, it is in order to suggest people with whom they might confer on the choice of a physician. If the parents are totally without funds, an outside source or sources must be found. Several could be considered:

1. Official funds (e.g., Crippled Children's Fund)
2. Voluntary health agency funds (e.g., The National Foundation)
3. Shriners' Hospital
4. Service organizations (e.g., Rotary, Lions, Kiwanis)
5. Parent-Teacher Association
6. Labor union
7. Church group
8. Private individuals
9. Children's clinic

However, before any of these sources are contacted, the school representative, together with the parents, should confer with the designated physician and inform him or her of the willingness of the school to be of assistance. Often, when the physician knows of the financial difficulties of the family, there is no charge for services. No children will go without needed medical service just because their parents lack financial means. The medical profession will make provision for any worthy case. This does not mean that persons with funds for everything except medical service will be permitted to impose on the medical profession, but physicians will always see that worthy persons, especially children, receive the necessary medical care.

When all arrangements between the family and physician have been made and the fee and hospital costs determined, the teacher, the nurse, and other associates can proceed to find the necessary funds. Some schools wisely have stand-by arrangements with organizations and individuals in the event that such funds are needed. Whatever the approach, ingenuity and promotion are essential, but dedication to a worthwhile cause is the indispensable element for success. This dedication projects itself to others and enlists the necessary support.

Many examples are recorded in which teachers, individually and collectively, paid the cost of correction for a child. In some instances the student body has contributed the funds. Perhaps under certain circumstances these measures are acceptable, even commendable, but they would not serve the purpose of an established workable program and may invite some difficulties and even unpleasantries.

It is often a frustrating task to assist children and their families to obtain these specialized services, but most of life's worthy tasks are difficult. The challenge and the gratification of achievement will repay the teacher fully for all the difficulties and sacrifices involved. Every avenue of assistance should be exhausted before the school gives up the attempt to aid a child who is in need of medical care.

Perform corrective functions. Corrective work that no one else seems concerned about and that the school staff is qualified to do offers numerous opportunities for service to pupils. Many deviations from the normal would go unnoticed, unheeded, and unaided except for the assistance the school staff gives. Most of these conditions are minor, but important. A physician is never consulted, and often physicians have little interest or time for these conditions.

Members of the school staff may be competent to aid children with poor posture, poor body mechanics, foot difficulties, malnutrition, and low vitality. In addition, through a modified program for the handicapped the school plays a secondary role in aiding the correction of defects.

Assist in adaptation to noncorrectable defects. It has been the plea of parents and the admonition of physicians that the school help children adapt to noncorrectable defects. It is an assignment the teacher accepts with the knowledge that perhaps no one is in a better position to do the job than the school personnel.

First, the school should accept the task only if it is capable of the assignment and no extreme demands are made of either the staff or other pupils. Second, the school should require a written statement from the supervising physician, which indicates the nature of the child's condition and the role of the school in helping the child to adapt. This should be an established and publicly known

policy. Third, whenever there are indications that the program is not working out as it originally was planned, the physician and parents should be asked to reappraise the original plan. These are steps to protect the teaching staff in the event of serious mishap. Although tragedies or even near tragedies rarely occur, instances of chronic cardiac patients who die on the school premises are solemn reminders that the school needs to anticipate such mishaps and protect itself accordingly.

Usually the major concern for a school-age child with an uncorrected disability is not survival. The problem is to get the child to assume a normal role in the life of the school. If the child cannot attain normal status, then the goal should be as nearly normal as is practical.

Adjustment physically, emotionally, socially, and academically must be fostered. These are not separate entities, but are integrated in the whole child. Adjustment involves many things, but all aspects of adjustment depend on the child's attaining status in school. When he or she gains satisfaction from self-status, the door to adjustment is open.

Nothing is gained by pretending before these children that they do not have a disability; they know that they have one. It is important that they acquire an acceptable understanding of the disability. All of us have shortcomings; ours are just different from theirs. They have to learn to adjust to their problems, just as all of us must adjust to ours. An understanding insight on their part is important. To see themselves fully, they must also be helped to appreciate their assets, capabilities, and outstanding qualities. They should strike a balance between emphasizing their assets and understanding their disability. This approach was indirectly expressed when a high school sophomore remarked, "But I am lame in my left leg," to which his instructor replied, "Yes, but not lame in the head like a lot of people in this world." A single incident rarely has the effect on a person's life that this timely remark had on that boy, who rose to outstanding academic heights.

Often ingenuity is required to satisfy children that they are normal members of the group. The old ruse of having them keep score neither fools nor pleases them. To find some spark of interest and ignite it challenges the best of teachers. Perhaps the child may get personal gratification from being outstanding in some activity or enterprise that others are less skilled in. The crippled boy whose model airplanes were the admiration of all his associates was accepted and held in special esteem. The girl with the cardiac disorder whose skill on the piano made her of special importance in her class was well adjusted and thoroughly enjoyed her role in the school. The school may find it necessary to provide extraschool aid for the child's benefit. Arranging for piano lessons from a private teacher may be the cardinal factor in adjustment and may provide the self-gratifying skill that will enable the child to attain the self-status for which the school is striving.

While one member of the school staff establishes rapport with the child and serves as counselor, several members of the teaching staff may contribute to the child's adjustment. If the aid of selected classmates is enlisted, the school may be able to carry out certain desirable measures and activities that otherwise would not be possible. All that can contribute constructively to the adjustment of a disabled child, including the services of classmates, school personnel, and teaching staff, should be incorporated into the school's plans for the child.

Some schools err in trying to do too much for children who can and want to do things for themselves. If their self-propelled activities do not transcend the acknowledged bounds of their capacities, they should be encouraged in the wholesome interests they manifest.

Rehabilitation after corrective work. Rehabilitation of children who have undergone correction for a defect really consists of effective counseling. First, there should be a thorough study and understanding of children as they are when they reenter school. The child's physical, emotional, intellectual, and academic states should be well understood. Parents and the family physician are the most fruitful sources of information. A school rightfully should expect the physician and parents to provide a comprehensive appraisal of the child. Second, there should be a well-defined course of action that is based on the appraisal of and is the result of a conference with the physician, the parents, and the school. If the physician is not available for such a conference, he or she should either send recommendations to the school or give approval to the plan agreed on by the parents and the school.

Selection of a counselor is imperative. The child will need guidance, which will be considerable at first, but can be reduced as the child is able to assume self-direction. Although the greatest attention must be given to the child's major handicap, rehabilitation includes readjustment of the whole child. Usually the child reentering school has been absent from school because of the correction of a major disability. Adjusting to the physical condition is a major consideration, but rehabilitation will also mean being restored to his or her entire former status.

Rehabilitation can be rapid and uneventful, but usually some difficulties are encountered. The path may be punctuated with setbacks, and progress may be disappointing. A child who has been out of school for months may feel like an outsider and, because of the associated timidity, may not respond to the friendliness of his or her classmates. Some children would never become fully rehabilitated if left to their own resources. More effort is needed for rehabilitation than for normal adjustment. The teacher must use ingenuity to create situations that literally push children into the normal channels of life. Usually they are better able to do things than they think they are. Suggestions and expressions of confidence by the teacher can give the encouragement necessary for satisfactory progress. If children understand their progress, they will be stimulated to further attainment.

Some plans for rehabilitation will prove to be inadequate, and a reappraisal is in order. The reason for the failure of the program may well provide the key to what needs to be done. Change that will yield results, rather than change for the sake of change itself, must be the guide. A modification of the first plan or a new plan that will be more effective may be devised. Or the conferees may be unable to devise a satisfactory plan of action. Before deciding that an agency other than the school must effect the rehabilitation, the teaching staff must agree that the school has exhausted its means. Occasionally the school is unable to rehabilitate a child who has suffered a disability.

DEFECTS THAT ARE THE PROVINCE OF THE PHYSICIAN OR ORTHODONTIST

Every human being is imperfect, but most schoolchildren have imperfections that are negligible in terms of effective, enjoyable living. However, a small percentage will have deviations of consequence, which a skilled physician or orthodontist can correct or relieve. If the teaching staff is familiar with the types of defects of children that physicians and dentists treat, the role of the school in initiating medical treatment and helping in readjustment will be fulfilled more enthu-

siastically and effectively. Understanding both the possibilities and the limitations of professional skills, the school will be in a position to makes its service more realistic and effective.

Orthopedic defects. Literally the term *orthopedic* means straight child (Gr. *ortho*, straight; *paidos*, child), but in its generally accepted sense it refers to conditions of the bones and joints. In their work, orthopedic surgeons are obliged to deal also with muscles, tendons, and ligaments in giving the patient functional joints, proper use of limbs, and a proper skeletal alignment. Although surgery is frequently the method used in correcting orthopedic defects, muscle training as well as mechanical appliances that provide for calculated stresses and strains may be utilized. Orthopedists must implement their scientific background and surgical skill with ingenuity to solve the particular orthopedic problem of each patient.

Fundamentally, the objective of the orthopedist is to restore function to a part compatible with the importance of the need and the risk involved. At times, parents and teachers are disappointed that a child did not benefit more from surgery. Even the finest orthopedic surgeons are not miracle men. They strive to make the most of what the condition offers. If a 20% increase in the use of a joint or a limb is considered in terms of 60 years of usefulness, the true value of the surgery can be appreciated.

About 400,000 school-age children are handicapped by orthopedic impairments. Some are congenital defects that occurred as a result of conditions of the environment before or at the time of birth. An unrecognized and uncontrollable condition present in the body of the mother or an injury at birth accounts for these defects. Congenital defects include clubbed feet (talipes), clubbed hands, and dislocations such as dislocation of the hip. Some disorders may be the result of incomplete development, the cause of which is not known. Among the more common developmental defects are harelip, cleft palate, failure of the vertebrae to fuse (spina bifida), and displacement of internal organs. Most of these prenatal (congenital and developmental) defects are amenable to treatment and usually have been corrected before the child enters school.

The school should assume some responsibility for the early detection of crippling conditions and should see that the child is directed to the proper source for thorough examination. Some of the signs (stigmata) of orthopedic defects the teacher can readily recognize are as follows:

Tilted head
Wryneck
Elevated shoulder
Hollow chest
Narrow chest
Round shoulders
Limp arm
Deformed fingers
Humped back (kyphosis)
Sway back (lordosis)
Backache
Bowleg
Knock-knee
Limp
Unusual gait
Walking on heels or toes
Weak ankles
Toes pointed in or out
Pain in the legs or feet
Calluses, corns, and other growths

It is not the task of the teacher to determine why a child's shoulder is elevated or why a child limps. The function of the school is to identify those children who appear to deviate from the normal. By the early discovery of an incipient defect the teacher and the school can help prevent increased deformity.

Poliomyelitis accounts for about one tenth of the orthopedic defects in school-age children. For practical purposes, children with less than a 20% functional loss in a single muscle or even a muscle group have no limiting handicap. They probably perform within the normal range of physical activity and skill, although they may not be near the top of their group. Children with considerably more functional loss are somewhat handicapped, but compensations can be developed. Children with extreme loss of function in one or more limbs may have to adapt to their physical limitations because the surgeon is not likely to have much to offer. Appliances, muscle training, and even muscle transplants will be of some help in selected cases, but even here an improvement—not a correction—is the best that can be expected.

Cerebral palsy, paralysis as a result of injury of the brain, accounts for about one tenth of the orthopedic disorders in children of school age. It is characterized by irregular gait, awkward movements, lack of balance, and guttural speech. Loss or impairment of control may be in the arms, legs, speech mechanism, or eye movements. There may also be a disturbance of vision, hearing, or other sensory perception and of the intellect. The condition may be caused by injury to the brain before, during, or after birth. Prematurity and congenital malformation of the brain may be factors. Head injuries and diseases such as diphtheria, encephalitis, German measles, scarlet fever, and whooping cough can be postnatal causes. If the damage to the brain is small and does not affect important motor action, the child not only can attend school, but also can be aided by the school activities.

Since muscle training will improve the efficiency of the neuromuscular patterns a child possesses, the school can be highly valuable in the program of muscle training. By supplementing and compensating for the lack of normal action, the child can improve his or her coordination measurably. Here the stimulation and challenge of the school situation are ideal for the development of the motor potential that the child may have. The school can do more therapeutically for some of these children than can the surgeon.

Muscular dystrophy is a biochemical disease characterized by a progressive weakness and wasting away of the muscles. In the United States about 50% of the 200,000 persons with muscular dystrophy are between the ages of 3 and 13 years. The cause is a biochemical irregularity of unknown nature. No pain exists, but certain indications, such as frequent falls, waddling gait, and difficulty in climbing stairs and in assuming a standing position are usually apparent. The pseudohypertrophic type is most common. It begins between the ages of 3 and 10 years, progresses rapidly, and occurs three times more often in males than in females. The onset of the juvenile type may occur during late childhood or even youth. It progresses more slowly, and the incidence for both sexes is about the same. A child with muscular dystrophy can attend school and be happy in the school situation. He or she may need considerable help in moving about. Classmates are usually pleased to be of assistance. The child may pass successively from difficulty in walking, to the use of a wheelchair, and finally to confinement in bed. Muscular dystrophy in itself is not fatal, but death may be due to related disturbances such as weak chest muscles, which affect breathing.

Muscular dystrophy has a genetic basis and can be sex linked. However, a test exists that will determine whether a woman harbors the gene for the defect. If she harbors the gene, half of her sons will have muscular dystrophy. From the standpoint of eugenics, an identified carrier of the trait would choose not to have children.

Accidental injury (trauma) is the cause of about one tenth of the orthopedic impairments present in the school population. Immobile joints, deformed limbs, and amputations usually cause the child's classmates to call him or her a "cripple." It is the difficult task of the school to see that all the children accept the crippled child as a normal member of the group. Most children are solicitous of the one who is handicapped, but a small group will delight in treating the defective with derision. This can best be handled by conferring with the gang and appealing to their sense of fair play. That the teacher expects them to show the way in accepting responsibility for the welfare of the handicapped classmate will appeal to their feeling of importance and social status. Besides aiding the handicapped child, the teacher will be guiding the gang in wholesome development.

Osteomyelitis is an infection of bone usually caused by the staphylococcus organism. It frequently occurs before the age of 10 years and may either develop from an injury or without any known injury. The large bone (tibia) of the lower leg is frequently involved. Early symptoms are pain and inflammation at the site of infection. Early diagnosis and medical care are highly important because in the early stages antibiotics and sulfonamides can be highly effective in eradicating the infection. Later the condition may be intractable and persist as a recurring infection for years.

A child's physician may recommend that the child return to school, even though the infection is not eradicated. The condition is not communicable, and experience indicates that the child may be able to carry on the normal activities of childhood. Indeed, athletes with chronic osteomyelitis have successfully pursued professional careers. An afflicted child will likely give little attention to the infection; therefore the teacher may be helpful in guiding the child in the regimen prescribed by the physician. When the child limps or otherwise favors the diseased member, the matter should be called to the attention of the parents. Renewal or change in treatment may be necessary, and the family physician should be consulted.

Torticollis (wryneck) may be of either prenatal or postnatal origin and is caused by contracted cervical muscles, injury to a neck muscle (sternocleidomastoid), hematoma, or muscle inflammation. Some wryneck conditions are minor and temporary, corrected by medication, heat, and stretching exercises. Others will respond only to surgery. Yet physicians frequently advise against surgery because the wryneck condition has no appreciable effect on general health. If the teacher knows that a child with wryneck has had the benefit of medical counsel, he or she should assume that the condition does not warrant surgery, and the child should be treated as a normal member of the group. When the child has not been examined by a physician, the teacher may be of assistance in obtaining a physician's opinion of the condition.

Other orthopedic disorders of school children also occur. It is important that the school have a medical history as well as the physician's instructions to the school. The school should report to the parents any observable change in the child's condition. Surprisingly often a child with an orthopedic defect develops an abnormal gait or posture. Early recognition by the school of this tendency may enable a physician to correct the abnormality.

Cardiovascular conditions. Correction of heart disorders is definitely limited. Using surgery, a physician may correct a cardiac valvular stricture. Because constriction of the valvular orifice is gradual, this disorder occurs most often in adults. Occasionally, surgery is necessary if a child is to survive. Some heart irregularities can be aided by medication, but the supervising physician is obliged to check the patient closely.

Although total correction of cardiac disorders is infrequent, successful treatment is possible for most patients. Basic to the program of treatment is a daily routine in keeping with the child's capacity. The former concept that a person with a cardiac condition should remain totally inactive has been displaced by a newer belief that these persons should engage in definite but limited activity. With old people the task is to get a person with cardiac disease to be active enough, but with children the task is to prevent the child from becoming too active. The school should have on file a set of instructions from the supervising physician for all children with cardiac disorders. The school would be wise to err on the side of conservatism in order to safeguard against overexertion. Yet the child should have opportunities for normal participation in school pursuits.

Teachers are often surprised when physicians tell them that a child has a murmur but not a defective heart and is not restricted in activities. On the other hand, an organic murmur acquired as a result of infection does limit the cardiac capacity of the child and calls for a restricted regimen. The school can carry out the physician's instruction without isolating the child or causing him or her to feel subnormal.

High blood pressure (hypertension) is usually caused by overstimulation of the constrictor nerves to the arteries. The resulting constriction of the arteries forces the pressure upward. Hypertension is rare in children, but occurs occasionally in high school students, usually in boys. Physicians may prescribe ordinary activities for hypertensive students, but exclude vigorous athletics. Some of these students are permitted to participate in athletics. Whatever the decision of the physician, the school is obligated to carry out his or her written instructions.

Defects of vision. Almost all defects of vision in a school population are amenable to correction. Errors of refraction can be corrected by proper prescriptions for glasses. Thus myopia, hyperopia, and even astigmatism can be corrected. In this instance a mechanical device is the correcting factor. Only a licensed practitioner should prescribe lenses for a child. Occasionally total correction cannot be prescribed. For these children the practitioner prescribes lenses that give the optimum benefit for their most frequent and important needs. Since the condition in a child is not caused by a rigid crystalline lens, as it is in late adulthood, bifocal and trifocal (continuous vision) lenses are of no particular value. Contact lenses can be especially valuable in the treatment of astigmatism.

Although prescription of lenses is in the province of the ophthalmologist, the school can serve in four capacities in the program for correction of defects in vision. First, teachers can refer new students they have reason to believe should have a thorough vision examination. Second, they can assist in obtaining professional service and glasses if needed. Third, teachers can see to it that children wear their glasses. Fourth, they can observe a child who wears glasses, continues to have difficulty in seeing, and should be rechecked by the person who prescribed the glasses. Occasionally a child may need a new prescription in less than a year's time.

Although surgery can correct many eye abnormalities, not all are correctable. Sometimes, if strabismus (squint or cross-eye) is not corrected early, it is not easily remedied after the child has entered late childhood. Eye exercises under the supervision of a specialist in eye alignment (orthoptics) can be helpful. If the dominant eye is covered, the child may be able to focus the squint eye normally. In convergent strabismus (esotropia) or true cross-eye, the short inferior oblique muscle may be lengthened by surgical means, but not all strabismus disorders are operable, even by the most skilled surgeon.

Whenever the school has any doubt about the visual capacity of a child, the parents should be notified and be urged to have the child's vision checked by a licensed practitioner. The school should follow up the referral and request a report of the practitioner's recommendations. Once teachers fully understand the vision range of a child, they can accomplish more effective guidance and can include him or her in the normal routine of school life.

Hearing impairment. To persuade a child that wearing a hearing aid is not a disgrace requires the ingenuity of the best of counselors. Yet it is the key to the remedial program for hearing impairments. When the hearing screening conducted by the teacher or school audiometrist indicates that a child has an appreciable hearing loss, the resistance to an examination by a physician is based on apprehension of a hearing aid and of possible ridicule. Once this resistance has been overcome and the otologist has prescribed a hearing aid, it may be necessary to reinforce the original counseling. Since most childhood hearing loss is the result of rigidity of the conducting apparatus (conduction deafness), a hearing aid is the usual means of correction. A person is fortunate if his or her only defect is one for which a mechanical device can compensate.

Some hearing disorders can be aided by surgery, some even by medication. Obstructions or partial obstructions may be removed, with improvement in hearing. Children who are under continuing treatment for chronic infection of the middle ear or who have a chronic discharge of the ear can attend school without jeopardizing others or themselves. Their physician may instruct the child and the school to avoid certain hazards. These hazards may include showers, swimming pools, chalk dust, vigorous contact play, and exposure to drafts.

Some children with hearing loss may fatigue easily. Both the physical and mental strain imposed by the hearing difficulty will predispose the child to fatigue. As a result, a routine classroom schedule may be sufficiently fatiguing to the child to warrant a special rest period. All factors must be considered in deciding the course of action for the hard-of-hearing child who is unduly fatigued by the day's activities.

Dental defects. It is readily recognized that dental cavities should be corrected by the dentist. Less commonly acknowledged is the urgent need for dental services for the treatment of malocclusion. A child with improper alignment of the dental arches should be treated by an orthodontist before the tooth-bone relationship is permanently established. To wait until a person is 20 years of age may be too late. To shift the teeth at that age may so disturb the alveolar (spongy) bone of the jaw that the teeth will never be well embedded, and both the teeth and the bone are exposed to serious disturbance.

All gum inflammations should be treated by a dentist. Whether the condition is caused by a vitamin C deficiency, accumulation of tartar, or infection, the dentist is best qualified to give the child the needed care. Perhaps the school can be most helpful by reemphasizing preventive measures through health instruction.

Neurological disorders. A child with a serious organic nervous disorder is not likely to be attending school.

St. Vitus' dance (Sydenham's chorea) appears to be the result of toxin that affects centers in the brain. The condition may be associated with rheumaatic fever. Chorea is characterized by involuntary, irregular jerky movements, facial grimacing, irritability, and depression. Although the child may be normal in most respects, other children are distracted by these actions. More important,

the child needs and should have the services of a physician who can do much to relieve the condition.

A *highly nervous child* is not normal and doubtless has a remediable condition. To accept the condition as being merely characteristic of the child is to take a neutral course. The highly nervous child is that way for a reason. Likely the cause can be diagnosed and successful treatment instituted by a physician. If the condition is functional, the school—under the physician's direction—may be especially valuable in helping the child dispel tenseness and attain a normal level of ease and relaxation.

Tic is the designation given to spasmodic movements or twitchings of the face, the head, the neck, the shoulder, or other limited area. These spasmodic peculiar twitchings attract the attention of others, but an afflicted child may be unaware of this peculiarity. A tic usually develops early in life and occurs among school populations. Some tics are psychologically conditioned responses; others have a true neurological basis. Some have no associated emotional complement; others are fundamentally a psychoneurosis. Whatever the cause or nature of the disturbance, a condition exists that demands the best of medical competence.

CORRECTIVE WORK OF THE SCHOOL

Ideally all children with remediable defects should have the benefit of medical advice and care. We live in a realistic world in which the ideal serves as a guide very much as a star serves the mariner for navigation purposes. For various reasons, children with defects or disorders do not always receive medical care. In some instances medical services are not available. In others the available physician does not consider such conditions as mild malnutrition, faulty posture, or sore feet of any great consequence or may consider the condition beneath his or her professional dignity. However, in still other instances the physician may brief the family on what may be done, but they, because of indifference or ignorance, do nothing.

When a child with these apparently minor disorders obviously will receive no help elsewhere, the easiest course for the school is to disclaim any responsibility. Yet the teacher who accepts the fundamental ethics of the profession will do everything possible to promote the best development of the child. Many teachers in this situation, eager to be of some help, have been frustrated by a lack of understanding of what can be done. A working knowledge of some of the more common conditions and of the relatively simple measures that can be highly helpful is all teachers need for the confidence and self-assurance to help children help themselves.

Examples of schools that have undertaken to help children with malnutrition, low vitality, poor posture, and foot conditions are many. In no instances were the results spectacular. In some cases the improvement was relatively small, but nonetheless valuable. In many instances the improvement was considerable. In terms of the long-range effects, even a small health improvement during childhood will assume value of immense proportions in terms of benefit projected over many years.

Malnutrition. Gross malnutrition is rare in the United States school population. However, mild and even moderate nutritional deficiency occurs with greater frequency than is commonly supposed. From a practical standpoint the school is concerned with two basic nutritional problems—obesity and a deficiency of protein and vitamin B_1 and C. Occasionally there will be children with an apparent deficiency in caloric intake, but usually they are deficient in proteins and vitamins, also. An increase in calories can be incorporated into a diet to increase the intake of vitamins and proteins.

Kwashiorkor is a disorder caused by a pronounced protein deficiency and is characterized by muscular weakness, undue fatigue, retarded growth, digestive disturbances, skin pigmentation, and apathy. Symptoms and signs may not be pronounced, but these symptoms indicate a possible need for supplemental protein in the diet.

In *obesity* the basic problem is to decrease the intake of calories or increase the number of calories the body uses in a day. Vigorous prolonged exercise is required to increase the amount of fuel the body burns, a discouraging task for children. In addition, their physical condition may preclude vigorous prolonged activity. A less difficult, but not easy, way to reduce weight is to reduce the daily caloric intake. The assistance the school gives to the child may mean the difference between success and failure. The school merely assists the child. Responsibility rests with the home, and the parents should be urged to seek the services of a physician.

Obese children must be motivated to want to lose weight if they are to overcome the many trials and difficulties of weight reduction. An appeal to their pride in terms of appearance, performance, and self-mastery is important. The reasons for their overeating must be analyzed. Many factors or combinations of factors may contribute to the overeating:

1. A family custom of overeating
2. A release from tension
3. A low blood sugar level that produces constant hunger
4. A poorly balanced high caloric diet

Next, the daily caloric intake must be calculated. From these data the program of action can be formulated.

Obviously the child must understand the plan fully and be impressed with the necessity for adhering to it closely. The basic principle of the plan is to reduce the daily intake by at least 600 calories. Since 4000 calories represent approximately a pound of body weight, the child will average a loss of a pound per week. Several measures can be helpful to the child:

1. The number of meals per day remain the same, the change being a reduction in the amount of food for each meal.
2. As far as possible the fat intake is reduced; otherwise the customary items in the meal are retained.
3. Proteins are substituted for carbohydrates.
4. The water intake at mealtime is reduced.
5. Low calorie wafers, raisins, water, or unsweetened grapefruit halves are used to relieve between-meal hunger.

Always remember that there is no easy, safe way to lose weight.

A sample high protein–low calorie diet indicates that a reducing diet can be reasonably balanced in vitamins and minerals. Sugar, salt, and fats should be omitted. Although this appears to be a spartan diet, it can satisfy hunger. Two weeks on this diet should be sufficient. At that time the child can shift to a diet that is more varied, but has low calorie value.

Breakfast
Grapefruit (no sugar), 2 eggs (not fried), dry toast, skim milk

Lunch
2 eggs (not fried), tomatoes, green vegetable, dry toast, skim milk

Dinner
Steak (not fried), celery, tomatoes, toast, skin milk

Alternate lunches
Fruit salad, toast, skim milk
Combination salad, toast, skim milk, grapefruit
Cold chicken, vegetable salad, skim milk

Alternate dinners
Fish, salad, toast, skim milk, grapefruit
Chicken (not fried), beans, tomatoes, celery, skim milk
Lamb chops (broiled), cabbage, carrots, toast, skim milk

The general condition of the student should be followed. Some uneasiness may occur, and the child will experience a feeling different from normal. Because of a tendency for some bodies to displace burned fat with water, which is heavier, there may actually be an increase in weight at the third day. A new water balance is soon attained, and a sudden drop in weight occurs.

Usually schoolchildren do not display pronounced symptoms of *deficiency disease*. General weakness, chronic fatigue, lack of normal endurance, poor muscle tone, protruding abdomen, sagging posture, strained facial expression, listlessness, irritability, and lack of appetite may indicate inadequate nutrition. These characteristics may be the result of other causes, but in the absence of knowledge of any other cause the need for an improved diet is indicated. When no physician has been engaged and all efforts have failed to have the parents obtain medical counsel for the child, the school—through counseling and the school lunch—should make an effort to help.

First a study of the family's day-to-day menus may be revealing. If the child's diet is deficient, it will likely be inadequate in protein and vitamins B_1 and C. A starting point is to encourage the home to provide foods high in these constituents. Through the parent-teacher association or other source, it may be possible to provide a supplementary lunch program at school. Special midmorning, noon, and midafternoon lunches, high in proteins and vitamins B_1 and C, will likely provide adequate amounts of all nutritional elements.

Sources of protein include eggs, cheese, milk, meat, fish, poultry, nuts, peanut butter, dried beans and peas, bread, and cereals. Sources of vitamin B_1 include liver, lean meat (especially pork), milk, eggs, whole-grain and enriched bread and cereals, wheat germ, nuts, beans, and peas. Sources of vitamin C include citrus fruits, tomatoes, raw cabbage, raw apples, potatoes, and other raw vegetables. Patent vitamin preparations should not be taken except on a physician's prescription.

Child with low vitality. Some children who have no organic defects of any kind seem to lack the vitality necessary for the normal activities of school. They have no outstanding symptoms, but display such general characteristics as listlessness, irritability, short attention span, nervousness, tenseness, frequent illness, frequent absence from school, fatigability, digestive difficulties, and frequent headaches. One or two or several of these factors may be present. Life seems to be a trial, and these youngsters do not seem to be able to function at a maximum rate.

Several factors or combinations of factors may account for the sluggishness. Habit, lack of rest, poor nutrition, lack of interest in school life or life in general, natively slow reactions, general depression, constitutionally sluggish response to fatigue conditions, imitation of members of the family or others as an attention-getting device, or even an escape mechanism—all may be involved. It is almost impossible to single out one factor as *the* factor. To reduce the cause to two or three factors would be excellent progress. As far as possible, the best approach is to remove or to modify these factors. A duty-obsessed teacher may make the child's school life unbearable. To drive this type of youngster is rarely successful. Situations that will modify the deficiencies through a gradual process can produce tangible results. Stimulation, encouragement, patience, and appreciation of the child's success will be helpful.

Vitality is a psychophysiological pattern, and both the psychological and physiological aspects must be considered. It may be helpful to reschedule the daily routine, including shorter sessions with television, a new sleep cycle (perhaps with a noon-hour rest), and new diet and meal habits (with midmorning and midafternoon snacks). A physical activity such as table tennis could be helpful. Participation in school activities such as dramatics may challenge the child. Setting realistic deadlines may speed up the work pace. He or she may never attain a satisfactory level of vitality, but an acceptable level can be attained with diligence and persistence.

Posture defects. A defect of posture caused by a structural disorder certainly is a problem for the orthopedic surgeon. If the bony architecture is out of alignment or a skeletal malformation exists, immediate referral to the parents and then to the surgeon is in order. However, most poor posture observed in schoolchildren is not caused by skeletal disorders.

Slovenly habits in standing and sitting can be responsible for poor posture. An appeal to pride in personal appearance and a plan for improvement can be initiated through counseling. If the whole class develops a consciousness of posture, it will lend support to a child who needs especially to improve his or her posture. The group effect is motivating to all. It sincerely is hoped that there will be no best posture contests.

Poor muscle tone following the effects of illness, malnutrition, focal infection, or inadequate rest will cause poor posture. The first step must be to correct the basic cause. Muscle tone can be built up gradually through planned activity.

Round shoulders is the most common posture defect among schoolchildren and is particularly prevalent among junior and senior high school students. The condition results from continuous activities in which the arms are held in front of the body. Most normal activities require the arms to be in front of one. The shoulders and arms are held forward by the continuous contraction of the muscles (pectoralis) of the chest. As a result, the relatively powerful pectoral muscles gradually shorten, increase in strength and bulk, and develop a tonus out of all proportion to the light muscles that draw the shoulder blades back. The strong muscles of the chest thus keep the shoulders drawn forward. The pectoral muscles must be stretched in order for the condition to be corrected.

The *gravity method* for the correction of round shoulders aims primarily, by an easy and simple process, to stretch the chest muscles and thus permit the architecture of the shoulder to assume its normal form. This is done by applying the force of gravity in such a way that the body weight produces the muscle strain.

First, the teacher measures the distance between the inner borders of the child's shoulder blades when they are drawn back moderately. Then a wooden block, 3 inches wide, is cut to a length ½ inch greater than the distance measured between the borders of the shoulder blades (Fig. 10-1). The *thickness* of the block will depend on the size of the child and the severity of the condition. The block should be somewhat thinner than normal for a severe condition and somewhat thicker for a mild condition:

> Senior high school age, 1¾ inches
> Junior high school age, 1½ inches
> Intermediate school age, 1¼ inches

The block is placed flat on the floor, and the subject lies so that the inner borders of the shoulder blades rest on the ends of the block, the block overlapping about one fourth inch on each shoulder blade. If the head rests on the floor and the arms are bent slightly and raised above the head, the pectoral muscles will be stretched (Fig. 10-2). The subject should feel a decided pull on the chest muscles. In the first trial the child

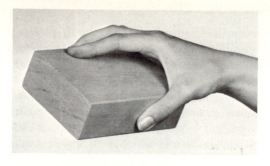

Fig. 10-1. Wooden block. For this particular subject a block 5 inches long, 3½ inches wide, and 1½ inches thick served perfectly.

should not remain in position for more than 3 minutes because a soreness will develop in the chest area. Each day the time is increased about 1 minute until the period reaches about 10 minutes.

If no pull is felt on the pectorals, the block is too thin or too long. As the round shoulder condition improves, the block must be made thicker by the addition of a one fourth inch piece to the bottom of the block. In some cases it is necessary to cut the block shorter as the condition improves.

Experience has demonstrated that morning, immediately after one arises, is the most convenient for lying on the block. More than 10 minutes on the block at a time is neither advisable nor necessary. The merit of the gravity method lies in its simplicity; yet it yields a maximum result, with a minimum of time and effort.

Foot conditions. Gross foot deformities require orthopedic care, and through one of the many channels available an affected child should receive orthopedic treatment. Gross abnormalities of the foot are usually corrected. It is the so-called nuisance types of foot conditions that never receive professional attention. Most physicians have very little interest in corns, calluses, perspiring feet, tender feet, or low arches. Podiatrists are professionally prepared to care for foot

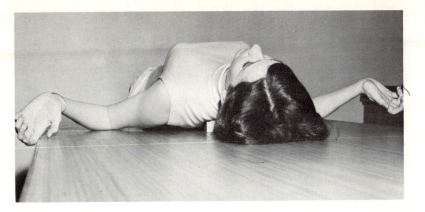

Fig. 10-2. Position of subject while resting on the block. The chest is arched, the shoulders do not touch the floor, and the weight of the arms stretched above the head exerts a pull on the chest muscles.

disabilities, but their services are available in few communities outside of metropolitan areas. In consequence, both adults and children frequently suffer from foot difficulties that would readily respond to treatment, but no service is available.

It is surely not the function of the school to treat foot disorders. Yet the school can be of service to children with foot difficulties by helping them obtain professional treatment from a physician or a podiatrist. Examination by a physician first is logical. If the condition is one for treatment by a podiatrist, the physician will recommend that course of action. If it is not, he or she will recommend treatment that is in the best interests of the child.

A teacher with a working knowledge of common foot disabilities will have a better appreciation of the problems involved and the essential action that should be undertaken. A painful condition of the feet markedly reduces effective and enjoyable living, causes general bodily fatigue, and contributes to premature aging. An informed teacher may help children to better health by helping them solve their foot troubles.

Foot strain involves the muscles, tendons, and ligaments essentially. The foot may appear to be normal, but be tender and painful on walking. Or there may be acute marked swelling, pain, tenderness, and spasm (cramp). If the condition is to be relieved, improper weight-bearing, faulty posture, improper shoes, or other causes must be eliminated. If the cause is improper weight-bearing, a person should walk as little as possible and keep the feet elevated as much as is practical. Severe strain may mean that one must remain in bed until the swelling and pain have disappeared. Contrast baths (30 seconds warm alternated with 30 seconds cool) or whirlpool baths are helpful. All exercise should be at a minimum during the painful period.

Morton's painful foot is characterized by cramps or sharp pains at the ball of the foot because of a fallen metatarsal arch. Any condition that throws the weight forward on the transverse arch may cause it to become concave and thus pinch nerves. As a first measure it is necessary to correct the cause of the forward weight-bearing. Artificial support for the fallen arch relieves the pain. Piano felt pads or commercial pads serve. Any child with a fallen metatarsal arch needs immediate care. Because of the flexibility of youthful structures, corrective measures can be highly effective. If it is permitted to persist, a fallen arch can mean lifelong foot trouble.

Plantar callus may form under the metatarsal arch as a result of constant rubbing caused by ill-fitting shoes or foot imbalance. In its early stage the callus is a symptom of an abnormal condition and a warning of trouble ahead. To remove the callus by medicated applications is advisable, but to correct the cause of the callus is the important thing.

A *plantar wart* is a wart on the sole of the foot. If the wart is on a weight-bearing area of the foot, a child may suffer intense pain. Since a wart can persist for years, immediate means should be taken to remove it. If a podiatrist is not available, the application of salicylic acid in colodion twice daily will destroy the wart in about 2 weeks. If the wart is embedded in a heavy callus, three weeks or more may be required to remove it. A sterile gauze-adhesive pad over the wart will help to prevent infection. Constant vigilance should be exercised to prevent infection, and immediate attention is imperative if it appears.

Pes planus is a condition in which the arch is low, but the foot is normal. Contrary to popular belief, a low arch can be an excellent arch.

Pes cavus is a condition in which the arch is high and the foot is normal. The arch is excellent in this condition, also.

Weak arches tire because of weak musculature. Exercises that flex the arches are helpful. An excellent exercise is to roll the arch over a 4-inch roller and attempt to grasp the roller with the arch and toes. An equally good exercise is to attempt to pick up a marble or a pencil with the toes. Wrapping the arch with a stirrup bandage could be a temporary measure. The integrity of the foot should be attained as soon as possible.

Tender feet can be relieved by contrast baths followed by covering the foot with tincture of benzoin compound. This is a sticky fluid that should be covered with clean white cotton socks and is highly effective in toughening the skin.

A *corn* is an accumulation of dead cells piled on one another. It results from friction and pressure that irritate the skin and cause an increase in the rate of cell division. Pressure on the sensitive nerves beneath the corn gives rise to the pain. Corns themselves have neither nerves nor roots. Most corns are on top of the toes, but soft corns form between the toes and seed corns form on the sole.

Corns are important as an index of foot imbalance, improperly fitting shoes, or other condition that calls for correction. A corn should never be cut with a knife or other instrument. Danger of infection is too great. Common medicaments are acceptable, but, after the corn has been lifted and until firm tissue forms at the site where it was lodged, a gauze pad should be applied to prevent infection. Podiatrists remove corns easily and safely.

Achilles bursitis is an inflammation of a fluid-filled sac along the tendon of Achilles. It results from overexertion and the resulting strain or from trauma. The condition is usually temporary and can be readily corrected if the foot is rested as much as possible, preferably in an elevated position.

Speech defects. Various studies reveal that about 1,000,000 children in United States schools have speech defects. Generally speech is considered to be defective when it deviates sufficiently to attract the attention of others or causes some difficulty in communication. Many persons have speech defects that are so minor as to be negligible. Yet if correction of the defect is possible, the individual should have the benefit of the correction. However, many youngsters have serious speech impediments, and, because speaking is very important in academic, social, and other relationships, the school should make every effort to assist in correcting these impediments. If the school does not help, in most cases there is no other recourse.

The mental health rather than the physical health of the child is of concern here. Of itself, a speech impediment can be an obstacle to normal mental health. Combined with one or more other factors, it can be an insurmountable handicap to wholesome adjustment.

Speech examination for every schoolchild by a qualified examiner is the ideal. Except for metropolitan areas few schools have such a service. As a consequence, classroom teachers must recognize speech difficulties. It is fortunate if as a part of their professional training teachers have had work in the recognition of speech disorders. After the teacher recognizes that a child has a speech difficulty, an examination by a speech clinician or speech correctionist should follow. A correctionist or teacher with special training should carry out the recommendations of the examinations. This is a task for a specialist, not for an unqualified person.

If a speech clinic or speech correction specialist is available, even at some distance, a diagnosis and suggested training program can be extremely valuable because the parents and teacher can carry out the necessary training under the supervision of the specialist. An effective program can be devised for almost every child with a speech impediment if the school is resolved that something shall be done for him or her.

MODIFIED PROGRAM FOR THE HANDICAPPED

In discussing the school's role in educating the handicapped, it should be recognized that the focus here is on the follow-up and remedial services for the so-called "normal" or typical child. However, it is very important to call attention to Public Law 94-142, the Education for All Handicapped Children Act, and the implications that this legislation holds for the total school health program, including health instruction, health services, and the healthful school environment.

Specifically, the legislation requires that every state educational agency provide for the education of children with special needs. Without regard as to the cause of those handicapping conditions, whether the result of physical, mental, or social problems, communities must provide for "free, appropriate" public education for all handicapped students. Moreover, it is required that the program be specifically planned to meet the unique needs of the individual student, and that the educational programs be provided in the "least restrictive" environment possible.

Many states have a crippled children's commission and have established schools to give the special training handicapped children often require. Although nobly conceived, these schools do not solve the problem even in the most populous states. Many parents will not permit handicapped children to leave home to be domiciled at these schools, which are usually located in a central section of the state.

In large school systems special programs and even special schools, staffed with qualified experts, have been established for the handicapped. Small systems as well as those of moderate size do not feel financially able to support such a program. Yet every school can do something for handicapped children. Numerous possibilities are open. Many states subsidize the program for the handicapped of local school districts. This subsidy usually applies to any standard local program of special classes, home instruction, or modification of the regular classroom program.

Special classes, particularly on the elementary school level, have been effective. Specialists in various phases of education, including occupational therapists, have been engaged for these classes. In some situations a single teacher is used to fulfill the requirements of the children. This is exceptional, since a teacher-student ratio of about 10 to 1 is usual. Ramps, wheelchairs, cots, and other special provisions may have to be supplied. Special lighting may be necessary. The needs of some handicapped children can best be met by these special classes, but other handicapped children such as those with a heart condition or hearing impairment may resent the class. From the mental health aspect the special class could be a liability for certain children. Selection of students for the special class must be a carefully considered process.

Home instruction can be made effective for many handicapped youngsters. Capable visiting teachers and a good home situation can provide an adequate education. However, home instruction is not always satisfactory. Poor light, distractions, inadequate ventilation, and lack of sanitation are not conducive to effective learning. In addition, the child is there 24 hours a day, which tends to produce a monotonous, stultifying atmosphere that only outside diversion can pierce.

It is apparent that with modifications most handicapped children can be fitted into the regular school organization. What should these modifications be and how are they to be determined? An effective plan can be based on individualization of instruction. A counseling team sets the basic policies. Using these policies, the team with the assistance of other teachers makes a thorough study of each case that involves a handicapped child. The collective judgment of this group produces a proposed program for the child in question. The teacher or teachers who will be in day-to-day contact with the child should be given a complete picture of the counselors' recommendations. After this review the final program is put into operation, with reappraisals as necessary from time to time.

As far as possible handicapped children should be accepted as normal members of the group and should live a normal school life. Adjustments should be made in accordance with their assets and liabiilties. Goals and standards should be realistic. Children must have reasonable insight into their abilities and limitations; otherwise they may be too ambitious, with resulting disillusionment. Or they may lack incentive to reach the standards of which they are capable.

The situation requires a teacher who is adept at adjustment and improvisation and is skillful in dealing with problem situations. A confidential relationship with the child is especially important. To make necessary adaptations in terms of the child's capacities while retaining the child's feeling of being a normal member of the group challenges the most ingenious of teachers.

Modification of any one phase or all phases of the program for the benefit of a handicapped child should not be made at the expense of all other children. This is both unnecessary and unjustified. When a handicapped child upsets or seriously affects the normal program, a thorough reappraisal is necessary. There may be agencies other than the school or persons other than the teachers who have more to offer a particular handicapped child than does the school and the teacher. When the child is a constant disrupting element in the classroom, in justice to the 30 or more other children, outside agencies or persons should be requested to assume the guidance of the handicapped child. This action should be taken only after the school has exhausted all its resources.

QUESTIONS AND EXERCISES

1. How can a physical defect adversely affect mental health?
2. What can be the relationships between a physical defect and academic performance?
3. If full restoration of function is not possible, why should measures be taken to achieve partial recovery of function?

4. Lack of family financial means should but increase the determination of the school to obtain the necessary medical services for the child needing correction of a defect. Explain the implications of this statement.

5. In advance of any need for providing medical corrective services for a child whose parents are without funds, what can a school do in the way of setting up a program and procedures for taking care of this type of situation?

6. Are there any circumstances in which a teacher should pay for medical correction for a child in the school where he or she teaches?

7. What can be done for children with noncorrective orthopedic defects to help them be normal members of their class and to give them the type of self-gratification from accomplishment that all normal youngsters want and need?

8. In any rehabilitation why is it important that one person have primary responsibility, even though the services of many persons may be utilized?

9. When a teacher recognizes that a child has a physical disorder, why should the teacher relate this to the school nurse and then to the school principal before anything is done on behalf of the child?

10. In a program to help a student adjust to a physical defect, why is it important to have the student develop a strong insight in terms of his or her status, needs, and progress?

11. How would you get a child to wear prescribed glasses when he or she does not want to wear them?

12. A high school junior is somewhat bitter and resentful that he has a hearing loss requiring the use of a hearing aid. How would you counsel with the youth to help him see the situation in a more wholesome light?

13. How would you convince high school students of the importance of dental examinations and immediate correction?

14. If the only persons dieting to reduce their obesity are those under the supervision of a physician, there would be very few people trying to lose weight. What are the implications of this statement?

15. A person must be highly motivated to stay on a reducing diet. What are some of the factors that can be used to motivate an obese high school girl to stay on a diet?

16. How would you impress on high school students the importance of having a high-protein breakfast every day?

17. Which usually is first—poor posture or poor health?

18. "Round shoulders" is a common posture defect of junior high school girls. Set up a program to improve the posture of the girls in a junior high school.

19. Why are girls more frequently bothered with foot problems than are boys?

20. What can a small school system do to provide a modified program for the handicapped pupils?

REFERENCES AND SELECTED READINGS

American Association of School Administrators: Health in schools, twentieth yearbook, Washington, D.C., 1957, National Education Association.

American Alliance for Health, Physical Education, and Recreation: Appraisal of school children, ed. 4, 1970, Washington, D.C., The Alliance.

Archer, E.: Let's face it: a guide to good grooming, ed. 2, Philadelphia, 1968, J. B. Lippincott Co.

Bach, M.: The power of total living, New York, 1977, Dodd, Mead & Co.

Barrett, M.: Health education guide, ed. 2, Philadelphia, 1974, Lea & Febiger.

Beyer, M. K., et al.: Positive health: designs for action, ed. 2, Philadelphia, 1976, Lea & Febiger.

Blumenfeld, A.: Heart attack: are you a candidate? New York, 1971, Pyramid Publications, Inc.

Dalzell-Ward, A. J.: A textbook of health education, ed. 2, New York, 1975, Barnes & Noble Books.

Daniels, A. S., and Davies, E. A.: Adapted physical education, ed. 3, (School and public health education), New York, 1975, Harper & Row, Publishers.

Gabrielson, I. W., et al.: Factors affecting school health follow-up, Am. J. Public Health **57** Jan. 1967.

Hanson, D.: Health-related fitness, Belmont, Calif, 1970, Wadsworth Publishing Co., Inc.

Jenne, F. H., and Greene, W. H.: Turner's school health and health education, ed. 7, St. Louis, 1976, The C. V. Mosby Co.

Jones, K. L., et al.: Principles of health science, New York, 1975, Harper & Row, Publishers.

Licht, S. H., editor: Therapeutic exercise, ed. 2, New Haven, Conn., 1961, Physical Medicine Library.

Mayshark, C., Shaw, D. D., and Best, W. H.: Administration of school health programs: its theory and practice, ed. 2, St. Louis, 1977, The C. V. Mosby Co.

Montoye, H. J.: Physical activity and health, Englewood Cliffs, N.J., 1975, Prentice-Hall, Inc.

Nemir, A.: The school health program, ed. 4, Philadelphia, 1975, W. B. Saunders Co.

Oberteuffer, D., and Beyrer, M. K.: School health education, ed. 5, New York, 1972, Harper & Row, Publishers.

Physicians and schools, report of the 1967 National Conference on Physicians and Schools, Chicago, 1967, Department of Health Education, American Medical Association.

Rathbone, J. L.: Corrective physical education, ed. 7, Philadelphia, 1965, W. B. Saunders Co.

Rathbone, J. L., and Lucas, C.: Recreation in total rehabilitation, Springfield, Ill., 1975, Charles C Thomas, Publisher.

Suggested responsibilities of the administrator, teacher, medical advisor, and nurse for the health of school children, Sacramento, 1953, California State Department of Education.

Wallin, J. E. W.: Education of mentally handicapped children, New York, 1965, Harper & Row, Publishers.

Wheatley, G. M., and Hallock, G. T.: Health observation of school children, ed. 3, New York, 1965, McGraw-Hill Book Co.

PART FOUR

Health instruction

CHAPTER 11

Health education and health behavior: the foundation of health instruction

Health educators and other health professionals have long called for a national commitment to good health as a way of life. Hilleboe (School Health Education Study, 1967), former New York State Director of Public Health, felt that achievement of this goal would require the implementation of a comprehensive program of health education beginning in the early years of school and extending throughout the entire life span. Health education should be one of the most dynamic components of the entire school curriculum, a program to achieve the goals of both education and public health.

The American public is evidencing a new awareness of health education and its potential for improving the nation's health. *Forward Plan for Health* (U.S. Department of Health, Education and Welfare, 1975), stated that "it has become apparent that the best hope of achieving any significant extension of life expectancy lies in the area of disease prevention." In 1978, Joseph Califano (Nightingale et al., 1978), then Secretary of the Department of Health, Education and Welfare, stressed the importance of emphasis on disease prevention and called attention to the potential of school health education in this regard.

It has become increasingly evident to medical researchers and the general public alike that many of today's health problems are caused by factors that are not responsive to medical solutions. For example, at this time there is no vaccine to prevent heart disease and no cure for the problem of alcoholism. Short of a dramatic breakthrough, such as the development of a cure for cancer, it is becoming apparent that further expansion in the nation's health care system will produce only marginal improvements in the health status of Americans. Although it is obvious that providing the best health care for all citizens is of great importance, it is also apparent that, in the long run, the greatest benefits to the health of the public are most likely to come from efforts to improve the life-style and the environment in which they live and work (U.S. Department of Health, Education and Welfare, 1975).

As a result of this thinking, a new emphasis is being placed on the behavioral aspects of health. Richmond (Nightingale, et al., 1978), on taking the oath of office as the nation's highest ranking health officer, stated that the importance of behavioral research must be recognized so that we can:

. . . discover how to enlist people into preventing disease and in promoting their own health. This means that health education encompasses not only the transmission of knowledge but also the full range of activities designed to provide the skills, the interest and the motivation to help make people's lives more fulfilling and free from disease and disability.*

PURPOSE AND ETHICS OF HEALTH EDUCATION

Over the years, members of the field of health education have attempted to develop a philosophy or point of view and have articulated a set of goals or a statement of purpose. These definitions not only reveal the intent of the particular time but also illustrate the growth and change in purpose that has occurred.

In 1934, the Joint Committee (NEA-AMA) on Health Problems in Education proposed the following definition: "Health education is the sum of all experiences which favorably influences habits, attitudes, and knowledge relating to individual, community, and racial health." This statement recognized that all of life's experiences, both in and out of school, contribute to the individual's attitudes toward health as well as patterns of living. Any formal health education planned by the school must recognize those forces outside of the school that shape the health behaviors of children and youth.

The 1948 Joint Committee (NEA-AMA) statement emphasized that ". . . health education is the process of providing learning experiences for the purpose of influencing knowledge, attitudes, or conduct relating to individual, community, and world health."

This definition stresses the role of the school in providing learning experiences through a formal and planned program of health instruction. The statement also provides guidance as to the purpose of the curriculum. For classroom learning to have a positive effect on what students think, feel, and do about health in the community and the world at large, it must deal with contemporary problems of society.

The inclusion of world health in this definition reflects awareness of the World Health Organization, which had been created during this period. The World Health Organization (WHO) issued its widely quoted definition on health as a state of complete physical, mental, and social well-being and not merely the absence of disease and disability. In 1954, WHO (Expert Committee, First Report, 1954) addressed the subject of health education with the following statement:

The aim of health education is to help people achieve health by their own actions and efforts. Health education begins, therefore, with the interests of people in improving their condition of living . . . in developing a sense of responsibility for their own health betterment and for . . . the health of their families and governments.*

This statement has proved especially useful to health educators working in countries other than the United States, enabling them to relate more effectively to people of different cultures and ethnic groups. It has served as a reminder to public health and school officials that health education is not something to be done for or to be given to people. Rather, if it is to be truly educational, it is a process that causes change within the person through changes in knowledge and attitudes. In turn, health education is reflected in what

---

*From Nightingale, E. O., et al.: Perspectives on health promotion and disease prevention in the United States, Washington, D.C., 1978, Institute of Medicine, National Academy of Sciences.

*Expert Committee on Health Education of the Public: First Report, World Health Organization Technical Report Series No. 89, Geneva, Switzerland, 1954, World Health Organization, p. 4.

the individual does for himself or herself and for others in order to promote well-being and prevent illness and injury.

With the upsurge of public interest in health education in the 1970s, more statements have been issued. Like the earlier statements, these served to clarify the evolving and emerging role of health education. The statement of the President's National Committee on Health Education (1973), issued in 1972, is illustrative.

Health education is a process that bridges the gap between health information and health practices. Health education motivates the person to take information and do something with it, to keep himself/herself healthier by avoiding actions that are harmful and by forming habits that are beneficial.*

Here again, the emphasis on process is apparent, speaking to the relationship between health information and health education. Only after health information is translated into health knowledge, understanding, and action does it become health education. In the schools the process of health instruction translates health information into health outcomes.

Following the President's Committee statement, the Joint Committee on Health Education Terminology (1972-1973) issued a revised definition of health education as:

. . . a process with intellectual, psychological, and social dimensions relating to activities which increase the abilities of people to make informed decisions affecting their personal, family, and community well-being. This process, based on scientific principles, facilitates learning and behavioral change in both health personnel and consumers including children and youth.†

*President's Committee on Health Education: The report of the president's committee on health education, New York, 801 Second Ave., 1973.
†Report of the 1972-1973 Joint Committee on Health Education Terminology prepared by representatives of the American Academy of Pediatrics, American Association for Health, Physical Education, and Recreation, American School Health Association, American Public Health Association, and Society for Public Health Education.

This statement also emphasizes the idea of process, but it recognizes that education is more than an intellectual experience. Emotional and social factors also shape health understandings and behaviors. But perhaps the part of the definition that is of most importance in the development of a philosophy of health education is the expression "the abilities of people to make informed decisions." This suggests that enabling the individual to make an informed decision about health is the central purpose of health education. Moreover, it implies that decision making is the prerogative of the individual. Although it is the teacher's responsibility to create the opportunities for decision making through the health instruction program, students must be given freedom to make decisions. If children and youth are to grow to full maturity, and if they are to become health-educated citizens of tomorrow, they must be allowed to make decisions, choices, and even mistakes in the realm of health. The challenge of the health teacher and of parents in matters affecting health is to know when to lead, when to guide or control, and when to let the young person make the choice.

Sullivan (U.S. Department of Health, Education and Welfare, 1977), in writing for health planning agencies, has suggested that a program of health education should meet the following criteria:

1. It should be consistent with current knowledge about how people learn.
2. It should be consistent with the rights of individuals to make their own decisions about health practices as long as these practices do not infringe on the rights of others.
3. The definition should be readily understood not only by the health educator specialist but also by the public at large.*

*U.S. Department of Health, Education and Welfare: Educating the public about health: a planning guide, Washington, D.C., Oct., 1977, Public Health Service Health Resources Administration.

The fact that these criteria apply primarily to programs geared to the health needs of the adult population suggests the need for an additional criterion. It should emphasize that adults must accept responsibility for the health and safety of the young and immature. For example, it is one thing for college students to make decisions and choices about their diets or about their physical exercise program, but it is quite another matter for primary grade children to make a choice about crossing the street. Health-related decisions and actions are highly specific to the individual and to the social and environmental setting. It must also be emphasized that in defining any program in health education, the information presented must be consistent with the scientifically established knowledge.

CODE OF ETHICS

Health educators, in addition to establishing criteria for health education, have attempted to clarify the relationship between the health educator and the student or client. The Society for Public Health Education, Inc., has adopted the code of ethics given below to guide health educators in their efforts to promote the health of all people through education.

THE CONTRIBUTION OF HEALTH EDUCATION TO HEALTH

The American Public Health Association, at its annual meeting in 1977, formally acknowledged the essential relationship of health education to the achievement of the association's goals of optimum health for the

---

CODE OF ETHICS*

Health educators, in utilizing educational processes to influence human well-being and to change health behavior, take on profound and grave responsibilities. Although ethical beliefs are a matter of personal choice, the values we have selected for ourselves must be constantly re-examined and modified. The nature, importance, and magnitude of health education is such that there is a potential for ethical abuse. To reduce the chances of abuse in health education and to guide professional behaviors of health educators toward the highest standards, the following code of ethics is adopted by and for the profession.

Principles

1. Health educators do not discriminate because of race, color, religion, age, sex, national ancestry, or socio-economic status in rendering service, hiring, promotion, or training.
2. Health educators observe the principle of informed consent with respect to individuals and groups served.
3. Health educators value privacy, dignity, and worth of the individual, and use skills consistent with these values.
4. Health educators maintain their competence at the highest levels through continuing study, training, and research.
5. Health educators foster an educational environment which nurtures individual growth and development.
6. Health educators support change by choice, not by coercion.
7. Health educators as researchers or practitioners report activities and findings honestly and without distortion.
8. Health educators accurately represent their competence, education, training, and experience and act within the boundaries of their professional competence.
9. Health educators are aware of unprofessional practices, and are accountable for taking appropriate action to eliminate these practices.

*Courtesy Society for Public Health Education: Code of ethics, San Francisco, Oct. 15, 1976, Society for Public Health Education, Inc.

nation's population. Today, more than ever, methods of improving the public's health status focus on health education. The conviction is growing among health professionals that major advances in health status will come from changes in the life-styles of individuals and from the control of health hazards in the environment. It is through the process of education that citizens in a democratic society are alerted to the personal and societal obstacles to good health. Health education offers a channel for achieving the needed changes.

Because of the complexity of factors that interact to affect health, including the environment, social conditions, and institutional and economic politics (Fig. 11-1), the solving of health problems often requires coordinated action on the part of informed citizens. From the public health perspective, then, the goal of health education is

the health-educated consumer-citizen who adopts a health-promoting life-style and wisely selects and uses health care resources, products, and services. Ideally, this citizen will actively participate in the formulation of public policy and planning on health care issues and in the larger environmental matters that affect health (American Public Health Association, 1977).

One of the most useful of statements issued thus far on the goals of consumer health is that of the Task Force Report on Consumer Health Education (Preventive Medicine USA, 1976). This report, one of eight provided by the American College of Preventive Medicine and the Fogarty International Center for Advanced Study in the Health Sciences, has served as the basis for the Department of Health, Education and Welfare *Forward Plan for Health*, FY 1976-80. According to the Task Force, the term *con-*

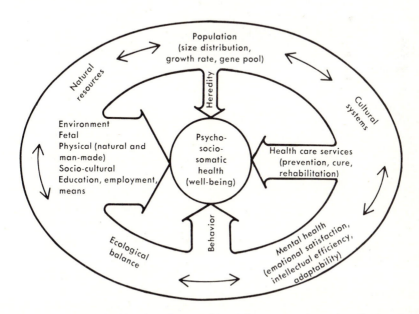

Fig. 11-1. Blum's inputs to health. The relative widths of the arrows indicate the relative importance attached to the various inputs. By inference, health education (behavior) is seen to make a major contribution to health. (From Blum, H. L.: Planning for health: development and application of social change theory, New York, 1974, Human Sciences Press.)

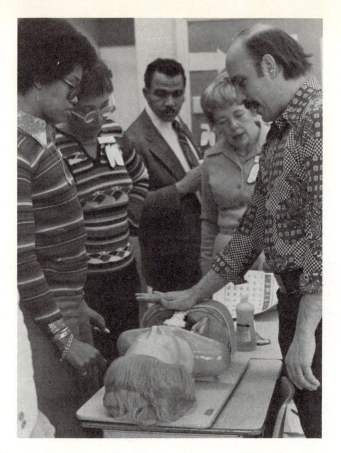

Fig. 11-2. Health educator explaining cardiopulmonary resuscitation (CPR) technique to a group of fellow teachers.

sumer health education subsumes a set of activities that serve to:

1. Inform people about health, illness, disability, and ways in which they can improve and protect their own health, including more efficient use of the delivery system;
2. Motivate people to want to change to more healthful practices;
3. Help them to learn the necessary skills to adopt and maintain healthful practices and lifestyles;
4. Foster teaching and communications skills in all those engaged in educating consumers about health;
5. Advocate changes in the environment that facilitate healthful conditions and healthful behavior; and
6. Add to knowledge via research and evaluation concerning the most effective ways of achieving the above objectives.

In brief, consumer health education is a process that informs, motivates, and helps people to adopt and maintain healthy practices and lifestyles, advocates environmental changes as needed to facilitate this goal, and conducts professional training and research to the same end.*

If the American Public Health Association statement provides the broad general goal for health education, the Task Force statement

---

*Preventive Medicine USA: Health promotion and consumer health education, A Task Force Report sponsored by the John E. Fogarty International Center for Advanced Study in the Health Sciences National Institutes of Health and the American College of Preventive Medicine, New York, 1976, Prodist.

spells out the details and activities that characterize an effective action program. The specificity of these activities makes it clear that health education includes informing, motivating, and helping people to acquire the skills needed to protect and promote health and to recover from illness. The program pertains to people of all ages and levels of health—the young, the aged, the handicapped, and the healthy. It covers more than academic, scientifically derived knowledge, including actions and practical skills ranging from the principles of diet selection to the life-saving skills of cardiopulmonary resuscitation (CPR) (Fig. 11-2). For the professional health educator, this statement carries a special message: to function effectively, teaching and communication skills are essential. Moreover, like any other successful program activity, health education must rest on a scientific basis of on-going research and evaluation.

A THEORETICAL BASIS FOR HEALTH EDUCATION

A theoretical statement involves terms that cannot be observed directly but that are inferred from a great deal of data. According to Snow (Travers, 1978), what first may be considered a theoretical term later may be found to refer to real objects or events. An abstract idea or theory may become fact. This relationship between theoretical statements and factual reality is well illustrated by Darwin's early ideas about evolution. Two theoretical statements, the theory of "natural selection" and the "survival of the fittest," served to guide his observations and collection of data. Darwin observed that many more individual organisms were born that could survive. Among those that survived, Darwin noted that some were born stronger, swifter, with more protective coating, or with less conspicuous marking, blending more readily into their natural surroundings.

Those born stronger, swifter, and more suited to their environments were more likely to survive, thus perpetuating those organisms having the more favorable variations (Moore and Editors of Life, 1964). Hence through evolution the surviving species or organism becomes ever more attuned to the environment.

A theory is a set of interacting, interlocking, or independent principles designed to account for a wide range of observations or facts (Bugelski, 1971). Travers (1978) contends that the behavioral sciences have been much less successful than the physical sciences in developing theories that eventually can be proved in the real world. In fact, many of the behavioral science theories have remained just that—theoretical abstractions, with little or no progress toward predicting real events. This discouraging fact does not diminish the importance of theories in science, for no science of any consequence has yet been built without employing theoretical terms. Therefore it becomes necessary to develop a productive theory of health behavior change on which to base health education programs.

What purpose does theory serve and how does it serve the field of health education? In the broadest sense, a theory is a way of interpreting knowledge. The interest in theories reflects a desire for unity and simplicity (Hill, 1963). Theories provide the individual with useful ways of conceptualizing his or her world. For the health educator, theories can provide an orientation, a systematic interpretation of the field, as well as a rational approach to the practice of health education.

Researchers are rarely content merely to collect more and more facts about learning. To satisfy the individual's desire for understanding, knowledge must be organized. Broad, general laws or principles from which specific principles may be deduced or related organize facts into knowledge. Unlike research in physical science, which utilizes general acceptance and understanding of concepts such as mass, space, and time, research in education offers no comparable agreements or general understandings on which to base a theory of learning. It is necessary to examine terms such as health and education in order to establish a common ground.

Theories of learning

A theory of learning is concerned with describing how learning takes place. As defined by Hilgard (1971), learning is a relatively permanent change in behavior that occurs as the result of practice. Establishing the desired changes and bringing them about constitutes the role of schools and education. It follows, then, that schools are interested in both theories of learning and theories of teaching or instruction. A theory of learning describes what happens when learning occurs, whereas a theory of instruction is concerned with the teaching methods and the instructional material required for something to be learned.

According to Hill (1963), most of the different theories of learning, no matter how diverse, derive from two general sources, the connectionist and the cognitive theorists. The connectionists or associationists, as they are sometimes called, view learning as a matter of making connections between stimuli and responses. This theory assumes that all responses are caused by stimuli. Other terms used to describe these connections are habits, stimulus-response bonds, and conditional response. Research is conducted on the responses that occur, on the stimuli that elicit the response, and on the ways by which experience affects these relationships.

Those employing a cognitive theory of learning are concerned with the perceptions or attitudes and beliefs that an individual has about his or her environment and the ways these cognitions affect behavior. Attention is directed to these cognitions to define and describe them and to determine how they are modified by experience.

Of course, there is no "either-or" approach to learning. Both kinds of interpretations are used. The connectionist's interpretation of learning can often be identified by comments such as, "I have developed a bad habit," or "His long hours of practice produced a flawless performance." Statements such as, "He has a very positive attitude about school," reveal a cognitive interpretation of learning.

Connectionist theory. Preference for one theory over another may relate, in part, to the nature of the learning task. For example, the connectionist theories lend themselves to greater precision and are utilized when there is need to define learning in objective and quantifiable terms that can be measured. The applied psychologists or the educational psychologists are more apt to employ the cognitive interpretation. Learning, in this sense, refers to the concepts of beliefs and purpose. This interpretation holds that behavior change results from a change in what one knows or from a change in cognition. Such learning is more likely to deal with complex problems and behavior.

Whereas learning theorists may be strongly biased toward one or the other of the major learning theories, it is apparent that no one approach is followed when theories are applied in the field. A review of educational research shows how the different learning theories are reflected in educational developments. In the early 1930s, when the progressive education movement had identified "critical thinking" as an outcome of major importance for schools, Tyler (Travers, 1978) led the way in writing behavioral objectives that were detailed, objective, and explicit. His purpose was to clarify the goals of education that had been, until then, so vague that it was virtually impossible to determine whether or not schools were accomplishing their intended purpose. Tyler's objectives were written in behaviors that could be observed, measured, and evaluated. On this basis Skinner developed operant psychology and insisted on definitions of behavior that met the standards of objectivity and accuracy necessary for laboratory research. This trend characterized the period of the 1960s and 1970s, when great emphasis was placed on the precision of objectives as illustrated in Robert Mager's (1961, pp. 314-315) behavioral objectives.

Concepts such as readiness, motivation, and stimulus are central features of the connectionist approach, as is the importance of practice (Fig. 11-3). Thorndike, in his "laws of exercise" (Hill, 1963), stated that one learns by practicing the correct response or skill. Through repetition and practice the behavior to be learned is strengthened or is "stamped in" to the individual's neurological

processes. A key concept in the learning theory is recognition of the importance of rewarding the learner's correct or desired responses. This principle is expressed in such terms as reinforcement, operant conditioning, and feedback, which is derived from cybernetics and from the study of control mechanisms, as in engineering. Reinforcement, or positive feedback, used in today's classrooms, rewards the student for giving the correct response to a classroom learning activity, such as answering a question, solving a problem, or demonstrating the appropriate behavior, as in performing a skill in first aid. Providing students with immediate and positive feedback has proved itself to be very effective in influencing student learning (Fig. 11-4). Examples of positive feedback would include the teacher's written comments on students' papers, class work assignments, and comments on examinations. The value or benefits of negative reinforcement, where the stimulus to an undesired response is removed, is

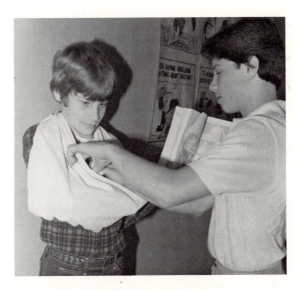

Fig. 11-3. Following directions. Gaining valuable learning experience in trying to figure out how to make a sling for a broken arm by reading directions from a first-aid manual and learning an important skill through practice. (Courtesy Corvallis Public Schools, Corvallis, Ore.)

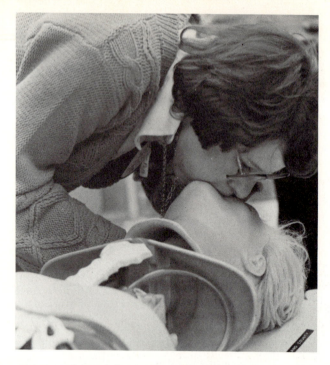

Fig. 11-4. Girl practicing mouth-to-mouth resuscitation illustrates the importance of repetition and feedback in learning a skill. (Courtesy Corvallis Public Schools, Corvallis, Ore.)

less clear. However, negative feedback, as displayed in the learning of a skill when the individual observes his or her error of performance and is able to make the necessary adjustments to achieve correct performance, is also widely accepted in educational practice.

Much of the connectionist theories, as revealed in the works of Thorndike, Watson, and Skinner (Zais, 1976), has influenced present-day curriculum planning. For example, principles derived from these theories advocated the subdividing of curriculum content and learning activities into their most elemental components. Once separated into the basic parts, content and activities then can be restructured or arranged into an optimum sequence for learning. According to this approach, the student learns by being taught first the simplest learning task and then the more difficult. By building on prior learning, complex learning is attained.

In addition, the process of bringing the curriculum together with the learner illustrates the classic stimulus-response (S-R) principle of the connectionist theory.

Although this development helped to overcome the vagueness of earlier educational thinking and goals, it did not produce the hoped-for advances in education. A chief criticism of the connectionist approach to learning is that it is too mechanistic and simplistic. According to Travers (1978), the problem with this approach is the fact that it never succeeded in providing an adequate description of human intellectual performance. Although it is useful in rote-type learning tasks, it does not contribute to the higher levels of intellectual learning and to general understanding.

Cognitive theory. The cognitive learning approach, as represented by those who accept the Gestalt and field theories, holds that

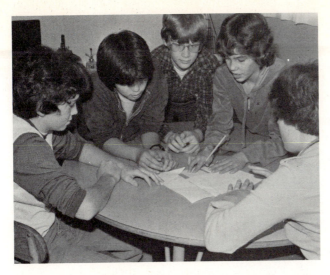

Fig. 11-5. Communication and mental health. Without talking, students are trying to put a puzzle together to illustrate nonverbal communication and interaction. (Courtesy Corvallis Public Schools, Corvallis, Ore.)

learning is determined by one's perceptions. One perceives in terms of a pattern or in dynamic, structured wholes. For example, according to this theory, the listener is not aware of all the separate tones when listening to a musical performance but rather perceives the whole or the melody. Nor does one perceive each separate skill of all the many related skills in observing an athletic performance. Instead, one perceives the total configuration of integrated skills in a gymnastic stunt.

Lewin (Hill, 1963), a leader among the field theorists, argues that a clear picture of learning cannot be attained unless the entire complex, psychological world that he calls the "life space" of an individual is considered. According to Lewin, the life space includes all the forces within which the individual operates. These include both internal forces, such as the basic psychological drives for food, water, and sex, and external forces such as the interaction with people met, objects encountered and used, and geographical places within which the individual moves. It must be stressed that life space means

those forces recognized by the individual's psychological perceptions. If an individual does not perceive an object in the environment, then it simply does not exist, insofar as that individual's life space is concerned.

Lewin contends that there are four different kinds of changes that compose the process of learning. These include changes in (1) cognitive structure, (2) motivation, (3) group membership, and (4) voluntary muscle control, such as in skills and motor performances (Fig. 11-5). Of central importance to Lewin's field theory is perception and motivation. He argues that the connectionist theory of learning is inadequate to explain the different types of learning. For example, he contends that the learning of a skill is not the same as learning to like a person or learning to live without alcohol.

Applying Lewin's principles to teaching and curriculum planning would involve giving increased attention to the relationships of the individual and studying the individual's motivation and behavior in the school. Small classes would be important in order for the individuals to know each other and to empha-

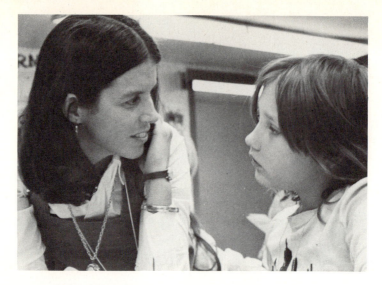

Fig. 11-6. Cognitive theory of learning emphasizes motivation and the importance of interpersonal relationships.

size those classroom activities that would place greater stress on interpersonal class activities. This approach recognizes the importance of motivation in learning and makes a distinction between the goals of the curriculum and the individual's psychological goals (Fig. 11-6).

HEALTH EDUCATION APPLICATION: THEORIES AND MODELS

Every health education program has as its major, long-range objective the outcome of health behavior change: the development of a life-style that will lead to good health. Traditionally, these objectives have been defined in terms of health knowledge, health attitudes, and health practices. However, health educators have long been aware of the troublesome gap that often exists between health knowledge, health attitudes, and health practices, or between what the individual knows about health and what he or she does about it. The physician who fails to care for his or her own health is an often-cited exam-

ple, as is the obese nutritionist, the physical educator who fails to exercise, and the health educator who smokes.

Despite this evidence, the pressure of the public's growing interest in health education as a method for preventing disease, eliminating social problems, and achieving better health often causes schools to adopt unrealistic and unattainable objectives for their health education program. As Kreuter and Green (1978) have warned, it is naive to expect health education to produce health behavior changes that result in significant improvements in health. Instead, school health education can make its most important contribution in the development of specific knowledge and skills. The school's health instruction program, since it is directed to healthy children and youth, is designed to intervene in or to prevent illness and disease before signs or symptoms are apparent.

Health behavior change is not a favorable goal or objective for schools because of the very complex nature of health behavior. Even in a situation offering optimum control,

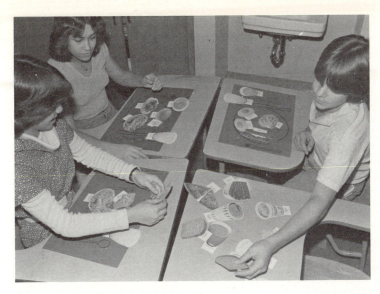

Fig. 11-7. Nutrition. Designing menus for breakfast, lunch, and dinner using models from the American Dairy Association. (Courtesy Corvallis Public Schools, Corvallis, Ore.)

such as in an experimental study, it is very difficult to determine which influences of many affecting children are causally related to health behavior. Although children do spend a considerable portion of their lives in school, its influence is relatively weak compared to pressure exerted by their homes, their neighborhoods and communities, and particularly their peer group. Under optimal conditions, such as an ideal school health instruction program, the time available for formal health instruction is relatively limited.

Therefore it becomes apparent that the major role of health instruction is to develop health knowledge and positive health attitudes (Fig. 11-7). Additionally, certain health behavior skills are taught, such as those related to hygienic measures, personal and interpersonal skills, selecting nutritious diets, selecting health care, participating in fitness and exercise activities, and acquiring the skills necessary to apply first aid and emergency care procedures. It is assumed that this approach will provide the develop-

ing students with the basis for making wise decisions and appropriate choices about healthful life-styles and behavior patterns that will contribute to their health and well-being.

Clarification of health behavior goals

With the development of health education and its expansion into a variety of settings outside the schools, such as public health, health care, rehabilitation, and occupational centers, it becomes important to recognize that objectives and approaches will differ. Professionals in health care settings have called attention to the need for making distinctions in the health behavior outcome in order to clarify the program objectives and related activity. This behavior can be classified as (1) health behavior—that which is related to the prevention of illness and disease, (2) sick role behavior—that which occurs after the appearance of symptoms of illness, and (3) illness behavior—that which occurs following the diagnosis of disease (Society for Public Health Education, 1976).

In light of these distinctions, the school's health instruction program will, to a large extent, focus on health behavior. Schools must also give some attention to sick role behavior, helping individuals to understand their own feelings and to know how to care for themselves when symptoms appear. Also, learning how to use health services and how to relate to health service personnel is an important aspect of health instruction. Illness behavior, although it may be beyond the scope of the school, is within the realm of health education. It has long been recognized that a sick person is much easier to motivate to adopt a recommended health practice or to accept medical advice than is a well person. A task force of the American College of Preventive Medicine (Preventive Medicine USA, 1976) concluded that the most effective health education programs have involved individuals who already had strong motivation, such as chronic illness or disability, an acute crisis such as surgery, or a job-threatening condition such as alcoholism. It is out of this experience of working with the ill that the logic of health education seems most appealing. If the individual understands his or her disease, recognizes how to control the disease, and understands why the medication should be taken or why the treatment should be followed, then he or she is more likely to comply with the physician's recommendations (Podell, 1976).

Although health education is involved with the total spectrum of the population, the three general arenas where it takes place may include only a portion of the whole. School health education deals with young people in a generally healthy state. Therefore the instructional emphasis is on primary prevention, and the curriculum covers a wide range of topics. The objectives of school health education would emphasize specific knowledge and attitudes, with health behavior change receiving much less emphasis. This is not because the health outcome is less important, but because, practically speaking, the opportunity to practice the health outcome is not always present.

Community health education covers the widest range of subjects, since it includes the total community: old, young, sick, and well. The instructional objectives for community health, however, are quite specific, focusing on programs such as glaucoma screening or measles immunization campaigns. There is greater emphasis on health behavior change, with specific actions being required to carry out the program.

Health care education deals with a narrow spectrum of subjects—sick people. The instructional objectives are very specific, concerning patient education on a particular disease, diet, or medical therapy. There is great emphasis on health behavior change, involving actions required by specific treatment, diet, or follow-up procedure.

Health belief model

How have the connectionist and cognitive theories affected the field of health education? The health belief model represents the most extensive work done thus far in an effort to develop a theory and a science of health behavior change. This model was influenced by the theories of Kurt Lewin and his phenomenological orientation, which holds that it is the individual's perception or psychological environment that determines what his or her action will be (Rosenstock, 1974). This complex of psychological forces, which Lewin calls the life space of the individual, explains how learning takes place. The life space includes regions of positive and negative valence that exert forces causing the individual to move away from negative and toward positive forces. Lewin considers motivation to be very important to learning, explaining that learning involves changes in both cognition (knowledge) structure and motivation (Zais, 1976).

Fig. 11-8 illustrates the health belief model and the three distinct phases leading up to a health action. The three phases are individual perceptions, modifying factors, and likelihood of action.

Individual perceptions. Individual perceptions include the individual's subjective risk of contracting the disease. For example, consider the issue of teenage smoking. The disease in question is a smoking-related disease such as lung cancer, emphysema, or heart disease. According to the principle of this model, the teenager's smoking behavior will be influenced away from smoking to a reduced or nonsmoking state or will continue in a nonsmoking state if the teenager perceives the effects of smoking as presenting a serious threat to health and perceives that conditions such as lung cancer, emphysema, and heart disease are very serious diseases. In addition, cigarette smoking must be perceived as behavior that greatly increases the likelihood of developing one of these diseases. Thus the two perceptions, personal susceptibility to the disease and the severity or seriousness of disease as a personal threat, are interacting perceptions that are the necessary conditions for modifying the smoking behavior or maintaining the nonsmoking behavior.

Modifying factors. Assuming that the foregoing perceptions or conditions are present, the ultimate decision of the individual to change or maintain his or her smoking behavior depends, to a great extent, on the various modifying factors present in the teenager's situation. For example, if the individual comes from a home where smoking has not been part of the family culture and if his or her peers are nonsmokers, the prospects of changing smoking behavior to nonsmoking or for continuing as a nonsmoker

are greatly enhanced. If, also, this young person has just gained knowledge from the high school health science course that further demonstrates the hazardous effects of smoking on health, the change in the student's cognitive structure (knowledge) adds an important factor to behavior change. The combined influence of the home, peer group pressure, and health knowledge gained at school act either to modify the teenager's smoking behavior or to reinforce the continuation of nonsmoking.

The calls to action issued by the mass media and other sources are interpreted in the context of these perceptions. If the cues encourage smoking, the individual is more apt to reject them because they are inconsistent with the major predisposing forces identified in this situation. Nonsmoking media presentations and similar advice from friends and respected adults is interpreted as consistent with the many other factors that support the nonsmoking position.

Likelihood of action. According to the health belief model, individual action is determined by the balance or imbalance between the individual's perceived positive and negative forces affecting his or her health behavior. In the foregoing example, the action of stopping smoking or continuing nonsmoking wins approval for the individual from family and friends. This action also assures consistency with the knowledge (cognitive structure) that the individual has acquired in the school health education course.

• • •

Admittedly, this example illustrates a situation in which all of what Lewin describes as the complex of psychological forces favor nonsmoking. In terms of the health belief model, the modifying factors and the perceived benefits favor nonsmoking. Another example might show the major forces in the student's life space as encouraging the con-

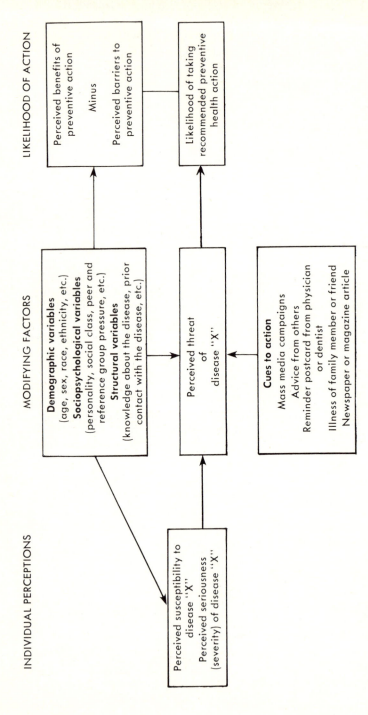

Fig. 11-8. The health belief model as predictor of preventive health behavior. (From Becker, M. H., editor: The health belief model and personal health behavior, Thorofare, N.J., 1974, Charles B. Slack, Inc.)

tinuation of smoking or encouraging its initiation. A more true-to-life example would show both negative and positive valences (values), some favoring and some opposing smoking, that combine to pose a genuine dilemma for the teenager. In this situation the student's health education experiences can play a major role in decision making. Obviously, the quality of this instruction, the preparation of the teacher, and the teacher's sensitivities to the student's dilemma are of critical importance.

Behavior modification

The behavior modification approach is a direct application of the connectionist theory of learning and emphasizes relating observable activity or responses to antecedents and subsequent events or stimuli. The stimulus-response association and the reinforcement of the desired activity or behavior compose essential elements.

One concept that has emerged from the behavior modification approach is contingency management, which is based on the experimental observations that the consequences of behavior, the reinforcing stimuli, determine the pattern of behavior. The reinforcer is a consequence that has the effect of making the behavior that preceded it more likely to be repeated. For example, if praise (reinforcement) is given to a boy for washing his hands before eating, he is more likely to repeat this act in the future.

The second important concept of behavior modification is stimulus control. This involves an analysis of how a stimulus provides the context for ongoing behavior. According to Bass (1976), a stimulus can affect behavior either because the stimulus has been associated with a reinforcer or because the stimulus signals a situation where the behavior has been associated with a reinforcer. Stimulus control analysis is used in many behavior applications to determine exactly how the en-

vironment controls a particular problem behavior. Such an analysis usually begins with the keeping of a detailed record of the times when the behavior occurs, the physical location, the current mood, and the social context of the behavior. For example, the characteristics of each occurrence of an unwanted behavior such as overeating or cigarette smoking would be carefully defined.

Bandura (1969) has developed a five-part process for applying a behavior modification approach that includes the following:

1. Analyzing existing relevant behavior and developing behavioral objectives
2. Modeling of the new behavior by the instructor
3. Providing guided practice of the new behavior by the learners
4. Providing for reinforcement of the new behavior
5. Being able to maintain the new behavior without further assistance from the instructor

Of these five parts, reinforcement devices for new behavior are particularly important. Changes in diet, smoking, and exercise, for example, might develop such reinforcements as encouragement from the instructor, support from family members, and approval from friends and peers.

A recent development that has made behavior modification more acceptable to the health educator is self-control behavioral strategems. As expressed in the code of ethics statement for health education, self-control is in keeping with the principle of fostering an educational environment that nurtures individual growth and development. It is also consistent with the idea of helping people to make behavior changes by conscious choices rather than by coercion.

In behavior modification, changes are often brought about by environmental manipulations that force the individual with the problem to modify or change his or her behavior.

Examples of such manipulation include putting a substance in the cigarette to create an unpleasant taste to the smoker, thus causing the smoker to consider stopping smoking, or, in an effort to get the automobile driver to wear safety belts, installing a device that creates a loud, unpleasant noise when the key is inserted into the starter switch and the seat belt is not fastened. Such environmental manipulation is designed to force compliance rather than to help the individual make a conscious choice of health actions.

Under a self-managed approach, the individual with the problem behavior becomes an active participant in changing or modifying his or her own behavior.

Although educators find the self-control strategem a more acceptable method than environmental manipulation, it often proves unsuccessful because of vague or poorly defined instructions. Also, as Bandura (1969) contends, such instructions may have no immediate implications. In addition, persons using this approach have often failed to provide the necessary support that comes from reinforcement. In order to assure the success of self-managed behavioral change, research has demonstrated the importance of the following steps:

1. Both immediate and long-range goals require carefully defined objectives. In keeping with the self-control approach, the individual involved should choose the objectives or goals.

2. Adopting contractual agreements is an important means of increasing the individual's commitment to goal achievement. For example, an agreement recommended for smoking behavior change would call for gradually restricting cigarette smoking by reducing the number of times and places where smoking is permitted. To succeed, individuals must personally set the objectives and then voluntarily commit themselves to attaining these immediate objectives on a day-to-day basis.

3. Negative self-evaluations that result from deviation from the individual's contractual agreement are an important element in helping counteract the undesired behavior.

4. The satisfaction resulting from an agreement and receiving a favorable social reaction from family and friends for adopting the new health behavior represents an important source of reinforcement.

5. Keeping a detailed record of behavior changes is an additional source of reinforcement, since it provides a tangible and objective measure of the progress. Experience has shown that those who record their daily activities continue to work toward achieving objectives until they have exceeded preceding performances, thus ensuring continued improvement.

The altering of stimulus conditions under which the maladaptive or undesired behavior occurs is an effective technique in changing or modifying behavior. For example, research has shown that the problem of overeating often arises in situations where appetizing foods are prominently displayed. In order to counteract this influence, altering the stimulus condition by storing foods out of sight and in less accessible places is effective. Another way of helping control the overeating problem involves limiting the circumstances under which the individual eats. Special efforts are made to avoid eating in nondining settings (e.g., while watching television, reading, or listening to the radio).

It must be recognized that many of the undesired behaviors, such as smoking, overeating, and drinking, provide immediate gratification or reinforcement to the individual. Since these behaviors occur in many and diverse situations and times, it is necessary for the individual to narrow this stimulus control over his or her behavior.

The need for developing self-reinforcing techniques must also be recognized in self-control behavior modification. To do this, individuals are taught to arrange for contingencies that serve as reinforcements. This is done by selecting a variety of activities that they find rewarding. For example, after refraining from smoking for a certain period of time, individuals then reward themselves by engaging in an enjoyable activity, such as taking a recreational break or watching a favorite television program.

The Stanford Heart Disease Prevention Program

The Stanford Heart Disease Prevention Program experiment is an example of behavior modification, using three California towns employing two different experimental conditions, while the third town served as the control. The study sought to produce changes in people's cognitive structure, motivational structure, and behavior skills in order to reduce their risks of heart disease. The specific program objectives were to produce both knowledge and behavior changes relating to diet, exercise, and smoking. The study compared the effectiveness of mass media used alone and with a personal instruction, including a self-control behavior modification approach. It is interesting in the context of learning theory, since both cognitive learning strategies and connectionist learning theory were employed in the personalized behavior modification phase of the study.

Results from the study showed that the mass media approach produced almost as much information gain as did the personalized instruction and, also, was effective in changing simple behaviors. However, in order to achieve complex behavior change, it was necessary to have the reinforcement or social support that was supplied by the personal instruction or self-control behavior modification approach (McAlister and Berger, 1979). The implications to be drawn from this study are that in order to achieve significant long-range health behavior outcomes the schools must play a major role in complementing mass media instructional programs. Schools can provide personalized instruction about health hazards and can help children develop the necessary knowledge and the self-help, self-management behavior skills needed to sustain health action that will lessen the risk of future chronic diseases.

Fishbein's behavioral intention theory

Although it is helpful to simplify the analysis of learning theories by grouping them into one of two broad categories—cognitive and connectionist or associationist learning theory—further attempts have been made to combine the advantages of these two theories. Many researchers have been attracted by the connectionist's objectivity in identifying behavior and precision in measuring behavior, but others have been dissatisfied with a stimulus-response analysis of behavior. These researchers have argued that in addition to this effect the individual's behavior is also a result of his or her beliefs, attitudes, and desires to achieve a goal. The Fishbein conceptual framework is one example of the attempt to combine cognitive and connectionist approaches to learning.

According to Fishbein's (Fishbein and Ajzen, 1975) theory, beliefs are the fundamental building blocks. The individual, through direct observation or by other methods such as receiving information from an outside source, as in health instruction, learns or forms a number of beliefs about a particular object. The individual also develops beliefs about the various attributes of the object. Through this process, beliefs about health, illness, cigarettes, food, physicians,

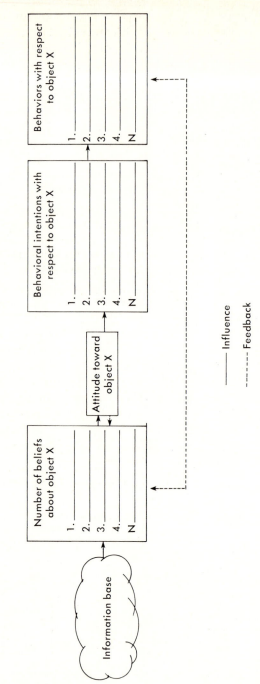

Fig. 11-9. Fishbein's conceptual framework. Adapted from Fishbein's conceptual framework relating beliefs, attitudes, intentions, and behaviors with respect to a given object. (From Fishbein, M., and Ajzen, I.: Belief, attitude, intention and behavior: an introduction to theory and research, Reading, Mass., 1975, Addison-Wesley Publishing Co., Inc., p. 15.)

hospitals, health behavior, and many other things in life are acquired. The totality of a person's beliefs serves as the information or knowledge base that ultimately determines the person's attitudes, intentions, and behavior. This approach views the individual as an entirely rational being, one who uses the information available to make judgments, to form evaluations, and to arrive at decisions. An adapted and simplified illustration of the behavioral intentions model is presented in Fig. 11-9.

Formally stated, the theory holds that an individual has many beliefs about a given object. Moreover, the object is seen as having various attributes or characteristics. For example, the object *cigarette* may be seen as having various attributes, such as the cigarette smoke that may represent odor, the cause of disease, and an offense to friends. If these beliefs about the attributes of cigarettes are associated with unfavorable attitudes, then, through the process of conditioning, the attitude of the individual toward cigarettes and smoking is likely to be negative. According to this theory, attitudes toward an object are conditioned by beliefs

about the attributes of the object and by evaluation of those attributes. Also, according to this theory, an individual's attitude toward an object is related to his or her intention to perform a variety of behaviors relating to the object, in this case, cigarettes. If the individual's overall attitude toward cigarettes is negative, his or her intention to perform certain behaviors with respect to cigarettes may be something like the following:

1. To decide against smoking a cigarette
2. To continue not smoking
3. To avoid areas where cigarettes are smoked

Fishbein points out that there may not be a direct and consistent relationship between beliefs, attitudes, and behavioral interactions. He contends that a person's intention to perform a particular behavior is a function of two basic determinants, one attitudinal and the other normative (Fig. 11-10). The attitudinal component refers to the person's attitude toward performing the behavior in question. The normative component (subject norm) is related to the individual's beliefs about people who are very important to him or her and what such people's expec-

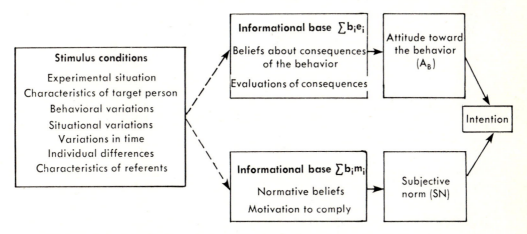

Fig. 11-10. Fishbein's behavioral intentions model. (From Fishbein, M., and Ajzen, I.: Belief, attitude, intention and behavior: an introduction to theory and research, Reading, Mass., 1975, Addison-Wesley Publishing Co., Inc., p. 334.)

tations of him or her are. For example, if the individual sees all the attributes of cigarettes as being bad or negative (attitude) and believes his or her parents and friends (subjective norm) do not want him or her to smoke, it is more likely that he or she will *intend not* to smoke.

In summary, a person's intentions (to smoke or not to smoke) are a function of two variables intervening between the stimulus conditions and the intention. These variables are (1) attitude toward the behavior and (2) the subjective norm. The individual's attitude is determined by the stimulus conditions, by beliefs about what others think he or she should do, and by his or her own desire to comply with their standards of behavior. Fishbein's general framework for behavior change with its stimulus conditions, intervening variables, and behavioral intentions response is clearly in the connectionist tradition of learning and its well-known model of stimulus-response. However, many of the precepts from the cognitive theory of learning have also been included in Fishbein's model. For example, the intervening variables of knowledge, beliefs, attitudes, and the influence of others on the individual's decisions are closely related to cognitive theories and Lewin's concept of life space.

School Health Education Study (SHES)

Health Education: A Conceptual Design for Curriculum Development is an example of learning theory applied to curriculum planning in health education. Oftentimes such projects are eclectic, using several different principles of learning rather than following a particular approach. The School Health Education Study (SHES) is an example of this in some respects, drawing on principles derived from both the cognitive and the connectionist traditions. Whereas school practitioners have sometimes been criticized for failing to adopt a consistent overall theory to guide the instructional program, common sense may dictate the use of both kinds of interpretations in certain instances. As Hill (1963) has observed, some principles of learning appear to apply in all situations while others are germane only in particular circumstances.

However, examination of the SHES conceptual model for curriculum design reveals that it is more characteristic of the field or cognitive theory of learning. The SHES model is based on the concept of health that serves as the focal point in formulating a structure of health and from which the model for health education is derived (Fig. 11-11).

The term *health* implies a wholeness or, as modern-day philosophers and scholars have contended, a dynamic process in which the individual is functioning in harmony both with his or her total self and with the total environment. The next step undertaken is to determine what constitutes the principal ideas to be elaborated on if a structure is to be devised that is at once logical for curriculum development, meaningful to the learner, and a valid representation of ideas held to be true by the scientist and the philosopher.

Health is the comprehensive, unified concept at the apex of the hierarchy developed for the conceptual model for health and health education. It has three dimensions—physical, mental, and social. More specifically, physical health pertains to the structure and function of the biological organism, mental health pertains to the behavior and personality patterns, and social health includes the complex of interpersonal and societal forces. Health is a quality of life involving dynamic interaction and interdependence among the individual's physical well-being, his or her mental and emotional reactions, and the social complex in which he or she exists. Any one dimension may play a greater or lesser role than the other two at a given time, but the interdependence and interac-

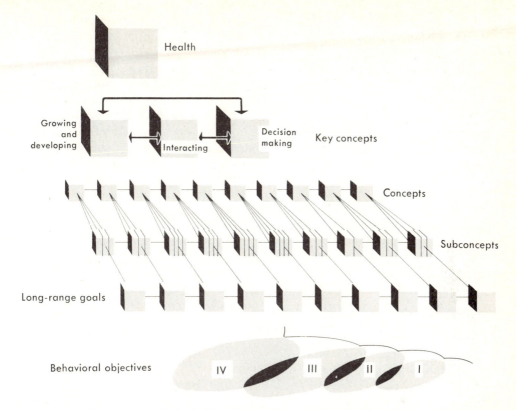

Fig. 11-11. The SHES model for health education, kindergarten through grade 12. (From School Health Education Study, Inc.: Health education: a conceptual approach to curriculum design, Washington, D.C., Copyright 1967, p. 27. Published by 3M Education Press, St. Paul, Minn., 1968.)

tion of the three dimensions still hold true (School Health Education Study, 1967).

This view of the individual and his or her health parallels closely Lewin's (Zais, 1976) contention that learning refers to a multitude of different phenomena. He argues that we cannot have a clear understanding of learning unless we take into account the entire complex psychological world that he calls the life space of the individual.

The hierarchy of concepts portrays the unified concept of health at the apex or highest order in the model. Following immediately are the three key concepts of growing and developing, interacting, and decision making, which are considered to be the unifying

threads of the curriculum (Fig. 11-12). These three features are peculiar to all human beings, and from the standpoint of health education are essential to the understanding of the individual's health problems and the forces affecting health behavior. Thus they are considered to be the processes that underlie health.

These three concepts are consistent with the cognitive theory of motivation that may be regarded as a theory of preferential choice or of decision making. The decision to become involved in it is made on the basis of cognitive considerations (Hill, 1963). For example, consider the importance of the key concept of growth and development to the

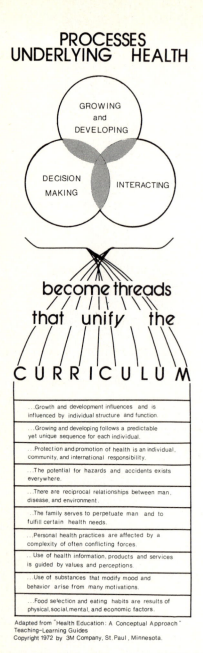

PROCESSES UNDERLYING HEALTH

GROWING and DEVELOPING

DECISION MAKING

INTERACTING

become threads that unify the

C U R R I C U L U M

...Growth and development influences and is influenced by individual structure and function.

...Growing and developing follows a predictable yet unique sequence for each individual.

...Protection and promotion of health is an individual, community, and international responsibility.

...The potential for hazards and accidents exists everywhere.

...There are reciprocal relationships between man, disease, and environment.

..The family serves to perpetuate man and to fulfill certain health needs.

...Personal health practices are affected by a complexity of often conflicting forces.

.. Use of health information, products and services is guided by values and perceptions.

...Use of substances that modify mood and behavior arise from many motivations.

...Food selection and eating habits are results of physical, social, mental, and economic factors.

Adapted from "Health Education: A Conceptual Approach" Teaching–Learning Guides
Copyright 1972 by 3M Company, St. Paul, Minnesota.

Fig. 11-12. SHES three key concepts. (Modified from School Health Education Study, Inc.: Health education: a conceptual approach to curriculum design, Washington, D.C., Copyright 1967, p. 20. Published by 3M Education Press, St. Paul, Minn., 1968.)

curriculum planner and health education teacher in the case of a teenage boy of 14 years whose pubescence is late in developing. Frequently, such a boy suffers severe emotional disturbances because his associates of the same age are not only sexually more mature but are also bigger and stronger than he is. Consider the impact of his state of growth and development on his social interaction with boys and girls of his same age. What kind of effect will his physical development have on his choices and decisions about participating in sports and physical activity? Will it affect his decision about diet?

Next come the 10 concepts and subconcepts that represent the scope of the subject matter treated in health education. The 10 concepts, according to Goodlad's (1963) curriculum nomenclature, are the "organizing elements" of the curriculum. According to this scheme, the concepts and subconcepts include some 31 different health topics.

These broad content areas have been phrased in conceptual statements in order to give more meaning and direction to the teaching-learning process. For example, instead of using the term *accident prevention*, the following conceptual statement is given: "The potential for hazards and accidents exists, whatever the environment." This is considered to be more descriptive as well as prescriptive, insofar as health education is concerned.

Located at the two lower levels of the model are the long-range goals and behavioral objectives. These are derived from the conceptual structure representing that which is to be learned. The goals and behavioral objectives represent the educational outcomes that are being sought. These represent various health behaviors, including the way students think, feel, and act with regard to health. The goals are long-term, general outcomes, whereas the behavioral objectives are specific outcomes. Similarly, goals are the end result of the total health education experience, whereas behavioral objectives are those designed for a particular educational level.

These characteristics of the SHES curriculum point to other similarities of the field or cognitive theories approach. For learning to occur, it is essential that the student pursue goals that the individual considers to be his or her own. Adopting affective as well as cognitive goals with constant attention to the three unifying key concepts serves as a constant reminder to the curriculum planner to be ever aware of the individual student's needs.

In order to apply the SHES conceptual model to teaching, each concept was analyzed and translated into priority behavioral objectives at four different educational levels beginning with level I and progressing through level IV. Here the SHES model draws on the connectionist theory of learning that calls for the writing of objectives in precise, observable, and measurable behaviors. Behaviors considered appropriate to the desired outcomes must be identified and carefully arranged in a progression of increasingly complex behaviors. This is similar to the approach used by the advocates of behavior modification, based on the principles developed by Thorndike, Guthrie, Watson, and Skinner. According to the behaviorists, establishing complex social behavior and modifying existing response patterns can be achieved most consistently through a gradual process in which the person participates in an orderly learning sequence that guides him or her stepwise toward more intricate or demanding performances (Bandura, 1969).

To illustrate how this progression is developed in the SHES model, behavioral objectives developed from the concept *food selection and eating patterns are determined by physical, social, mental, economic, and* *cultural factors* (p. 264). Behavioral objectives from each of the four educational levels are illustrated to show the sequences and progressions of these behaviors.

Behavior modification applied to school health education

Golaszewski (1979) has developed an innovative composite behavior modification model for use in school health education programs. His proposal, similar to previous efforts to apply learning theory in schools, draws to some extent on both the connectionist and cognitive traditions of learning. This composite model provides a good example of behavior modification as the application of connectionist theory to school health education. As Golaszewski points out, in any attempt to develop an ideal program, the following points should be considered: (1) a multitude of environmental influences shape the child's behaviors; therefore the tendency to take an overly simplistic view of learning and behavior must be avoided; (2) many individual variations exist, resulting from ethnic and cultural differences; and (3) the constraints of school finances, school policies, and biases of the health educator affect curriculum decisions.

The three steps of the composite model include the following:

1. Providing for student participation through appropriate laboratory experiences. For example, in teaching a unit on heart disease, activities such as an exercise stress test, serum lipid evaluations, blood pressure measurements, and growth measurements might be included. Such measures can be related to results taken from actual student surveys of behavior, such as eating, exercise, and smoking habits. Data from this step can be used as the basis for developing goals for behavior change.

2. Providing students with the information necessary for them to build a knowledge base

required for rational decision making. This procedure draws on the cognitive theory of learning for behavior change. Since the objectives of this unit are to reduce the risk of heart disease, information to be included should relate to the need to eat a nutritious diet low in fats, to avoid cigarette smoking, to exercise regularly, to control blood pressure, and to make appropriate use of health care services. A variety of teaching aids, including multimedia tapes, film reports, and guest appearances of experts is needed in order to assure the validity of the content material and to stimulate the students' interest.

3. Providing value clarification activities that delineate actual and ideal behavior patterns aimed at preventing disease and promoting health. A major purpose of this step is the use of student participation in the setting of personal goals. Each student is expected to formulate a written plan of action to meet this goal. The goal selected should be measurable, related to a specific time period, and realistic for the student. In keeping with the self-management or self-care approach, the student should provide a plan for monitoring progress and a system of rewarding or reinforcing the desired behavior.

To help assure the success of a behavior modification approach in school health education, the following procedure for the teacher is recommended:

1. Review all student plans to determine their appropriateness as well as feasibility.
2. Follow a contract grading procedure, where each step of progress is appropriately rewarded.
3. Organize the class into small groups of students having similar goals. Encourage students to make a group commitment and to share their progress as well as their problems.
4. Include the technique of mental imagery in student learning activities. This encourages the student to visualize goal achievement, such as losing 20 pounds of weight, being able to jog 3 miles, or stopping smoking. The student then imagines being rewarded for achieving the goal and receiving compliments on the results.
5. Provide opportunities for the students to give a public demonstration following goal achievement. For example, a diet group might give a "health meal" demonstration, an exercise group might sponsor a special road race, and an anti-

---

PROGRESSION OF BEHAVIORAL OBJECTIVES BY EDUCATION LEVEL

Concept 1: Food selection and eating patterns are determined by physical, social, mental, economic, and cultural factors

Level I   *Identifies* —many different kinds of foods
                  ↓

Level II   *Illustrates*—that a variety of foods are necessary in maintaining a balanced diet
                  ↓

Level III   *Describes*—the relationship between nutritional status and disease
                  ↓

Level IV   *Applies*   —criteria for selecting foods and planning meals that provide for a balanced diet

smoking group might give a special class presentation to younger students in the school.

6. Arrange special booster sessions or programs that will provide reinforcement for student progress toward goal achievement, for example, giving awards to students for adopting a new behavior or recognizing students reducing weight.

School Health Curriculum Project (SHCP)

The School Health Curriculum Project represents an innovative approach for health instruction at the elementary and middle school levels. The curriculum originated as an experimental project in California during the early 1960s and initially was taught to intermediate grade school children as an indepth study of the heart and circulatory system. It was first known as the "Berkeley Project" but later was given the title of the School Health Curriculum Project (SHCP). Its general purpose is to help children learn how their bodies function in a normal, healthy state and the changes that occur when disease strikes. The effects of the environment and living habits on the body are stressed.

The goal of the SHCP is to help the child realize that the body is each person's great-

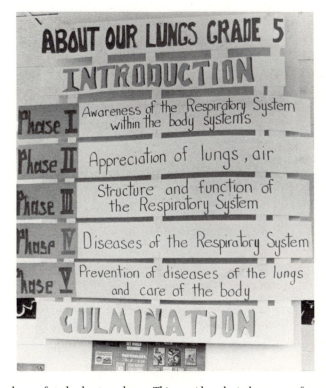

Fig. 11-13. Five phases of study about our lungs. This provides a logical sequence for understanding the progression of disease. (From School Health Curriculum Project, Pub. No. (CDC) 78-8359, Atlanta, 1977, Public Health Service, Center for Disease Control, U.S. Department of Health, Education and Welfare.)

est natural resource in life, is uniquely one's own, is exquisitely beautiful and complex in its structure and function, and is affected by the choices one makes throughout life (U.S. Department of Health, Education and Welfare, 1977). From a health perspective, children are taught about the importance of controlling events in their lives that might create a serious health problem, such as heart disease or cancer. In brief, the SHCP is (1) a curriculum, (2) a method of teaching, and (3) a training program for classroom teachers in health education. The curriculum focuses on the healthy body and ways of maintaining it. Activities are designed to involve and motivate a wide range of persons associated with the school, including students, teachers, school administrators, school health staff, community resource people, voluntary agencies, and parents.

The curriculum plan is designed for the elementary school, kindergarten through grade seven. The primary grades (K-3) unit studies the senses, while successive grade levels from four through seven develop study of a different organ system at each level, including units on digestion, the lungs, the heart, and the brain.

UNIT 5—ABOUT OUR LUNGS*

Introduction: Curiosity arousal about air

The existence of air
The body's need for air
Life needs air
Artificial resuscitation demonstration
Your breath can save somebody's life

Phase one: Overview of the body's systems

Skeletal system	Excretory system
Muscular system	Endocrine system
Respiratory system	Reproductive system
Circulatory system	Nervous system
Digestive system	

Phase two: Appreciation of air and lungs

Essence of air
Properties of air
Functions of air
How the human body uses air
Pollution and its effects on the respiratory system

Phase three: Structure and function of the respiratory system

Nasal passages, trachea, bronchial tubes, bronchioles, alveoli, lungs, diaphragm, rib cage, cells

Phase three: Structure and function of the respiratory system—cont'd

Inhalation, exhalation, oxygen-carbon dioxide exchange with blood, cleansing of system

Phase four: Diseases and problems of the respiratory system

Communicable diseases: colds, flu, pneumonia, bronchitis, etc.
Noncommunicable diseases: allergy, asthma, emphysema, lung cancer, heart disease

Phase five: Care of body and prevention of respiratory diseases

Clean air/pollution
Effects of tobacco smoke
Good and harmful effects of drugs
Nutrition
Rest
Exercise

Culmination: The respiratory system

Activities planned and executed by children, including skits, games, poster presentation, etc., presented to class or to the total school community, including parents.

---

*From The School Health Curriculum Project, Washington, D.C., DHEW Pub. No. (CDC) 78-8359, U.S. Department of Health, Education and Welfare Public Health Service Center for Disease Control, Bureau of Health Education, Atlanta, 1977, HEW Publications.

The curriculum employs a common organization (Fig. 11-13 and box, p. 268) for each of the units that includes the following:

Introduction: Curiosity arousal and motivation of students

Phase one: Overview of the body's system

Phase two: Appreciation of one of the body's systems and its unique function

Phase three: Structure and function of the body system

Phase four: Diseases and problems of the body system

Phase five: Care of the body and prevention of disease

Culmination: Synthesis, through group presentations of the previous phases

Developers of the curriculum contend that using the same teaching approach serves to reinforce the children's understanding of the concept that all body systems are related and that any single event affecting a part of the body affects the whole body and the total health of the person.

Audiovisual materials, including films, film strips, slides, tape recorders, and records, are used extensively to stimulate the children's interest. Models and dissection and analysis of animal organs make the study of health more realistic. Such concrete experiences help the student to personalize the relationship between living habits and their effect on the body.

This curriculum involves the use of a learning center of five or six stations, enabling children to participate in several different learning activities simultaneously (Fig. 11-14). Children study in small groups, rotating through each of the stations in the learning

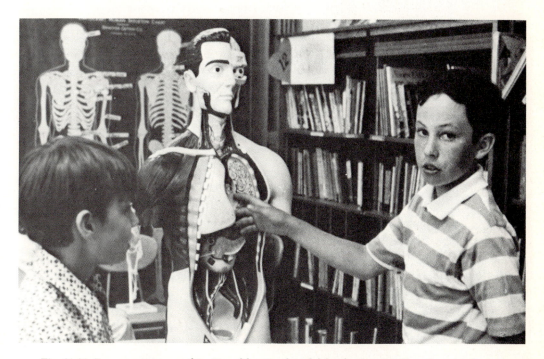

Fig. 11-14. Boys examining manikin. Use of functional model fortifies learning from the printed page. (From The School Health Curriculum project, Pub. No. (CDC) 78-8359, Atlanta, 1977, Public Health Service, Center for Disease Control, U.S. Department of Health, Education and Welfare.)

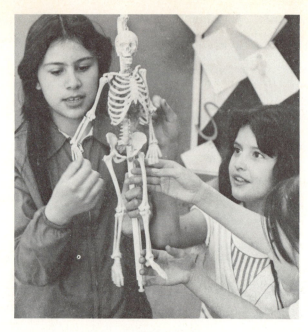

Fig. 11-15. Girls examining skeleton illustrate students' active involvement in learning. (From The School Health Curriculum Project, Pub. No. (CDC) 78-8359, Atlanta, 1977, Public Health Service, Center for Disease Control, U.S. Department of Health, Education and Welfare.)

center, actively involved in the learning process (Fig. 11-15). For example, a series of activities might be developed around the study of circulation, including tracing the locations of arteries and veins, examining red blood cells under the microscope, and learning to take blood pressure. Groups rotate every 30 minutes or at the end of each period, depending on the complexity of the task.

Schools wishing to initiate the curriculum are required to send a team of four or five members to a special training center. The team is composed of at least two classroom teachers who will teach the unit at a particular grade level. Other members of the team include the principal and two other persons such as a nurse, a health educator, or a curriculum specialist. These teams participate in a training session of 60 hours for each unit. During this intensive training workshop, teachers are introduced to each step of the unit exactly as it will be taught to their classes. After the teacher has successfully taught the program, he or she then must conduct a training session for other teachers in the school district in order to assure the dissemination of the model throughout the school system.

Strengths of the SHCP approach include clear definition of each unit, which facilitates the classroom teacher's understanding and preparation. The variety of audiovisual aids, teaching materials, and learning activities makes the curriculum interesting to both students and teachers. The active participation of the student in his or her learning, the involvement of community health agencies in providing resources for the curriculum, and the interest of parents in the health problem being studied not only facilitate learning, but also provide a broad base of support and reinforcement to the student.

This curriculum has not been identified with a particular learning theory, but is based on principles that have evolved from a distillation of empirically tested school practices. Widely accepted principles of instruction evident in the project include the following: (1) the active involvement of the learner, (2) the extensive use of concrete learning activities, (3) the use of cooperative group learning activities, and (4) the structured yet flexible program that allows for variation in student abilities. Several of the principles derived from the cognitive learning theory are employed in the emphasis on motivation and the recognition of structure and its interrelationship in the study of body systems. Perhaps the characteristic that would most closely relate this curriculum to connectionist theory is its recognition of individual differences and its use of a variety of individual learning activities.

GUIDELINES FOR THE HEALTH INSTRUCTION PROGRAM

In theory, well-designed health instruction programs can make significant contributions toward the prevention of health problems. However, school officials and especially health educators should guard against unrealistic expectations of the results of such programs. An individual's health behavior results from many interacting forces. Among the influences affecting the child are his or her family, neighborhood, and peer group, as well as school experiences. For these reasons the school should resist the temptation to join the bandwagon by launching a crash program in an effort to solve a particular health problem. Instead, schools are in a better position to respond to individual and community health needs through an existing comprehensive and systematically planned program of health education. Such a program in the school can respond effectively to new problems or crisis situations. In developing the school health instruction program, the following principles should be considered:

1. The health education program should be recognized as a distinct instructional area of the school curriculum.
2. The program of health instruction should be comprehensive in its scope and organized sequentially, beginning with the child entering school and continuing through senior high school.
3. The curriculum plan for health instruction should reflect the health needs and concerns of students, of the family, and of the larger community.
4. Health instruction, like any other subject in the school curriculum, requires an adequate budget to provide for those elements that are considered essential for any instructional program, such as the following:
   a. A carefully organized and written curriculum plan
   b. An ample supply of current materials and library resources
   c. Classroom facilities and equipment that are conducive to a variety of teaching methods
   d. Sufficient time to achieve the instructional objectives
   e. Teachers who are prepared and interested in health education
5. The correlation and integration of health instruction into other subject areas should supplement and not substitute for the formal or special health course.
6. The scheduling of the health course should follow the pattern established for other subjects in the curriculum. In this regard, experience and research have shown that a block of time equivalent to a minimum of one semester's instruction at both the junior and senior high school levels has produced superior results. Schedule pat-

terns may vary from condensed modules of frequently recurring instruction to longer time periods such as 9-week or semester-long blocks of instruction.

7. A comprehensive and ongoing evaluation plan for the health instruction program should be employed. Such a plan would involve the assessment of both short-range and long-range objectives. Short-range objectives might include such elements as student health interests, attitudes, knowledge, and practices. Long-range objectives should be evaluated in terms of their effect on the health of the students.

8. Students should be evaluated and should receive credit for health instruction consistent with the policies and practices established for other school subjects.

9. A qualified person with specialized graduate preparation in health education should be appointed to assume the responsibility for developing, coordinating, and implementing the school health instruction program.

10. School districts should provide for teachers a regular program of in-service education on current developments relating to health education and school health services.

QUESTIONS AND EXERCISES

1. What evidence is there to indicate that the nation's health programs are giving more attention to prevention and education in health care?
2. Contrast the definitions of health education offered by the President's Committee and the definition offered by the Joint Committee on Terminology. What implications do you draw from these definitions? How do they differ?
3. How might the code of ethics statement adopted by the Society for Health Education affect one's choice of health education definitions?
4. What criteria do you consider most important in adopting a definition of health education?
5. What new roles for the health educator are identified in the consumer health education task force statement on health education?
6. George enrolled in a 5-day program to break his habit of smoking. What kind of learning theory is most likely to have been employed in this program?
7. Contrast the two broad learning theories: (1) cognitive and (2) connectionist or associationist approaches. How do they differ?
8. What learning theory do you favor for school health instruction? Why?
9. How might the objectives for health education in school differ from the objectives of patient education and community health education?
10. What criticisms would you offer of the following statement? Schools' health instruction programs should be expected to reduce the number of cases of venereal disease, the prevalence of drug dependence, and the incidence of unwed pregnancies among youth.
11. Assume you were teaching a unit on the role of exercise in health, how would you introduce this unit if you were using the health belief model to guide your teaching?
12. What is the role of attitudes in Fishbein's theory of behavior change?
13. What advantages and disadvantages do you see in using a behavior modification approach in health instruction?
14. Contrast the School Health Education Study with the School Health Curriculum Project. What strengths and limitations do you see in these two approaches to health teaching?
15. What are the differences between immediate and long-range objectives in school health education?

REFERENCES AND SELECTED READINGS

The American Health Foundation: KYB teacher's guide, the know your body disease prevention program, New York, The American Health Foundation.

American Public Health Association: Toward a policy on health education and public health, position paper adopted by the governing council of the American Public Health Association, Washington, D.C., Nov. 2, 1977.

Bandura, A.: Principles of behavior modification, New York, 1969, Holt, Rinehart & Winston.

Bugelski, B. R.: The psychology of learning applied to teaching, ed. 1, Indianapolis, 1971, The Bobbs-Merrill Co., Inc.

Creswell, W. H., Jr.: Theoretical propositions of a curriculum design for health education, The Academy Paper, No. 2, Oct. 1968, The American Academy of Physical Education.

Expert Committee on Health Education of the Public: First report, World Health Organization Technical Report Series No. 89, Geneva, Switzerland, 1954, World Health Organization, p. 4.

Fishbein, M., and Ajzen, I.: Belief, attitude, intention, and behavior: an introduction to theory and research, Menlo Park, Calif., 1975, Addison-Wesley Publishing Co., Inc.

Givner, A., and Grantard, P. S.: A handbook of behavior modification for the classroom, New York, 1974, Holt, Rinehart & Winston.

Golaszewski, T. J.: Influencing behavior through instruction: methodology in health education, Washington, D.C., Feb., 1979, ERIC Clearinghouse on Teacher Education.

Goodlad, J. I.: Planning and organizing for teaching. Project on Instruction, Washington, D.C., 1963, National Education Association.

Hilgard, E. R., Atkinson, R. C., and Atkinson, R. L.: Introduction to psychology, ed. 5, New York, 1971, Harcourt, Brace, Jovanovich.

Hill, W. F.: Learning: a survey of psychological interpretations, Scranton, Pa., 1963, Chandler Publishing Co.

Joint Committee of the National Education Association and the American Medical Association on Health Problems in Education.

Kreuter, M. W., and Green, L. W.: Evaluation of school health education: identifying purposes, keeping perspective, J. School Health. 48(4):228-235, April, 1978.

Mager, R. F.: Preparing objectives for programmed instruction, Belmont, Calif., 1961, Fearon Publishers.

McAlister, A. and Berger, E. D.: Media for community health promotion. In Lazer, P. M., editor: The handbook of health education, Germantown, Md., 1979, Aspen Systems Corporation.

Moore, R., and the Editors of Life: Evolution, Life Nature Library, New York, 1964, Time Incorporated.

Nightingale, E. O., et al.: Perspectives on health promotion and disease prevention in the United States, Washington, D.C., Jan., 1978, Institute of Medicine, National Academy of Sciences.

Podell, R. N.: Appendix V: Physician's guide to compliance in hypertension. In Preventive Medicine USA: Health promotion and consumer health education, New York, 1976, Prodist, pp. 209-255.

President's Committee on Health Education: The report of the President's Commitee on Health Education, New York, 1973, The Committee.

Preventive Medicine USA: Theory, practice and application of prevention in personal health services: quality control and evaluation of preventive health services, Task Force reports sponsored by the John E. Fogarty International Center for Advanced Study in the Health Sciences National Institutes of Health and the American College of Preventive Medicine, New York, 1976, Prodist.

Report of the 1972-1973 Joint Committee on Health Education Terminology, prepared by representatives of the American Academy of Pediatrics, American Association for Health, Physical Education and Recreation, American School Health Association, American Public Health Association, and Society for Public Health Education, Washington, D.C.

Rosenstock, I. M.: Historical origins of the health belief model. In Becker, M. H., editor: The health belief model and personal health behavior, Thorofare, N.J., 1974, Charles B. Slack, Inc., pp. 1-8.

St. Pierre, R., and Lawrence, P. S.: Reducing smoking using positive self-management, J. School Health 45(1):7-9, Jan., 1975.

School Health Education Study: Health education: a conceptual approach to curriculum design, St. Paul, 1968, 3M Education Press.

Society for Public Health Education: Code of ethics, San Francisco, Oct. 15, 1976, The Society.

Travers, R. M. W.: An introduction to educational research, ed. 4, New York, 1978, Macmillan Publishing Co., Inc.

U.S. Department of Health, Education and Welfare: Educating the public about health: a planning guide, Washington, D.C., Oct., 1977, Public Health Service Health Resources Administration.

U.S. Department of Health, Education and Welfare: Forward plan for health FY 1977-1981, Washington, D.C., June, 1975, U.S. Government Printing Office.

U.S. Department of Health, Education and Welfare: The school health curriculum project, Public Health Service Center for Disease Control Bureau of Health Education, Atlanta, Dec., 1977, U.S. Government Printing Office.

Zais, R. S.: Curriculum principles and foundations, New York, 1976, Thomas Y. Crowell Co.

The journey of a thousand miles begins with one step.

Lao-Tse

CHAPTER 12

Elementary school health instruction

The school is not the sole agency that contributes to the health education of a child. However, the core of health instruction must come from the school. Other health instruction should not be considered an embellishment of the program of the school, but an intensification and extension of what the school is doing. The school must proceed on the principle that it will provide the best possible health instruction for the pupils and that other sources of health instruction will add to it. This is altogether sound because some children have limited opportunities for health instruction outside of school.

In the elementary school, health instruction, like all other instructional areas, should be a meaningful experience of permanent value, not an activity to occupy time. In an effort to make health interesting and enjoyable, the means should not become so important that they obscure the real purpose of the activity. Poster construction, puppet shows, and plays can be effective vehicles for health instruction, but, when the poster, the puppets, or the play becomes the purpose of the experience, little in the way of health education is derived. Health instruction must be an effective experience, not a delightful diversion. An elementary school teacher

should resolve to affect the health of each child favorably.

ORGANIZING FOR EFFECTIVE HEALTH INSTRUCTION

Once the health curriculum or course of study has been established, the next logical step is the organization of the implementation of the curriculum. Health instruction must be fitted into the total school schedule. More than time is involved. Effective instruction requires that all possible teaching opportunities be included in the class organization. The schedule for health instruction should allow for planned teaching, incidental learning, correlation, and integration. Although flexible, the schedule must be sufficiently definite to ensure effective health instruction. Certain current practices in education indicate the principles that will guide scheduling for health instruction:

1. A weekly schedule provides for extended time periods and allows for necessary flexibility.
2. A daily health period is not required for health instruction.
3. Two fairly extended periods per week may be sufficient for health instruction in the primary grades and three periods

274

a week can serve the intermediate grades.

4. A flexible schedule allows for continuation of an activity that is particularly challenging.
5. Opportunities should be provided for the varieties of activities health instruction entails.
6. When special health needs or interests require it, the schedule should be arranged. Extra time invested in health instruction during one week can be followed by incidental instruction in the following week or weeks.
7. Opportunities for incidental and integrated health instruction should not be sacrificed to maintain a rigid schedule.
8. Correlation of health with other areas, to be effective, must be given a definite place in the organization for health instruction.

Health director's role. Properly the health director should be thought of primarily as a supervisor. Recent studies reveal that competent supervision more than justifies its cost in the added effectiveness that it gives to the school program. A supervisor who can help each teacher improve his or her services by 5% has made a considerable contribution.

As a supervisor, the health director helps teachers do a more effective job. In helping teachers organize their health instruction program, the director gives them the benefit of his or her own professional preparation and experience as well as knowledge of the total school health program. The health director becomes the key to the grade-to-grade integration of health instruction and is also familiar with state requirements and resources. The health director does not hand classroom teachers a schedule or plan for organization, but works the plan out with them or reviews their proposals with them and makes suggestions for improving the program. An experienced health director recognizes individual differences in teachers and accordingly recognizes that each teacher tends to organize the program in a pattern that best fits his or her particular abilities. Variation from grade to grade in the organization of health instruction is an indication of a vitalized program.

During the course of the year the director serves as a consultant for the teacher, aids in working out problems, and suggests new approaches that might be introduced. The director appraises the program both during the year and at the conclusion of the year.

Administrator's responsibility. If there is no health director, the principal should serve as a resource person for organizing health instruction. Some elementary school principals have an excellent health background and can provide highly valuable health supervision. However, principals with a very limited health background can be of assistance to the classroom teacher in resolving specific problems that may be particularly vexing.

Health resource person or coordinator. Some elementary schools have regular staff members serve as resource people in music, art, geography, health, and other areas. Elementary school teachers with a minor in health are prepared for this. Some elementary teachers return to college during summer sessions to obtain a minor in health. This health resource person serves as a health consultant for the other teachers in the building. In some school systems such a resource person may serve more than one building, and some have eventually become health directors for the whole school system. The advisability of such a health resource person in an elementary school is obvious. If the present trend continues, most elementary schools will have a recognized health resource person on their staffs.

Classroom teacher's function. Minimum health preparation of the elementary school teacher should be course work in general hygiene, school health services, and health instruction. Further health preparation would be highly desirable, but the many competencies expected of the elementary teacher leave little room for electives in the college curriculum. However, in-service preparation could include such course work as the health of the school-age child, physical growth and development, and mental health, as well as other courses.

Classroom teachers are the key persons in the organization and implementation of elementary school health instruction. Others may advise teachers and assist in various ways, but, because of their strategic location, only teachers are in a position to appreciate the total situation and the health implications inherent in it. Because they will direct children in learning, it is essential that they have a complete grasp of the health instruction plan and organization. If an inflexible plan and organization are handed to them, they are not likely to do an effective job of health teaching. On the other hand, if they have been a prime figure in the development of a health instruction plan and organization, their familiarity with the *what*, *how*, and *why* of the program should make their contribution a more meaningful and more effective one.

When teachers are left to their own resources, they are justified in utilizing plans and programs that have been developed by others, and then modifying and adapting them to their own classroom situations. These standard or developed programs should be a guide, not inflexible, unalterable procedures to be accepted in toto. The use of several sources may provide teachers with the substance from which to organize their own health instruction. Whatever the approach or source of reference, the health needs and interests of the children in a particular classroom should be the focal center

from which the program emerges. The health concerns and outcomes in terms of the students are the vehicle that propels the program. The guiding motive in the organization of health instruction is to provide students with opportunities to explore health concerns and to solve vital health problems.

Certain universal health needs and interests of pupils make it possible for teachers to utilize available materials and to apply them effectively to the immediate situation. Yet each group of children has need for special health emphasis or the consideration of a different type of health problem. For this reason, in a new situation an elementary schoolteacher might consider the organization of health instruction for a half year. A reappraisal at that time will indicate the strengths and weaknesses of the program and the modifications that are in order.

CLASSROOM INSTRUCTION

Motivating pupils sufficiently so that they want to establish desirable health practices is the basis for all health instruction. Motivation is the catalyst of all teaching, but most essentially so in health teaching.

Fundamental to motivation in elementary school health instruction is giving each pupil status in the classroom. A *team* concept—*us, we, all of us*—must permeate the atmosphere. This relationship within the group should be supported by a strong teacher-pupil relationship. Active participation in health projects is needed for all pupils. Neither passive nor vicarious participation will establish health practices. Above all, an organic relationship of pupil to group and group to pupil must be maintained for effective health instruction.

Pride in oneself, in one's own accomplishments, and in one's own progress is basic to all of us. Developing this pride constitutes a most effective means for initiating a health practice and for continuing the practice until it becomes ingrained in the pupil's mode of life. Appeal to pride in personal appearance can be as effective at the elementary school level as at adolescence if attention and praise are properly distributed.

Self-progress reinforced by an understanding of that progress motivates pupils in their quest for advancement. Competition with themselves can be wholesome motivation for pupils when realistic standards are the guide and when counseling in appraisal of their advances, plateaus, and failures is offered. Achievements that are visible to children can stimulate them to further achievement. It may be necessary to help them see their achievements.

Unless children internalize health instruction themselves, the whole opportunity for education has been missed. They must be the center of action—the vital element of greatest consideration. Moreover, they should feel this and be stimulated by it. This, of course, is necessary for any teaching situation to be effective.

At all times the elementary school teacher should direct health instruction toward the establishment of certain desirable health practices. Knowledge and attitudes can grow out of the establishment of health practices, contributing to their formation and permanence. These practices should be related to recognized factors in health such as play and rest, vision promotion, hearing protection, care of the teeth, cleanliness, general appearance, use of the toilet, avoiding infection, work practices, sleep, safety at school, safety at home, going to and from school, bicycle safety, fire safety, water safety, courtesy, self-reliance, self-discipline, and social adjustment. Specific practices will be listed in units and other sources that follow, but the teacher with some degree of ingenuity can develop a list of practices suited to the particular group of youngsters in the room.

In a well-organized system-wide health program, certain specific health practices should be common to all elementary schools as a guide in health education. This common core of practices will provide continuity and intensification. It will assure some measure of performance in health practices. In an elementary school where teachers agree on health practices to be established, the health program is assured of reasonably effective long-term results. Besides the reinforcing effect of such an established program, the likelihood of omissions is reduced, if not eliminated.

Various approaches to health instruction are in general use. Each has merit and can be used to advantage when adapted to particular needs and situations. Four approaches are of special interest:

1. Integrated living as health instruction
2. Planned direct formal and informal instruction
3. Incidental instruction
4. Correlated health instruction

Since all four approaches have special attributes and merits, the prudent elementary schoolteacher utilizes all four in conducting an effective health instruction program. Together the four approaches tend to ensure the maximum in effective health instruction.

INTEGRATED LIVING AS HEALTH INSTRUCTION

Life is not cast in a mold of isolated islands or separate compartments. Interwoven in each child's daily activities are health implications, values, and factors. All adaptation that pupils make has implications of either mental or physical health. In some activities health occupies a prominent role and in others assumes a lesser role. Yet whether it occupies a major or minor role, if the opportunity for health instruction is fully developed, the resulting health education can be both effective and lasting. If learning is a meaningful function experience, it becomes an established integral part of the mode of living of a child—the true goal of the school.

Pupil-teacher relationships. No one has objectively measured the specific influence of a particular teacher on a given pupil. Yet there is ample evidence that the teacher can modify the child in a beneficial way. Perhaps no phase of the school health instruction program can have a more beneficial lasting effect than the teacher's interest in and encouragement of each child's health. The approval of the teacher can develop the self-interest in health that is necessary to the promotion of personal health. From such experiences will develop worthy health goals, which, because of self-esteem, each person will strive to maintain. Teachers make a lasting wholesome impression when they recognize and commend the child's cleanliness, appear-

ance, dental care, posture, safety measures, dietary practices, courtesy, thoughtfulness, social adjustment, vitality, buoyancy, and general development. To the child, health truly becomes a matter of personal concern and gratification. It is the seed from which will develop a lifelong interest in personal health promotion.

Most teachers are interested in the well-being of schoolchildren. However, this interest should be expressed by interest in the child's health and his or her efforts in its behalf. Could there be a more worthy outcome of the total program of the school than students with a wholesome concern for their own health and with the necessary preparation to make the decisions that relate to their health and to that of their families? Pupil-teacher relationships provide the most effective means for motivating children to accept

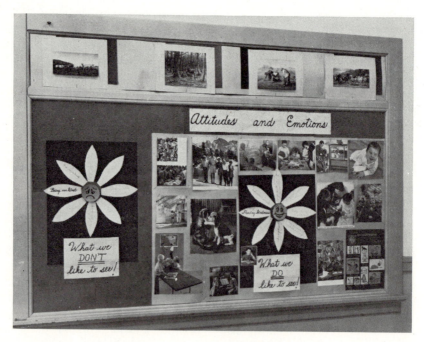

Fig. 12-1. The positive and the negative. Mental health can be portrayed pictorially with a little ingenuity. This bulletin board is more than clever. It is intensely meaningful as well as artistic. (Courtesy Corvallis Public Schools, Corvallis, Ore.)

responsibility for the promotion of their own health.

School experiences. Many school activities with health aspects provide opportunities for effective education. At times the instructional opportunities are missed completely. Perhaps more frequently, the experience is given cursory treatment. An alert teacher not only utilizes the unusual event for instructional purposes, but also recognizes opportunities for health instruction in the regular program (Figs. 12-1 and 12-2).

There are many opportunities in daily school experiences to apply health knowledge. The acts of coming to school and going home involve problems in safety for pedestrians, for bicycle riders, for general traffic, and for bus riders. Within the school, safety is an ever-present problem. Lighting, ventilation, cleanliness, dental health, posture, activity, rest, lunchroom practices, and social problems provide a diversity of opportunities for learning and its application.

Unusual experiences can have health implications of instructional value. The illness of a child can have learning value for classmates if the teacher directs the learning into constructive channels. An appendectomy can be discussed in terms of early indications, the desirability of avoiding self-diagnosis and self-medication, the need for immediate medical care, the effectiveness of modern medicine, and the importance of relying on the physician to restore health. Thus the fact that it is the individual who promotes health and the physician who restores health can be reemphasized.

If a child in the class wears glasses because of a physician's advice, the wisdom of wearing glasses can be emphasized by a class

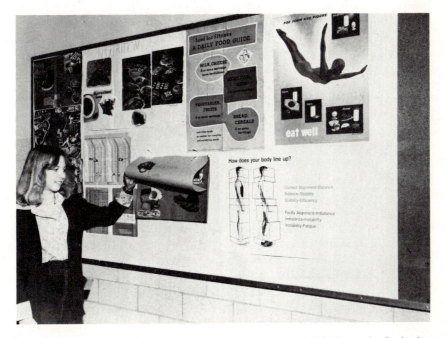

Fig. 12-2. Nutrition project in the intermediate grades. Posted on a hall bulletin, the display becomes available to all students in the school. (Courtesy Salem Public Schools, Salem, Ore.)

study of the problem. If the situation is dealt with openly, the supposed onus that youngsters may associate with glasses is removed. The children can learn that wearing glasses is not a stigma, but the badge of a person who is wise enough to use the fruits of modern science, just as a wise person uses other modern inventions.

Occasionally sensitive circumstances that relate to health arise in the school. Discretion would indicate that the teacher consider the situation carefully. After extended deliberation a means of using the event for instructional purposes may be devised. Perhaps the solution will be to consider related problems rather than the specific event. If a child has been hospitalized with influenza, a discussion of the measures for control of communicable disease rather than of influenza alone may be less disturbing but educationally just as valuable.

Many school experiences merit repeated consideration. A single discussion may create an interest but may not result in effective learning. Correlation of the factors in two or more experiences adds interest to the discussion and provokes thinking.

Community experiences. Events in the community may be a concern of schoolchildren. In the primary grades pupils have only slight community interest, which tends to develop as they reach the intermediate grades. Expansion of the municipal water facilities, construction of a sewage disposal plant, restaurant inspection, control measures for communicable disease, medical services, air pollution, safety programs, industrial health, recreation, and special health drives should be of interest to the future adults of the nation. Community health personnel can serve as a resource for stimulating the interest of children in community health.

Interest in local health can be projected to the state and nation. Children can acquire health understanding from epidemics, disasters involving health problems, new health experiments and discoveries, reports on the conquest of disease, extension of life expectation, and population growth. Indeed, international health can become interesting.

PLANNED DIRECT INSTRUCTION

With the elementary school program fragmented, as it tends to be, a scheduled time for health instruction is helpful. Doubtless a few teachers, highly skilled in incidental, correlated, and integrated health instruction, may do an effective job of health teaching without a scheduled period for health, but most teachers will need definite scheduled time to provide the necessary core instruction. A daily period is not necessary, but a fairly extended period of 30 minutes twice a week for primary pupils and three periods a week for intermediate children should serve as a minimum for core health instruction if supplementary health teaching makes a reasonably strong contribution. Such scheduling does not make an inordinate demand on school time.

Direct teaching is the core of the instructional program. Other procedures can supplement it advantageously, but the base of the instruction pyramid should be direct teaching. It serves many purposes and has definite advantages, such as the following:

1. Direct teaching gives status to health as a subject area.
2. It assures at least a minimum of emphasis on teaching.
3. It provides an organized approach.
4. It deals with realistic specific needs.
5. It makes effective results possible for a teacher of average ability.
6. It tends to emphasize the positive aspects of health.
7. It can be applied even with incidental teaching.
8. It can emerge from correlated teaching.
9. It can be channeled into integrated and other approaches.

10. It provides for outcomes in terms of interpretations, values, and other worthwhile attributes.

The imaginative teacher can use direct teaching as an adventure in health education, as effective as it is interesting.

Allocation and gradation. Emphasis for areas of special teaching should be allocated in the overall plans for health instruction. The key must be the interests and needs of the children at each age level. Health instruction is effective when it begins with children and their concerns or problems. If they can identify with a health problem and associate themselves with it, it takes on a personal meaning. The most effective health education is achieved when it seems to emanate from children rather than to be imposed on them from above. Complexity of treatment is adjusted to the psychological level of the pupils. Interests of the students indicate levels of maturity.

Areas of emphasis. Teachers can obtain an overview of the health needs, interests, and problems from observing the children; from their questions; from observing school, home, and community life; from statements of parents; from suggestions of health personnel; and from school records. Teachers will note that children in their early years tend to be individualists, which is reflected in their health interests. Starting in about the fifth grade, the tendency toward gangs begins to be expressed in an interest in group and community health.

Several studies have revealed the almost universal health interests and needs of children at various levels. An elementary schoolteacher can be guided by these studies if no other data are available. Where allocations of areas have been made on a school basis, results of these studies have frequently been used as a guide. Usually kindergarten and grades 1, 2, and 3 are grouped and grades 4, 5, and 6 given individual assignments of areas. It will be noted that the health of the individual is emphasized in the early years and community health is emphasized beginning with the fifth grade. Repetition and duplication are not necessarily objectionable. Certain duplications are inevitable, even desirable, but specific emphasis changes with the maturity of the pupil. Nutrition in the primary grades deals with a few simple dietary practices. In the intermediate grades an understanding of the *how* and *why* of certain nutritional needs is of interest to the pupils (Tables 12-1 and 12-2).

Table 12-1. Areas of emphasis, kindergarten and primary grades and grade 4

Kindergarten and primary grades	Grade 4
Physical health	
Personal cleanliness	Vision and hearing
School cleanliness	Illumination
Rest and sleep	Ventilation
Eating practices	Clothing
Posture	Cleanliness
Play practices	Activity
Dental health	Dental problems
Lighting	Nutrition
Common cold	Preventing infection
Safety to and from school	Illness
Schoolroom safety	Avoiding poisons
Playground safety	Fire prevention
Home safety	Traffic safety
Body growth	
Mental health	
Sharing	Sportsmanship
Working together	Self-direction
Kindness	Confidence
Being friendly	Our friends
Orderliness	Being grown up
Depending on ourselves	Courtesy
Attaining goals	Accepting disappointments
Community health	
Home life	Family health
Sources of water and milk	Helping the neighborhood
Sunshine and health	Improving the neighborhood

Table 12-2. Areas of emphasis, grades 5 and 6

Grade 5	Grade 6
Physical health	
Appraisal of personal health	Bicycle safety
Personal health promotion	Safety patrol
	Health examination
Balanced diets	Body function
Food preparation and care	Growth and development
	Grooming
Communicable diseases	Posture
Recreation needs	Rest and sleep
Developing skills	Communicable diseases
Body development	Home and farm safety
Relaxation	Emergency care
Types of school accidents	First-aid procedures
Playground accidents	Safety patrol
Fire prevention	
Fire drills	
Mental health	
Family relationships	Interesting people
Peer groups	Personality
Loyalties	Emotional adjustment
Social status	Life goals
Emotional maturation	Self-improvement
Community health	
Home sanitation	Community disease control
Health advertising	
Community safety program	Community water supply
	Milk control measures
School sanitation	Community sanitation

Motivation. A cue to all motivation in education is the natural human desire for self-status through attention, achievement, advancement, improvement, superiority, praise, and recognition. Motivation in health instruction should be relatively simple because health deals directly with a pupil's own welfare, but the whole experience must begin within the child if encouragement and direction are to be given him or her.

To promote self-identification in health, effort should be made to introduce each topic as a problem that is the concern of all who are present. By using a question as the ve-

hicle, the problem should be launched with emphasis on *you, we, all of us,* or *you* and *I.* The question should include or imply self-improvement. How can *we* keep clean so that *we* always look nice? Out of this appeal to appearance and improvement will emanate subquestions of keeping the hair clean, having clean fingernails, and other specific activities. How can *you* keep *your* teeth healthy and looking nice? The approach can apply equally to *our* school, *our* community, and *our* nation.

Questions can serve various purposes in making the instruction effective, such as the following:

1. Arouse curiosity, stimulate interest, and develop purpose
2. Prepare pupils for learning by leading them to draw from their experiences what they need and are concerned about
3. Cause the student to think and evaluate
4. Understand the pupil's thinking
5. Help the student discriminate
6. Direct the pupil's attention to significant elements
7. Bring about new concepts
8. Lead the pupils to give expression to their thinking
9. Help pupils see the pathway that might be taken

Once the project is launched, guidance and particularly recognition are necessary. Since children are gratified by their achievements, they have something to live up to, something to improve. Self-status becomes a wholesome motivating force. Every child can achieve some degree of success in feeling well, in improving personal appearance, and in following recognized health practices.

Methods. The versatile teacher uses a diversity of methods and adapts teaching to the needs and purposes of the situation. Certain teaching procedures are especially adaptable to the elementary school level. These include group discussion, lecturette, counseling, construction, independent study, oral presentation, problem solving, project method, reports, demonstration, dramatization, exhibits, field trips, and audiovisual aids.

In kindergarten and the primary grades the health instruction program can be based effectively on the development of desirable health practices. "Things We Do" is the theme:

1. Wash the face, neck, and ears every morning.
2. Wash hands before and after eating.
3. Wash hands before leaving the toilet room.
4. Keep the fingernails clean.
5. Wash the scalp at least once a week.
6. Keep the hair well groomed.
7. Take a cleansing bath at least once a week.
8. Stand, sit, and walk tall.
9. Get to bed on time each night: kindergarten and first grade, 8:00 P.M.; second and third grades, 8:30 P.M.; fourth grade, 9:00 P.M.; and fifth and sixth grades, 9:30 P.M.
10. Drink at least a half pint of milk with each meal.
11. Eat fruit at least twice a day.
12. Eat at least one green vegetable each day.
13. Eat one other vegetable in addition to potatoes each day.
14. Include proteins in each day's diet.
15. Brush the teeth immediately after eating and before going to bed.
16. Visit the dentist at least twice a year.
17. Keep fingers and other objects out of the mouth.
18. Use a clean handkerchief to cover a sneeze or cough.
19. Remain at home when ill.
20. Be alert for hazards that may cause accidents.
21. Follow all safety rules.
22. Use proper lights for all needs.
23. Provide proper ventilation without drafts.
24. Keep things orderly.
25. Hang up wraps.
26. Play out of doors at least 1 hour each day.
27. Work together with others.
28. Be friendly.
29. Accept disappointments cheerfully.
30. Finish tasks that are begun.

In the intermediate grades the health instruction program can be effectively incorporated into the general theme of daily living. This is functional instruction at its best.

The use of health texts or health readers and other written materials can be effective when these materials serve as a source of knowledge for pupils and do not constitute the total sum of the health instruction.

Materials. The busy elementary school classroom teacher must obtain instruction materials for a multitude of purposes. To assemble materials for health instruction poses an especially difficult task because of the diversity of topics encompassed by the term *health instruction.*

In order to assist the classroom teacher, several examples of health instruction units have been included in this chapter. Appendix A contains a listing of commercially published textbooks suitable for health instruction at the different grade levels. In addition to the commercially published materials, a number of new and experimental materials sponsored by private, voluntary government, and nonprofit agencies are now available to schools. An example of the latter are the American Health Foundation's Know Your Body Program and the Elementary School Health Project (Chapters 11 and 13).

Classroom teachers and school administrators may contact their state department of education regarding federal funds available to local schools for the development of curricular materials for health teaching. Such legislation as the amendments to the Child Nutrition Act and the Health Education Act of 1978 (an amendment to the Elementary and Secondary Act) are designed to help local schools improve their health instruction programs.

Two problems may be especially difficult for the elementary classroom teacher: What text should be used? Should commercially prepared materials for health instruction be used?

A textbook should be regarded as a reference. If textbooks are to be used in health instruction, certain standards in relation to health needs should then be met, in addition to the general criteria for all textbooks:

1. Primary emphasis should be on normal well-being.

2. Health principles should be stressed.
3. Discussion should be directed to the interests and needs of the pupils.
4. Personal appearance, physical health, and mental health are essential in the primary grades.
5. Community health should be included in the intermediate groups.
6. Very little physiology and less anatomy are needed.
7. An overview of each section can be of special value.
8. The literary style should be lucid and interesting.
9. Stimulating examples and original approaches add to the book's value.
10. Vocabulary should be adapted to the grade level.
11. A variety of suggested activities for pupils should be included.
12. Illustrations should be meaningful.
13. Graphs and charts should be such that the pupils can use them.
14. Suggestions for evaluation should be presented.

Commercial firms have turned out mountains of health instruction materials. Obviously the motivating factor has been the promotion of sales for their merchandise. Yet much of this material has been excellent— accurate, reliable, and well presented. If the firm has national operations and promotes its name and sales incidentally, teachers should feel free ethically to use the material if it serves their purposes. The use of commercial health instruction materials that are produced or distributed locally may lead to certain complications. Local competitors may accuse the school of partiality and of advertising commercial products.

Evaluation. In the final analysis the effectiveness of the health instruction program should be measured in terms of improved health of the pupils. This can be done to a limited degree both objectively and subjectively. Beyond this the teacher can observe and measure the effect of health instruction in terms of the child's conduct. Health attitudes, health knowledge, and health practices can be appraised in a practical way. Instruments for measurement will be presented in Chapter 17. Even in considering specific evaluation of the health instruction, the teacher can ask one cardinal question: Is each child building an *estate of health understanding* that will enable him or her to make the decisions necessary for health?

GRADE-TO-GRADE INTEGRATED RESOURCE UNITS—GRADES K, 1, 2, 3

Sex education in the primary grades properly is education in interpersonal relationships that is the core of all sexual expression. All sex education should be geared to the child's level of maturation, and these units take this into consideration (Fig. 12-3). Until about 9 years of age children are sexually neutral. There is no stronger an attraction to members of the opposite sex than to members of their own sex. This sexual neutrality stems from the child's constitutional biochemistry. Until about 10 years of age the boy's output of male sex hormones (androgens) is but slightly greater than his output of female hormones (estrogens). In the girl the output of estrogens is little more than the output of androgens. Thus to talk about sex to youngsters under 10 is to puzzle the youngsters with something they have not experienced and that would have little meaning to them. Certain social conditioning has helped the boy and girl develop their roles as male and female.

Human interrelationships
OVERVIEW

At this stage of life children are neutral in sexuality and have no particular interest in anything of a sexual

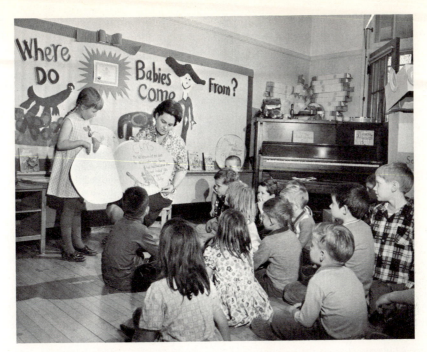

Fig. 12-3. Teaching concepts on reproduction in the kindergarten. Elements of reproduction can be taught in a wholesome manner, which will satisfy the curiosity of the children. Advance support of the school patrons is essential before reproduction is taught at any level. (Courtesy Portland Public Schools, Portland, Ore.)

nature because it is a feeling or concept they have never experienced and thus is completely foreign to them. However, this is a most opportune time for the child to acquire an understanding of wholesome, effective human relationships that, after all, are the basis of wholesome sex relations in maturity. Children benefit from an early knowledge of how to relate to other people, what society accepts and expects in one's relationship to others, and what to expect in return. Children who early in life acquire the attitudes, the knowledge, and the practices essential to a high level of interpersonal relationships will possess assets of lifelong value. In these early grades the school can lay the foundations on which wholesome adjustments, including sexual adjustments, will be made in the youth and adult periods of life.

AIM OF THE UNITS

Develop in children those qualities of personal worth that will command a high level of respect from others and will have an equally high respect for others.

OBJECTIVES

Develop in children attributes of:
1. Wholesome pride in self
2. Respect for parents
3. Respect for brothers and sisters
4. Respect for classmates
5. Respect for teachers
6. Respect for other people
7. Respect for authority
8. Respect for the rights of others
9. Respect for privacy
10. Respect for property
11. Thoughtfulness
12. Kindness
13. Fair play
14. Sharing
15. Obedience
16. Cooperation
17. Honesty
18. Courteousness
19. Responsibility
20. Consideration

21. Neatness

Through practice acquire knowledge of:
1. Personal care
2. Social customs
3. Social manners
4. Making introductions
5. Conversation courtesies
6. Proper dress
7. Relating to others
8. Making apologies

KINDERGARTEN
Unit title—Every boy and girl a friend

CONCEPT

I. Friends
  A. Discussion
    1. What friends are
    2. How we make friends
    3. Why we need friends
    4. Why friends need us
    5. How we are nice to each other
    6. Partners in play and work
    7. Sharing
    8. Taking turns
    9. Helping each other
    10. Being careful not to hurt anyone
    11. Returning things we have used
    12. Returning things we have borrowed
    13. Saying, "Thank you"
    14. Fun of being nice to everyone
    15. People who make us happy
    16. People we make happy
  B. Construction
    1. Bulletin board of pictures of friendship
    2. Pictures of kindness to animals
    3. Pictures of kindness to boys and girls
  C. Dramatization and other activities
    1. Act out proper ways to be polite to others
    2. Act out how to let the other person go first
    3. Act out safety rules outside of the schoolroom
    4. Act out safety rules in the schoolroom
    5. Act out situations in which courtesy is involved
II. Cleanliness
  A. Discussion
    1. Why we should always try to be clean
    2. When we should wash our hands
    3. When we should wash our face
    4. When we should bathe
    5. Keeping teeth clean
    6. Combing our hair
    7. How we can keep our clothes looking neat

8. Taking care of our clothes
9. Keeping our shoes clean
10. Helping our parents by keeping ourselves clean
11. Keeping all of our things in the right place
12. Why people like boys and girls who are clean and neat
  B. Construction
    1. Have a corner grooming stand with mirror where children can check their grooming
    2. For inclement weather have a mat or other device for cleaning off shoes
    3. On bulletin board, post pictures of children properly dressed for different purposes
    4. Have a plan so every child has a place for his or her coat, umbrella, and other possessions, and puts things in their proper place
  C. Dramatization
    1. Demonstration of how to wash and dry hands properly
    2. Wash parade before lunch
    3. Demonstration of proper brushing of teeth
    4. Demonstration of hair grooming
    5. Showing how to help each other put on and take off coats

EVALUATION

Periodically observe children regarding their:
  1. Relationship with one another
  2. Improvement in sharing
  3. Improvement in working with others
  4. Courteousness
  5. Neatness
  6. Personal care
  7. Pride in appearance
  8. Orderliness
  9. Ability to adjust to different types of children and situations
  10. Apparent desire to get along with everyone

GRADE 1
Unit title—Social development activities

CONCEPT

I. Respect for parents, brothers, and sisters
  A. Discussion
    1. Discuss what parents do for us
    2. What can we do for parents?
    3. What do brothers and sisters mean to us?
    4. What do we do to be nice to brothers and sisters?
    5. What does it mean to have respect for people?

B. Construction
1. Cut out pictures showing parents and children
2. Collect pictures showing brothers and sisters

C. Dramatization and practices
1. Oral reports on examples of being kind and helpful to parents
2. Skit in which one child after another relates different things a child can do to help his or her parents
3. Dialogue between four pupils telling how they help their brothers and sisters and also play with them

II. Making friends

A. Discussion
1. Sharing
2. Why we share
3. What friends are
4. How to earn friends
5. Why we like to be nice to people
6. Why we want friends
7. Fair play
8. Honesty
9. Kindness
10. Helping others
11. How to make up when there has been a misunderstanding
12. What to do when a stranger speaks to a child

B. Construction
1. Make a list of your friends
2. Collect color ads showing friendship
3. Cut out pictures showing children helping someone
4. Make a drawing of friendship as a tree with branches named for each of your friends
5. Make drawings of some friends

C. Dramatization and practices
1. Each child describing a special friend and explaining the reason for the friendship; others guessing who the friend is
2. Skit showing how to greet people
3. Skit showing thoughtfulness toward others
4. One child serving as master of ceremonies and asking others to explain why friends are important

III. Having good manners

A. Discussion
1. Why we should learn to do things correctly
2. Being polite to other children
3. Being polite to teachers
4. Being polite to parents
5. Being polite to brothers and sisters
6. Saying, "Thank you"
7. Saying, "You are welcome"
8. How and when to say, "Excuse me"
9. How and when to say, "Pardon me"
10. Good manners in the schoolroom
11. Good manners in the halls
12. Good manners on the playground
13. Good manners on the bus
14. Good manners at home
15. How to show appreciation
16. Being obedient
17. Boys letting girls go first
18. Being orderly
19. What good sportsmanship means

B. Construction
1. From magazines cut out pictures showing politeness
2. Paste cutouts showing table manners
3. Have a bulletin board of pictures showing good manners
4. Have children keep order going to lunch, to the playground, or elsewhere
5. Have a plan for greeting visitors with children having roles

C. Dramatization and practices
1. Demonstrate making and accepting introductions
2. Demonstrate how to offer apologies
3. Demonstrate how to show appreciation for a favor
4. Have a small table set for luncheon with a boy and girl to serve as models, and demonstrate good table manners

IV. Looking neat and clean

A. Discussion
1. Why we should try to be clean
2. Why we should keep our clothes neat and clean
3. Keeping hair combed
4. Washing hands before meals
5. Washing hands after the toilet
6. Keeping fingernails clean
7. Keeping shoes clean
8. Proper dress at different times

B. Construction
1. Collect colored pictures showing children who are appropriately dressed
2. Have children bring snapshots showing themselves appropriately dressed
3. Collect pictures showing good grooming
4. Have a bulletin board showing children looking attractive
5. Girls bring dolls dressed neatly and cleanly

C. Dramatization and practice
1. Wash parade before going to lunch

2. Cleaning fingernails using toothpicks
3. Keeping hair combed or brushed
4. Wiping off shoes before coming into classroom
5. Keeping wraps in order and in assigned place

EVALUATION

Periodic checkups of children relating to:
1. Manners
2. Appearance
3. Politeness
4. Consideration of others
5. Sharing
6. Respect for wishes and property of others
7. Acceptance of responsibility
8. Relating to others
9. Respect for adults
10. Growth in social maturity

GRADE 2
Unit title—Social, emotional growth

CONCEPTS AND ACTIVITIES

I. Importance of friendships
  A. Discussion
    1. Meaning of growing up
    2. Number of ways of growing up
    3. How making friends helps us grow up
    4. What a friend is
    5. Three characteristics you would look for
    6. How to make friends
    7. Meaning of making people happy
    8. How to help a friend be happy
    9. Meaning of being sad
    10. Meaning of being angry
    11. What to do if a friend is angry
    12. What to do if a friend is sad
    13. What to do when a friend makes a mistake
    14. What is meant by helping a friend who is in trouble
    15. How a child in second grade shows courtesies to grown-ups
    16. Some problems we might have with friends
    17. Being honest
    18. Being thoughtful of the child who is alone
    19. Why being selfish does not make friends
    20. How to get along with one person
    21. How to get along with a group of people
    22. Talking things over
    23. Reporting good deeds that a friend does
    24. What to do when we are disappointed
    25. Being helpful to others
  B. Construction
    1. Have children keep track of good deeds they see in others

2. Make a chart listing mistakes to be avoided
3. Show pictures of facial expressions and have the children identify the feelings (e.g., joy, anger, sorrow, hunger, fear, jealousy)
4. Make a chart of feelings, both helpful and harmful, in making friends
5. Post pictures showing friendship among children of other lands
6. Post pictures showing friends at play
7. Draw pictures showing children playing together
8. Make a list of the way your friends differ
  C. Dramatization and other activities
    1. Give a problem in child-to-child relations to groups of six children and ask each group to work out a best solution (e.g., both children claiming ownership of a book or other object; deciding who should go first; deciding which of two things should be done)
    2. Devise a situation involving a conflict and have the class help the child or children find the best solution; bring attention to the procedures used to decide the matter
    3. Have a small group work up a skit using different ways to greet a friend

II. Courtesy
  A. Discussion
    1. Courtesy in public
    2. Courtesy to policemen
    3. Courtesy to teachers, custodians, lunchroom people
    4. Why we need rules
    5. Traffic rules
    6. School rules
    7. Rules at home
    8. Who goes first
    9. Letting others go first
    10. When we should give our name to strangers
  B. Construction
    1. Bulletin board with list of polite words
    2. Display of pictures showing politeness
    3. Display list of kind things to do for others
    4. Display pictures of children doing kind things for their parents
    5. List of good things children have done the past week
  C. Dramatization and other activities
    1. Act out courteous behavior through skits, role-playing, or pantomimes
    2. Act out a situation in which someone misunderstands (e.g., taking out bats and balls or other equipment without permission, or not returning something borrowed)
    3. Children tell ways to be helpful at home
    4. Children tell of volunteer services, those

performed by their parents and other grown-ups

5. Act out discourteous behavior followed by the right behavior

III. Human life
A. Discussion
1. What makes people different from animals?
2. Why do animals as well as people have to take care of the young?
3. What can people do that animals cannot do?
4. What makes plant life different?
5. Why do people live in cities?
6. What do families do for other families?
7. Why should we help each other?
8. Why should we help animals?
B. Construction
1. Display pictures of animal families
2. Display pictures of family life
3. Display pictures of grown and young plants
4. Plant seeds in a planter and tend the growing plants
5. Display pictures of the different jobs people do to help other people
6. Make booklets showing different kinds of people that are in the world
C. Dramatization and other activities
1. Bring baby pictures and try to identify
2. Bring pictures of churches, synagogues, and other important community buildings and explain why they are important
3. Report on community activities important for human life (e.g., hospital, fire station, police force, water department, health department)
4. Display pictures of families from other lands and explain how they live
5. Display and explain pictures of people at different stages of life (e.g., babyhood to old age)

EVALUATION

From time to time check on pupils regarding:
1. Adjustment of their classmates
2. Acceptance of tasks cheerfully
3. Participating in group activities
4. Consideration of rights of others
5. Adjustment to disappointment
6. Courteousness
7. Consideration of the feelings of others
8. Regard for the child who is sad or alone
9. Conformity to traffic rules
10. Conformity to rules within the school
11. Increased social sensitivity
12. Dependability
13. Willingness to do their share
14. Pride in their families and homes

GRADE 3
Unit title—Growth and maturing

CONCEPT AND ACTIVITIES

I. Life and growth
A. Discussion
1. All life has a beginning, grows, changes, matures, and eventually dies
2. In what ways are plants and animals alike and different?
3. All life reproduces itself
4. How do plants reproduce themselves?
5. What do plants need to keep alive and where do these things come from?
6. Plants grow, change, and carry on certain activities
7. How important are plants to the lives of all of us?
8. Animals have young that are hatched from eggs or borne by the mother
9. Care of the young is important for all of the animal species
10. Care of their babies is important to our parents, too
11. Discuss the nature of human growth
12. How do we change from babyhood through each stage to adulthood?
13. Discuss how boys and girls differ in their growth patterns
14. All life needs nourishment for what purposes?
15. How does what we feed the baby differ from what children of 8 or 9 years old are fed?
16. Discuss what is meant by a well-balanced diet
17. How does the school lunch provide for growth?
18. Evaluate personal diets
B. Construction
1. Have an aquarium or terrarium in the room to demonstrate the "web of life"
2. Grow plants from seeds and seedlings
3. Make a chart of the four basic food groups
4. Plan a single meal such as breakfast
5. Plan a menu for a day
6. Make a chart of stages of growth using cutouts as models
7. Make a bulletin board or mural titled, "What helps us grow?"
8. Make lists of how children differ: physical characteristics, manners, grooming, speaking, opinions, interests
C. Dramatization and other activities
1. Get information from parents on family growth characteristics and report to the class

2. Report on human growth differences throughout the world
3. Using a veterinary resource, report on rate of animal growth over a period of several weeks
4. Have a nurse, physician, or other resource person talk on human life, growth, and well-being
5. Bring baby pictures to school and have children guess who each is

II. Maturing

A. Discussion
   1. How does maturing differ from growth?
   2. What does it mean to act grown up?
   3. What feelings or emotions do we have?
   4. How do we control the emotion of anger?
   5. How do we control selfishness or meanness?
   6. Why do people dislike us if we cheat?
   7. What is meant by:

      | Happiness | Respect |
      | Honesty | Forgiveness |
      | Courage | Responsibility |

   8. How do our thoughts about ourselves influence the way we think about others?
   9. Why does self-respect promote respect for others?
   10. Why should we always try to have more friends?
   11. How do we get more friends?
   12. What qualities do you like in others?
   13. What do we mean when we say a certain third-grader acted like a first-grader?
   14. What do we mean when we say a certain third-grader acted like a fifth-grader?
   15. Note individual differences and qualities
   16. How do we show others we value their friendship?

B. Construction
   1. On the blackboard each week have a question relating to behavior asking if all students have exhibited a certain quality each day (e.g., "Am I courteous?" "Am I thoughtful?" "Am I dependable?"
   2. Post pictures displaying desirable mature conduct
   3. Have children keep records of their good deeds
   4. Have children make an appraisal of their best qualities and those in which improvement is needed

C. Dramatization and other activities
   1. Read the book, *Laugh and Cry,* by Gerrold Beim, which explains that emotions are natural
   2. Tell stories to the class about people with ex-

ceptional courage, thoughtfulness, dependability, or other qualities
3. Have children report an exceptional case of helpfulness, courtesy, industriousness, or other quality they observed
4. Have a skit that demonstrates courtesies of boys toward girls and of girls toward boys
5. Demonstrate courteous conduct toward adults in various walks of life
6. Have each of a panel of five give a description of some junior high youngster who is unusually mature and explain why he or she is regarded as unusually mature

EVALUATION

Observe class members regarding:
1. Interest in life about them
2. Concern for life
3. Interest in their own growth
4. Interest in children in other parts of the world
5. Nutrition interests and practices
6. Concern about growth of others
7. Desire to improve relations with other children
8. Interest in expanding friendships
9. Respect shown for adults and pupils
10. Increased sense of responsibility
11. Honesty
12. Obedience
13. Ability to make amends for mistakes

RESOURCE UNIT—GRADE 2

As a vehicle for direct health instruction the integrated unit permits the use of various teaching procedures that grow out of recognized interests and needs of the pupils. If the unit is constructed for the primary purpose of establishing certain health practices, it will include health attitudes and knowledge (Fig. 12-4). The representative unit presented is designed primarily to establish certain nutritional practices, but cleanliness, dental health, and table manners are associated with the experiences in eating, which can fortify the nutrition practices and, in turn, can be established as part of a total aspect of life.

The unit can be introduced by questions that deal with feeling well, looking well, and growing (Fig. 12-5). Out of the preliminary discussion will evolve the question, What foods help us feel best and grow best?

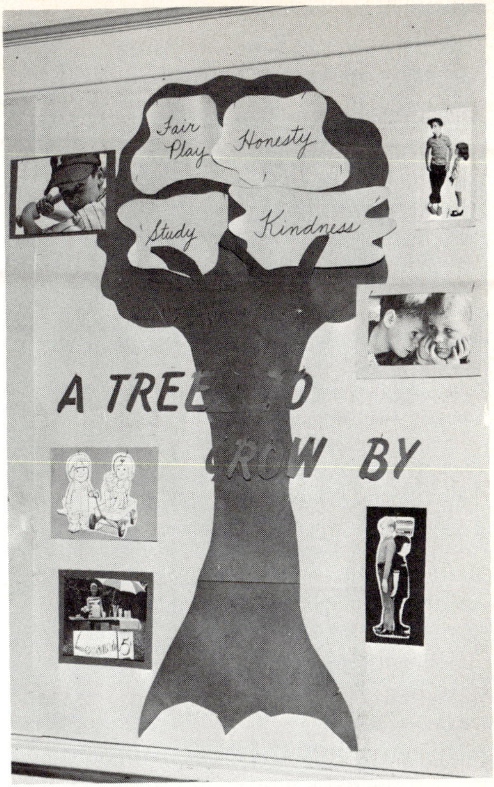

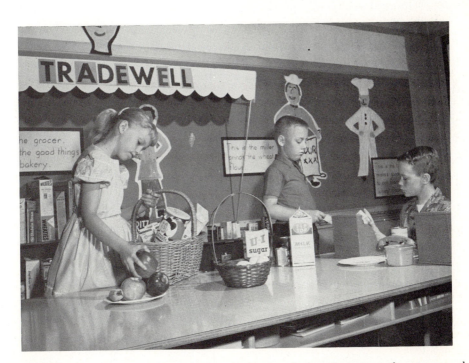

Fig. 12-4. First-grade health bulletin board. Attributes such as kindness, fair play, honesty, and study may be rather abstract, but the highly impressionable children, through an attractive visual display, can begin to incorporate these ideas into their thinking and conduct.

Fig. 12-5. Selecting food for a balanced diet. A grocery store mock-up gives practice in the primary need in nutrition education—the selection of food. (Courtesy Portland Public Schools, Portland, Ore.)

Unit title—What foods help us feel best and grow best?

OBJECTIVES

Establish the practice of washing hands before and after eating

Keep the fingernails clean

Establish importance of regularity of mealtime

Practice drinking at least a half pint of milk with each meal

Eat fruit at least twice a day

Eat one green vegetable each day

Eat other vegetables every day

Eat whole-grained cereals and bread

Eat meat, eggs, or dairy products each day

Brush the teeth immediately after each meal and before going to bed

Visit the dentist at least twice a year

Choose a wholesome breakfast, lunch, and dinner

Use proper table manners

Promote an active interest in personal growth in height and weight

Create a pride and interest in personal well-being, appearance, and conduct

ACTIVITIES
Group discussion

Why we all like to feel well

Why we all want to look nice

Why we all should learn to do things correctly

Getting ready for a meal

Why we should always try to be clean

Eating meals at regular times

Mealtime

Milk and growth

Milk and feeling well

Amount of milk to drink with each meal

Why coffee and tea are not good for children

Source of milk for each home

Care of milk

Cereals and whole-grained bread

Kinds of fruits—name all we know

Favorite fruits

Amount of fruits we should have each day

Learning about new fruits

Why babies should have orange and tomato juice

Kinds of green vegetables

Other vegetables

Favorite vegetables

Vegetables that should be eaten each day

Learning about new vegetables

Kinds of meat and dairy products

Meat, eggs, or dairy products every day

Meat, eggs, dairy products, and growth

Weight and height as signs of growth

Foods good for teeth

Why we should brush our teeth right after eating

How to brush the teeth

Toothpaste

How we care for our toothbrushes

Seeing the dentist

Construction

Collecting color advertisements on cleanliness

Color advertisements on milk

Color advertisements on fruits

Color advertisements on vegetables

Color advertisements on meat, eggs, and dairy products

Color advertisements on care of the teeth

Making posters

Color fruit and vegetable outlined forms

Cutouts of sample meals

Exhibits of fruits and vegetables

Make toothbrush holders

Model of a dairy

Make a clock to indicate mealtime

Make a card shaped like a milk bottle or carton to record height and weight

Dramatization

Have a wash parade before lunch

Demonstrate hand washing

Clean the nails (with toothpicks)

Have a toothbrush parade

Have a fruit party

Have a vegetable party, with raw vegetables that can be eaten

Plan breakfast, lunch, and dinner

Play cafeteria

Play store

Buy food

Have a host and hostess at each table at lunchtime

Field trips

Dairy

Grocery

Market

Farm

EVALUATION

Periodic survey of health practices

Observed attitudes of children toward
    Cleanliness
    Milk
    Fruit and vegetables
    Meat, eggs, and dairy products
    Care of the teeth

Knowledge test
    Oral
    Chalkboard with yes and no answers
    Vocabulary

Many elementary schools are departing from the practice of using one central lunchroom, and instead all children eat their lunches in their respective classrooms. This arrangement has excellent possibilities for health instruction. A wash parade before lunch, white napkins at the table or desk at lunchtime, and a host and hostess each day have a marked effect on table practices.

RESOURCE UNIT—GRADE 3

Teachers frequently encounter a situation that involves a single highly important aspect of child health behavior. Such a special demanding health topic frequently requires a conference of all teachers in the school. The conference is desirable to review what must be taught and in what grade or grades the special emphasis is to be applied. An example is the problem of cigarette smoking.

Some years ago the schools recognized that they could and should make a supreme effort to deal with this highly important health topic. Teachers decided that smoking was a senior high school problem and consequently almost all emphasis was directed to the senior high schools. Teachers soon recognized that they were too late. Students coming up from the junior high were already smokers. Further study of the problem indicated that the junior high school was too late and that students were experimenting with smoking in the fifth and sixth grades. So down to the third and fourth grades a program to prevent smoking seemed logical. It also became apparent that a concise, student-involvement program be developed.

Such a teaching unit, preferably directed to the third grade, could be highly effective in the prevention of smoking. It should be recognized that pupils must be personally involved and that the discussions and activities must make all students associate this prevention of smoking with themselves. This unit is designed to aid the teacher in this highly important aspect of student behavior.

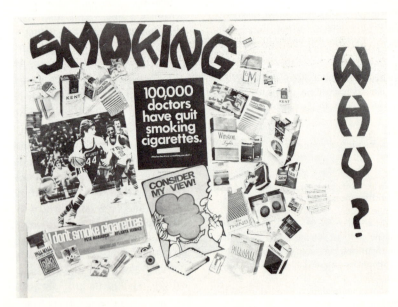

Fig. 12-6. Resisting the temptation to smoke. A bold frontal attack on the dangers of smoking perhaps will have its greatest impact on the elementary school students. (Courtesy Salem Public Schools, Salem, Ore.)

It also illustrates one type of resource unit that can be highly effective in the development of desirable attitudes (Fig. 12-6).

Unit title—Resisting the temptation to smoke

OVERVIEW

Children are first tempted to smoke when they are in the fifth or sixth grade and are tempted by members of their peer group. Children do not know how to cope with this new situation because they have never associated themselves with the use of cigarettes. This curiosity, coupled with peer group pressure, entices them to try it. Giving children advance knowledge of this confrontation and what to expect can prepare them to meet this very critical stage in their lives. If they know the answers to these questions and have this knowledge fortified by concern for their own welfare, they can build up a resistance or inhibition that will serve them in their moment of need.

AIM OF THE UNIT

To develop in third-graders an effective barrier against trying that first cigarette by giving these youngsters the know-how to deal with the temptation to smoke.

OBJECTIVES

Develop self-pride
Develop appreciation of people who do not smoke
Develop appreciation of right and wrong
Develop experience in being able to face up to difficult situations
Respect wishes of parents
Develop appreciation of harmfulness of smoking
Explain how smoking detracts from a person
Develop experience in how to go against people who are wrong
Learn to say no
Resolve not to smoke until after the age of 21 years

ACTIVITIES

A. Discussion
  1. Why cigarettes are not our friends
  2. Why people smoke
  3. What to say when someone offers you a cigarette
  4. How do you tell a classmate he or she should not have cigarettes
  5. Why we should be proud that we do not "try" a cigarette
  6. Why we should not plan to smoke before we become adults
  7. Why there is no value in smoking
  8. What makes us liked by others
  9. How to deal with all temptations
  10. How we feel proud when we do the right thing
  11. Why some boys and girls smoke
B. Construction
  1. Bulletin board with people enjoying themselves without smoking
  2. Pictures of nonsmoking families
  3. Pictures of prominent people who do not smoke
  4. Pictures of well-groomed, attractive nonsmokers
C. Dramatization
  1. Demonstrate how to refuse a cigarette
  2. Demonstrate how to tell classmates they should never smoke
  3. Panel: why boys and girls should not do things they must hide from their parents
  4. Tell someone that you do not smoke

LEARNING ABOUT YOUR ORAL HEALTH, LEVEL II: 4-6

This unit illustrates another way in which the subject matter (content) of health education can be organized. The unit of human interrelationships or sex education for kindergarten through third grade presents a grade-by-grade progression of the social, emotional, and physiological aspects of sex education. The oral health unit, however, presents a horizontal structure emphasizing a particular sequence of topics—integrating dental health with other health topics such as nutrition, health services, disease, safety, and consumer health. The unit offers an in-depth study of dental health, focusing on preventing dental disease by controlling plaque in the mouth through oral hygiene (flossing and brushing) and proper diet. In addition to the benefits afforded by integrated learning, the unit provides a number of classroom activities designed to stimulate student interest and understanding of the importance of dental health to total health.

When curriculum materials such as the American Dental Association's oral health program are used, teachers must make special adaptations for the particular school system and give careful study to the materials in order to understand the guiding philosophy

Text continued on p. 305.

TO THE TEACHER

Dental disease is the leading morbidity problem in America today. It affects practically everyone.

By the time he starts school, the average child has at least three decayed primary teeth. With development of permanent dentition, decay attacks the teeth at the rate of about one tooth per year. By age 20, the average young adult has 14 decayed, missing or filled teeth. While neglect of oral hygiene during early years takes a heavy toll in tooth decay, many people do not realize that it also sets the stage for an even higher toll from gum disease in adulthood. This illustrates vividly the need for education of our country's children in methods for preventing decay and gum disease. To do this requires the development of appropriate knowledge, skills and attitudes.

As an elementary school teacher, *you* are in a unique position to help prevent dental disease among your students. With your guidance, effective oral hygiene habits can be established that will benefit them all their lives.

Classroom instruction in flossing and brushing is the first objective of the program. This is essential to ensure habit development and positive behavioral change.

Once the children have demonstrated their ability to control plaque mechanically, they should study the relation of diet to oral health. Additional portions of the program are important to strengthen awareness and appreciation for oral health.

Many local dental societies and women's auxiliary groups are interested in assisting with prevention-oriented dental health education in the schools. You may wish to explore the possibility of cooperation with these groups, especially in classroom teaching of flossing and brushing.

BASIC CONCEPTS

The underlying philosophy of the program is summarized by the following statements:

1. "Health is a state of complete physical, mental and social well-being, not merely the absence of disease and infirmity." (World Health Organization)
2. Optimum oral health is an integral part of general health.
3. Acceptance of oral health information, practices and services is the result of interaction between various forces, often of a divergent nature.
4. Developing and maintaining optimum oral health is the responsibility of:
    a. The individual
    b. The family
    c. The dentist and the dental professional team
    d. The community
5. Most dental disease is preventable by:
    a. Correct, thorough and consistent oral hygiene procedures
    b. Proper diet
    c. Use of accepted therapeutics
    d. Professional supervision at appropriate intervals
6. Many oral injuries are preventable through observance of safety precautions.
7. Dental diseases and problems should be treated to develop optimum possible function of oral structures.
8. Optimum oral health in part depends on knowledge of the structure and function of oral tissues, and the causes and treatment of various oral diseases.
9. Optimum oral health in part depends on a positive attitude toward oneself, oral health practices and products, as well as professional dental health services.
10. Optimum oral health in part depends on each individual's acceptance of his responsibility to promote programs of community dental health.

Continued.

Learning About Your ORALHEALTH

THE WHY AND HOW OF PLAQUE CONTROL

Goals: To develop the knowledge, skills and attitudes needed for prevention of dental disease.
To develop an understanding of the role of plaque in dental disease.
To develop acceptance of personal responsibility for daily plaque removal.
To develop abilities needed for daily plaque removal.

Behavorial Objectives	Content	Suggested Activities	Related Activities in Other Classes
The pupil can define plaque in simple words. The pupil can recognize plaque in his own mouth.	**Plaque defined** Plaque is a sticky, colorless layer of harmful bacteria. Plaque sticks to teeth, especially near the gum line. It forms constantly on everyone's teeth. If plaque is not removed, it can harden (become mineralized) and is then called calculus. Calculus can only be removed by the dentist or one of his assistants. Calculus will not form if plaque is removed daily.	Ask pupils what they would like to know about their teeth and gums. List their questions on the chalkboard. Retain a copy for reference during oral health instruction. Have each pupil chew a disclosing wafer (see "Cleaning Your Teeth and Gums" for method). Have pupils examine their teeth and gums using small mirrors brought from home. Explain that the red-stained areas are plaque which needs to be removed. (This activity may be conducted separately, or may be combined with the first in-class cleaning time.)	**Drama:** Have pupils develop a skit, playlet or puppet show about the dangers to teeth and gums, and how teeth and gums can be protected by good personal oral hygiene practices. **Art:** Have pupils make charts or posters to use at home, to remind them to disclose, floss and brush. **Art:** Have pupils make their own floss and brush holders. A thoroughly rinsed milk carton covered with construction paper is the holder. A "door" can be made for floss to go through, and the brush is the chimney. This container can also hold disclosing tablets and a small mirror.
The pupil can describe the process of development of tooth decay, with emphasis on the role of plaque.	**Plaque and decay** When sugar is eaten, bacteria in plaque form acid. Plaque holds acid to the tooth surface. Acid eats holes in the tooth surface, causing decay. The body cannot repair this damage by itself. If not treated by a dentist, decay will spread throughout the tooth. The tooth might ultimately have to be removed.	Demonstrate to pupils the decalcifying effect of acid by soaking an uncooked egg in vinegar for 6 hours. As acid decalcifies the shell, it will become soft and the egg can be pushed through an opening too small for it prior to acid exposure. Explain that what acid does to the egg shell, it can also do to teeth. Obtain an unbruised apple. Make a hole in it, one inch deep. Set it aside for several days, protected from view in a paper bag. Cut through the place where the hole was made and have the class observe the effect of decay. Explain that this illustrates the way decay spreads through a tooth. Obtain some extracted teeth from a dentist. Protect a portion of each tooth with wax. Place the teeth in various solutions, such as saliva, sugar water, sugary soft drink, acid (vinegar), salt water, etc. Observe changes for two weeks. (3rd grade)	

A preventive approach to dental health as recommended by American Dental Association oral health teaching-learning specialists, program level II.

Behavorial Objectives	Content	Suggested Activities	Related Activities in Other Classes
The pupil can describe the development of gum disease, with emphasis on the role of plaque.	**Plaque and gum (periodontal) disease** Bacteria in plaque secrete substances which irritate the gums (gingiva), causing inflammation. When plaque is not removed and calculus forms, more plaque forms on top of the calculus. Bleeding when teeth are flossed and brushed is one sign of gum disease. Inflammation can progress to formation of pockets between teeth and gums, loosening of teeth and their eventual loss. Pressure caused by thickening calculus helps separate the gums from the teeth.	Ask pupils how many have had bleeding when they clean their teeth. Explain that this is a sign of gum disease, and that they can help prevent gum disease by daily removing the plaque from their teeth.	
The pupil shows improvement in the amount of plaque removed. The pupil can specify the periods set aside each day in his routine for plaque removal. The pupil demonstrates continued ability to remove plaque, as measured by periodic spot checks with a disclosing wafer.	**Removing plaque** Plaque is disclosed, then flossed and brushed away. To help prevent disease, children should brush after eating, brush and floss before bed.	Ask pupils to name ways to clean teeth and gums, listing reported suggestions on the chalkboard. Have pupils attempt to remove stained plaque by: a. eating crisp food (celery, apple). b. rinsing the mouth with water. c. chewing sugarless gum. d. brushing. e. flossing. This experiment is designed to destroy the myths related to detergent foods, rinsing and gum chewing as helping to clean the teeth and will reinforce the need for brushing and flossing.	
	Disclosing Plaque may be made visible by coloring it with a wafer made of harmless dye. Consult "Cleaning Your Teeth and Gums" for a description of the procedure.	If possible, involve parents in the classroom plaque removal program. The Plaque Control Kit contains copies of "Happiness is a Healthy Mouth" to send home for parents of 35 pupils. Parents may be invited to participate in plaque removal sessions. Or an evening program for pupils to demonstrate plaque control techniques may be planned.	
	Flossing Flossing is necessary to remove plaque from the sides of teeth. Consult "Cleaning Your Teeth and Gums" for a description of the procedure.	**Introduction to flossing** To demonstrate the need for flossing, cover your hand with thick tempera paint. Then use a toothbrush to clean off the paint, holding fingers tightly together. The brush will not remove material from between the fingers. The comparison with plaque on the sides of teeth can then be made. Have the class study the transparency, "Where Plaque Hides."	

Continued.

A preventive approach to dental health as recommended by American Dental Association oral health teaching-learning specialists, program level II.

Behavioral Objectives	Content	Suggested Activities	Related Activities in Other Classes
	A method of holding floss which may be easier for children is: Tie a knot in the ends of 12-14 inches of floss to form a circle. Hold the circle with 3rd, 4th and 5th fingers of each hand. Use thumbs and forefingers to guide floss.	**Flossing practice** Issue floss to each pupil. Have pupils floss their teeth, starting with the back of the back tooth and working around the arch in a regular pattern. The prepared drawing, "Flossing Your Teeth," provides an illustration for each pupil.	
	Brushing Consult "Cleaning Your Teeth and Gums" for a description of a brushing method frequently recommended for plaque removal. Use of a dentifrice is not required for classroom plaque removal. However, use of a toothpaste containing an effective fluoride compound is recommended for brushing at home.	**Introduction to brushing** Have the class study the transparency, "How to Brush Your Teeth." Distribute a toothbrush to each pupil. These should be marked with pupils' names. Brushes should be returned following each session. (Egg cartons with holes punched in each segment can serve as storage racks.) Demonstrate the correct brush position. A clean comb can represent teeth and gums. Show the back-and-forth wiggle of the brushing motion. The prepared drawing, "How to Brush Your Teeth," provides an illustration for each pupil.	
		Brushing practice Have pupils stain plaque. Pupils then attempt to remove all plaque by brushing, working in a regular pattern around the mouth. Pupils can check their progress with mirrors. Floss will be needed to remove plaque from the sides the brush cannot reach. (Water can be used for rinsing, but is not necessary. If water is used, a paper cup to hold water and another cup to catch rinsings will be helpful.) Brushes will need to be rinsed daily.	
	Note: Some pupils may have been taught other cleaning methods by their dentists or dental auxiliaries. They should, of course, continue to follow the instructions they have been given. Some pupils may have special problems with flossing because their teeth have little space between them, are crooked, or contain fillings which have overhanging portions. They should ask a dentist or dental auxiliary to suggest a solution to the difficulty. If the school does not furnish additional disclosing wafers when the sample contained in the Plaque Control Kit has been used, pupils may be asked to provide them.	**Note:** Learning experiences with flossing and brushing should take place each day for at least a week, for maximum effect. Thereafter, supervision and reinforcement may be less frequent—perhaps once or twice a week during the rest of the semester or year. If pupils eat lunch at school, they can use this opportunity to clean their teeth daily. Have each pupil make a large construction paper toothbrush, label it with his name, and wind some string around the handle to represent floss. On each day he can report thoroughly removing plaque from his teeth, he can hang his toothbrush on a long "toothbrush holder" that stretches across a wall. From time to time during the year, conduct an unannounced spot check of each pupil's oral hygiene, using a disclosing wafer. This will help to reinforce the need for thorough removal of plaque.	

A preventive approach to dental health as recommended by American Dental Association oral health teaching-learning specialists, program level II.

Resources:

Awareness films:
"Dudley the Dragon"
"Merlin's Magical Message"
"Teeth are Good Things to Have"

Teaching film:
"Showdown at Sweet Rock Gulch"

Plaque Control Kit

Pamphlet for the teacher:
"Cleaning Your Teeth and Gums"
(Resource for plaque removal methods.)

Pamphlets for pupils:
"Dudley the Dragon"
"Casper Presents Space-Age Dentistry"

Transparencies:
"How to Brush Your Teeth"
"Where Plaque Hides"

Spirit masters:
"How to Brush Your Teeth"
"Flossing Your Teeth"

DIET AND DENTAL HEALTH

Goals: To develop an awareness of foods containing and not containing table sugar (sucrose).
To develop an awareness of foods needed for general good health.

Behavioral Objectives	Content	Suggested Activities	Related Activities in Other Classes
The pupil can name six to eight foods which promote decay. The pupil can name six to eight suitable snack foods which do not promote decay.	**Sugar** Many common snack foods contain sugar. Examples include cake, candy, pie, sweet rolls, ice cream, cookies, doughnuts, sugared gum, sugar-containing soft drinks, chocolate milk, sugar-containing gelatin desserts. Bacteria in plaque make acid when sugar is in the mouth. Each time sugar is eaten, the bacteria continue to make acid (perhaps for about 30 minutes). Snack foods which do not contain table sugar include meat, nuts, cheese, fresh fruits and vegetables, fruit and vegetable juices, sugarless soft drinks, milk, plain yogurt, hard-boiled eggs, popcorn, pretzels, potato chips.	Have pupils bring to class magazine pictures of a variety of different foods. Have pupils cut out pictures, and separate into foods containing and not containing sugar. Construct a "Smart Snacks for Me" poster or bulletin board display with the pictures of non-sugary foods. Have a party at which only non-sugar-containing snacks are served. Have a tasting party. Blindfold pupils and have them eat small pieces of foods which do not contain sugar, such as oranges, apples, carrots, celery, cheese, crackers, etc. Have pupils tell what the foods are by taste and texture. Using the prepared sheet, "Smart Snacks for Me," have pupils indicate those foods containing and not containing sugar.	
The pupil can name the four food groups and describe a balanced meal plan for one day.	**The four food groups— a guide to good nutrition** Milk and dairy products— 3-4 cups milk (or the equivalent) per day. Meat and fish—2 or more servings daily. Fruits and vegetables—4 or more servings daily. Bread and cereals—4 or more servings daily.	Have the class study the transparency, "The Four Food Groups." Have pupils name foods to fit into each group. Have pupils write a class story about a trip to the grocery store. Describe selection of foods from each group, emphasizing the groups as a guide to good nutrition. Using the prepared sheet, "What's Missing?" have pupils tell what food groups are included, which are omitted, from pictures of meals.	**Art:** Have pupils make posters from cutout magazine pictures, showing an acceptable breakfast, lunch, snack, and dinner.

Continued.

A preventive approach to dental health as recommended by American Dental Association oral health teaching-learning specialists, program level II.

Behavioral Objectives	Content	Suggested Activities	Related Activities in Other Classes
		Using the prepared sheet, "The Four Food Groups," have pupils indicate to which group each pictured food belongs.	
		Using the prepared outline drawings, "Foods to Color and Cut," have pupils color them, or cut them out to use as guides for making food shapes from construction paper. Finished work may be used for display purposes.	

Resources:

Teaching film:
"The Munchers: A Fable"

Pamphlet for the Teacher:
"Diet and Dental Health"

Transparency:
"The Four Food Groups"

Spirit masters:
"Smart Snacks for Me"
"What's Missing?"
"The Four Food Groups"
"Foods to Color and Cut"

TEETH: WHAT THEY ARE AND WHAT THEY DO

Goals: To develop understanding of the three basic functions performed by teeth.
To develop familiarity with the structure and function of teeth and surrounding tissues.
To develop understanding of the primary and permanent dentition.

Behavioral Objectives	Content Functions	Suggested Activities	Related Activities in Other Classes
The pupil can name the three basic functions of teeth and tell why each is important.	Chewing food—teeth are needed for adequate nutrition. Clear speech—teeth are needed for communication. Pleasant appearance—teeth are important for mental well-being and social development.	Ask pupils to tell what they like to eat for dinner. Make a list of foods mentioned which could be eaten without teeth; which must be chewed. Have pupils with infant siblings tell how many teeth the siblings have, and what kinds of food they can eat. Ask pupils to bring magazine pictures of smiling people to class. Display them, discussing the importance of teeth in facial expression. Then black out some of the teeth with crayon, to demonstrate the effect of missing teeth on appearance.	**Art:** Have pupils draw or paint pictures showing the functions of teeth in eating, speech and pleasant appearance. **Music:** Have the class sing "All I want for Christmas is My Two Front Teeth." **Reading (phonics):** Have pupils say the alphabet, noting which sounds must be formed by contact of teeth with tongue and lips. Have the class develop a list of words which are hard to say if the incisors are missing. (If there is a speech teacher available, she may assist.)

A preventive approach to dental health as recommended by American Dental Association oral health teaching-learning specialists, program level II.

Behavioral Objectives	Content	Suggested Activities	Related Activities in Other Classes
The pupil can identify the crown and root, and discuss their respective functions.	**Parts of a tooth** Crown—the visible part, which bites, tears or grinds food. Root—the part which anchors the tooth in the jawbone.	Have pupils label the crown and root on the prepared drawing, "A Molar Tooth." Below the drawing, have them write a sentence describing the function of the crown, and a sentence describing the function of the root.	
The pupil can name the tissues which surround the tooth and describe their function.	**Surrounding tissues** Gums (gingiva)—soft tissue covering the bone in which the teeth are anchored. Bone (alveolar bone)—surrounds and supports the roots of the tooth. Periodontal ligament—attaches the tooth to the bone.		
The pupil can describe the specialized functions of incisors, cuspids, molars and bicuspids.	**Specialized jobs of different types of teeth** Incisors 4 center front teeth in each jaw. Especially shaped for biting and cutting. Cuspids 2 in each jaw, one on either side of upper and lower incisors. Shaped for tearing. Bicuspids (permanent teeth only) 8 teeth, between cuspids and molars. Shaped for tearing and grinding. Molars 8 primary, 12 permanent, farthest back in the jaw. Shaped for grinding.	Have pupils eat apples and discuss the ways different types of teeth function in the biting and chewing process. Have pupils bring pictures of animals, showing the animals' teeth. Conduct a class discussion of the difference between animal and human teeth, and how various types of animal teeth function in relation to the type of food eaten. A bulletin board display might be developed from the pictures. Using the prepared drawing, "Types of Teeth and Their Jobs," have pupils indicate the function of each type of tooth by noting the kind of tool which performs a similar function.	
The pupil can indicate the number of primary teeth. The pupil can describe the process of eruption and shedding of primary teeth. The pupil can discuss reasons primary teeth are important.	**Primary teeth** There are 20 primary teeth 8 incisors. 4 cuspids. 8 molars. They begin to erupt at 4-8 months and eruption is usually complete at 24-30 months. Shedding begins at about 6 years and is complete by about 11 years.	**Suggested Activities** Have the class view the transparency, "How Teeth Grow." Point out different types of primary teeth and discuss the order in which they are usually shed. Point out permanent teeth preparing to erupt. Have pupils bring shed teeth to class. Have the class examine them for vestiges of roots, if any.	

Continued.

A preventive approach to dental health as recommended by American Dental Association oral health teaching-learning specialists, program level II.

Behavioral Objectives	Content	Suggested Activities	Related Activities in Other Classes
	Primary teeth (continued) Lower incisors are shed first, then upper incisors, lower cuspids, first molars, second molars, upper cuspids. Before primary teeth are shed, their roots begin to disappear (resorb). Primary teeth are very important as guides for the position of permanent teeth.	Ask pupils to tell how many and which primary teeth they have shed, and when shedding occurred (2nd and 3rd grades). Draw a 3-foot wide smile with teeth. Every time a class member loses a tooth, put his name on any tooth, along with the date the tooth was lost (1st grade).	
The pupil can explain that eruption and shedding of teeth are part of natural human growth and development.	**Permanent teeth** There are 32 permanent teeth 8 incisors. 4 cuspids. 8 bicuspids. 12 molars. **Eruption** Begins at about age 6, and is complete by 12-13 years, (except for third permanent molars, which erupt at 17-21). Starts with first molars, then lower incisors, upper incisors, lower cuspids, bicuspids, upper cuspids, second molars, third molars.	Have pupils make a model of permanent teeth of one or both jaws, using navy beans as teeth and modeling clay, modeling dough or wallpaper cleaner as the gums and surrounding structures.	
The pupil can explain why first permanent molars are particularly important and must be cared for especially well.	**First molars—because they are the first permanent teeth to erupt, they are** Especially important as guides for the position of the rest of the permanent teeth. Especially vulnerable to decay. Often thought to be primary teeth which will soon be shed.	Point out the first permanent molars on the transparency, "How Teeth Grow." Have pupils look at their first permanent molars in their mirrors, using tongue depressors to point them out. Discuss with the class the guidepost functions of these teeth.	

Resources:

Pamphlets for the teacher:
"Your Child's Teeth"
"The Care of Children's Teeth"

Transparency:
"How Teeth Grow"

Spirit masters:
"A Molar Tooth"
"Types of Teeth and Their Jobs"

A preventive approach to dental health as recommended by American Dental Association oral health teaching-learning specialists, program level II.

THE DENTIST AND HIS HELPERS

Goal: To develop understanding of the role of dental professionals in the prevention of disease.

Behavioral Objectives

The pupil can describe briefly the role of the dentist and his auxiliaries in prevention and treatment of dental disease.

Content

The dentist
Teaches people how to prevent dental disease.
Examines teeth to see if they are developing normally or if they are diseased.
Treats decayed teeth, gum disease and other oral diseases.

The dental hygienist
Teaches people how to prevent dental disease.
Cleans teeth, removing calculus and stains.
Takes X-ray pictures.

The dental assistant
Helps to teach people how to prevent dental disease.
Helps the dentist examine and treat teeth and gums.
Takes X-ray pictures.

The pupil can describe the function of the common pieces of equipment in the dental office, such as the dental chair, X-ray machine, mouth mirror, explorer, examination light.

Examining teeth
The dental chair is adjustable to fit people of different sizes and can be raised and tilted so that the dentist can work easily.

The dentist uses a small round mirror to see the backs of teeth.

He uses a metal probe called an "explorer" to help find decay.

The X-ray machine is a camera which uses radiation to take pictures of teeth and bones, revealing conditions which cannot be seen by looking in the mouth.

The examination light can be focused to light up all parts of the mouth.

Suggested Activities

Set up a "pretend" dental office. Make a mock-up of an X-ray machine. Have pupils role-play dentist hygienist, assistant, parents and patient.

Ask pupils who have been to the dentist to describe their experiences. Discourage exaggerated descriptions of pain and fear.

Arrange a field trip to a dentist's office so that the dentist, hygienist, and assistant can explain their roles and epuipment.

Have pupils color the pictures, "Susan and the Dentist," "Danny and the Hygienist."

Related Activities in Other Classes

Art: Have pupils make pretend dental instruments for the dental office.

Language Arts: Have children solve the crossword puzzle, "Crossword Tooth," as a class project.

Continued.

A preventive approach to dental health as recommended by American Dental Association oral health teaching-learning specialists, program level II.

Behavioral Objectives	Content	Suggested Activities	Related Activities in Other Classes
The pupil can describe in simple terms why professional cleaning of the teeth is necessary.	**Cleaning teeth (prophylaxis) at the dental office** For most people, a periodic professional cleaning is necessary to help prevent disease. Calculus is removed by scraping with a special instrument. The teeth are polished with a revolving rubber cup and special toothpaste. Air and water sprays help remove debris and help to keep the tooth cool.	Ask a hygienist to visit the class and explain professional cleaning of the teeth.	

Resources:

Film:
"D is for Dentist" (K only)

Spirit Masters:
"Susan and the Dentist"
"Danny and the Hygienist"
"Crossword Tooth"

Pamphlets:
"D is for Dentist" (K only)
"I'm Going to the Dentist"
"A Visit to the Dentist"

KEEPING TEETH SAFE

Goals: To develop an awareness of potential hazards to teeth and gums.
To develop an awareness that hazards can be avoided.
To develop understanding of first aid procedures.

Behavioral Objectives	Content	Suggested Activities	Related Activities in Other Classes
The pupil can list at least three types of activities which may be hazardous to teeth, and tell how dangers may be avoided.	**Accidents to teeth commonly occur as a result of** Rough play at drinking fountains. Thrown baseball bats. Falls from bicycles. Carelessness around hard-seated swings, teeter-totter boards and other playground equipment. Falls caused by objects lying on floor or sidewalk. Failure to wear seat belts when riding in an automobile. **Teeth and gums can be injured** If pencils, hard objects or other foreign objects are placed in the mouth.	Have pupils role-play situations in which teeth and other oral structures may be injured and ways in which accidents may be avoided. Develop a class list of safety do's and don't's for home and school. From your dentist, obtain some pictures of chipped teeth before and after restoration. Show them to the class. These can be reassuring to the child who, despite precautions, does suffer a chipped tooth. Have pupils make a display of items which should not be placed in the mouth.	**Art**: Have pupils draw posters or pictures of situations in which teeth are likely to be injured, and pictures of how injury might be avoided in each situation. These could be displayed in the classroom or placed in the corridor for the benefit of the entire school.
The pupil can tell what to do if a tooth is loosened, chipped or fractured, and if a tooth has been knocked out.	**First Aid** If a tooth is loosened, chipped or broken, it should be examined by a dentist as soon as possible. If a tooth is knocked out, find it, place it in water or wrap it in a clean, wet cloth, and take child and tooth to the dentist at once. *Do not clean the tooth*. The dentist may be able to replace the tooth in the jaw.		

A preventive approach to dental health as recommended by American Dental Association oral health teaching-learning specialists, program level II.

of the developers. This unit is designed as a health instruction resource for children in the intermediate grades (4 to 6). The teacher must decide which grade level is most appropriate for teaching the unit. Regardless of the grade level selected, experience suggests that the oral health program should be taught as a unit and that the topics covered should be presented in the sequence suggested by the guide.

Research experience at the University of Illinois has demonstrated that fifth-grade teachers with a minimum of preparation can use this program to achieve effective results with their fifth-grade students.

RESOURCE UNIT—GRADE 6

A unit developed primarily to emphasize the prevention and control of communicable diseases can logically incorporate sanitation practices in a functional way. Since youngsters in the sixth grade are beginning to have an interest in group and community affairs, emphasis can be placed on community and also personal responsibility for disease prevention and control as well as for sanitation.

Unit title—How can we prevent disease?

OUTCOMES
Knowledge

Nature of infectious disease
Characteristics of disease-producing organisms
Modes of disease spread
Routes over which diseases travel
Common respiratory diseases and their prevention
Common skin infections and their prevention
Infections of the digestive system
Special infections transmitted by food
Immunization
Isolation and quarantine
Food sanitation

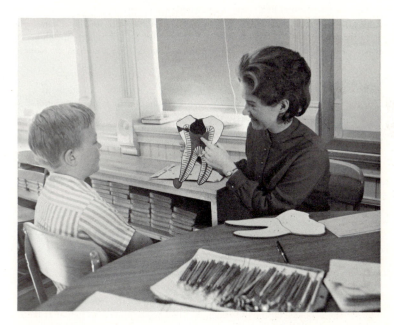

Fig. 12-7. Dental hygienist as a health educator. The effectiveness of individualized health instruction is best exemplified in the relationship of the dental hygienist to the pupil. (Courtesy Denver Public Schools, Denver, Colo.)

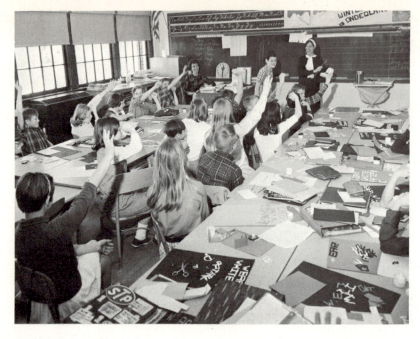

Fig. 12-8. Guest teacher. Dental hygienists, nurses, physicians, nutritionists, sanitarians, and other specialists can contribute immeasurably to the health education program. Such appearances are much enhanced if the teacher lays the advance groundwork before the guest teacher appears and then reviews the presentation after the guest has left. (Courtesy Denver Public Schools, Denver, Colo.)

Restaurant sanitation
Milk sanitation
School sanitation
Water purification
Pupil's responsibility in sanitation practices
Cooperation in sanitation and prevention of disease spread
Home sanitation
Boiling and refrigeration as disease prevention measures
Community disease control problems and measures
Value of laboratories in disease control
Responsibility for sanitation in the community
Federal control over food, drugs, cosmetics, and biological products such as vaccine
Effectiveness of sanitation measures

Attitudes as expressed in

Willingness to undergo inconvenience for the protection of others
Reliance on scientific sources of knowledge
Willingness to cooperate in disease prevention efforts
Desire to contribute to the welfare of others
Preference for prevention

Pride in a healthy environment
Caution in drinking water or milk from unknown source
Need for investing public funds in disease control and sanitation
Appreciation that disease prevention demands constant vigilance
Positive attitude toward community health regulations
Eagerness to cooperate in efforts to improve the health of all

Practices

Avoid exposure to known infection or contamination
Take measures to help others avoid infectious disease
Voluntary isolation when ill
Follow health authorities' recommendations on immunization
Maintain sanitary school environment
Practice approved sanitation in the home
Cooperate in community health efforts
Drink water only when from known safe sources
Check on the source of milk before drinking it
Look for sanitation approval certificate in restaurants
Report health hazards to responsible persons

Read newspaper and magazine reports and articles on communicable diseases

Read available articles on scientific sanitation practices

ACTIVITIES
Discussion

What is the nature of infectious disease?

What are the characteristics of disease-producing organisms?

How are respiratory infectious diseases spread?

What are some of these diseases?

How can their spread be prevented?

What is the nature of immunization?

What are the dangers of self-diagnosis and self-medication?

Why do we need isolation and quarantine?

What are community requirements for isolation and quarantine?

How can we cooperate as a school?

How can we help as individuals?

How are diseases of the skin acquired?

What are some of these diseases?

How do we prevent skin infection?

How does food transmit these diseases?

What are some other diseases spread by food?

How do we get infections of the digestive system?

What are some of these infections?

What diseases are spread by milk?

What are some diseases water can spread?

How does our community provide water that does not spread disease?

How does sanitation prevent disease spread?

What other purposes does sanitation serve?

Why is restaurant sanitation important?

What does the community do in sanitation measures?

What are good home sanitation practices?

What are the things that make good school sanitation?

What is the responsibility of students and teachers in school sanitation?

What sanitary measures should be taken while camping?

Reports

Respiratory diseases
  Common cold
  Influenza
  Poliomyelitis
  Rheumatic fever
  Sore throat
  Tuberculosis
Skin diseases
  Boils
  Impetigo contagiosa
  Ringworm
  Scabies

Diseases of digestive system
  Dysentery
  Typhoid
Other diseases spread by food
  Trichonosis
  Undulant fever
Special disease
  Tetanus (lockjaw)
Immunization
Isolation and quarantine
Community garbage disposal
Federal control of foods, drugs, and cosmetics

Guest participation

Public health nurse
Sanitarian
X-ray technician
Laboratory technician

Projects

School patrol for school cleanliness
Clean up school grounds
Keep toilet rooms and fountains clean
Keep record and causes of absence

Field trips

Visit to a model home
Locker plant
Water plant
Restaurant
Bakery

Exhibits

Labels on food and drug containers
Communicable disease charts
Tables and graphs on state-reported communicable diseases
Posters on sanitation practices

EVALUATION

To measure the effectiveness of instruction of this unit, the knowledge, attitudes, and practices in the proposed outcomes should be the guide for evaluation procedures. Knowledge can be evaluated in a preliminary way by oral examination of the entire class. Following the oral practice test, written objective and essay tests can give the instructor a more definite evaluation of the knowledge each student has gained. Vocabulary and spelling tests should be included. Attitudes can be judged by the teacher. Practices can be evaluated by surveys or by observation of the youngsters (Fig. 12-9).

In adapting this resource unit to a particular classroom situation, the teacher in charge should be ex-

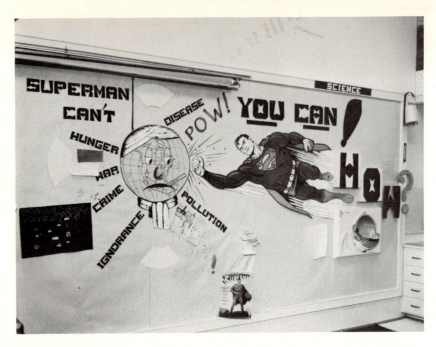

Fig. 12-9. Even Superman can be topped. The study of health need not be stodgy and dull. Ingenuity on the part of the students can be a most meaningful and enjoyable academic exercise. (Courtesy Salem Public Schools, Salem, Ore.)

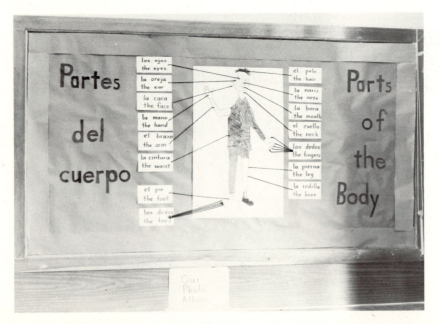

Fig. 12-10. Bilingual health instruction: in a class composed of half English-speaking and half Spanish-speaking students, the teacher wisely used both languages as vehicles for teaching health along with the second language. (Courtesy Salem Public Schools, Salem, Ore.)

pected to omit, change, and add, in terms of the interests and needs of the group. A unit developed for one situation is not likely to be 100% suitable for use in some other classroom (Fig. 12-10). Indeed, for their own classroom needs, sixth-grade teachers often wisely develop a resource unit so broadly inclusive that the person who developed the unit may not use everything the unit provides.

INCIDENTAL INSTRUCTION

Opportunities and a need for casual or incidental health instruction arise naturally in the course of a school day. Some phases of health teaching may best be handled by such incidental instruction. Problems that are of deep personal concern to a particular pupil or particular types of pupils may be dealt with most effectively by incidental treatment. However effective such instruction may be for certain purposes, if the teacher relies entirely on incidental health instruction, a decidedly limited health instruction program results, regardless of how skillful the teacher may be.

Pupil-teacher conferences and counseling frequently include incidental health instruction. When a teacher discovers the particular needs and problems of a child, the person-to-person relationship promotes a clarifying discussion of the problems. The conference may proceed beyond the original problem and

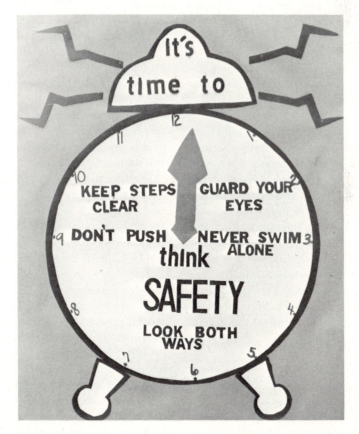

Fig. 12-11. Novelties can be effective. Devices that command attention are highly recommended when a central idea needs emphasis. (Courtesy Corvallis Public Schools, Corvallis, Ore.)

explore related problems of interest and importance.

In class a pupil's question on a health matter may be an occasion for the whole class to learn. At times a discussion of a question considerably removed from health may gradually shift to its health aspects. An alert teacher utilizes expressed class interests and explores a whole area of health, perhaps leaving the class with several questions to ponder over, and concludes the discussion at a later date.

Simple incidents in school can have meaning in health terms, and the teacher can make effective use of such realistic teaching situations. Health terms occasionally are used in areas aside from health instruction, and opportunities are presented for the pupils to expand their vocabulary. Examinations usually offer opportunities for incidental health instruction. This is particularly true during the review of the examination after the tests have been scored and returned.

Daily newspaper, radio, and television reports frequently have health topics of interest to the pupils. A new health discovery, an epidemic, a person who has reached the age of 100 years, and a physician who has practiced for 50 years are examples of news items that provide both the opportunity and necessity for consideration in the classroom.

Opportunities are plentiful for the alert teacher who utilizes incidental instruction to fortify and amplify planned health instruction (Fig. 12-11). Spontaneous live instruction is usually most stimulating to the pupils.

CORRELATED HEALTH INSTRUCTION

Correlation is a reciprocal relationship, and a kindred relationship or alliance exists between health and other cognate areas, which provides opportunities for effective instruction. Health aspects can enrich other fields and make experiences more stimulating and rewarding for the child. There are many opportunities in health for instruction in the basic academic skills as well as in the field of life experiences. In health instruction, diction, pronunciation, spelling, coherence, and clarity are important. In a very real sense health involves history, art, and the people of other lands.

Reading. Health readers are available at various levels. They are interesting, are written with regard for comprehension by children, and can be used to encourage general supplementary reading. For the teacher who seeks to enrich the curriculum of the superior pupil, health readers as well as health projects offer a fertile field of exploration (Figs. 12-12 and 12-13).

Language arts. In writing and speaking assignments, health topics are a frequent choice of pupils. Reports on special health topics, field trips, and health experiences are used. Articles on health in the school may be written for newspapers. Letters asking agencies for health materials and requests to the health department provide correlated health and writing experience.

Spelling also can be included. Of the 2,000 basic words in common usage, which are the core of instruction in elementary school spelling, many are in health literature. From classroom health study an instructor can find ample material for spelling purposes.

Art. Paper cutting, crayon fill-in, and free drawing can deal with health topics. Paste-on or original posters can be health posters. Health report cards can be a health project.

Music. Implications of mental and physical health in vocal and instrumental music are of interest. Many musical compositions have references to health. Health parodies on recognized songs should be avoided.

Arithmetic. Keeping records of changes in height and weight, attendance, and illness provides problems in arithmetic. Calcula-

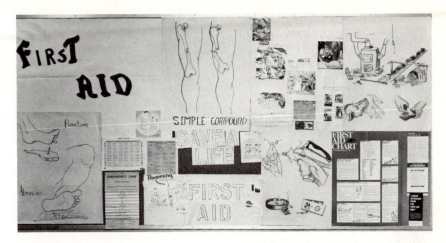

Fig. 12-12. First aid: this type of activity can be highly thought provoking because it provides wide participation. From the central core, additions may be made as each student gets ideas for the board. (Courtesy Salem Public Schools, Salem, Ore.)

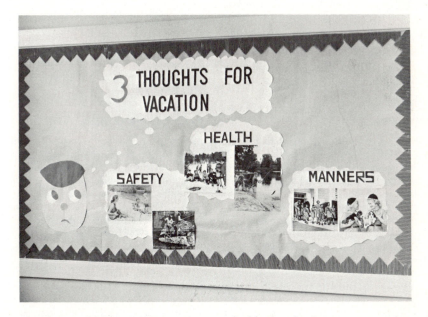

Fig. 12-13. Timing in health instruction. Appropriate health ideas for the vacation period just ahead project health education into the everyday lives of the pupils. (Courtesy Corvallis Public Schools, Corvallis, Ore.)

tion of sleeping time and the amounts of certain foods consumed in a given period of time can be interesting experiences in arithmetic. The intermediate grades may be interested in rates for various health factors.

Geography. Health customs, life span, health problems, and dietary practices of peoples of other lands can be of interest to pupils. How other people live usually interests children.

History. The influence of health and disease on history challenges the imagination of youth. Health problems of different periods in history and health problems of famous historical figures are of special interest. Celebrated men and women health heroes live in historical perspective.

Nature study. The life and habits of lower animal forms have health implications. Feeding habits are particularly germane. The interrelationships that exist between humans and the plant and animal world are concepts that children should acquire as fundamental education.

Children must be helped to see relationships in life. Especially important are the relationships of health to the many aspects of everyday living.

QUESTIONS AND EXERCISES

1. What are the possible sources of health learning available to elementary school pupils?
2. How is it possible for the learning activity itself to be so fascinating to the elementary school pupil that very little is learned about health?
3. What is the responsibility of the elementary schoolteacher for the health education of the pupils?
4. For the elementary grades what scheduling for health instruction do you advocate and why?
5. How can the health coordinator be most effective in an elementary school?
6. What people are conveniently available to serve as health resource people for the elementary schoolteacher?
7. What is the role of the elementary schoolteacher in health counseling?
8. To the elementary schoolteacher what are the advantages in having ready-made health resource units?
9. Why is the home background of elementary school pupils an important consideration in determining what should be taught in the health program?
10. What means can be used to motivate learning in health instruction in the elementary grades?
11. Why is the child-centered classroom especially important in health instruction?
12. What are the merits of building an elementary school health education program around desired health practices?
13. What is meant by integrated school living as health instruction?
14. Why is a positive interest by the teacher in every child's health important to effective health education?
15. Why must special care be taken in using a child as an example in the course of health instruction?
16. Appraise the statement, "It is desirable to plan for coordination and progression of health instruction from grade to grade, but not all duplication is objectionable."
17. "Mental health instruction in the primary grades is a matter of teaching interpersonal relationships." Explain the implications.
18. How much truth is there to the contention that in school we teach youngsters to understand everything but themselves?
19. Every day hundreds of elementary schoolteachers miss hundreds of opportunities for effective incidental health instruction. Why?
20. In the third grade how can health be correlated with reading?

SELECTED READINGS

American Association of School Administrators: Health in schools, twentieth yearbook, Washington, D.C., 1951, National Education Association.

American Dental Association: Learning about your oral health: a prevention-oriented school program, Level II: 4-6, Chicago, 1973, American Dental Association.

Barrett, M.: Health education guide, ed. 2, Philadelphia, 1974, Lea & Febiger.

Children and fitness: a program for elementary schools, Washington, D.C., 1960, National Conference on Fitness of Elementary School-Age Children, Alliance for Health, Physical Education, and Recreation.

Cornacchia, H. J., Smith, D. E., and Bentel, D. J.: Drugs in the classroom: a conceptual model for school programs, ed. 2, St. Louis, 1978, The C. V. Mosby Co.

Cornacchia, H. J., and Staton, W. M.: Health in elementary schools, ed. 4, St. Louis, 1974, The C. V. Mosby Co.

Davis, R.: Quality in school health administration, National Elementary Principal 39:6, Feb., 1960.

Dutton, W. H., and Hockett, J. A.: The modern elementary school, New York, 1960, Holt, Rinehart & Winston.

Elementary teachers guide to free curriculum materials, Randolph, Wis., published annually, Educators' Progress Service.

Grout, R. E.: Health teaching in schools, ed. 5, Philadelphia, 1968, W. B. Saunders Co.

Health education in the elementary school, The National Elementary Principal 48:2, Nov., 1968.

Health in the elementary school, twenty-ninth yearbook, National Elementary Principal—Bulletin of the Department of Elementary School Principals, Washington, D.C., 1950, National Education Association, no. 1.

Humphrey, J. H.: Child learning through elementary school physical education, ed. 2, Dubuque, Iowa, 1974, William C. Brown Co., Publishers.

Humphrey, J. H., Johnson, W. R., and Moore, V. D.: Elementary school education, New York, 1962, Harper & Row, Publishers.

Instruction material for elementary schools, thirty-fifth yearbook, Washington, D.C., Department of Elementary School Principals, National Education Association.

Irwin, L. W., et al.: Health for better living, ed. 2, Columbus, Ohio, 1972, Charles E. Merrill Publishing Co.

Logan, L., and Logan, V.: Teaching the elementary school child, New York, 1961, Houghton Mifflin Co.

Los Angeles City School Districts, California: Health in the elementary schools, publication No. EC-201, 1959, Office of the Superintendent of Schools.

Ridenour, N.: Mental health education, New York, 1969, Mental Health Materials Center.

Schneider, R. E.: Methods and materials of health education, ed. 2, Philadelphia, 1964, W. B. Saunders Co.

Stoll, F. A.: Dental health education, ed. 4, Philadelphia, 1972, Lea & Febiger.

Stone, D. B., O'Reilly, L. B., and Brown, J. D.: Elementary school health education: ecological perspectives, ed. 2, Dubuque, Iowa, 1980, William C. Brown Co., Publishers.

The elementary school health program, National Elementary Principal 39:1-48, Feb., 1960.

United States Public Health Service: Teaching poison prevention in kindergartens and primary grades, Washington, D.C., 1962, U.S. Government Printing Office.

Vannier, M.: Teaching health in elementary schools, ed. 2, New York, 1972, Harper & Row, Publishers.

Vaughn, G.: A pictorial guide to common childhood illnesses, New York, 1972, St. Martin's Press, Inc.

Willey, R. D.: Guidance in elementary education, rev. ed., New York, 1960, Harper & Row, Publishers.

Willgoose, C. E.: Health education in the elementary school, ed. 4, Philadelphia, 1974, W. B. Saunders Co.

Yost, C. P.: Teaching safety in the elementary school, Washington, D.C., 1962, American Alliance for Health, Physical Education, and Recreation.

CHAPTER 13

Junior high or middle school health instruction

Junior high or middle school is a transition from the self-contained classroom in the sixth grade to departmentalized instruction in the seventh grade. It represents a change in the relationship between students and teacher. Junior high school teachers usually do not have the opportunity to establish the degree of rapport with students possible in the elementary grades. However, when the seventh grade curriculum is modified by large core areas, the transition for the students is easier, and teachers have a better chance to establish a close relationship with students. Health instruction, as all other instruction at this stage in school, must recognize the factors that motivate students and account for their interests and conduct.

Students between the ages of 12 and 15 years include children who are in the homophilic or gang period, a few who have not yet reached that stage, and perhaps one fifth who can be classed as adolescents. To complicate the picture, physiologically and socially a 12-year-old girl is almost 2 years ahead of a boy.

During the homophilic period girls are arm-in-arm with girls and boys tend to gang up with boys. Group loyalty is exceedingly important. The teacher should capitalize on the strong desire for approval by their associates and the tendency toward united action by directing health instruction into channels of group approval and action. Group interest can mean group accomplishment and community interest.

BASIC OBJECTIVES OF HEALTH INSTRUCTION

Health practices previously established will continue to be fortified in the junior high school, and new practices, particularly those associated with group health responsibility, will be established. Knowledge to promote understanding of health measures and procedures will be provided in the junior high school. However, greatest attention should be given to the development of attitudes that are essential to provide the necessary intensity to health practices and to assure the fullest utilization of health knowledge.

Many health attitudes, in terms of certain concepts of ideal personal and community attainments, will prove to be the most lasting and valuable in terms of the individual's lifelong health measures. Among these will be attitudes that are directed toward the following:

1. Resolution to attain a high level of health
2. Pride in high quality of well-being

3. Application of reasoning to health problems
4. Conviction that only established health principles should be utilized
5. Acceptance of responsibility for the health of others
6. Ideals of citizen responsibility
7. Cooperation with community health efforts
8. Insistence on high community health standards
9. Pride in community assets

The knowledge of health that the junior high school student should acquire is expressed in the areas of primary interest at this level.

AREAS OF PRIMARY INTEREST

Certain health interests are virtually universal for children of this age, and instructional planning can be based on these major interests as the central core. Participation of students in planning the classroom instruction brings out their special health interests (Fig. 13-1). Health needs and interest surveys can be highly revealing.

Physical health

Personal health standards
Periodic health examination
Choice of a physician and dentist
Medical and hospital insurance
Biological changes between the ages of 12 and 20 years
Adjustments to sexual and reproductive changes
Body care and grooming
Activity, fatigue, and rest
Tobacco, alcohol, and other harmful drugs
Noncommunicable diseases
   Acne
   Anemia
   Cancer
   Diabetes mellitus
   Heart conditions
   Tuberculosis

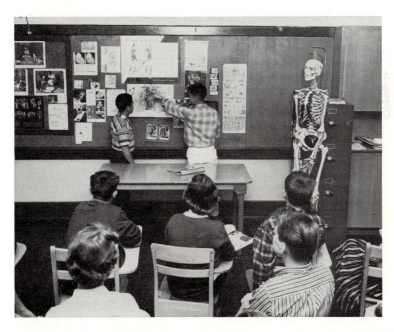

Fig. 13-1. Upgrading the level of health instruction. Junior high school students are not bored by a level of health teaching that challenges them.

Mental health

Social conduct
Personality adjustment
Adapting to common frustrations

Community health

Health superstitions, fallacies, and quackery
Fraudulent health advertising
Patent medicines
Community health services
   Water
   Sewage disposal
   Garbage collection
   Insect and rodent eradication
Medical, dental, and hospital services
   Community health projects
     Helping the disabled
     Mobile x-ray units
     Safety program
     American National Red Cross
Voluntary health agencies
   Local health department
   State health department
   United States Public Health Service
   World Health Organization

CORRELATION OF HEALTH AND OTHER SUBJECT FIELDS

Because of the departmentalized organization in the junior high school, there is difficulty in correlating health and other subject areas (Figs. 13-2 and 13-3). In the self-contained classroom of the elementary grades it is both easy and natural for the teacher to recognize and use these correlations for more effective teaching. Because correlated instruction is also important at the secondary school level, Chapter 15 is devoted entirely to what should be done in health instruction through other subject fields. The discussion applies to junior and senior high schools alike.

INTEGRATED AND INCIDENTAL HEALTH LEARNING

The daily experiences of junior high school students are rich in health implications. Opportunities for integrated health instruction are plentiful, but usually only the health

instructor capitalizes on them. However, if the organized health class does its work effectively, the students will be alerted to the health significance of everyday occurrences. If students are stimulated and challenged by a competent health instructor, a considerable amount of integrated health learning will go on.

In-service preparation of all the school staff in the possibilities and value of integrated health instruction is an ideal that rarely becomes a reality. Yet the health director or health instructor may enlist the cooperation of other staff members, particularly those who have a reasonably good background in health training.

Incidental health instruction arises from student-teacher conferences, questions from students in the classroom, injuries to students, news reports, tests, and as an outgrowth of some topic outside of the health field. Incidental instruction should not be superficial teaching. Any topic under consideration should be developed sufficiently so that the students understand and appreciate it.

Various activities in the regular program of the school provide health learning opportunities. Assemblies, lunchroom service, projects of the student council, announcements on the bulletin board, safety drives, and health examinations all contribute to the understanding, appreciation, and practice of health.

ORGANIZING FOR HEALTH INSTRUCTION

Health instruction is a recognized area in the curriculum of the junior high school, and there are very few junior high schools that do not offer formal classroom instruction in health. The scheduling of health instruction follows a variety of patterns. Unfortunately in some junior high schools health can truly be labeled an orphan. It is included if the

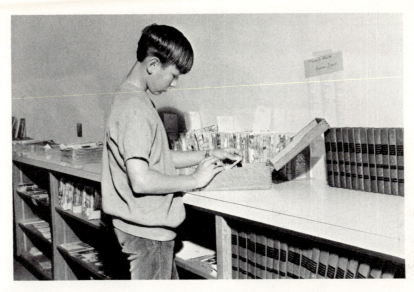

Fig. 13-2. Card file of health materials. This junior high school health classroom has shelves of all the school's health publications and gives students the added advantage of learning how to use a card file system. (Courtesy Salem Public Schools, Salem, Ore.)

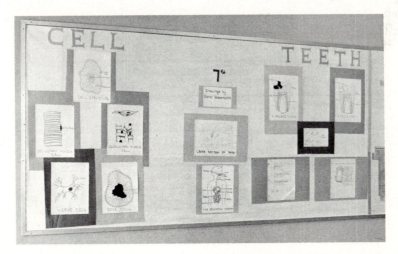

Fig. 13-3. Correlation of biology and health. Health as applied biological science can be impressive to the seventh-grader, who revels in his or her newly found knowledge and appreciates opportunities to demonstrate understanding. (Courtesy Salem Public Schools, Salem, Ore.)

schedule of a particular section or class has a place for it and someone is available to "take" the class. In such schools there is an urgent need to apprise the responsible administrators of the importance of health and what an effective health instruction program can do for students.

Few subject areas offer the student as much in a functional way as does health. Several factors determine the schedule and emphasis assigned to health instruction. The traditional background of the school, state requirements, community demands, the general pattern of the curriculum, the understanding of the administrators, and the competence of the health instructors all affect the nature of health instruction programs.

Health incorporated into general science. In a crowded curriculum it is understandable that the uniting of subject areas can be justified for expediency and possible integration. Unfortunately too frequently the marriage of two disciplines is a kind of shotgun wedding, which does not always turn out successfully. Biologists frequently regard instruction in physiology as health teaching (Fig. 13-4). It is granted that physiology is a foundation on which to build health instruction, but it is extremely limited in teaching functional health.

A composite course of health and general science can be mutually beneficial. To be successful, such a course must have an instructor interested and professionally prepared in both fields. Some specialists in school health

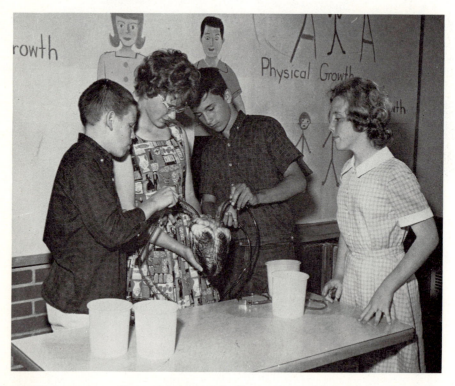

Fig. 13-4. Demonstration of human circulation. A beef heart, plastic tubes, and red and blue fluids are used to demonstrate the course of blood through the body. (Courtesy Portland Public Schools, Portland, Ore.)

work consider this arrangement the most commendable and satisfactory design for health instruction.

Health incorporated into social studies. A frequent tendency to treat health too superficially and to deal exclusively with the social aspects of health is a common deficiency in this type of arrangement. Even in dealing with community health, the social scientist tends to emphasize government organization and gives very little consideration to real health problems.

An instructor prepared in both social science and health is rather unusual. In a sense public health practice is social engineering. The combining of health with social studies has been successful, although it is the individual classroom instructor who is the key to a successful health instructional program (Fig. 13-5).

Health alternated with physical education. As a matter of scheduling convenience, administrators alternate health with physical education. The plan is to teach physical education on Monday, Wednesday, and Friday and health at the same hour on Tuesday and Thursday. During the next week 3 days are devoted to health and 2 days to physi-

cal education. Unless the instructor in charge is well prepared and highly interested in the health field, health instruction becomes an ugly duckling. Situations of this type have caused students to develop a distaste for health instruction. A disinterested instructor creates the impression generally that the whole thing is a waste of time and not worthwhile. It would be better not to schedule health than to foster this type of situation. Even when the instructor is interested in health and is competent to teach it, the three-two scheduling arrangement is generally unsatisfactory.

In some junior high schools, physical education is conducted during the fall and spring months. During the inclement weather of winter, health is taught.

To schedule health for a half year and physical education for a half year during each of the 3 years of junior high school is to allot more time to health than is needed or justified. A highly satisfactory plan is to schedule two half years of health instruction on this basis during the junior high school years.

Health as a quarter-year–three-year course. Too much fragmentation of the health instruction program detracts both

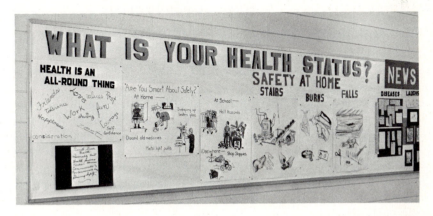

Fig. 13-5. Self-evaluation in health. A ninth-grade display aimed at making each student involved in personal health is both a superb work of art and an effective health education device. (Courtesy Salem Public Schools, Salem, Ore.)

from the stature of health as an area and from the effectiveness of the teaching. Rather than integrate health with general science, social science, or any other field, some administrators prefer to assign definite time blocks to health instruction. Occasionally classroom space and available faculty are considerations. A quarter year of health instruction in each grade under the direction of a competent teacher will provide excellent health instruction.

Health as full-year course. A frequent administrative practice is to schedule health for a full year in the eighth grade. This has proved to be an excellent plan, whose excellence is perhaps exceeded only by scheduling a half year of health instruction in each of 2 years. An ideal schedule of health instruction is to teach it in the second semester in the seventh grade and the first semester in the ninth grade.

Health as half-year course. The recognized minimum of time devoted to health instruction in the junior high school is a daily period for a half year. When the elementary school has an excellent health program and a full academic credit of health is required in the senior high school, a half year of health instruction in the junior high school can be adequate.

INSTRUCTIONAL PERSONNEL

Since the recognition of the importance of health instruction, state certification has required preparation for health teaching comparable to preparation in the traditional classical fields. In harmony with state requirements, colleges have provided the necessary offerings in their curriculums to prepare the health instructor adequately.

Teachers who are inadequately prepared when first assigned to health instruction have become fully qualified through work in in-service courses, through attending summer sessions at college, and through growth in their classroom role. An interest in health, a good general education background, and good scholastic ability constitute an adequate foundation on which to begin building the necessary qualifications for teaching health in the junior high school. Biology instructors, social science instructors, home economics instructors, and other members of the staff may be prepared adequately for health instruction. Competence in one field can be combined with competence in another field.

METHODS OF INSTRUCTION

As in the other fields, an almost unlimited number of methods and combinations of methods can be used in health instruction, but certain methods appear to be in special favor with health instructors: surveys of health needs and interests, projects, group discussion, panels, symposiums, buzz sessions, lecturettes, reports, demonstrations, presentations of sociodramas, field trips, textbook assignments, reference work, and the use of audiovisual aids. Emphasis on total participation of students, utilization of group interests and recognition, and motivation through self-achievement and self-improvement are the barometers that indicate the essential methods.

KNOW YOUR BODY (KYB) RISK FACTOR UNITS, LEVELS I AND II

The American Health Foundation, a nonprofit health organization in New York City, has developed a health education program for schools that is aimed at reducing the risk of heart disease, cancer, and stroke. These diseases are responsible for a great majority of the adult deaths in America and in other industrialized nations of the world.

Medical and public health scientists have helped to develop the Know Your Body

(KYB) Program in order to provide school-age youth with the most recent scientific knowledge on the prevention of these diseases. Through research, it has become evident that a number of risk factors are directly related to unhealthy habits of living, such as cigarette smoking, eating too much fat, and the lack of exercise. The KYB Program employs health screening for risk factors as a means of personalizing the health instruction. The students learn more about the interrelationship of their bodies, their habits, and the environment.

The KYB Program has three main components: (1) health screening, (2) providing the results of screening to the student, and (3) health instruction. The screening is done annually and consists of measures of height, weight, and blood pressure; blood tests, including cholesterol, glucose level, and hematocrit; a test of physical fitness; a health knowledge questionnaire, and a health habits survey. The KYB health education curriculum consists of units on the following topics:

(1) risk factors; (2) smoking; (3) nutrition, including principles of prevention, behavior and change, and fat in the diet; (4) blood pressure; (5) physical fitness/exercise; and (6) primary cancer prevention. The units are designed to be taught at level I for grades 6 to 8 and level II for grades 9 to 10. Each level I unit contains background information for the teacher that may be used for teaching both level I and level II units. The KYB units are intended to be used as an enrichment program for existing curricula or, according to the developers, may stand alone as a 10-week course of study.

The level I and II units have been planned to provide an articulated progression in the student's learning from one step to the next. Level I instruction focuses on the individual with personalized learning activities, whereas level II instruction is focused on the student as a member of the family unit. To illustrate the KYB programs, the two risk factor units, levels I and II have been included here.

Text continued on p. 336.

Philosophy

The American Health Foundation is a voluntary, non-profit health agency dedicated to advancing interest and action in preventive medicine. AHF believes that preventive medicine will hasten the day when every American will not only live longer, but will gain useful longevity, unencumbered by the destructive effects of chronic illnesses. Our slogan has always been: "To help people die young — as late as possible."

Underlying the Foundation's objectives is the fact that disease prevention is as scientifically sound as our knowledge of disease treatment. And, since the medical profession readily admits it sees little hope for solving the major problems of degenerative diseases by curative medicine alone, the upgrading of disease prevention should be a necessary, if not urgent, national priority.

Generations of neglect of preventive medicine cannot be wiped out in a few short years. But the guidelines for changes to come have been drawn. The movement to make preventive medicine an integral and vital part of America's health care delivery system is clearly underway.

Continued.

Risk factor education, level I. The Know Your Body Disease Prevention Program. Further information may be obtained by writing The American Health Foundation, 1370 Avenue of the Americas, New York, N.Y. 10019. (Courtesy The American Health Foundation.)

Philosophy—cont'd

Today, in the face of a crisis affecting all aspects of health care in the United States, it has become increasingly apparent that attempts to treat disease are simply not enough. There also is greater awareness that we cannot solve our nation's health problems merely by pouring more billions of dollars into our present health care system.

Under this "too much, too late" approach, the burden on society in suffering and economic cost is too great. In addition to an estimated annual cost of more than $63-billion, deaths and disability from chronic diseases are taking a tremendous toll on the nation's resources and energies.

Cancer, heart disease and stroke, the leading causes of premature death among American adults, are often rooted in childhood. These roots, commonly known as risk factors, relate to personal health habits and lifestyles and include smoking, high blood cholesterol level, high blood pressure, overweight and physical inactivity. The American Health Foundation has been a leader in developing and implementing programs designed to lower the incidence of cancer and heart disease in the United States.

The American Health Foundation believes in the promotion of healthier lifestyles among people of all ages — especially the young. Disease prevention cannot wait until adulthood; it must begin early in life when life-long attitudes and health habits are being formed. Based on this belief, *Know Your Body* was developed.

The American Health Foundation is dedicated to advancing interest and action in preventive medicine. *Know Your Body* is a product of that dedication.

Risk factor education, level I. The Know Your Body Disease Prevention Program.

RISK FACTORS

Introduction

Extensive research studies have identified several factors as contributing to an increased risk of cardiovascular disease. Some of the major risk factors have been determined to be high blood pressure, cigarette smoking and high blood cholesterol. This unit is intended to provide KYB students with an overview of the relationship between disease risk factors and personal health behavior.

People often acquire their personal habits early in life: overeating, smoking cigarettes, developing a liking for fattening foods and avoiding strenuous exercise are examples of habits that relate to risk factors. By the time they reach middle-age, people usually find it difficult to change these ingrained risk behavior habits.

The activities in this section are focused on increasing student knowledge about disease risk factors and helping students understand the importance of establishing positive health habits in their early years. It is hoped that the classroom experiences will motivate students to undertake preventive measures to reduce their own risk factors.

Although this unit is probably best covered in a health education or science course, teachers of all subject areas are encouraged to seize opportunities to integrate instruction on risk factors whenever and wherever appropriate. Suggested learning activities for correlating this topic with various subject areas are available (Appendix 1).

Teachers will find supplementary information for their use on the leading causes of death in the U.S., and the extent to which particular factors increase the risk of the number one killer, cardiovascular disease.

Risk factor education, level I. The Know Your Body Disease Prevention Program.

BACKGROUND INFORMATION
RISK FACTORS IN CHRONIC DISEASE

LEADING CAUSES OF DEATH   United States: 1973

Heart disease remains the Number one cause of death in the U.S. today. About 1,000,000 Americans have heart attacks each year, and more than 660,000 individuals die from them. In New York State, 200 individuals die of heart disease each day. Cancer is the second leading cause of death in the U.S., with lung cancer among men having the largest incidence. There are more deaths attributed to lung cancer yearly than to any other type of cancer.

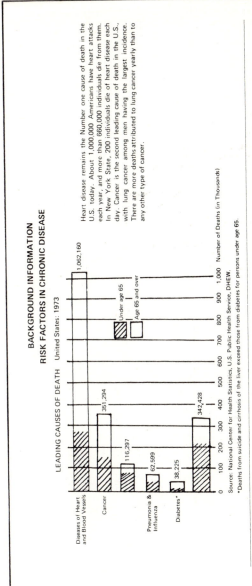

Source: National Center for Health Statistics, U.S. Public Health Service, DHEW.

*Deaths from suicide and cirrhosis of the liver exceed those from diabetes for persons under age 65.

*The following charts show the extent to which certain risk factors increase the risk of heart attack and stroke in a male population (ages 30-62).

A man with a blood cholesterol measurement of 250 or above has about three times the risk of heart attack and stroke as a man with a cholesterol below 194.

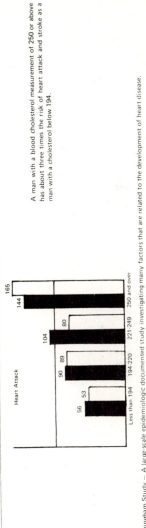

*Framingham Study – A large-scale epidemiologic documented study investigating many factors that are related to the development of heart disease.

Continued.

Risk factor education, level I. The **Know Your Body** Disease Prevention Program.

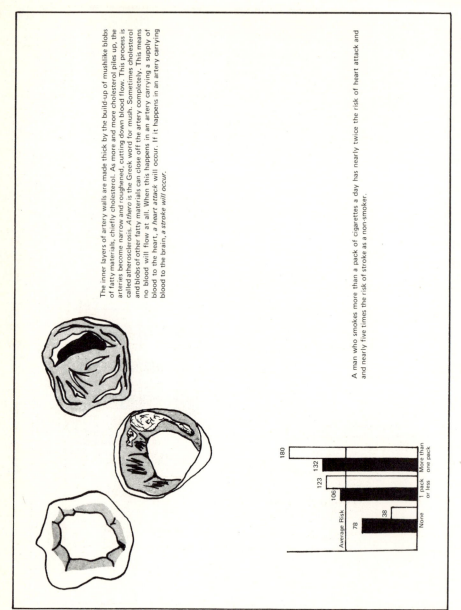

The inner layers of artery walls are made thick by the build-up of mushlike blobs of fatty materials, chiefly cholesterol. As more and more cholesterol piles up, the arteries become narrow and roughened, cutting down blood flow. This process is called atherosclerosis. *Athero* is the Greek word for mush. Sometimes cholesterol and blobs of other fatty materials can close off the artery completely. This means no blood will flow at all. When this happens in an artery carrying a supply of blood to the heart, *a heart attack* will occur. If it happens in an artery carrying blood to the brain, *a stroke will occur.*

A man who smokes more than a pack of cigarettes a day has nearly twice the risk of heart attack and and nearly five times the risk of stroke as a non-smoker.

Risk factor education, level I. The Know Your Body Disease Prevention Program.

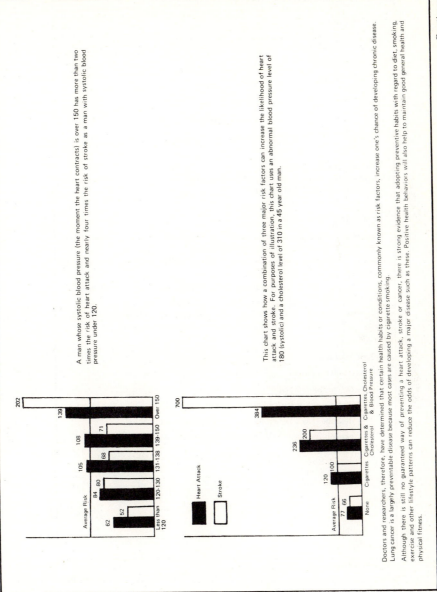

Risk factor education, level I. The Know Your Body Disease Prevention Program.

Continued.

RISK FACTORS

UNIT GOALS:

Students gain an understanding of the relationship between chronic disease risk factors and personal health habits.

CONCEPTS:

Individuals should be informed about the nature and degree of certain risks before deciding whether they are worth taking.

Research studies have identified certain factors which place an individual at increased risk for cardiovascular disease.

Reducing the risk of cardiovascular disease often requires changes in basic health behavior.

Research studies indicate that risk reduction measures should be undertaken early in life in order to prevent cardiovascular disease in later years.

OBJECTIVES:

Students will be able to:

- define risk factors.
- identify risk factors of cardiovascular disease.
- describe how risk factors relate to personal health habits.
- explain the need for establishing good health habits early in life.

Risk factor education, level I. The Know Your Body Disease Prevention Program.

LEVEL I ACTIVITIES

UNIT GOAL: Students gain an understanding of the relationship between chronic disease risk factors and personal health habits.

OBJECTIVE: Define risk factors.

CONCEPT	SUGGESTED LEARNING ACTIVITY	RESOURCE
Individuals should be informed about the nature and degree of certain risks before deciding whether they are worth taking.	Have students discuss what we mean when we say we will take a risk. Ask them to name some risks or risky things they have done or have heard about (e.g. riding in a car or bicycle, not studying for a test, participating in a sport). Ask them what was being risked in each case. Discussion Questions: — Why do we take risks? — When would it be unwise to take risks? When we say cigarette smoking is a risk or a "risk factor," what is it that we are risking? Have class develop a definition for risk factors of disease. Definition: A risk factor is a health habit or condition which increases a person's chance of developing disease. (Some risk factors may also be described as "silent warning signals" that the body gives to indicate that diseases may develop if individuals continue to practice risky health habits.)	Book: Hochbaum, Godfrey M., *Health Behavior*.

Risk factor education, level I. The Know Your Body Disease Prevention Program.

Continued.

UNIT GOAL:	Students gain an understanding of the relationship between chronic disease risk factors and personal health habits.	
OBJECTIVE:	Identify risk factors of cardiovascular disease.	

CONCEPT	SUGGESTED LEARNING ACTIVITY		RESOURCE
Research studies have identified certain factors which place an individual at increased risk for the development of cardiovascular disease.	Assign students research to do and come up with a list of risk factors of cardiovascular disease (heart disease and stroke). Have them put a star next to the three major risks. Compare their list to the following:		Film: *Heart Sweet Heart* (10 minutes) N.Y.U. Film Library
	*Cigarette Smoking	Diabetes	Pamphlet: *Seven Ways to Prevent a Heart Attack* New York State Department of Health
	*High Blood Pressure	Over 40 years old	
	*High Blood Cholesterol	Family History of Heart Disease	Pamphlet: *Reduce Your Risk of Heart Attack* American Heart Association
	Overweight		
	Inadequate Exercise		Film: *Our Way of Life* (27 minutes) American Heart Association
	Excessive Stress		Publication: *Heart Facts, 1975* American Heart Association

Risk factor education, level I. The Know Your Body Disease Prevention Program.

UNIT GOAL: Students gain an understanding of the relationship between chronic disease risk factors and personal health habits.

OBJECTIVE: Describe how certain risk factors relate to health habits.

CONCEPT	SUGGESTED LEARNING ACTIVITY	RESOURCE
Reducing the risk of cardiovascular disease often requires changes in basic health behavior.	Write the nine risk factors (listed above) on separate slips of paper and throw them into a hat. Call on students to pick one out, read it aloud and tell the class whether that particular risk factor is related to personal health habits. Use the following chart to discuss with your students the preventive measures which may be taken to reduce these risk factors.	Book: Brinney, Kenneth, *Cardiovascular Disease: A Matter of Prevention*

RISK FACTOR — **PREVENTIVE MEASURES**

Cigarette Smoking — Avoid cigarettes — if you do smoke, make an attempt to quit.

High Blood Cholesterol — Food choices can be made to lower blood cholesterol. This means decreasing intake of foods high in saturated fat and cholesterol and increasing those high in polyunsaturated fats.

High Blood Pressure — Know your blood pressure and have it checked regularly. Weight and excessive salt intake can increase blood pressure.

Overweight — Know your weight and know how to control it through proper diet and exercise.

Inadequate Exercise — Find an activity that you like such as jogging, swimming, bicycling or walking and do it on a regular basis.

Excessive Stress — Know Your Body. Identify what causes excessive stress and attempt to find solutions to stressful situations in your lifestyles.

Risk factor education, level I. The Know Your Body Disease Prevention Program.

Continued.

UNIT GOAL: Students gain an understanding of the relationship between chronic disease risk factors and personal health habits.

OBJECTIVE: Explain the need for establishing good health habits early in life.

CONCEPT	SUGGESTED LEARNING ACTIVITY	RESOURCE
Research studies indicate that risk reduction measures should be undertaken early in life in order to prevent cardiovascular disease in later years.	Have students suggest reasons why a study comparing Wisconsin school children with Mexican children found that 1/3 of the American children had cholesterol levels above what was considered top normal (200 mg%), whereas none of the Mexican children exceeded this level. Compare the typical Mexican diet to that of Americans. Have students review the overall KYB screening results for their school (e.g. percentage of the participating students who were found to be overweight, have cholesterol levels 180% or higher, have high blood pressure, have a recovery index rating of fair or poor, etc.). Have students discuss the benefits of identifying risk factors in their pre-adolescent and adolescent years.	Article: Golubjatnikov, R. et al, "Serum Cholesterol Levels of Mexican and Wisconsin School Children."

Risk factor education, level I. The Know Your Body Disease Prevention Program.

APPENDIX 1

INTEGRATION OF RISK FACTOR EDUCATION
WITH
DIFFERENT SUBJECT AREAS

Teaching about risk factors need not occur in isolation in a health education or science course, but should be supported and reinforced in as many subject areas as possible. It is strongly recommended that teachers of all subjects seize every opportunity to integrate content and classroom experiences on risk factors whenever and wherever appropriate.

The following are suggested learning activities for correlating risk factor education with various subject areas.

Continued.

Risk factor education, level I. The Know Your Body Disease Prevention Program.

INTEGRATION OF RISK FACTOR EDUCATION

English

Students will:

- Prepare debates, compositions, speeches, research reports, etc. on risk factors.

  Suggested Topics:

  Cholesterol: Is elevated blood cholesterol the primary villain of heart disease?

  Smoking in Public Places: Is this an invasion of privacy?

  High Blood Pressure: Is excessive tension the primary cause?

- Develop short scripts or skits for television to market low-cholesterol foods, non-smoking, blood pressure check-ups.

- Write persuasive essays convincing teenagers to smoke or not to smoke, to maintain or change current American eating habits, to maintain or change exercise habits.

- Research and discuss what trends, if any, are apparent with regard to teenage smoking and teenage diets in modern literature.

- Write critique on books about nutrition, smoking and physical fitness. Recommend and obtain books for a school book fair (see section on "Resource Center").

- Conduct a spelling "B" on risk factor related words (e.g. cholesterol, emphysema, hypertension, atherosclerosis, sphygmomanometer (see "Glossary").

Mathematics

Students will:

- Use the current price of cigarettes to calculate the total cost of smoking one pack of cigarettes a day for a week, a month, one year, five years, etc. Discuss what this money can be used for instead.

- Compare, graph, and comment on national expenditure for tobacco, education, cancer research, hospitals, etc.

- Analyze their family's food budget. Figure out what percent of the total cost is spent on protein foods, fatty foods, "junk" foods, etc.

- Determine ratio of incidence of lung cancer in cigarette, cigar, pipe and non-smokers.

- Survey the smoking habits of students and their parents. Collect, tabulate and analyze data to determine any link between teenage smoking and parental smoking.

Risk factor education, level I. The Know Your Body Disease Prevention Program.

INTEGRATION OF RISK FACTOR EDUCATION

Social Studies

Students will:

— Compare today's leading causes of death to those 100 years ago.

— Research and use a world map or a globe to point out countries with high incidence of heart attacks, stroke and certain types of cancer (e.g. lung cancer, colon cancer).

— Research and compare the fat content of diets and the average cholesterol levels of different cultural groups (e.g. Japan vs. United States).

— Discuss different cultural and social forces that influence smoking and eating habits and customs.

— Suggest action the government might take to protect the public from the dangers of smoking, high fat diets, high blood pressure, inadequate exercise.

— Debate whether the government should ban all cigarette advertising or ban smoking altogether.

— Act as congressmen and prepare and present legislative bills on school lunches, food labeling, smoking prohibition.

Home Economics

Students will:

— Discuss the effect of smoking on family budget.

— Discuss and recommend specific ways of changing to a low-cholesterol diet and how those changes can save money.

— Bring to class original low-cholesterol snack recipes and prepare them for tasting in class.

— Compare life insurance premium rates for persons with desirable weight vs. persons who are overweight, persons with normal blood pressure vs. those with high blood pressure.

— Discuss how different methods of food preparation affect blood cholesterol levels and weight.

— Bring to class food labels and discuss their nutrient content. Suggest how reading food labels can help to reduce weight and cholesterol levels.

— Discuss whether smoking behavior and physique are important considerations in choosing a date.

— Write an article on "What can I do personally to help solve the cigarette smoking problem?"

Continued.

Risk factor education, level I. The Know Your Body Disease Prevention Program.

INTEGRATION OF RISK FACTOR EDUCATION

Science

Students will:

- Participate in KYB Teacher's Guide classroom learning activities.
- Perform experiments, demonstrations and design exhibits on the effects of smoking, high blood pressure and high cholesterol levels on human physiology. (See Appendices in Section on "Classroom Learning Activity Units.")
- Discuss how the scientific method may be applied to do research on the bodily effects of smoking, elevated blood cholesterol, high blood pressure, overweight and inactivity.
- Research and explain the different types of medical evidence that shows a relationship between risk factors and chronic disease.

Physical Education

Students will:

- Investigate and compare the physical fitness of American youth with that of other countries.
- Identify and practice exercises which are most beneficial to the heart (i.e. endurance-type such as jogging, cycling, swimming).
- Discuss why athletes, in particular, are encouraged not to smoke.
- Discuss the affect of exercise on weight control.
- Identify a recommended diet for athletes.
- Discuss what types of exercise and how much is required to burn up the calories of different foods.

Art

Students will:

- Design posters, collages, sculptures, cartoons, etc. on KYB themes and display them throughout the school.
- Develop advertising slogans and layouts to "sell" preventive measures related to high blood pressure, high blood cholesterol and smoking.

Risk factor education, level I. The Know Your Body Disease Prevention Program.

RISK FACTOR BIBLIOGRAPHY

Books

Brinney, Kenneth L.
Cardiovascular Disease: A Matter of Prevention.
Wadsworth Publishing Company, Inc., Belmont, California, 1970.

Hochbaum, Godfrey, M.
Health Behavior.
Wadsworth Publishing Company, Inc., Belmont, California, 1970.

Films

"Heart Sweet Heart"
NYU Film Library
New York University, N.Y., 1972.

"Our Way of Life"
American Heart Association, 1975.

Pamphlets

American Heart Association
Reduce Your Risk of Heart Attack.
American Heart Association, Inc., 1974.

New York State Department of Health
Seven Ways to Prevent a Heart Attack.
New York State Department of Health, Albany, N.Y., 1975.

Periodicals

Golubjatnikov, R., et al.,
"Serum Cholesterol Levels of Mexican and Wisconsin School Children."
American Journal of Epidemiology, 96:36-39, 1972.

Publications

American Heart Association
Heart Facts — 1976.
American Heart Association, Inc., 1975.

Risk factor education, level I. The Know Your Body Disease Prevention Program.

RESOURCE UNIT—TOBACCO, ALCOHOL, AND OTHER HARMFUL DRUGS

Some instructors in the school health program prefer to defer a consideration of tobacco, alcohol, and other drugs until the last 2 years of senior high school. However, both observation and organized study have revealed that adults who use tobacco, alcohol, and other harmful drugs do not lack knowledge of the effects of these products. They lack the kind of attitudes that will cause them to refrain from the harmful use of these products. If the school is to help individuals acquire certain desirable attitudes toward the use of harmful products, the junior high school will provide the most fertile soil for effective results (Fig. 13-6). Proper attitudes established in junior high school, fortified by the acquisition of further supporting knowledge in senior high school, constitute the most effective type of program of instruction about tobacco, alcohol, and other harmful drugs.

Unit title—Tobacco, alcohol, and other harmful drugs

OVERVIEW

Much of what has been said and written on this subject has been of doubtful value because of the bias of individuals who tend to overstate or understate to serve their own prejudices. Individuals with something to sell or those imbued with a missionary zeal to reform everyone who uses tobacco, alcohol, or other harmful drugs present a greatly distorted view of the question. The need is for an objective presentation of what is known and what is not known on the subject so that each youngster can formulate his or her own conclusions and establish personal values and standards.

Presentation of the subject as a physical, mental, and social health problem primarily, rather than a moral or legal problem, will establish the unit on a sound foundation. Youngsters who have learned to prize their

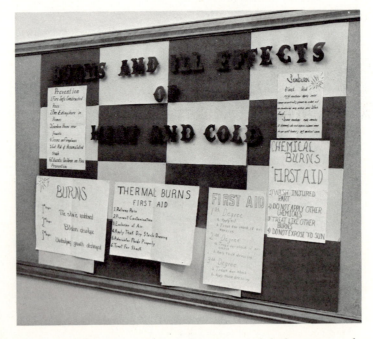

Fig. 13-6. Glass-covered display board. Students with ingenuity made both an artistic and an educational display by the clever use of the glass cover. This bulletin board is revised with each new health area being studied. (Courtesy Salem Public Schools, Salem, Ore.)

health highly will reject anything likely to jeopardize that health. When they understand why people use these products and the psychological aspects of habituation, they will tend to develop attitudes that reject the use of tobacco, alcohol, and other harmful drugs.

The instructor should recognize that many students come from homes in which tobacco and alcohol are used regularly. Data need not be feathered for their benefit. These children can face and accept reliable unadulterated data. Yet as health instructors we should not create the impression that all people who drink alcohol will become alcoholics. We also need to make crystal clear that it takes about 20 years for tobacco smoke irritants to have an effect in creating cancer and that, because individuals vary in susceptibility, some persons may be entirely immune to the production of cancer of the respiratory system.

Controversial questions should be analyzed systematically and thoroughly by the whole class. The teacher can help to guide the thinking of the class, particularly in weighing the reliability of data. Not all questions will be resolved satisfactorily. Perhaps further exploration will be indicated.

Junior high school students need and are interested in fundamental questions and problems, not detailed data. It is necessary to guard against consuming valuable class time with questions of minor significance or voluminous details. A straightforward consideration of the main

factors in the study will make the unit comprehensible, meaningful, and impressive to the youngsters (Fig. 13-7).

OBJECTIVES
Knowledge

Composition of tobacco smoke
Action of nicotine
Effect of smoking on respiratory system
Effect of smoking on digestive system
Effect of smoking on circulation
Effect of smoking on thyroid gland
Length of life and smoking
Motherhood and smoking
Why people smoke
Nature of ethyl (grain) alcohol
Absorption of alcohol
Intoxication as indicated by blood-alcohol concentration
Alcoholic malnutrition
Effect of alcohol always narcotic
Effect of alcohol on circulation
Effect of alcohol on nerve conduction
Effect of alcohol on physical health
Relationship of alcohol and mental disorder
Alcohol and the length of life
Absence of a hereditary basis for alcoholism
The social drinker
Why people drink alcohol

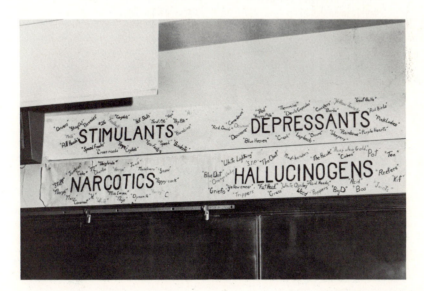

Fig. 13-7. Subtle message, effective education. Originally designed to create attitudes of aversion to drugs by means of ridicule, this clever display carried a simple, effective message that did more than teach facts. (Courtesy Salem Public Schools, Salem, Ore.)

Weekend and aggressive drinkers
Addiction as physiological dependence
Habituation as psychological dependence
The path of alcoholism
Alcoholism as a problem of the individual
Alcoholism as a family problem
Alcoholism as a community problem
Curing alcoholism
Preventing alcoholism
Community responsibility
Marihuana as a threat to youth
Sources of marihuana
Methods employed to recruit users
Action of marihuana
Measures to control marihuana
Why people take morphine
Action of morphine
Measures to control morphine
The problem of sleeping pills (barbiturates)
Action of barbiturates
Measures to solve the barbiturate addiction problem
Hallucinogens
Amphetamines
Importance of substituting a healthful practice for an unhealthful one

Attitudes as expressed in

Desire to conserve and protect personal health
Desire to avoid those factors that injure health
Conviction that prevention is better than cure
Recognition that smoking adds nothing of value to a person
Self-reliance in refusing to begin injurious practices
Reliance on one's own ability to adjust, not on a crutch such as tobacco
Self-gratification through wholesome achievement
Realization that pupils must make their own decisions
Insistence on having facts before making decisions
Refusal to go along blindly with a popular practice
Pride in the ability to be master of one's actions
Acceptance of inconvenience resulting from nonconformity
Respect for the right of others to choose their practices
Support of worthy recreation outlets for youth
Promotion of wholesome school atmosphere
Support of community efforts to control use of tobacco, alcohol, and other harmful drugs
Recognition of social pathology of alcoholism and drug addiction
Acceptance of responsibility for dealing with the problems of smoking, alcoholism, and drug addiction
Acceptance of the alcoholic and drug addict as ill persons
Need for constant vigilance in preventing marihuana peddlers from recruiting students

Avoid use of drugs, including barbiturates, except on prescription

Practices

Be guided by established health principles
Engage in wholesome recreation outlets
Conform to community laws and regulations
Follow positive mental health principles
Take drugs only on a physician's prescription

CONTENT AND ACTIVITIES
Tobacco (Fig. 13-8)

What is the nature and action of nicotine?
What irritants are present in tobacco tar?
What is meant by differences in tolerance?
What causes smoker's cough?
How does smoking affect nutrition?
How does smoking affect the heart and blood pressure?
Why does smoking cause a tremor in some people?
What is the evidence that smoking is related to cancer of the respiratory system?
How does smoking affect the length of life?
Panel discussion on the topic *Why Do People Smoke?*
Symposium on the topics *Smoking and Athletics, Popularity,* and *Cost?*
Sociodrama to illustrate life situation of refusing a cigarette
Ask the class to list disadvantages of smoking, with help of chairman and recorder
Panel discussion of the topic *Why Should the Expectant or Nursing Mother Refrain from Smoking?*
Buzz session on the topic *How Would You Persuade a Person to Quit Smoking?*
Assignment, written report, on the subject *Why I Would Be Wise Not to Smoke*
Current film on effects of alcohol and tobacco on the body.

Alcohol (Fig. 13-9)

Why is alcohol called the benevolent tyrant?
What are some valuable uses of alcohol?
What is meant by ethyl alcohol?
How is a laboratory test of blood used to determine drunkenness?
How does alcohol affect circulation?
Why do alcoholics suffer from poor nutrition?
What effect does alcohol have on general health?
How does alcohol affect the length of life?
Why is alcohol called a narcotic?
What mental changes does alcohol cause?
Why does a person take the first drink of alcohol?
What is a social drinker?
How extensive is the problem of alcohol in the United States?
How does a person become an alcoholic?

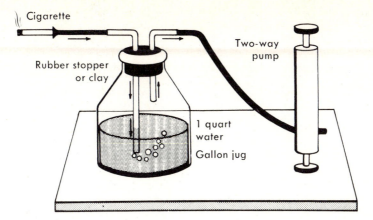

Fig. 13-8. Mechanical smoker. Pumping slowly will wash the cigarette smoke through the water. First smoking two regular cigarettes, then through a new quart of water smoking two filter cigarettes, should provide a comparison of interest to the students.

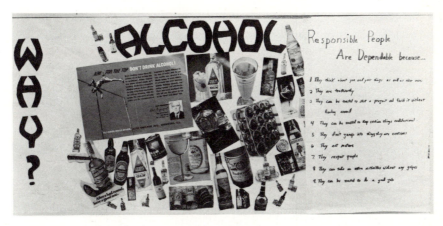

Fig. 13-9. Positive approach to the alcohol problem. By identifying the attributes of the nondrinker, students acquire a pattern of life that can be wholesome and highly productive. (Courtesy Salem Public Schools, Salem, Ore.)

What is the community's responsibility to the alcoholic?

Why must alcoholism be regarded as an illness?

Sociodrama to illustrate the situation of refusing an alcoholic drink

Symposium on the topic *Effect of Alcoholism on the Individual, the Family, the Individual's Employer, the Community*

Guest participation by a representative of Alcoholics Anonymous

Written reports on the subject *Why the Group I Belong to is so Important to my Health and Well-Being*

Select current films to be shown in relation to the effects of alcohol on the body

Conduct a survey on the sale of alcohol in the community

Report on the community program to reduce consumption of alcohol

Keep a clipping booklet of convictions for drunken driving

Why do people abuse drugs?

Escape from problems and frustrations

Need to be accepted by peers

Experimentation
Desire for a new experience
Curiosity
Glamor
Excitement
Emotional instability
Attain status

What teachers must look for

Sudden and dramatic change in attendance, discipline, academic work
Changes in neatness and caliber of work
Unusual degree of activity or inactivity
Sudden and irrational flare-ups
Neglect of personal appearance
Furtive behavior
Borrowing money from several sources
Stealing items easily converted to cash
Wearing sunglasses at inappropriate times
Finding student in unusual places (to take drugs)
Association with known drug users

Marihuana (Fig. 13-10)

Hallucinogen but legally classed as a narcotic
Not addictive but psychological dependence can result

Usually smoked as a cigarette
Use puts person in a drug environment
Cost of marihuana is minimal
Effect is that of distortion of judgment, time, and place; may produce feeling of irresponsibility and silliness by reducing inhibitions
Class activities for study of marihuana:
    From where is marihuana obtained?
    How is it used?
    How is it peddled?
    How does it affect a person?
    How is it related to crime?
    What do government agencies do to control it?
    Report on topic, *Marihuana and Youth*
    Obtain a picture of the *Cannabis sativa* plant

LSD-25 (lysergic acid diethylamide)

Hallucinogen affects individuals differently
Not addictive but dependence may occur
Visual and auditory centers affected
    Swirling colors and movement of fixed objects
    Walls sway and ceilings breathe
    Time and place distorted
    Incoherent speech, laughing and crying
    Suicide and homicide episodes

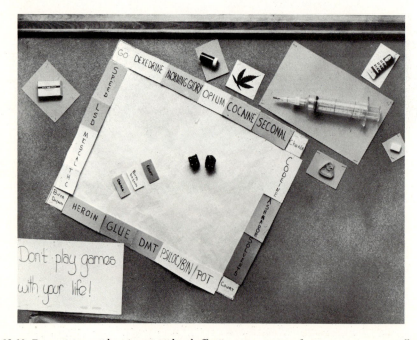

Fig. 13-10. Dramatizing an idea. An original and effective presentation of an important concept illustrates the old adage that one picture can be worth a thousand words. (Courtesy Salem Public Schools, Salem, Ore.)

Brain damage such that recurrences of disturbances occur even though the drug is no longer being used

Long-time effect may be that of lifelong psychosis and hospitalization

Class activities for study of LSD-25:

1. Any LSD available to the public is impure and the potency unknown. Why is this a special danger?
2. Taking LSD for kicks is like playing Russian roulette. Why?
3. Try to find out how many persons under 20 years of age have LSD psychosis and are in mental hospitals in this state.
4. What kinds of persons would experiment with LSD?

Morphine (or heroin)

Narcotic

Addictive

Derivative of opium, properly used by the medical practitioner to relieve pain

In powder, pill, or capsule form

Swallowed or injected under the skin or into a vein

Relieves pain, gives a sense of well-being

Produces addiction with great inner distresses if withdrawn

Physical, mental, moral, and social deterioration

Crime involved to obtain funds for purchase of morphine on the black market

Class activities for the study of morphine:

Justify the medical practice of prescribing morphine

Why are most morphine addicts in the lower socioeconomic groups?

Why would a person take morphine without a prescription?

Have guest participation by physician, police chief, or social worker to discuss drugs and control measures

Use sociodrama to illustrate how youth may be lured into the use of drugs

Barbiturates (sleeping pills)

Legally obtained only with a physician's prescription

All names end in *al;* thus, barbital, phenobarbital, secobarbital (Seconal)

Swallowed or injected

Induce sleep and symptoms similar to intoxication

Users in a groggy state and go into deep sleep

Addictive

May cause death

Class activities for the study of barbiturates:

What are the causes of sleeplessness?

What is the wisdom of consulting a physician?

What kind of people rely on barbiturates?

What measures should these people take for wholesome living?

Conduct a survey to determine whether in the community a prescription is necessary to obtain barbiturates

Collect newspaper and other clippings of deaths and near-deaths from an overdose of barbiturates

Amphetamines (pep pills)

Stimulants—increase activities of all neural centers

Amines such as Benzedrine, Dexedrine, D amphetamine

Swallowed as tablets

Relieve depression and anxiety

Can cause talkativeness, excitation, and elevation of mood

Disguise the feeling of fatigue

Create false sense of mental alertness

Psychological dependence can occur

Drug psychosis can be developed

Overdose may be lethal

Identification of amphetamine user

Excessive activity

Irritable, argumentative, jittery, nervous

Dilated pupils

Bad breath without other reason

Dryness of mouth, licking of lips

Rubs and scratches nose because of itching

Goes for long periods without eating or sleeping

Class activity for study of amphetamines:

What kind of people are likely to use amphetamines?

What measures should these people take to attain wholesome living?

Inquire of pharmacists whether amphetamines can be obtained without a prescription

Why should a person take only medicine that has been prescribed by a physician?

Why have amphetamines been found to be of no value in improving athletic performance?

What can be done to prevent the use of amphetamines except when prescribed by a physician?

Evaluation

Attitude of students toward drug abuse is the important outcome of this unit. In the absence of a valid, reliable instrument for measuring, the teacher will have to depend on his or her observations for appraisal of attitudes. During class discussions students will best reveal their attitudes toward the various drugs. Particularly significant are student reports of drug incidents with disastrous effects. *Drugs are not for me* is the expression of the cardinal attitude to be desired. From this it is apparent that class discussion is the method of choice in developing and bringing out attitudes while certain knowledge is being acquired.

Class discussion questions

1. What is the most serious drug problem in the United States?
2. Why are laws relating to drugs difficult to enforce?
3. How are others affected when a person becomes a drug addict?
4. Under what conditions will a person try marihuana for the first time?
5. What kinds of persons experiment with drugs?
6. Why will young people be attracted to LSD when they know it is so dangerous?
7. Not all poorly adjusted people resort to drugs. Why?
8. For a person with personality problems, what does our community have to offer as an alternative to drugs?
9. Is drug abuse a medical, legal, social, religious, economic, or educational problem?
10. Survey the drug addiction prevention, control, and treatment facilities of this community and recommend some desirable improvements.
11. Who usually introduces a student to drugs?
12. How can a student resist pressures such as being called "chicken" for not trying drugs?

EVALUATION

In evaluation it is most important to determine whether students have acquired the attitude that drugs are injurious to physical, mental, and social health and should never be used, except when prescribed by a physician. Knowledge is important to support these attitudes and prepare the student to evaluate the desirability of never starting an undesirable practice. "This will not be me," should be the cardinal attitude. Knowledge of individual and community responsibility is important. Avoiding certain practices is a negative approach, but has value in this area. Engaging in wholesome activities, following positive mental health principles, and conforming to community laws should be observable outcomes.

RESOURCE UNIT—MENTAL HEALTH

To prepare the junior high school student for the social adjustments life will demand, a teaching unit must deal with the specifics of social conduct to give students the self-confidence that comes from knowing what is accepted in social relationships. To be effective, teaching in this area must deal with one's own feelings, failures, and successes. Students should learn early in life that a good social personality is the result of working at developing such a personality. First, the student should learn what is proper in social conduct and, second, apply himself or herself to practicing this conduct, reviewing failures and successes, and then improving over previous performances. The importance of social confidence to one's level of mental health is self-evident.

Unit title—Mental health

GENERAL PURPOSE

To increase in depth the information presented in former grades and to aid early teenagers to accept themselves and to adjust to new responsibilities and experiences of which they are becoming aware. Increased emotional tension associated with glandular changes needs both explanation and knowledge as to how it can best be channeled. This unit could stimulate inquiry in pupils and help them to find their own answers concerning their emotional needs and the emotional needs of those about them. When aware of these needs, adjustment is greatly aided.

PUPILS SHOULD

A. Learn to make friends with members of the same sex
   1. Choice of friends
   2. Meeting social needs
   3. Developing a pleasing personality
   4. Cliques versus a large circle of friends
   5. Development of independent thought and action
B. Learn to make friends with members of the opposite sex
   1. Choosing friends
   2. Corecreational activities
   3. Dating
      a. What is a date?
      b. Etiquette
      c. Standard of conduct
      d. Going steady
      e. Age and maturity
      f. Kinds (single, double)
      g. Expense
      h. Gifts
      i. Conversation
C. Learn to get along with family members
   1. Understand the viewpoint of parents
      a. Finances, allowances
      b. Hours
      c. Chaperones

    d. Home tasks
    e. Friends
    f. Clothing
  2. Learn responsibilities of increasing independence
  3. Understand consideration for other members of family
    a. Show respect for rights and belongings
    b. Accept differences in ability and interest in siblings
D. Demonstrate courtesy and good manners
  1. Grooming
  2. Telephone etiquette
  3. Acceptable behavior
    a. School
    b. Home
    c. Public places
    d. Extracurricular activities
E. Demonstrate responsibility in the community by
  1. Increased awareness of its problems
  2. Increased appreciation of its services
  3. Awareness of their role in the community
  4. Increased awareness of
    a. World problems
    b. Responsibilities in world affairs
    c. Health attitudes toward world conditions
    d. Abilities necessary for meeting crises (e.g., nuclear attack, floods, hurricane)

PUPILS MAY

A. Use a question box in which they deposit questions they have regarding friends
B. Develop a bulletin board display with pictures of outstanding men and women who exemplify pleasing personalities
C. Evaluate themselves on a personality checklist
D. Discuss ways in which pupils, teachers, and parents might help make sure that boys and girls have plenty of opportunities to participate in group activities for making friends; the PTA may help, too
E. Have a panel discussion on good manners. Talk about ways of applying good manners to their relationships with each other
F. Make posters and cartoons depicting good manners at home, at school, and at church
G. Demonstrate and discuss table manners at home, in a restaurant, and at school
H. Report on Helen Keller and other outstanding individuals who have adjusted successfully to some handicap
I. Have a discussion on why good mental health cannot be separated from attractive personality development
J. Take a census of hobbies enjoyed by members of the class; this may serve as a basis for a hobby day

or a hobby show in which various class members tell about and show results of their hobbies
K. Collect advertisements about care of the skin and treatment for blackheads, pimples, and dandruff; the class then evaluates claims of the products in the light of research
L. Discuss current events, both local and world; write letters to the United Nations concerning mental health or areas where assistance is needed in world projects (e.g., CARE, UNICEF)
M. Have a debate or panel on local curfew regulations or other teenage problems
N. Dramatize going on a date; follow this with questions such as: What is a date? How do you ask for a date? How do you act on a date? Should you go steady?

EVALUATION

The effectiveness of a program for health instruction in junior high school must be measured in terms of the extent to which it has changed the individual student. That change will be in the understanding of health, in health practices, and most important in health attitudes.

Health understanding that is based on fundamental health principles, not infinitesimal detail, is the important knowledge that should be evaluated. Ability to interpret and evaluate health factors is important in understanding. Knowledge of sources of health data, health resources, and methods for dealing with health problems should be an outcome of health instruction. An understanding of community health and united efforts in behalf of health are important results of effective health instruction on the junior high school level.

Health practices should expand from those for sheer personal benefit to practices in behalf of the group, the school, and the community as an outgrowth of health instruction in junior high school.

Attitudes that the student acquires are especially important at this level of health instruction. They are difficult to measure objectively, but a discriminating instructor can detect indications of student attitudes. Particularly important are the attitudes toward a high level of personal health, utilization of established health principles, application of reason in matters of health, responsibility for the health of others, and cooperation in community health standards and assets.

In a junior high school with an effective program in health instruction, students are conscious of the importance of personal and community health. The vitality of the students and the atmosphere about the school reflect the kind of health program in action. There will be ample evidence of its effectiveness.

QUESTIONS AND ACTIVITIES

1. What characteristics of the junior high school student should be taken into consideration in planning a health education program for the junior high school?
2. Why does the departmentalized organization of the junior high school call for a different approach to health education from what is customary in the elementary school?
3. In the junior high school why is so much emphasis placed on the development of health attitudes?
4. How can adjustments be made to compensate for the great advance for the junior high school girl over the junior high school boy?
5. Some educators advocate that ninth-grade girls go into the senior high school but that the boys should go into the senior high school in the tenth grade. What is your reaction to this proposal?
6. Appraise the statement, "The junior high school is the most propitious level at which to emphasize responsibility for the health of others and for community health."
7. In the junior high school how would you prepare students to react to health superstitions, fallacies, quackery, and fraudulent health advertising?
8. On the junior high school level what should be taught in the areas of sex and reproduction?
9. What are mental health needs of the junior high school students, and how can these be met in health education?
10. In some junior high schools health is taught 4 days a week and on the fifth day that period is used by the health teacher for health counseling. What is your reaction to this arrangement?
11. What are the opportunities in the junior high school for incidental health learning?
12. Appraise the contention, "Health teaching demands a wider, more diverse professional preparation than does any other subject in the junior high school curriculum."
13. What subject in the junior high school curriculum is more important than health?
14. Why is health instruction rarely adequate when combined with general science as one subject area?
15. Some aspects of health are socially oriented, yet health scientists contend that relying solely on social science courses to teach health is a mistake. Why?
16. Each year more and more junior high schools have abandoned the practice of correlating the scheduling of health and physical education. Why?
17. In the junior high what is the best pattern of health instruction scheduling in terms of effective health education?
18. What should be the minimum professional preparation of the junior high school health educator?
19. Having guest lecturers or resource people come into health classes can be highly beneficial, but what are some safeguards the teachers should take?
20. Controversial health issues must be dealt with on the junior high school level. Develop some guidelines for handling controversial issues.

SELECTED READINGS

Alder, S.: Health and education of the economically deprived child, Westport, Conn., 1968, Greenwood Press, Inc.

American Health Foundation: KYB teachers' guide: The Know Your Body Disease Prevention Program, New York, 1978, The Foundation.

Anderson, W. J.: How to explain sex to children, Minneapolis, 1972, T. S. Denison & Co., Inc.

Barrett, M.: Health education guide, ed. 2, Philadelphia, 1974, Lea & Febiger.

Billett, R. O.: Improving the secondary school curriculum, New York, 1970, Lieber-Atherton.

Billett, R. O.: Teaching in the junior and senior high schools, Paterson, N. J., 1963, Littlefield, Adams & Co.

Crawford, C. O., editor: Health and the family, New York, 1972, The Macmillan Co.

Dalzell-Ward, A. J.: A textbook of health education, ed. 2, London, 1974, Barnes & Noble Books.

Diehl, H. S.: Health and safety for you, ed. 4, New York, 1969, McGraw-Hill Book Co.

Faunce, R. C., and Clute, M. J.: Teaching and learning in the junior high school, Belmont, Calif., 1961, Wadsworth Publishing Co., Inc.

Faunce, R. C., and Munshaw, C. L.: Teaching and learning in the secondary schools, Belmont, Calif., 1964, Wadsworth Publishing Co., Inc.

Force, E.: Teaching family life education, New York, 1962, American Social Health Association.

Foster, J. C.: Teaching of health education in the junior and senior high schools, New York, 1968, J. Lowell Pratt & Co., Inc., Publishers.

Grout, R. E.: Health teaching in schools, ed. 5, Philadelphia, 1968, W. B. Saunders Co.

Haag, J. H.: School health program, ed. 3, New York, 1972, Holt, Rinehart & Winston, pp. 403-406, 417.

Hafen, B. Q.: Health for the secondary teacher, Dubuque, Iowa, 1972, William C. Brown Co., Publishers.

Hanlon. J. J., and McHose, E.: Design for health, the school, and the community, ed. 2, Philadelphia, 1971, Lea & Febiger.

Hanson, D.: Health-related fitness, Belmont, Calif., 1970, Wadsworth Publishing Co., Inc.

Herzlick, C., and Graham, D.: Health and illness, a social psychological analysis, New York, 1974, Academic Press, Inc.

Irwin, L. W., et al.: Health for better living, ed. 2, Columbus, Ohio, 1972, Charles E. Merrill Publishing Co.

Jenne, F. H., and Greene, W. H.: Turner's school health and health education, ed. 7, St. Louis, 1976, The C. V. Mosby Co.

Joint Committee on Health Problems in Education of the National Education Association and the American Medical Association (Russell, R. D., editor): Health education, Washington, D.C., 1975, National Education Association.

Kilander, H. F.: School health education, ed. 2, New York, 1968, The Macmillan Co.

Montoye, H. J.: Physical activity and health, Englewood Cliffs, N.J., 1975, Prentice-Hall, Inc.

Oberteuffer, D., Harrelson, O. A., and Pollock, M. B.: School health education, ed. 5, New York, 1972, Harper & Row, Publishers.

Rathbone, F. S., and Rathbone, E.: Health and the nature of man, New York, 1971, McGraw-Hill Book Co.

Sloane, R. M., and Sloane, B. L.: A guide to health facilities: personnel and management, ed. 2, St. Louis, 1977, The C. V. Mosby Co.

Stack, H. J., and Elkow, J. D.: Education for safe living, ed. 4, Englewood Cliffs, N.J., 1966, Prentice-Hall, Inc.

Star, S. W.: Here's to good health, New York, 1973, Cebco Standard Publishing.

Wheatley, G. M., and Hallock, G. T.: Health observation of school children, ed. 3, New York, 1965, McGraw-Hill Book Co.

Willgoose, C. E.: Health teaching in secondary schools, Philadelphia, 1972, W. B. Saunders Co.

CHAPTER 14

Senior high school health instruction

High schools of today encompass at least three broad purposes that seek to provide the student with (1) the skills and knowledge that are needed to continue further study at the higher education level, (2) basic preparation needed for a vocation, and (3) preparation for accepting responsibilities of adulthood. Health education at the senior high school level is most often considered to be one of the essential requirements in this preparation for adulthood.

To be effective, health instruction must be adapted to the distinctive characteristics of the high school age. At times the individual displays the consistency of maturity and at other times the inconsistency of immaturity. Youth is a period of transition from the dependence of childhood to the independence of adulthood. Self-assertion, determination, and independence reveal the desire of all young people for emancipation from adult domination and for recognition as competent, self-reliant individuals in their own right. They want to know the *how* and *why* as well as the *what*. High school students are imaginative, enthusiastic, sensitive, and idealistic. They seek status within their group and try to merit the respect of their instructors. They need to develop a mature standard of values that will provide a basis for positive motiva-

tion. Gaining self-esteem that grows out of successful and satisfying participation is essential to their ultimate well-being.

At the high school level, teachers are working with students who have virtually attained their maximum level of native intelligence. They will gain a great deal more knowledge from experience and from instructors who can challenge these young people by providing stimulating opportunities for learning. Their experiences can be most meaningful when students have a role in planning and implementing the instructional program. In education, as in self-growth, the individual must participate actively in the process whether the learning involves memorization, analysis, or creativity. Effective learning must develop as growth from within. The teacher guides this growth by providing motivation through wholesome experiences. While students will learn something about health without a teacher, a well-designed health instruction program increases both the quantity and quality of student learning.

BASIC OBJECTIVES OF HEALTH INSTRUCTION

High school students are on the threshold of adulthood and soon will have to rely on their own initiative in an adult world. To

346

enable young people to play their proper role in a complex society, schools have the obligation of helping the individual develop to full potential. Although high school students will continue to learn about health after graduation, the degree of observation, discernment, and interest they maintain in health areas will depend to a large extent on their school health education experiences. Therefore high school graduates should have a solid foundation of health knowledge, attitudes, values, and practices on which to build their life-long growth in health learning. Such a foundation will assist them in achieving that health education goal stated by the World Health Organization, the necessity for all people to meet their own health needs and to accept responsibility for the health of their families and of their communities.

By the time students enter senior high school they will have acquired some health knowledge as well as certain desirable health attitudes and practices. These practices and attitudes toward health can be reinforced by giving students an opportunity to extend their knowledge of the health sciences. A representative list of topics in each of the major health behavior categories is as follows:

Knowledge related to

Characteristics of optimum health
Methods of personal health promotion
Adjustment in marriage
Mental health principles
Biological bases of health
Heredity and eugenics
Growth and development
Personal grooming
Choice and use of health services and products
Nutrition
Health aspects of activity, fatigue, and rest
Sex and reproduction
Stimulants and narcotics
Common poisons
Communicable and noncommunicable disease control
Community health problems
Community health resources
Sanitation

Health aspects of air and sunlight
Safety
Emergency care and first aid

Attitudes as expressed in

Concern for the quality of one's health
Appreciation of the value of health
Appreciation of moderation and regularity in health promotion
Recognition of the importance of periodic health examinations
Attention to any deviation from normal
Utilization of professional services for restoring health
Concern for having disorders corrected immediately
Interest in new advances in health science
Eagerness to acquire mature understanding of health
Acceptance of only verified health information
Refraining from self-diagnosis and self-medication
Recognition of the value of prevention
Acceptance of responsibility for the health of others
Safety consciousness
Willingness to cooperate in health programs
Support of community health efforts
Appreciation of community health services
Interest in community health problems
Interest in state health problems and programs
Interest in national health promotion
Interest in international health promotion

Practices

Apply health principles to daily living
Apply reasoning to health problems
Use recognized nutrition practices
Engage in moderate activity daily
Avoid overexertion and extreme fatigue
Obtain adequate rest regularly
Refrain from self-medication
Refrain from the use of tobacco, alcohol, and other harmful drugs
Use preventive measures against communicable diseases
Have tests for tuberculosis when available
Impose isolation on self when communicable disease is suspected
Use recognized safety measures
Make wholesome adjustment to frustration
Participate in normal social activities
Adapt effectively to different individuals and situations
Recover quickly from emotional upsets
Use established sanitary measures
Assume responsibility for improving the environment
Follow all community health laws and regulations
Participate in school and community health promotion
Support special health projects

To be classified as successful, a health instruction program need not meet these objectives 100% for every student, but every graduate should have a substantial knowledge of fundamental health principles, a positive health awareness, and established health practices.

Although high school health instruction properly emphasizes the practical aspects of education, opportunities for cultural developments are always present. Pride in high standards of personal care, grooming, vigor, and appearance promotes the self-esteem that is essential to a high level of mental health. If such an attitude is properly cultivated, those high standards of personal well-being are projected to a desire for high environmental standards as well.

AREAS OF PRIMARY INTEREST

In accord with the current philosophy of secondary education, insofar as is possible the school should prepare the student for the demands of adult life. To discover which areas will be of primary interest to young people, it is both practical and educationally sound for the students to participate in planning the areas to be studied. Special health interests and needs of the group may be discovered through surveys and class discussion (Fig. 14-1). A committee of students can be used to identify those topics of greatest interest. Surveys of student health interests have identified the following health topics:

Indices of personal health
Personal health promotion

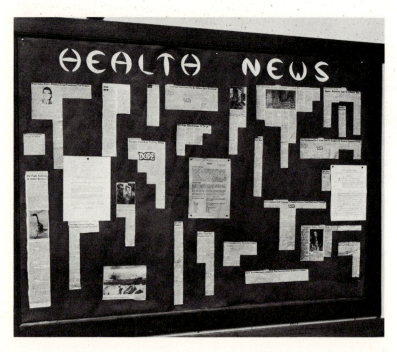

Fig. 14-1. Sustaining health interest. Being alert for news items of health interest to post on the bulletin board makes health a relevant subject and reinforces the planned, regular instruction. (Courtesy Salem Public Schools, Salem, Ore.)

Extension of the prime of life
Life expectancy
Use of medical and dental services
Use of health products
Body structure and function
Heredity and disease
Eugenics
Physical growth and development
Care of the skin
Care of the eyes
Dietary practices and weight control
Sex and reproduction
Health aspects of activity
Fatigue, rest, and sleep
Effects of drugs
Venereal disease
Cancer
Health aspects of air and sunshine
Bicycle safety
Emergency care and first aid
Emotional development
Attributes of a well-adjusted personality
Adjustment to common problems
Personality adjustment
Adjustment in marriage
Causes of mental illness
Causes of suicide
How to select a physician
How to select health insurance
Understanding aging and death

Initiating a course of study through a survey of student health interests illustrates an important principle in curriculum planning —relevance of the instruction. This principle recognizes that (1) learning is more efficient when the subject is of interest to the student and (2) information is more likely to be applied when it is of interest to the student. However, if the health education curriculum is to include the health content of greatest value to the student, it must draw on at least two additional sources of information. The foundation of the modern school health education curriculum should rest on (1) the health needs and interests of the student, (2) the health needs of the larger society, and (3) the body of health knowledge or the discipline of the health sciences. Examples of health topics or sub-

ject matter identified from each of these sources include the following:

A. Health topics identified by a study of the individual student.
  1. Growth and developmental characteristics
    a. Young children
      (1) Susceptibility to upper respiratory infections, the complications of which affect hearing
    b. Junior high school level
      (1) Sexual development causes the student to be very aware of bodily changes
    c. Senior high school level
      (1) Interest in the opposite sex provides incentive for developing responsible adult roles in preparation for marriage
      (2) Growing interest in adult consumer role and many existing misconceptions about medications
B. Health needs of society
  1. Morbidity and mortality data reveal the need to prevent such problems as deaths caused by accidents at all age levels
  2. Need for early detection and treatment of cancer
  3. Disease effects caused by smoking
  4. Disease and suffering caused by misuse of drugs
C. Data from health knowledge or the discipline of the health sciences
  1. Man's experiences and scientific research have created a body of information that has been organized into broad categories such as nutrition, environmental health, mental health, communicable and chronic diseases, family health, dental health, etc.

Two important developments have led to an improvement in the organization of the health education curriculum. First, the subject matter or content of health education has been organized into broad categories for ease of classification. Two such lists are selected to illustrate content areas used in California and Illinois state curriculum guides.

Content areas (California guide)

1. Consumer health
2. Mental-emotional health
3. Drug use and misuse
4. Family health
5. Oral health, vision, and hearing
6. Nutrition

7. Exercise, rest, and posture
8. Diseases and disorders
9. Environmental hazards
10. Community health resources

Content areas (Illinois guide)

1. Health and human ecology
2. Consumer health
3. Dental health
4. Drug use and abuse
5. Growth and development
6. Mental health and illness
7. Nutrition
8. Personal health
9. Prevention and control of disease
10. Public and environmental health
11. Safety education and disaster survival
12. Smoking and disease

Second, the concept approach has been used to give meaning to curriculum. This approach is designed to organize isolated facts and information into interrelated units. Although the identification of topic areas for classifying information is meaningful, the use of conceptual statements reveals relationships between broad areas. An example of the conceptual approach to curriculum planning in health education is that employed by the School Health Education Study Team. In this study the curriculum was organized in relation to the following conceptual statements:

1. Growth and development influence and are influenced by the structure and functioning of the individual
2. Growing and developing follow a predictable sequence, yet are unique for each individual
3. Protection and promotion of health are individual, community, and international responsibilities
4. The potential for hazards and accidents exists, whatever the environment
5. There are reciprocal relationships involving humans, disease, and the environment
6. The family serves to perpetuate humankind and to fulfill certain health needs
7. Personal health practices are affected by a complexity of forces, often conflicting
8. Utilization of health information, products, and services is guided by values and perceptions

9. Use of substances that modify mood and behavior arises from a variety of motivations
10. Food selection and eating patterns are determined by physical, social, mental, economic, and cultural factors

CORRELATION OF HEALTH AND OTHER SUBJECT AREAS

Reciprocal relationships exist between health and other curriculum areas in the high school, but are little used in unifying the student's learning experiences and knowledge. Health is a collective science that utilizes concepts, data, and materials from many sources. It is an applied discipline that devotes itself to human welfare and incorporates biological, psychological, social, economic, and physical aspects of human existence. Too frequently the health instructor does not adequately assist the student to see how knowledge in some other field is applied to health science. To point out such applications is to develop one of the fundamental characteristics of a well-educated person (i.e., the ability to see relationships).

Control of communicable disease is much better understood when the student has a grasp of the characteristics and function of disease-producing organisms. A study of the physiological basis of activity provides an understanding of the factors of exercise, fatigue, and rest. Social studies reveal the meaning of family relations and economic conditions in health terms. A foundation in nutrition and family life needs is obtained in home economics classes. A study of physical science provides the health field with the fundamentals of light and optics. Statistics permit meaningful presentations of ratios or relationships. The health instructor should help the students appreciate this use of knowledge from other areas of instruction.

Conversely, virtually all subject areas in the high school offer opportunities for incorporating health instruction into their classroom activities. To be aware of these opportunities and to utilize them, instructors in fields outside of health must have some preparation. Ideally this should be provided in the instructor's preparation for teaching, but it rarely is. In the absence of such background experience, in-service and postprofessional training should be provided. Administrative encouragement and health director leadership and assistance can make the necessary preparation possible.

The incorporation of health instruction into other subject areas is so important that Chapter 15 is devoted entirely to its treatment. If health is to be reflected in a young person's way of life, it should be a part of all possible aspects of school living. Such a school experience is most likely to provide the complete, unified health education that is the goal of all health instruction.

INTEGRATED AND INCIDENTAL HEALTH LEARNING

Incidental health learning is a by-product of various school experiences. The ability of the teacher to guide students in recognizing the health significance of the experience determines the degree of learning they derive from a given opportunity. Incidental health learning can result from accidents, student-teacher conferences, news reports, school and community incidents, and student questions on health. Incidental teaching should not be brushed off lightly. The question under consideration may be of deep concern to one or all of the students. It is imperative that any health question be pursued to a point at which the students will have a satisfactory grasp of the solution to the question.

Integrated health learning is functional learning. To gain health understanding from participation in the many school activities is to develop a type of ability for learning that should be invaluable in years to come. Persons who gain most from the various experiences of life are those with a mind-set that alerts them to the various implications of situations. They are able to gain insight into the operation of health phenomena in a diversity of experiences. Providing these opportunities for integrated health learning in school is half the task. The other half is to utilize these opportunities to the fullest. Health instructors are expected to make use of the health possibilities in any activity, but ideally all teachers should likewise be alert to the opportunities for health learning.

Some of the regular high school activities that provide possibilities for integrated health learning are assemblies, athletics, bulletin boards, proper illumination, lunchroom service, school newspaper, safety drives, student councils, example of teachers, ventilation, and the health council. This does not exhaust the possibilities. An alert health instructor can make a health learning experience out of almost any student activity.

ORGANIZING FOR HEALTH INSTRUCTION

It is an unusual senior high school today that does not offer classroom instruction in health. Some high schools offer health as an elective, but the present trend is to require one credit in health for graduation. In some instances this is a state requirement established by the state board of education or by statutory provision. However, many local school districts specify one or more credits in health as a requirement for graduation. This recognition of the importance of health instruction is in harmony with the present-day emphasis on a functional curriculum.

Occasionally health is included as a part of a larger core area. Completion of the work in the core area is thus recognized as meeting the health requirement for graduation. Health, which is taught as a phase of a larger area, can be taught effectively as an integrated learning experience. However, usually such instruction includes only a part of a total health education program. Emphasis may be given to one aspect of health while omitting other important areas. Social health may be developed fully, but physical health and even mental health may be given only cursory consideration. A balanced coverage of health topics must be presented if the health instruction program is to be considered adequate.

The separation of boys and girls for health instruction is gradually giving way to the more normal practice of assigning both boys and girls to the same class. When health is paired with physical education, boys and girls may be separated for health instruction. In some communities boys and girls are traditionally separated for health classes. However, for both legal and pedagogical rea-

sons, boys and girls should not be segregated for purposes of health instruction.

Health incorporated into biological science. Unification of health and biological science is entirely logical and could provide an excellent teaching situation for the instructor who is competent in both disciplines (Fig. 14-2). However, when such arrangements are made, the instructor may be well prepared for teaching biology but have little or no interest in teaching health or vice versa. An instructor interested in both fields and equally prepared can make the integrated offering an enrichment of both fields. Health provides for the application of fundamental biological principles, and, in turn, biological principles point up the why and how of health principles and practices.

If the two instructors plan and work together, separate courses of biological science

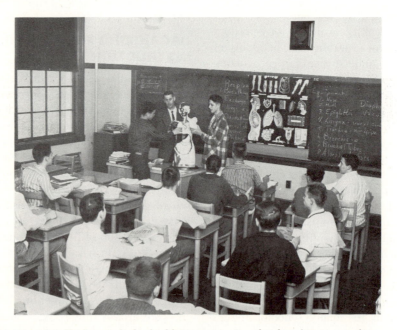

Fig. 14-2. Principles of biology applied to health instruction. Correlated teaching can result in more lasting learning.

and health can be coordinated and will virtually constitute an integrated offering. Such arrangements are not difficult and represent a widely accepted practice. The school should consider this arrangement unless an instructor who is capable of conducting the unified course is available.

Health alternated with physical education. In many high schools health instructors also teach physical education and the subjects are often paired when schedules are worked out. Available physical education facilities therefore affect the scheduling of health. It must thus be recognized that in some situations health class schedules must be adapted to physical education schedules.

One highly undesirable schedule plan is to alternate health and physical education daily. This is commonly referred to as the 3-2 plan and results in a dilution that makes health instruction a mere veneer. Surveys of entering college freshmen who have had high school health education reveal that those who have been on a 3-2 schedule score lowest as a group on standardized health knowledge tests. Even more significant, experience has shown that students taught on an alternating schedule tend to develop a dislike for health education. For these reasons, scheduling health instruction on an alternating plan with physical education is generally not recommended.

Health on a quarter-year basis. A fairly frequent practice is to schedule health for one quarter or a nine-week block of time in each of the 3 or 4 high school years. Usually physical education will be scheduled the other three quarters. Some physical education teachers object to this plan because students will have no physical education during an entire quarter. This objection is not serious unless the primary objective of physical education is to give the student a workout. Modern physical education is an instructional

program that is designed to develop skills, knowledge, and attitudes that will enable students to participate in physical activities and sports throughout their lifetimes. Although the physical fitness objective is important, it is a secondary objective, because one class period daily is not enough time to develop fitness per se.

The scheduling of health classes on a 9-week basis is acceptable, but not as satisfactory as utilizing a longer period of time. The 9-week period may effect too much segmentation. Although certain continuity is possible, some discontinuity is very likely to occur.

Full-year basis. Scheduling health in the junior or senior year on a full-year basis provides a concentrated study of health and permits the instructor to give proper time and emphasis to those health interests of most importance to the student. Since a full-year schedule is the usual pattern for traditional courses, offering health instruction for a full year is tacit recognition of health as a primary subject area.

Full-year scheduling of health does not necessitate a choice of either the junior or senior year as the preferred time. There are advantages to each. Instruction in the junior year permits application of learning for an additional year, and the health instructor is available for health counseling. In the senior year the added maturity and preparation for the years immediately ahead give added force and direction to health instruction.

Full semester in each of two years. Authoritative opinion generally supports the recommendation of the National Commission on School Policies that health be taught one semester in the ninth or tenth grade and another semester in the eleventh or twelfth grade. Experience indicates that three different combinations are satisfactory: ninth and eleventh grades, ninth and twelfth grades, or tenth and twelfth grades. Perhaps the combination of the first semester of the tenth grade and the last semester of the twelfth grade may have a slight advantage over other combinations.

Many advantages accrue from dividing health instruction between 2 years. The foundation laid down in the first semester will carry over into subsequent semesters and can give the student the awareness of health necessary for the fullest realization of health opportunities. The interim experience and maturation between the two semesters of health instruction produce a student who is more able to benefit fully from health instruction in the junior or senior year. Most important, as has been pointed out, the development of a confidential relationship between the teacher and student in the first semester provides a vehicle for health counseling throughout the high school life of the student. This is an important consideration for all students, but it is an invaluable service for students with serious health problems.

In the first semester of high school teaching, considerable emphasis should be given to the importance of health and the individual's responsibility for his or her own health. From this self-interest in health, a program of health promotion can be developed. Periodic evaluations and inventories complete the picture.

In the last semester of health instruction, reappraisal of the previous instructional semester and subsequent experience will lead directly to health needs and interests of deepest concern to the student. Student planning and participation are inevitable in such an approach.

TEACHER PREPARATION

Poor teaching in any field can be harmful to students, but incompetent teaching in the health field can actually be injurious. It would be better to cancel a scheduled health class

Table 14-1. Recommended health minor

Area	Hours
Personal health	3
Community health	3
Mental health	3
Family relationships	3
Nutrition	3
School health services	3
School health instruction	3
Safety education	3
First aid	3
TOTAL	27

than to turn it over to a person known to be incompetent to teach in the field. This is not to imply that only the great teachers of this generation should be entrusted with health instruction in the high school but that the necessary interest and preparation in health are essential. A recognized health teaching major or minor is acceptable as the initial preparation. The minor constitutes minimum preparation and should include at least 7 quarter-hours in the areas listed in Table 14-1.

Supporting preparation in biological science, social science, and psychology is usually an institutional requirement.

As more and more teaching candidates major in the health field, an increasing proportion of teachers come into the field with a major in the area of health. Others from related fields who have a health interest pursue a major in health on the graduate level. This is particularly true in states where a fifth year of study is required for a life certificate in teaching.

Selection of a group of courses constituting the best major in health is a difficult problem with many suggested solutions. It would be foolhardy to attempt to propose *the* curriculum for an undergraduate health major, but to propose *a* curriculum might be of some value as a guide (Table 14-2).

Table 14-2. Recommended curriculum for health major (by academic areas)

Subjects		Term hours
Humanities—social science		47
English composition	9	
Literature	9	
Speaking	3	
American government	3	
Sociology	3	
Anthropology	3	
Economics	3	
Philosophy	3	
Physical education	5	
General psychology	6	
Science		39
Physical science	12	
Biological science	12	
Human anatomy	6	
Human physiology	6	
Microbiology	3	
Education		24
Educational psychology	3	
Psychology of adolescence	3	
Special secondary methods in health	3	
Student teaching	12	
Seminar: student teaching	3	
Health		39
Introduction to health education	3	
Survey of health and health problems	3	
Nutrition	3	
School health services	3	
School health education	3	
First aid	3	
Safety education	3	
Communicable and chronic diseases	3	
Community health	3	
Sanitation	3	
Family relationships	3	
Health of the school-age child	3	
Driver education	3	
Electives		43
TOTAL		192

Most states require a fifth year of college preparation for life certification to teach in a recognized subject field in secondary schools. In any field the fifth year of preparation should supplement, intensify, and extend the baccalaureate program. Graduate study properly must be tailored to the candidate. This calls for some flexibility in the fifth-year program, and in no field is this more true than in health education.

It would be presumptuous to be specific in structuring a fifth-year curriculum, but some guidelines can be suggested. Depth in subject matter is an ever-present need in a field as broad and as rapidly developing as health. A logical corollary is further exploration into the understanding of students. All this must be cemented by an in-depth investigation of methods and techniques in health education.

Many delineations or classifications are possible, but the professional needs of the graduate student in health education can be classified simply into the areas of personal health, community health, and health education:

Personal health

Health and disease
Mental health
Nutrition
Physical growth and development
Genetics

Community health

Community health problems
Environmental health
Epidemiology

Health education

School health education
Sex education
Drug education
Guidance
Curriculum development in health
Evaluation in health
School health administration

No specific credit hours are suggested. Supporting work in cognate fields can fortify the candidate's professional preparation.

It must be emphasized that on-the-job professional growth and further formal study should strengthen and extend the qualifications of the health instructor. A considerable portion of the stimulation for growth will come from the students. Only an unresponsive instructor does not learn from students. Those who love the teaching profession most and thus are its severest critics regard such a person as unworthy of the teaching profession.

METHODS OF INSTRUCTION

Many teaching methods and combinations of methods are in use in high school health classrooms. Those best adapted to each specific problem or interest are the result of analysis, understanding of students, knowledge of the subject, and experience. Effective teaching requires adaptation, improvisation, and experimentation. The safe course is to use the methods that have proved consistently successful in past experience, but perhaps the instructor would be a better teacher, or at least a more interesting teacher, if he or she experimented with new procedures and techniques. Certainly there are many procedures adaptable to health instruction in the senior high school: surveys of health needs and interests, group discussions, buzz sessions, lecturettes, demonstrations, projects, field trips, reports, panel discussions, symposiums, sociodramas, textbook assignments, reference work, research, and audiovisual aids (including classroom and activity audiotape and videotape recordings). Group interests and needs are the hub of the instructional program. Student exploration and participation provide motivation and effective learning. This participation is particularly valuable when applied to student appraisal of progress. Establishing the practice of self-inventory or self-appraisal is especially important in the area of health.

Know Your Body (KYB) risk factor unit, level II

As explained in Chapter 13, the purpose of the *Know Your Body* (KYB) *Program* is to improve the health-related behavior of students. The program rests on the assumption that changing certain habits of living will reduce the possibility of later development of such health problems as heart disease, cancer, and strokes.

This instructional program is a direct outgrowth of the knowledge gained from major public health epidemiological research, such as the Framingham, Massachusetts, heart disease study. In such research, large groups of people are observed for a number of years, and data are collected on the incidence of a specific disease. By analyzing these data, it becomes possible to estimate an individual's risk of getting specific diseases. Although the science of this approach is not yet perfected, the preponderance of data collected suggests that taking steps such as reducing fat in the diet, reducing cigarette smoking, controlling hypertension, and increasing exercise will be beneficial to the individual's health.

The KYB *Program* is based on the beliefs that (1) many major health problems originate early in life and (2) it is much easier to change habits during the period of childhood and youth than in adulthood. Two hypotheses have guided the research on risk factors reduction. They are as follows:

1. Changing the prevalence of the risk factors associated with a particular disease (e.g., number of cigarette smokers among persons who have coronary heart disease) will reduce the incidence of the disease.

Text continued on p. 369.

RISK FACTORS—LEVEL II

Introduction

As discussed in Level I, extensive research studies have identified several factors as contributing to an increased risk in cardiovascular disease, cancer and other chronic illnesses.

In this unit, students will learn that certain risk factors are prevalent within families. Family members tend to have the same hereditary, as well as lifestyle patterns and thus often have similar risk factors.

Students will have the opportunity to gain an understanding of the relationship of their risk factors with the risk factors of other family members. They will be encouraged to identify family health behavior that contributes to family risk factors and describe ways that families can change their health behavior patterns to reduce their risk of developing chronic disease.

Present data indicate that the reduction of risk factors should be undertaken early in life in order to prevent the development of diseases later. It is easier to maintain patterns of behavior learned in the early years than it is to change old and ingrained habits. Students, therefore, will be encouraged to act as established role models in influencing family members to change health behavior patterns.

Continued.

Risk factor education, level II. The Know Your Body Disease Prevention Program. Further information may be obtained by writing The American Health Foundation, 1370 Avenue of the Americas, New York, N.Y. 10019. (Courtesy The American Health Foundation.)

LEVEL II—RISK FACTORS

UNIT GOALS:

Students become aware of the risk factors of all family members.

Students gain an understanding of the relationship between their risk factors and the risk factors of other family members.

Students learn ways to change family risk factor profiles.

CONCEPTS:

Research studies have identified certain risk factors that are prevalent within families.

Family members tend to have the same hereditary, as well as lifestyle patterns and thus, similar risk factors.

Once students have learned about their own risk factors and the risk factors of their family members, comparisons can be made.

Reducing the risk of chronic disease patterns in families often requires health behavior changes in all family members.

Risk factors can be changed more easily in younger family members than in adults.

OBJECTIVES:

Students will be able to:

— Define the terms "Family Risk Profile," "Fixed Risk Factor" and "Flexible Risk Factor."

— Identify what the risk factors are of all family members.

— Identify the health behavior habits that contribute to family risk factors.

— Describe ways that families can change health behavior patterns in order to reduce risk factors.

— Act as a role model in influencing family members to change health behavior patterns.

Risk factor education, level II. The Know Your Body Disease Prevention Program.

UNIT GOAL: Students become aware of the risk factors of all family members.

OBJECTIVE: Define the terms "Family Risk Profile," "Fixed Risk Factor" and "Flexible Risk Factor."

CONCEPT	SUGGESTED LEARNING ACTIVITY	RESOURCE
Research studies have identified certain risk factors that are prevalent within families.	Write the three risk factor terms on the blackboard. Ask students to identify the terms without looking at the definitions and chart. After students have done this, discuss the definitions with them. **Definitions are as follows:** *Family Risk Factor Profile*—An overview of a family's risk factors by using a chart to identify a set of factors which increase a person's chance of developing disease. *Fixed Risk Factor*—A risk factor that cannot be changed. *Flexible Risk Factor*—A risk factor that can be changed by modifying one's behavior or lifestyle. Have students look at the *Know Your Body Risk Score* and chart their own risk factors. (See Appendix 1) Have them discuss which risk factors they feel are most prevalent in their families.	Chart: *Know Your Body Risk Score* American Health Foundation

Risk factor education, level II. The Know Your Body Disease Prevention Program.

Continued.

UNIT GOAL: Students become aware of the risk factors of all family members.

OBJECTIVE: Identify what the risk factors are of all family members.

CONCEPT	SUGGESTED LEARNING ACTIVITY	RESOURCE
Family members tend to have the same hereditary, as well as lifestyle patterns and, thus, similar risk factors.	Ask students to look at the *Risk Factor Profile* published by the Santa Clara, California Heart Association for Adults. (See Appendix 2) Have them discuss some of the risk factors they might find within their families. Ask students to take copies of the *Risk Factor Profile* home and have their parent(s) and siblings fill out the profiles. (See Appendices 1 and 2) Have students summarize the findings from their families' risk factor profiles. **Suggestion for student summary:** Identify and research information on the most pronounced risk factor(s) within their family unit and report to class members what they learned.	Chart: *Adult Risk Factor Profile* Santa Clara Heart Association Article: Ball, Keith and Turner, Richard, "Realism in the Prevention of Coronary Heart Disease" <u>Preventive Medicine</u> December 1975 Article: Young, Patrick, "Predicting the Risk" <u>The National Observer</u> May 23, 1977

Risk factor education, level II. The Know Your Body Disease Prevention Program.

UNIT GOAL: Students gain an understanding of the relationship between their risk factors and the risk factors of other family members.

OBJECTIVE: Identify the health behavior habits that contribute to family risk factors.

CONCEPT	SUGGESTED LEARNING ACTIVITY	RESOURCE
Once students have learned about their own risk factors and the risk factors of their family members, comparisons can be made.	Have students fill out a Family Tree. (See Appendix 3) Have them identify which risk factors or diseases were prevalent in their family during past generations. Identify how many students can actually relate information about their families beyond parents or grandparents. Have students take home copies of the Family Tree and ask parents to fill in the missing information. Ask students to also identify what kind of lifestyle each generation lived. The following sample questions might be considered: — What kind of stress did past generations have? — What kind of diet did they eat? — What and how much did they smoke? — What kind of exercise did they do?	BOOKS: Berg, Alan, *The Nutrition Factor*, 1973 Tannahill, Reay, *Food in History*, 1973 Haenszel, William, *Tobacco Smoking Patterns in the U.S. 1880-1955,* U.S. Government Printing Office, 1956 Gottsegan, Jack, *Tobacco, a Study of Its Consumption in the U.S.*, 1940

Continued.

Risk factor education, level II. The Know Your Body Disease Prevention Program.

UNIT GOAL: Students learn ways to change family risk factor profiles.

OBJECTIVE: Describe ways that families can change health behavior patterns in order to reduce risk factors.

CONCEPT	SUGGESTED LEARNING ACTIVITY	RESOURCE
Reducing the risk of chronic disease patterns in families often requires health behavior changes in all family members.	Have students read some of the scientific research studies that focus on changing behavior patterns in order to reduce risk factor profiles. Divide students into five groups and have them research the following risk factors and the changes in one's lifestyle necessary to reduce the risk factors. • Blood pressure • Cigarette smoking • Obesity • Elevated cholesterol levels • Elevated glucose levels (diabetes) In addition, have them identify what other changes other than change in lifestyle or behavior may also be necessary in reducing the risk. For example: Taking medication is often necessary when a person has high blood pressure. After students have completed this activity, have them identify ways families in their community can change behavior patterns in order to reduce the risk factors mentioned in the previous activity.	ARTICLES: Wynder, Ernst L., "Nutrition and Cancer" Federation Proceedings May 1976 Podell, Richard N. et al., "Cardiovascular Nutrition Knowledge and Lipid Levels Among New Jersey High School Students" The Journal of the Medical Society of N.J. December 1975 (Reprint) Kotulak, Ronald, "The 'Good Life'—It Can Kill You" Chicago Tribune April 1976 Pomerleau, O. et al., "Role of Behavior Modification in Preventive Medicine" New England Journal of Medicine June 1975

Risk factor education, level II. The Know Your Body Disease Prevention Program.

UNIT GOAL: Students learn ways to change family risk factor profiles.

OBJECTIVE: Act as a role model in influencing family members to change health behavior patterns.

CONCEPT	SUGGESTED LEARNING ACTIVITY	RESOURCE
Risk factors can be changed more easily in younger family members than in adults.	A. Have students identify one risk factor out of the following that is prevalent in their family. ● Smoking of cigarettes ● Eating high fat, high caloric or high carbohydrate diets ● Obesity or overweight ● Lack of exercise ● High blood pressure B. Ask students to develop a strategy based upon motivating themselves to institute a change in their behavior that could influence the risk factor that they have identified. **Example:** The student is not at an ideal weight for his age/height. He eats many high fat/high caloric snacks at night time. This includes potato chips, fritos, ice cream and various types of pastries. The student identifies which of these snacks is highest in calories/fat and substitutes other less fattening snacks. He carefully looks at his behavior patterns and activities when indulging in these junk food items. Ask students to develop a similar strategy for other members in the family who may also be overweight.	ARTICLES: Williams, Christine and Wynder, Ernst L., "A Blind Spot in Preventive Medicine" Journal of American Medical Association November 8, 1976 Flaste, Richard, "Prevention of Heart Disease Can Start in Childhood" New York Times May 20, 1977 Pomerleau, O. et al., "Role of Behavior Modification in Preventive Medicine" New England Journal of Medicine June 1975 Publication: Atherosclerosis, MEDCOM, Inc., 1974 Pamphlet: You the Nutrition Expert, American Health Foundation, 1976

Continued.

Risk factor education, level II. The Know Your Body Disease Prevention Program.

APPENDIX 1

"KNOW YOUR BODY" RISK SCORE

PART I — FLEXIBLE SCORE

RISK FACTOR	0 POINTS	1 POINT	2 POINTS	
BLOOD CHOLESTEROL	139 mg% or less	140 — 179 mg%	180 mg% or greater	_____
CIGARETTE SMOKING	Never smoked	Smoked, but quit	Current smoker	_____
SYSTOLIC BLOOD PRESSURE (upper reading)	109 mmHg or lower	110 — 129 mmHg	130 mmHg or higher	_____
WEIGHT FOR HEIGHT	Underweight	Average weight	Overweight	_____
PHYSICAL FITNESS STEP TEST	132 or less	(133 — 149) (150 — 170)	(171 — 198) (199 or more)	

TOTAL — Flexible Score: _____

PART II — FIXED SCORE

RISK FACTOR	0 POINTS	1 POINT	2 POINTS	
HEREDITY (factors relating to parents, grandparents, parents' brothers and sisters)	Coronary Heart Disease (heart attack, angina— frequent chest pain) only in relatives over age 60	Coronary Heart Disease in relatives aged 50 to 59	Coronary Heart Disease in relatives under age 50	_____
SEX	Female	Male		_____

TOTAL — Fixed Score: _____

Add your Flexible Score from above: _____

TOTAL "KNOW YOUR BODY" RISK SCORE: _____

(c) 1976—American Health Foundation
Adapted for children ages 10 — 15

Risk factor education, level II. The Know Your Body Disease Prevention Program.

APPENDIX 2

*RISK-FACTOR PROFILE

SEX

If you're a man, give yourself one point. Before the age of 60, the average man has a higher risk of heart attack than the average woman.   (   )

AGE

If you're over 35, give yourself one point. The older you are, the greater your risk.   (   )

FAMILY

Give yourself one point if a member of your immediate family died of a heart attack before retirement age.   (   )

CHOLESTEROL

An average person eats five whole eggs a week, organ meats once a month and red meat almost every day. If you eat about the average amount of foods high in cholesterol give yourself one point. More? Two points. Substantially less? No points.   (   )

HIGH-FAT FOODS

The average person eats:
- sausage or bacon once per week
- lunch meats or cold cuts 3-5 times per week
- whole milk, cheese and ice cream 3-5 times per week
- deep-fat fried foods (french fries, doughnuts) 3-5 times per week
- butter, lard, shortenings and margarines made with hydrogenated oils 3-5 times per week

If you eat any or all of these foods, you are average. Give yourself one point; two if above average. No points if you eat non-fat or low-fat dairy products and restrict your consumption of high-fat foods.   (   )

SALT AND HIGH-BLOOD PRESSURE

If you know that your blood pressure is higher than it should be or if you use a lot of salt . . . take one point.   (   )

SUGAR

If you sugar your coffee, eat candy, or lots of sweets you can raise your level of triglycerides and you should take one point.   (   )

SMOKING

Give yourself one point for each half pack of cigarettes you smoke each day.   (   )

Continued.

Risk factor education, level II. The Know Your Body Disease Prevention Program.

RISK-FACTOR PROFILE (Cont.)

EXERCISE

If you get no real exercise . . . two points. Some . . . one point. No points if you exercise thoroughly at least three times a week. ( )

WEIGHT

If you are more than 10 pounds overweight . . . two points. Between 5 and 10 pounds over . . . one point. ( )

TENSION

One point if your life is constantly full of deadlines and time pressures. ( )

Total Score ( )

*Adapted from Santa Clara County Heart Association San Jose, California.

OK. ADD THEM UP

A score of 4 or less means a very low risk. Only about 5 out of 100 people in this group will suffer heart attacks before the age of 65.

5-7. Slightly below average. There is room for change.

8-10. Average risk. Too high for comfort. 20 out of 100 average men suffer heart attacks in middle age.

11-13. High risk. Make some changes in your lifestyle. Like today. If possible, get a medical checkup so that you can find out what your cholesterol level, triglyceride level and blood pressure are.

Over 14. One person out of every two in this group is likely to have a heart attack before the age of 65.

Risk factor education, level II. The Know Your Body Disease Prevention Program.

APPENDIX 3

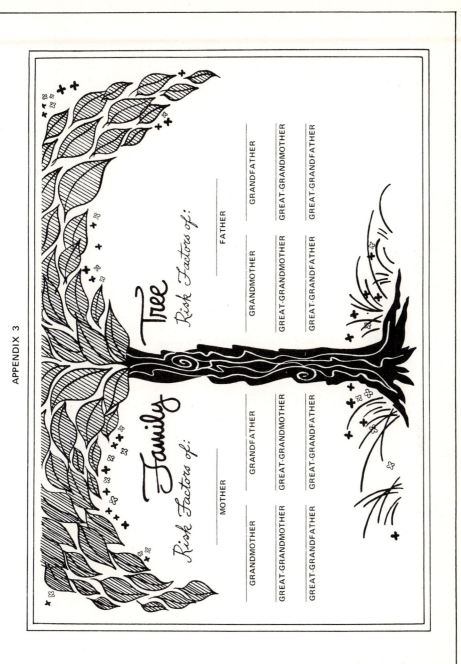

Family Tree

Risk Factors of:

MOTHER
_____

GRANDMOTHER

GREAT-GRANDMOTHER

GREAT-GRANDFATHER

GRANDFATHER

GREAT-GRANDMOTHER

GREAT-GRANDFATHER

Risk Factors of:

FATHER
_____

GRANDMOTHER

GREAT-GRANDMOTHER

GREAT-GRANDFATHER

GRANDFATHER

GREAT-GRANDMOTHER

GREAT-GRANDFATHER

Continued.

Risk factor education, level II. The Know Your Body Disease Prevention Program.

RISK FACTOR BIBLIOGRAPHY — LEVEL II

Books

Berg, Alan
The Nutrition Factor
The Brookings Institution, Washington, D.C., 1973

Gottesegen, Jack J.
Tobacco, A Study of Its Consumption in the United States
Pitman Publishing Corporation, New York, N.Y., 1940

Haenszel, William
Tobacco Smoking Patterns in the U.S., 1880-1955
Public Health Monograph No. 45
U.S. Government Printing Office, Washington, D.C., 1956

Tannahill, Reay
Food In History
Stein and Day, New York, N.Y., 1973

Charts

American Health Foundation
Know Your Body Risk Score
American Health Foundation, New York, N.Y., 1977

Santa Clara Heart Association
Adult Risk Factor Profile
Santa Clara, California Heart Association

Newspapers

Flaste, Richard, "Prevention of Heart Disease Can Start in Childhood,"
New York Times, May 20, 1977

Kotulak, Ronald, "The 'Good Life' It Can Kill You," *Chicago Tribune,*
April, 1976

Young, Patrick, "Predicting the Risk," *The National Observer,* May 23,
1977

Pamphlet

American Health Foundation
You,The Nutrition Expert
American Health Foundation, New York, N.Y., 1976

Periodicals

Ball, Keith and Turner, Richard, "Realism in the Prevention of
Coronary Heart Disease," *Preventive Medicine,* 4, 390-397, December, 1975.

Podell, Richard N., et al, "Cardiovascular Nutrition Knowledge and
Lipid Levels Among New Jersey High School Students," *The Journal
of the Medical Society of N.J.,* 72, 1027-1031, December, 1975.

Pomerleau, O., et al, "Role of Behavior Modification in Preventive
Medicine," *New England Journal of Medicine,* 292 (24), 1277-
1281, June, 1975.

Williams, Christine, Wynder, Ernst L., "A Blind Spot In Preventive
Medicine," *Journal of American Medical Association,* 236 (19),
2196-2197, November 8, 1976.

Wynder, Ernst L., "Nutrition and Cancer," *Federation Proceedings,*
35, 1309-1315, May 1976.

Publications

Medcom Learning Systems, *Atherosclerosis,* Publication No. WG 300
M 489a, New York, N.Y., 1974.

Risk factor education, level II. The Know Your Body Disease Prevention Program.

2. Informing individuals about their own risk of getting a particular disease will lead them to take actions (health-related behavior) that they believe will reduce their risk of getting the disease.

This latter hypothesis has been tested in a number of experimental studies conducted in schools. This approach involves three phases: (1) administering a number of screening tests, such as blood lipid measurement (amount of fat in the blood) to students; (2) providing results of this screening to the students, their parents, and their physicians; and (3) offering school health instruction such as KYB Risk Factor Unit, Level II, to help students develop new habits and more healthful patterns of living.

Physical and emotional growth issues and interpersonal relationships

A UNIT FOR HEALTH EDUCATION*

By: Tom Higgins and Candy Purdy

INTRODUCTION

As health educators at Maine Township South Senior High School, we were growing more concerned every year with the increasing apathy among our freshmen and sophomore students toward "drug-abuse" educa-

---

*This unit was developed by the Health Education Department faculty of Maine Township High School South in Park Ridge, Illinois. It was included as a part of the health instruction program during the school year 1974-1975. The form of the unit as presented here includes an introduction and a content outline, which is keyed to a list of teaching and learning activities. Other teachers wishing to make use of the unit will have to develop their own instructional objectives as well as educational materials and resources.

tion. It seemed that part of the problem was that we were separating drug use and abuse from other aspects of our curriculum in Health Education when we knew it was related to Mental Health and Sex Education or Family Living.

Consequently, the following teaching outline combines three units—Mental Health, Sex Education, and Drug Education. In this unit we attempt to discuss various aspects of drugs, mental health, and sexuality in what seems to us to be a logical progression.

Since the origin of the Health Education Department in our school in 1969, we have noted that students have had questions about alcohol while we were talking about dating or questions about psychosis when we were discussing LSD and we would find ourselves saying, "Wait until we get to our next unit." This new combined unit is written with these questions and the timing of these questions in mind.

We would like to stress the fact that the order of presentation is not inflexible. Nor do we suggest that it is the only possible order. We simply wanted to construct an outline that would allow for better discussion of physical and emotional problems our students are likely to face. It also permits more value clarification and discussion-type teaching.

The main limitation of a large unit like this one is coordination of films, but this is an organizational problem and can definitely be worked out. We feel the student interest that will be created will far outweigh the small organizational problems.

PERSONALITY DEVELOPMENT

A. Human needs
   1. What are man's physiological needs?
     a. Oxygen
     b. Food and water
     c. Sleep
     d. Activity
     e. Sex
     f. Shelter

2. What are some of the emotional and cultural needs of man?
   a. Belonging
   b. Success (1)
   c. Love
   d. Goal accomplishment
   e. Problem solving
   f. Self-esteem
3. Is delaying gratification of needs a sign of maturity?

B. Role development
   1. What is the age of earliest development?
   2. What are some of the contributing factors to role developments? (2)
   3. What are the psychosexual phases of development?
      a. Oral
      b. Anal
      c. Oedipal
      d. Latency
      e. Puberty
      f. Adolescence
   4. What were some role changes that occurred between 1800 and the present?
      a. Male behavior past and present
      b. Female behavior past and present (3)

C. Women's liberation
   1. What is women's liberation?
   2. What is the basis for argument? (4)
   3. Does women's liberation cause role confusion?
   4. What is the effect of the movement on male ego? (5)
   5. Is dominance a recipe for success?

D. Psychosexual differences
   1. Are psychosexual differences inherited or learned? (6)
   2. What would be the result of crossing-over in talent or behavior between male and female?

E. Personality structure
   1. What are Freud's theories of personality—id, ego, and superego? (7)
   2. What is transactional analysis and how is it used today?
   3. What is the effect of nurture and nature on personality?
   4. What is normal personality?
      a. Who is to judge what is normal?
      b. What is normal . . .
         (1) Background
         (2) Interests
         (3) Ability
         (4) Attitudes
         (5) Behavior
         (6) Intelligence

F. Emotional growth
   1. What accompanies normal social and physical growth?
   2. What are some milestones in emotional growth?
      a. The child's ability to withstand a separation from parents
      b. The child's ability to emotionally accept social setbacks such as group rejection, discipline, competition, and grades
   3. What emotional growth problems occur when the body develops ahead of the emotions?

G. Intellectual differences
   1. What is the use of the EEG?
      a. Reveals electrical energy from the brain
      b. Used to study sleeping and waking and epileptics
   2. What are the functions of the forebrain, midbrain, and hindbrain?
   3. Why does the brain need 24% of the total oxygen supply?
   4. What are the three basics of intelligence and learning?
      a. Registration
      b. Retention
      c. Retrieval
   5. What may determine one's occupation? (8)
      a. Intelligence
      b. Culture
      c. Education
      d. Religion
      e. Environment

H. Ordinary stress on the personality
   1. What is ordinary stress?
      a. Anything that pushes the body to its limit within normal activity
      b. May be pleasant or unpleasant, but the important thing is the intensity
   2. What is short-term stress?
      a. Brief startle reaction
      b. Beginning of startle reflexes
   3. What is chronic stress?
      a. A sustained series of shocks
      b. Psychological pressures of a marital, economic, or occupational nature
   4. What are some controversies about stress and its effects? (9)

I. Death as a cause of grief and a stress to man (10)
   1. What may be the reactions to the concept of one's own death?
      a. Recognize need to learn to feel comfortable with our own death
      b. Encourage children to discuss death early in life (11)
      c. Recognize the importance of living fully

2. What are the stages experienced by those dying of long illness and those experiencing the death of a loved one?
   a. Stage I—denial
      (1) Characterized by the statement, "Not me."
      (2) Individual may shop for a new physician who gives more hope
      (3) Individual tries to gain time to adjust to the shock
      (4) Suggested reaction to this stage is to avoid criticism or contradiction of their hopes
   b. Stage II—anger
      (1) Rage, envy, and resentment may be directed toward those closest
      (2) Worry about being forgotten
      (3) Individual often asks, "Why me?"
      (4) Suggested reaction to this stage is to help the person feel needed and allow him or her to make his or her own decision
   c. Stage III—bargaining
      (1) Individual operates on the idea, "If I'm good I'll get more time."
      (2) Individual may postpone treatment and make deals to go home
      (3) Sometimes stems from feelings of guilt or fear
      (4) Suggested reaction to this stage is to encourage the person to talk out fears
   d. Stage IV—depression
      (1) A sense of loss develops stemming from loss of appearance, weight, job, or a body part
      (2) A preparatory depression may develop sensing the loss of life and loved ones
      (3) This stage is often characterized by silence
      (4) Suggested reaction is to avoid trying to cheer them or to insist on constant talk, decrease visits
   e. Stage V—acceptance
      (1) A stage characterized by an absence of feeling
      (2) Person often desires to be alone
      (3) This stage is an acceptance of death; not because it is desired but because it is unavoidable
      (4) Suggested reactions are to allow silence, visit in the evenings, and not interpret this stage as rejection
3. What are the controversies concerning death?
   a. When does death occur?
      (1) Medical death
      (2) Biological death
      (3) Theological death
      (4) Legal death
      (5) Clinical death
   b. Death with dignity
   c. Euthanasia

J. Dealing with various types of stress effectively
   1. Should we flee, fight, or compromise? (**12**)
   2. What are some ego defense mechanisms used in times of stress?
      a. Compensation
      b. Conversion
      c. Denial
      d. Fantasy
      e. Identification
      f. Negativism
      g. Projection
      h. Rationalization
      i. Regression
      j. Substitution
      k. Sublimation
   3. How can we handle everyday stresses? (**13**)
      a. Balance work with play
      b. Try to avoid persistently taking on too much work
      c. Avoid excessive use of drugs of any kind
      d. Sidestep obvious stressful situations
      e. Keep changes to a minimum
      f. Loaf a little
      g. Get enough rest
      h. Physically work off tension (sports)
      i. Cultivate a hobby or pastime
      j. Be frank and open in discussing personal problems with members of your family
      k. Accept your limitations
      l. Seek psychological help if needed
      m. Learn to accept what you cannot change
      n. Avoid self-medication
      o. Have regular physical checkups
   4. What are some acceptable drug uses?
      a. Prescribed antidepressant drugs
      b. Social use of alcohol (**14**)
      c. Acceptable as defined by drug users
K. Ineffective reactions to stress
   1. What are some drugs that are used to combat teen stress and boredom?
      a. Alcohol
      b. Hallucinogens
      c. Stimulants
      d. Depressants
      e. Narcotics
      f. PCP
      g. Bonamine
   2. How do postteen stresses create alcoholic behavior?
      a. Early stages

b. Middle stages

c. Late stages

3. Does dealing with stress by drug use teach a person to deal with stress in constructive ways?

a. Legal use of antidepressants

b. Drugs affect the symptom, producing stress; it is not the situation that causes stress

c. Drugs' effect on one's self-concept

THE TROUBLED PERSONALITY

A. Role confusion

1. What may be the effect of an absent parent on the child?

a. The busy father and/or mother

b. The divorced family

2. What are the effects of traumatic shock?

3. What are some misleading roles in advertising, TV, and the printed media?

4. What may be the effect of parents wanting a child of another sex?

5. What are transexual changes (surgery and hormone therapy)?

6. What is homosexuality and is it physically or emotionally caused?

a. Identification in society

b. Changing views toward homosexuality (15)

c. Future trends in the incidence of homosexuality

7. What are some forms of sexual deviation? (16)

a. What is normal sexual behavior?

b. Laws regarding sexual behavior

c. Zoophilia

d. Bestiality

e. Voyeurism

f. Exhibitionism

g. Pedophilia

h. Fetishism

i. Sadism

j. Masochism

k. Incest

8. What are the causes and consequences of rape?

a. Severe emotional reactions of the female after rape

b. Legal aspects of rape (17)

c. The psychology of rape

d. Avoidance of rape

e. Procedure for reporting rape

B. Neurosis

1. How is neurosis defined?

2. What are obsessive-compulsive acts?

3. What is a depression reaction?

4. What is hysteria?

5. What are phobias?

a. Causes of phobias (18)

b. How phobias differ from fears (19)

c. Desensitization as a treatment of phobia

6. How do we view psychosomatic illnesses?

7. How serious is depression?

a. Defined as a serious, debilitating, and deep bout of gloom

b. For every man that seeks treatment for depression, three to four women do (20)

c. Balanced life is suggested as a preventive

d. Mood-elevating drugs are used as a treatment

8. What are some causes of suicide?

a. Suicide is the third most common cause of death of teens between 15 and 19 years of age; most common causes are cancer and accidents (21)

b. Suicides are not impulsive

c. Suicide people are not fully intent on dying (22)

d. People are not suicidal for life

e. Improvement does not necessarily mean the risk has passed

f. Suicide occurs among people of all economic and occupational classes

g. Suicidal tendencies are not inherited

h. Suicide often follows a double stress

C. Treatment of neurosis

1. Why does the family physician treat 99% of all neuroses?

2. How does medicine use antidepressant drugs?

INTERPERSONAL RELATIONSHIPS

A. Communication—a key to mental health

1. What is nonverbal communication?

a. Body language

b. Clothing styles

c. Parent-child nonverbal communication

d. Male-female nonverbal communication

e. Media communications of a nonverbal type

2. What are the purposes of verbal communication?

a. Needed for mental health

b. Societal limitations

c. Overcoming shyness

d. Indirect and direct communication

3. What are two types of sexual communication?

a. Nonverbal predominates early in a relationship (23)

b. Verbal later is less difficult and predominates (24)

4. What are some stages of family communications? (25)

a. Stages of parent-child relationship that create stress

  (1) Difficulty of parents "letting go"
  (2) Freedoms and responsibilities involve discipline and two-way respect
  (3) Major points of conflict in adolescence
  (4) Parental favoritism
  (5) Working out compromises
  b. Changing family communication
  (1) Use of transactional analysis
  (2) Opening lines of communication (**26**)

B. Dating
  1. When does interest in the opposite sex develop?
  2. What are some purposes of dating?
  3. How do students define sexual attractiveness? (**27**)
  4. What are some dating customs and expectations?
  5. Where to go and what to do?
  6. What are some advantages and disadvantages of going "steady?"
  7. How do people achieve popularity?
  8. What are some dating problems and how might they be solved? (**28**)

C. Drugs and sexual behavior
  1. What is the effect of alcohol on inhibitions? (**29**)
  2. What effect do depressants have on sexual responsiveness?
  3. What is the history of aphrodisiacs and how effective are they?
  4. What effect has the birth control pill had on sexual behavior?
  5. What is the relationship between drugs and sexual potency? (**30**)
  a. Alcohol
  b. Marihuana

D. The progression of sexual feelings
  1. How does puberty change sexual interest? (**31**)
  2. What is the physical progression of sexual feelings? (**32**)

E. Premarital sexual behavior and nonmarital sexual behavior
  1. What are society's four standards of sexual behavior?
  a. Abstinence
  b. Permissiveness with affection (emotional readiness)
  c. Double standard
  d. Permissiveness without affection and its affect on personality and reputation
  2. What is the relationship between love and premarital behavior? (**33**)
  3. How can sexual exploitation be recognized?
  4. What are some effects of premarital pregnancy? (**34**)
  a. Effect on female's mental health
  b. Effect on male's mental health
  c. Effect on family relationships

  d. Choices
  (1) Offer the child for adoption
  (2) Marriage with or without love
  (3) Keep the child
  (4) Abortion
  e. Effect on future relationships
  (1) Future husband's view of wife's previous experience
  (2) Dealing with guilt feelings
  f. Venereal disease (**35**)
  (1) Prevalence among promiscuous
  (2) Review effect on reproductive systems
  (3) Social effects and laws regarding treatment
  (4) Importance of naming contacts

F. Mate selection
  1. What are a few characteristics of mate selection?
  a. Background, economic similarities, social strata, family relationships, likes and dislikes, religious beliefs, values, in-laws, preferred family size (**36**)
  b. Emotional and economic readiness for marriage (**37**)
  2. How does one distinguish between infatuation and love? (**38**)

G. Marriage
  1. Are there societal pressures to marry?
  2. What are a few unsuccessful reasons to marry?
  a. Escape from home
  b. Sexual attraction
  c. As a utopia
  d. Because others are marrying
  3. Marriage and love—how are they related?
  4. What are the pros and cons of marriage and living together? (**39**)
  5. Is successful marriage a give-and-take arrangement? (**40**)

H. Genetics
  1. What can be accomplished through genetic counseling?
  a. Prediction of birth problems
  b. Prediction of birth defects
  2. What is new in genetic research?
  a. Extrauterine fertilization "test-tube baby"
  b. Cloning
  c. Genetic reconstruction
  d. Sperm banks and artificial insemination (**41**)
  e. Legal and moral implications of genetic research

THE FAMILY

A. Review of the male and female reproductive systems (**42**)
B. Family planning (**43**)

1. What is a definition of family planning? (**44**)
2. What are some of the historical attempts at family planning?
3. What are some of the basic purposes of contraception?
   a. Aid sexual adjustment to marriage
   b. To space pregnancies
   c. To limit family size for economic reasons
   d. To avoid aggravation of an existing disease
   e. To prevent perpetuation of inherited disorders
4. What are some of the types of contraceptives in order of effectiveness?
   a. Oral contraceptives
   b. IUD
   c. Diaphragm
   d. Cervical cap with gel
   e. Condom
   f. Chemical spermicides
   g. Coitus interruptus
   h. Rhythm
   i. Douche
5. What are some possible dangers of oral contraceptives?
6. What are some of the moral aspects of contraception?
7. What place does abortion have in controlling family size?
   a. Definition and history of abortion
   b. Therapeutic methods of abortion
      (1) X-ray
      (2) Laminaria
      (3) Dilatation and curettage
      (4) Salt injection
      (5) Menstrual aspiration
      (6) Prostaglandins
   c. Possible physical dangers of abortion to mother
      (1) Danger during twelfth to sixteenth week and after sixteen weeks
      (2) Difficulty in having children later
      (3) Increase in prematurity rate
      (4) Stillbirth increase
      (5) Ectopic pregnancy increase
      (6) Hemorrhage and infection
   d. Legal aspects of abortion
      (1) Current federal law
      (2) Current state law
8. What is the use and success rate of fertility medications?
C. The troubled marriage (**45**)
   1. What are the most common causes of troubled marriage?

   a. Money, children, in-laws, unfaithfulness, increasing job demands, sexual problems, boredom, guilt feelings, alcohol (**46**)
   b. Drug abuse within the family (**47**)
      (1) Effects of an alcoholic parent (**48**)
      (2) Effects of a child abusing drugs (**49, 50**)
      (3) Treatments for drug abuse (**51**)
2. Why are people motivated to abuse children?
3. What are some problems and options in unwanted pregnancies in a marriage?
   a. The option of abortion (**52**)
   b. Offering the child for adoption
   c. Keeping the child
      (1) The unwanted child
      (2) Psychological effects of an unwanted child on a marriage
4. What are some causes and effects of divorce?
   a. Legal grounds for divorce
   b. Current divorce rate
   c. Effect of divorce on children

SEVERE PERSONALITY DISORDERS

A. Psychosis—detachment from reality
   1. What is the difference between neurosis and psychosis?
   2. What are the three major types of psychosis?
      a. Schizophrenia (**53**)
      b. Manic-depressive
      c. Paranoia
   3. What are some of the causes of psychosis? (**54**)
      a. Faulty personality development
      b. Inadequate self-concept
      c. Traumatic experience
      d. Chemical imbalance (possibly hereditary)
   4. How can the effects of drugs be explained by neuroanatomy?
      a. Drug-induced psychosis and its relation to nondrug-induced psychosis
      b. Amphetamine psychosis compared to paranoia
      c. Alcohol psychosis and delirium tremens
      d. LSD and schizophrenic behavior
      e. Drug-related suicides
   5. How is mental illness of a psychotic nature treated today?
      a. Psychiatry and psychology
      b. Group therapy
      c. Psychoanalysis
      d. Drug therapy
      e. Mental health services in the community
      f. Hypnosis
      g. Hospitalization

METHODOLOGY

The methodology is coordinated with the outline. The numbers in parentheses located to the right of the outline indicate that information that may assist in teaching is included in the methodology under that number.

1. Ask students what reactions constant failure may cause in someone 5 years old and then in someone 16 years old.

2. Bring in some ads from magazines that appear to teach sexual roles and have some affect on our concept of male and female.

3. Prepare a list of various jobs and activities such as cooking, sports, medicine, etc., then have students rate them 1 thru 10, 1 being masculine and 10 being feminine. Discuss why these decisions were made. Was it on the basis of a need for physical strength or a culturally influenced decision?

4. Have the class list what they feel are legitimate "gripes" women have in regard to women's liberation.

5. Have the class prepare a list of things from which men need to be liberated.

6. A few psychosexual differences that could be discussed are:

Males	Females
Mature slower	Mature early
Adjust to change slowly	Adjust to change quickly
Work better with things than people	Work better with people than things
Are greater risktakers	Take fewer risks
Have few emotional outlets	Make use of many emotional outlets
Fail to seek medical care	Seek medical care regularly
Are restless sleepers	Sleep soundly
Tend to be overweight	Are more weight conscious
Have poor resistance to disease	Are more resistant to disease
Have shorter life span	Have longer life span

7. List four emotions on the board and ask students to choose one they have experienced and write a short essay about the incident. They should then try to decide what ruled their reaction in this situation.

8. Ask students whether they feel it would help or hurt mankind if parents were able to choose their child's I.Q.

9. Some possible controversies in regard to stress would be:

Do you inherit a tendency to suffer from stress?

Can you suffer from stress and not know it?

Does stress affect sleep?

Is stress contagious?

Does stress affect one's sex life?

10. Discuss Dr. Thomas Holmes' scale below, which assigns points to changes that cause stress. If over 300 points are accumulated within one year, depression may result. Have students analyze this chart in regard to their family life.

Life change	Points
Death of spouse	100
Divorce	73
Marital separation	65
Death of close family member	63
Personal injury or illness	53
Marriage	50
Fired from job	47
Retirement	45
Change in health of family member	44
Change in financial status	38
Death of close friend	37
Change in work responsibilities	29
Son or daughter leaving home	29
Wife beginning or stopping work	26
Trouble with boss	23
Change in schools	20
Vacation	13
Minor violations of the law	11

Note the number of stresses associated with death.

11. Ask students how death was explained to them as a child. How do they think it should have been explained?

12. Write out five situations involving stress. Have each student list what they would do and why. Then decide if they used an ego defense, fight, flight, or compromise.

13. Set up and discuss some everyday stresses in the life of a high school student and choose from the list the better possible responses.

14. Set up about ten situations where alcohol might be used. Then have the students rate each situation 1 through 10, 1 being acceptable and 10 being unacceptable. This will tell you how the students view drinking habits. Take note of their view of mood-change drinking, a prologue to alcoholism.

15. Ask students, "If you were the head of a company that sold used cars, and a prospective salesman applied for a job but admitted he was a homosexual, would you (a) hire him without any thought, (b) hire him but be reluctant, or (c) not hire him?"

16. Try using antagonistic statements to begin a discussion.

"Two consenting adults should be able to do anything sexually provided it is in privacy."

"We would be better off if we had total unisex—no distinction except childbearing, between the sexes."

17. What laws might be passed that may help cut down on rapes, or is rape the type of occurrence that is not solved by laws?

18. Give examples of parents' behavior toward children and explain how it might cause neurosis in the child.

19. Prepare a list of things people often fear, and poll the class to see which is most common. Then see if students know where they learned the fear.

20. It has been estimated in 1974 that about 125,000 Americans suffering from depression enter hospitals every year. Another 200,000 undergo treatment in outpatient clinics and another 4 million need psychiatric assistance. Refer to methodology number 10 and ask the class if these numbers could be reduced by stressing positive lifestyles.

21. In 1974 a Russian physician came out with a theory that chronic strain of everyday life is "overloading" the human brain. Of the 50,000 Americans who commit suicide every year, half are known to have suffered from depression. Ask students if they feel more time should be spent in school on learning how to "cope" and handle stress.

22. Pose this question to the class: "If someone comes to you and says they have given it a lot of thought and they want to commit suicide, should you stop them? Do they have the right to do what they want to do with their lives as long as they don't affect others?"

23. Have the class list the progression of a typical boy-girl relationship as to whether verbal or nonverbal communication predominates. Start with the first time the two meet at a concert or in a class together.

24. Role play some different types of nonverbal signals. For example, have a shy boy meet a girl for the first time but do not allow the actors to speak and see if the class can interpret their feelings.

25. Have each student write out one family problem. Then discuss a few of the problems in class or have other students write suggestions for solutions. The entire exercise can be done without names, but students benefit from hearing more than one way to solve their difficulties. The same thing can be done for dating problems.

26. Ask students who they bring most of their problems to at home and why they choose that person. If they do not discuss their problems at home, who do they discuss them with? Let students decide if discussing problems is a good idea in terms of mental health.

27. Prepare a dating questionnaire to be given to all students. Students should each write one question they would like to see on a questionnaire for students of the opposite sex. These questions may deal with physical attractiveness, the date itself, the physical relationship, or opinions on matters related to dating. Students submit questions in writing so that the teacher may organize the questionnaire and delete questions that are inappropriate. Then the questionnaires are typed (one for males and one for females) and each student fills one out. They do not have to include their names. Students may then tabulate the questionnaires and this serves as an excellent way to discuss current dating practices.

28. Discuss situations that students have had on a date that they found were hard to handle. These may be submitted on paper and then read in class so that many possible alternatives can be mentioned.

29. Discuss the meaning of the statement: "Candy is dandy but liquor is quicker."

30. Obtain statistics on the number of unwanted pregnancies that occurred when one or both people had consumed alcohol. Ask students why this occurs.

31. Discuss difficulties that arise during adolescence with the strong physical sex drive that could lead to emotional instability.

32. Discuss the following statements: "Petting is just a natural part of a date. If a couple doesn't pet, it shows that they are not really interested in each other." "Sure my boyfriend and I pet but we'll always stop before sexual intercourse."

33. Discuss whether two people could love each other without touching.

34. Have a few students write examples of relationships where premarital sex could take place. Then have students discuss the effects and the reasons why the relationship could run into difficulty.

35. Group the class into groups of five or six students each. Then tell them that they have

been granted the power to set up a plan for eliminating all venereal disease from the world. They may have any professional help or supplies now available to accomplish this task. Have each group set up a plan for stopping VD.

36. Have each student list on paper the characteristics they would look for and want their future spouse to have. Discuss which characteristics appear the most often and why.

37. Have the class debate whether sexual compatibility should be a criterion for selecting a mate. Compare this to whether the ability to shoot a basketball at age 7 years should be a criterion for whether the child will be a good basketball player at 16. The relationship between the two is that compatibility develops over a period of time.

38. Have students list the things in their background that they feel would influence their success in marriage. These things are the ones they should check out in selecting a mate.

39. Choose a panel of students to discuss the advantages of marriage and the advantages of living together. This could also be done in the form of a debate. Be sure children are considered.

40. To follow up the panel in the previous question, have the class get the groups and write their own laws governing male-female relationships in the United States. They may start fresh or revise the present system.

41. Discuss the following statement: "Soon sexual intercourse will be unnecessary because sperm banks and test-tube babies will be available. This is good because it lessens the chance of birth defects and VD."

42. Prepare some 3 × 5 cards with the names of various parts of the reproductive systems on them. Hand the cards out to students in the room. Tell them that if they think they have a part of the male system to sit on the right side of the room and if female on the left. Start with the female system and draw the parts on the board by having each student with a card come up and add a part. The same should be done with the male system.

43. Since this section of the unit may be new to some students and somewhat emotion-laden, provide a question box and instruct every student to write a question dealing with reproduction on a piece of paper and place it in the box as it comes around the room. Those students who have no question should put paper in the box as well so nobody will know whose question will be answered the following class period.

44. Be sure to check into your district's written policy as to what material may and may not be discussed during this unit. An approval list of audiovisual materials may also be available and should be consulted prior to teaching this unit.

45. Discussion question: "Of those married people that you know who are not getting along or who are divorced, do you think the divorce could have been avoided by picking a mate more wisely or by concentrating more on working out marriage disagreements?"

46. Discuss the effect of children on a husband-wife relationship. When might children enhance a marriage and when might they destroy it?

47. Ask students whether they feel alcoholism can be predicted by knowing a personality type.

48. Where can teens go if they have an alcoholic parent in your community? Make this information available to students.

49. Ask students whether they think parents should teach young people not to drink or how to drink. What do they plan to do when they become parents and their children are old enough to become interested in drinking?

50. Role play situations such as:
A parent confronting a child about pills in his or her room
A sister who knows her brother is abusing drugs and is afraid he might overdose

51. Discuss the progression from social drinker to alcoholic. Point out some of the milestones along the way and what might be done at those points to halt the progression. Mention various treatments for alcoholism such as Antabuse, Alateen, Alanon, and psychotherapy.

52. Have students discuss:
"Who should decide what happens to a child or whether an abortion should occur if the girl is 15 years old?"
"What if the woman is 20 years old and unmarried?"
"What if the woman is 35 years old and married?"

53. When describing manic-depressive psychosis, construct a pendulum to explain the shifts in mood. The pendulum is at one side or the other but fails to stop in between as it does with mentally healthy individuals.

54. Have the class prepare their own list of possible causes of mental illness. Try not to suggest too many yourself so the class will come up with their own. This may tell you what particular situations bother your students.

Evaluation

Appraisal of health instruction in the high school should be considered in its broadest sense. What has been the effect of the health program on the health status of the students? What has been the effect on the behavior of the students? What understanding of health have students attained?

Records, pretests, reports, and observations will reveal the health status, health behavior, and health understanding of the student when he or she first enters the high school health course. Standardized health knowledge tests may serve as pretests of knowledge. Thereafter progress tests, singular and collective observations, daily contact with the student, and observations by persons outside of the school will indicate the progress in health and health education of the students.

Such testing will help the student and his or her parents to appreciate the progress achieved thus far. These progress evaluations can be interviews, conferences, surveys, reports, records, questionnaires, self-appraisals, or tests. These tests may be combinations of essay tests as well as multiple choice, completion, matching, and other types of objective tests. In addition to evaluating health knowledge, the teacher should attempt to appraise health attitudes and practices.

Near the end of the semester, a final achievement test should be administered to assess the final level of health knowledge, attitudes, and practices. As part of the final appraisal, achievement in health knowledge may be indicated by repeating the standard health knowledge test. However, a battery of tests will probably yield a better measure of student attainment. Perhaps no better use could be made of the last week of the semester than to review the tests, item by item. Emphasis on the correct concepts by interpreting, evaluating, and expanding on ideas will help to crystallize the health experiences of the students and to reinforce their prior learnings.

QUESTIONS AND EXERCISES

1. Interpret the Emerson quotation, "The things taught in schools and colleges are not an education, but the means of education."
2. Should the senior high school health instructor regard high school education as termination?
3. What knowledge should high school gradua to make the necessary decisions relating to they will be called on to make as individuals and as parents?
4. Perhaps the most difficult task in health teaching is to develop an intense interest in personal health in a student who already has good health. What are some means that might be used to develop the student's appreciation of health and the need to safeguard and promote this asset?
5. If a considerable percentage of students in a high school exhibit a practice detrimental to health, how would you replace the undesirable practice with the proper health practice?
6. How can personal grooming be used as a motivation vehicle in high school health instruction?
7. Present some examples showing that health education in the high school can be cultural education.
8. Mental health instruction that gives the student wholesome insight can be extremely valuable education. Explain.
9. Mental health instruction that gives students tangible knowledge that will enable them to improve their personality and develop poise serves the intended purpose of mental health instruction in the high school. Evaluate this statement.
10. What is the merit in teaching mental health as a lead-up to sex education?
11. Why are interpersonal relationships the foundation of sex education?
12. In any high school there are likely to be students with inherited defects. How can heredity be treated in the health class without embarrassing those with hereditary disorders?
13. In secondary school health education today less and less emphasis is being placed on the study of anatomy. What is your evaluation of this trend?
14. What is meant by the statement that health is a collective science?
15. Other than the regularly scheduled course in health, what course in your high school contributed most to health education, and what was this contribution?
16. What is meant by saying that all knowledge should be integrated to be of most value to the student?
17. How can a high school health council be a valuable vehicle for health education?
18. Why is the 3-2 plan for scheduling health classes highly ineffective in terms of student learning?
19. Some health educators contend that a full year of health instruction in the senior year is the best

schedule plan for high school. Evaluate this statement.

20. Why is it important that only qualified, state-certified people teach health in the high school?

REFERENCES AND SELECTED READINGS

American Health Foundation: KYB teacher's guide, The Know Your Body Disease Prevention Program, New York, 1978, The Foundation.

Bossing, N. L.: Teaching in secondary schools, ed. 4, Boston, 1967, Houghton Mifflin Co.

Critical Health Problems and Comprehensive Health Education Act, 1971, The School Code of Illinois With Additional Acts Affecting Schools, Chapter 122, pp. 861-866.

Cushman, W. P., and Bennett, B. L.: Selected health problems, Columbus, Ohio, 1967, Charles E. Merrill Books, Inc.

Florio, A. E., Alles, W. F., and Stafford, G. T.: Safety education, ed. 3, New York, 1979, McGraw-Hill Book Co.

Fodor, J. T., and Dalis, G. T.: Health instruction: theory and application, ed. 2, Philadelphia, 1974, Lea & Febiger.

Grout, R. E.: Health teaching in schools, ed. 5, Philadelphia, 1968, W. B. Saunders Co.

Framework for health instruction in California public schools, Sacramento, Calif., 1972, Office of State Printing.

Haag, J. H.: School health program, ed. 3, New York, 1972, Holt, Rinehart & Winston.

Hanlon, J. J., and McHose, E.: Design for health, the teacher, the school, the community, ed. 2, Philadelphia, 1971, Lea & Febiger.

Jenne, F. H., and Greene, W. H.: Turner's school health and health education, ed. 7, St. Louis, 1976, The C. V. Mosby Co.

Kilander, H. F., editor: Preparing the health teacher, recommendations from five national conferences on professional preparation, Washington, D.C., 1961, American Alliance for Health, Physical Education, and Recreation.

Kilander, H. F.: School health education, New York, 1968, The Macmillan Co.

Manley, H.: A curriculum guide in sex education, St. Louis, 1964, State Publishing Co., Inc.

Mayshark, C., and Foster, R. A.: Health education in secondary schools, ed. 3, St. Louis, 1972, The C. V. Mosby Co.

Mayshark, C., and Foster, R. A.: Health education in secondary schools, ed. 3, St. Louis, 1972, The C. V. Mosby Co.

National Association of Secondary School Principals: Curriculum change in health education, The Bulletin of the National Association of Secondary School Principals, vol. 52, no. 326, March, 1968.

Oberteuffer, D., Harrelson, O. H., and Pollock, M. B.: School health education, ed. 5, New York, 1972, Harper & Row, Publishers.

Read, D., editor: New directions in health education, New York, 1971, The Macmillan Co.

Ridenour, N.: Mental health education, New York, 1969, Mental Health Materials Center.

School Health Education Study: Health education: a conceptual approach to curriculum design, St. Paul, 1967, 3M Education Press.

School Health Education Study: A summary report, Washington, D.C., 1964, National Education Association.

Simon, S. B., Howe, L. W., and Kirschenbaum, H.: Values clarification, New York, 1972, Hart Publishing Co., Inc.

Teaching about drug abuse, 1970, Illinois Interagency Drug Abuse Education Development Committee.

Willgoose, C. E.: Health teaching in secondary schools, Philadelphia, 1972, W. B. Saunders Co.

Williams, C. L., Arnold, C. B., and Wynder, E. L.: Primary prevention of chronic disease beginning in childhood: the know your body program: design of study, Preventive Med. 6:344-357, 1977.

For knowledge, too, is itself a power.

Francis Bacon

CHAPTER 15

Health contributions of high school subject fields

Health promotion, like the promotion of citizenship, is a function of all the school. In the high school health must be part and parcel of the school community and should be woven into its everyday fabric. It should be a concern of all the faculty as well as of all the students. It should be an integrated part of various activities and should be correlated with the several instructional fields. When health weaves a pattern through the woof and warp of the school fabric, it becomes an integrated part of the student's makeup. True education is a garment of seamless cloth. Health is not an accessory to be pinned on the garment where, in someone's opinion, it would look best. It is part of that whole cloth, which the loom of education weaves into a complete garment.

The overall purpose of the school, the best possible growth and development of all students, encompasses the mental and physical well-being of each student and is both the responsibility and the opportunity for all teachers.

Most secondary school instructors are willing to participate in the school health program and to contribute insofar as is possible to the general well-being of the students. With this potential contribution to the health program ready to be tapped, it would be a shortsighted school administrator or school health director who would not draw on this resource and put it to full use. It will truly yield an integrated overall health program and a correlated health instruction program.

HEALTH PREPARATION OF THE SECONDARY SCHOOL STAFF

Many secondary school instructors have some health background in their preservice professional preparation. In addition to general health, they have had work in child growth and development and in the general organization and function of the school health program. Their preparation for teaching frequently includes methods and techniques for correlating subject fields. All secondary school instructors should have a course of study in school health as part of their teaching preparation, which would increase their value to the students they serve.

On any secondary school instructional staff there will likely be some members who do not regard their health preparation as adequate for proper participation in the health program. Thus there is usually a need for an in-service program to give the entire staff the background and confidence necessary.

381

An in-service program can consist of a regular extension course that has been arranged by the director of health and the school administration. Such a course should not be limited to the instruction phase of school health. Because the whole staff has a direct contribution to make to the health of the students, the health of the individual child and the school health services aspect of the program should be given particular emphasis.

When an extension course is not available, other provisions can be made. A lecture series may be arranged or a symposium can be scheduled in which several persons present different aspects of the health program. A health institute at the beginning of the school year can emphasize key aspects of services, instruction, and living and provide resource material as a supplement for use by the teachers. These various plans are particularly effective when they are designed to incorporate the problems that are especially important to a particular high school. Visits to other schools can fulfill the purposes of in-service training, and observation of health work in the schools that are visited should be particularly valuable.

Most important is the inclusion of all staff members in the planning of the health program. All teachers should understand the objectives, organization, and procedures of the health program if they are to be effective in implementing the program. When the staff members understand the plan clearly and their role in the plan, they are more likely to be enthusiastic participants.

The administration, perhaps through the health director, should make clear to the staff the importance of student health appraisal, the channels and procedures for referrals, practices for control of communicable diseases, correlation of health instruction, and responsibilities for promoting healthful school living. As a part of the program, teach-

ers can bring to the attention of the health administrators certain problems and conditions needing attention. Suggestions of staff members can be exceedingly valuable.

HEALTH RESPONSIBILITIES OF ALL INSTRUCTORS

High school instructors are responsible for many duties other than those related to health. Thus health responsibilities should not impose a burden on the instructor. A staff member who is alert to health needs and opportunities will find that the program requires only a small proportion of time and effort. The teaching staff composes the lookout team for health, not the labor crew to carry out all the details and time-consuming tasks inherent in the complete program.

Cooperation with health program. All aspects of the school health program merit the cooperation of all faculty members. Only through teamwork can an effective program be attained. An obligation rests on the health director and administration to keep all instructors informed of health plans and developments. Periodic reports and announcements are particularly in order. An obligation also rests on the faculty to inquire of the proper persons when doubt exists about some phase of the program. Misunderstandings and disagreements can be resolved only when there is cooperation between faculty and health personnel.

Health status of students. An instructor who has developed a health awareness will tend to appraise and make a mental assessment of the quality of health of each student. Although ideally it would be laudable for every high school instructor to review the health condition of each child in class during the first period of the day, practical considerations rule it out. Constant observation during the day has been found to be an acceptable substitute. Teachers who are with students every day can get a reliable inventory of their level of health and the distinguishing characteristics of their endowment.

Once the instructor has an established assessment of each student's health, he or she should be able to recognize deviations readily. A slight transitory change may be only a signal to be on the alert for any further developments. Chronic or recurring deviations are the significant sources of concern. A conference with the student may elicit futher evidence of need for a follow-up. When this conference is unproductive, the observations of other instructors may be solicited. The instructor will have discharged his or her professional responsibility by referral to the director of the health program, the school nurse, or the administration. Personal interest may motivate the instructor to pursue the follow-up further.

Health problems of students. By noticing the questions students ask about health and the health problems they have, the instructor can guide students in solving their health needs. The only guidance necessary may be to help find an answer to the questions. Or it may be necessary to work out a projected course of action or to refer a student to another person. Whatever the health need, the instructor should be interested sufficiently to assure the student of a satisfactory solution.

School practices affecting health. Each instructor should be aware of the relationship of the organization of the school day, rest, relaxation, study, homework, and extracurricular activities to the health of the students (Fig. 15-1). It would hardly be consistent for a school to advocate home practices beneficial to health and itself be guilty of practices inimical to health. A crowded schedule, constant tension, and chronic fatigue may all be injurious to health. Practical considerations key the academic program to the needs and capacities of the general run of students. Yet the program must be adaptable to varying needs. However, both students who overconscientiously submerge themselves in the academic program and those who escape into extracurricular activities must be adjusted to the program.

Faculty meetings should consider the relationship of school practices to the health of the students. Homework assignments, class

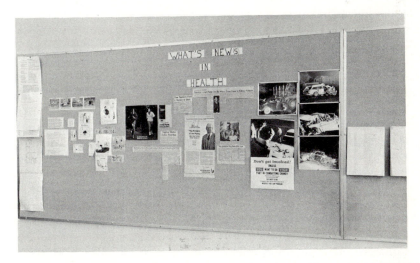

Fig. 15-1. Health as a day-to-day event. Keeping students alerted to health is greatly facilitated by this ingenious bulletin board.

period requirements, and the scheduling program must be worked out by joint faculty action. Student activities outside of school supervision must be considered in appraising the school's program in the light of student health promotion.

Control of communicable diseases. Each instructor should be familiar with the prodromal symptoms of communicable respiratory diseases and the indications of common skin infections and infestations. A tendency of high school students to refuse to accept the first slight symptoms of disease as significant emphasizes the need for staff members to be alert to early indications of respiratory disease. A quiet conference with the student can lead to a friendly suggestion that he or she lie down in the emergency rest room or go home for the remainder of the day. If these suggestions are not accepted, referral to the nurse, health director, or administration would follow.

When a student has been absent, each instructor routinely should require administrative clearance before readmitting the student.

Healthful school environment. Every conscientious faculty member intends to maintain a healthful environment in the classroom, the laboratory, and elsewhere in the school. Yet unless a planned step-by-step procedure is established, the instructor can overlook many factors that detract from a healthful environment. A systematic check of lighting practices, ventilation, cleanliness, and orderliness should be made. The mental health aspects of the classroom should be reviewed. Are the students at ease? Do they feel they are accepted by others? Are they confident they can succeed, attain success, and enjoy their experiences? How can the school life of students be more healthful? These are questions all instructors should ask, answer, and implement.

Healthful student living. Certain children may be in special need of help in health adjustment. A particular example is the student who returns to school after an absence because of illness. The return to school makes many demands on him or her. Guidance is probably needed, and its cardinal objective must be consideration of the student's health.

School can expect to have a few children who for health reasons must be given special consideration. Helping these students to live effectively and enjoyably in terms of their endowment is an obligation of all faculty members. More than this, the goal should be to help the child attain the normal level of health and general well-being.

Handling of emergencies. Every classroom teacher should know the basic fundamentals of first aid and emergency care. In practice, every instructor encounters emergencies that involve illness or injury. To be prepared for these duties is as logical as to be prepared for the subject field in which one is to teach.

Unusual mass emergencies such as fires involve school organization in which every faculty member must have a responsibility. If the teacher is an integral part of the entire school program rather than an isolated classroom drone, the vitality thus derived will doubtless be reflected in the instructional program.

Correlation of subject with health. All aspects of human experience that contribute to the development and maintenance of a high level of physical and mental function must be considered health activities. By their very nature all subject areas in the high school contribute in some form to the health of the student. In addition to the contribution to the student's immediate health through surveillance and guidance from the teacher, health education in some measure grows out of the classroom experiences of the year. Too often the teacher, unaware of the possibilities, passes up excellent opportunities for the development of certain health attitudes and the understanding of health relationships in the particular subject area.

Correlation of health with subject areas is surprisingly simple. It involves no elaborate sideline preparation. It demands no special procedures, calls for no disruption of normal plans, and requires no unusual teaching skill. All high school subject areas deal with the substance of life and living. Living always encompasses health or some phase of mental and physical well-being. It is a matter of the instructor's realizing the health implications and potentialities of the subject. Some subject areas have rather limited contributions to make to the health knowledge of the student, but other areas have extensive opportunities for health instruction as a phase of the subject itself. If health is incorporated in its framework, the subject field is not handicapped or deprived of anything. The subject itself is enriched from the experiences of the students. By thus revealing its vital applications as related to human health, the subject becomes a more meaningful and personal experience for the student. A greater appreciation of the subject field is a common outcome.

On an all-school basis several plans have been worked out to make correlation effective without unjustified duplications and flagrant omissions. Some schools have used a faculty curriculum committee to carry on the necessary cooperative planning. A modification of this approach is the use of joint curriculum planning by the instructors in the immediate subject areas, with the health director as consultant. In other schools the health instructor serves as an informal chairman of a group that includes instructors in the fields that particularly have contributions to make to health instruction. Out of these groups have come several plans.

Where a core curriculum is in use, health

materials are included in the basic studies. New, broader courses have made the allotment of health areas a relatively simple problem. Some schools have used the recognized health needs as a guide for all faculty members, who thus use their subject field as a vehicle for finding answers to these needs. In other schools, instructors have developed units, which are then compared for duplications and omissions. Many schools permit each instructor complete leeway in determining the manner in which health is developed in a particular subject field.

Perhaps, in harmony with the present trend toward complete integration and correlation of subject fields, a high school course in health could be dispensed with and health instruction could be carried out entirely through existing courses and the normal activities of the school. To date, even with outstanding correlation of other subjects with health, a marked deficiency in health education would exist if the health course were not a part of the curriculum plan. To make the health knowledge and understanding of the student complete and functional, the recognized health course in the high school is still indispensable.

ESSENTIAL SAFEGUARDS

In order that misunderstanding be precluded and correlation with health placed in its proper perspective, certain safeguards or limitations should be explored. An instructor with a totally inadequate health background would be discreet to limit health instruction in the classroom to the expressed interests and spontaneous activities of the students. Even in this event or situation the faculty member should seek the counsel of the health instructor or director on the appropriateness of the class approach and the accuracy of the content.

Health should not usurp a disproportionate part of the time in a class. Yet time devoted

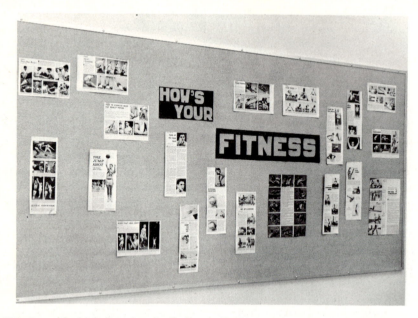

Fig. 15-2. Topical health bulletin board. All phases of health lend themselves to a program designed to interest students in looking for published health resources. (Courtesy Salem Public Schools, Salem, Ore.)

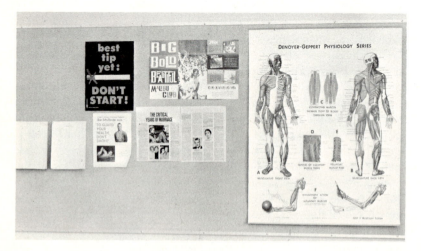

Fig. 15-3. Health interest display. A special interest for high school students is a collection of articles on various phases of health, which, besides providing the initial impact, can be discussion catalysts.

to a specific health question should be in proportion to its importance and the interest of the students. In the subject field a topic that has health significance merits the time necessary for its development.

To insert an isolated unit on health in some subject field is not a correlation of health with the subject field. The tie-in that expresses correlation will be the study of health within the subject field—not as an independent entity. The recognized scope of the subject includes areas with health implications or overtones. These areas can be studied and the health aspects developed simultaneously. Frequently the subject is the vehicle for health instruction. The mutual relationship that exists can make the entire activity a more meaningful experience (Figs. 15-2 and 15-3).

HEALTH IN ENGLISH OR COMMUNICATION FIELDS

Instructors in English long have recognized the motivating value of student interest in health as a fruitful resource for themes or compositions. A theme on the health of the community requires a preliminary study of aspects of government, social conditions, and public service. Hospital and medical facilities may be studied. Composing the theme is an important experience, but the by-products may be equally valuable. Vocabulary growth is not insignificant. Whether the composition calls for exposition, narration, description, or argumentation, health is a fertile field of subject matter. Every measure should be taken to assure accuracy and soundness in the material the student writes.

In speech activities that draw on the interests of students for subject matter, students frequently select health subjects. Controversial issues in the health field offer much material for both classroom and extracurricular debates. The question of a national health insurance program is an example.

Reading in the biographical field can include assignments on celebrated health figures. The adventures of Walter Reed, Louis Pasteur, Robert Koch, and even Hippocrates can be fascinating to inquisitive youth. Sir Alexander Fleming left a heritage that is stimulating to all who enjoy reading the exploits of the modern scientist.

Instruction in foreign languages can be vitalized and enriched by including the distinctive health problems, customs, and contributions of the people whose language is being mastered. The language of a nation becomes more functional as it is applied to the people and the problems of that nation. Health is universally both a personal and a public problem.

PHYSICAL EDUCATION

As in other fields, physical education makes a considerable contribution to the health program, but physical education per se does not constitute a total health program. More opportunities are presented for contributing to the health education of the student than in any other division of the school, with the exception of the health course proper. The list of these opportunities is considerable, and each activity in the list encompasses a number of possible procedures, activities, and outcomes:

1. Mechanics of bodily movement
2. Coordination and efficiency
3. Physiological effects of activity
4. Adaptation of activity to physiological capacity
5. Conditioning
6. Nature of fatigue
7. Rest and sleep
8. Relaxation
9. Nutrition and activity
10. Weight and activity
11. Promotion of personal health
12. Bodily cleanliness and grooming
13. Cleanliness and care of clothing
14. Proper dress
15. Mental health contributions of activity
16. Disease control practices
17. Responsibility for health of others

18. Promotion of safety
19. First aid and emergency care
20. Sanitation of locker rooms, shower rooms, swimming pool, gymnasium, and playgrounds

Any physical educator who does not utilize these opportunities for health instruction lacks a full appreciation of the true role of the physical educator. A unique opportunity is afforded the physical education staff to help the student integrate and apply health knowledge. Time and again the physical educator will be called on for counseling in health problems. The physical education situation provides an atmosphere that lends itself to a highly confidential relationship between student and instructor. Rapport of this type should be utilized in promoting the student's ability to understand and guide his or her own health.

BIOLOGICAL SCIENCE

Often regarded as the fundamental science on which health is based in both its fundamental principles and their application, biological science can contribute considerably to the student's understanding and appreciation of health. Teaching biological science as a fundamental health science provides additional motivation for learning. In addition to established biological principles, certain specific applications should be especially emphasized:

1. Application of the scientific method to the practical problems of health
2. Contributions of biologists to human welfare
3. Physical growth and development
4. Physiological needs
5. Physiological capacities
6. Biological adaptation
7. Reproduction
8. Genetics applied to health and disease
9. Analysis of fads and quackery
10. Health superstitions and fallacies
11. Biology of infectious disease
12. Biology of disease control
13. Body defenses, including immunity
14. Biological aspects of penicillin, Aureomycin, streptomycin, and other antibiotics
15. Physiological nature of injuries
16. Biological basis of first-aid measures

All these suggestions represent normal health interests of students. Biology teaching becomes more interesting to the students when it becomes more functional in terms of final outcomes.

SOCIAL STUDIES

A field as broad as social studies provides an almost limitless number of health implications. Practically all social problems have health overtones. This is particularly true not only in social pathology, but also in the positive aspects of social progress. Although disease with its social impact is important, the role of health in human social progress is at least equally important and interesting.

Health as a social factor can be considered from the standpoint of the individual, the family, the neighborhood, the community, the nation, and the world. Several vital topics are especially interesting to youth:

1. Role of health and disease in history
2. Present health status of the world
3. Health status of the nation
4. Health status of the community
5. Health and its social impact
6. Sociological aspects of disease and disability
7. Spiral of disease–poverty–further disease
8. Community health problems
9. Community health resources
10. Public health organization and service
11. Family health problems
12. Cost of medical care
13. Medical and hospital insurance
14. Sanitation problems
15. Protection of food
16. Patent medicines

Individual, family, and community health needs represent perhaps the core of any study of the sociological aspects of health. Recognizing, understanding, and working out solutions for these needs represent laudable outcomes of classes in social studies. Health problems can have a vital self-identification for the student.

HOME ECONOMICS

Correlating home economics with health is as logical and natural as correlating play with physical activity. A mutual relationship is inherent in the two fields. Both deal with effectiveness and enjoyment in living and with problems of personal and family concern. Many of the questions and problems of concern in the home economics field are significant in health terms:

1. Nutrition
2. Dietary problems
3. Purchasing food
4. Food preparation
5. Boy-girl relationships
6. Social behavior
7. Personal appearance
8. Courtship and marriage
9. Adjustment in marriage
10. Family life
11. Family resources
12. Child care
13. Care of the sick
14. Home nursing
15. Consumer education
16. Home safety

The present practice of scheduling home economics courses for boys as well as for girls is in harmony with the current philosophy of functional education. Adolescent boys as well as girls have a recognized need for education in family life in its broadest sense. That such a course includes health aspects of family living indicates that the course is realistic and the subject matter is integrated.

PHYSICS

Many high schools have developed a broad general course in physical science that integrates physics, astronomy, geology, chemistry, and even mathematics, rather than to offer distinct courses in the various branches of physical science. It is recognized here that such a broad integrated experience has considerable merit, but for the present discussion it is more satisfactory to consider physics, chemistry, and mathematics individually. An individual treatment serves schools with separate distinct courses; yet it permits the integration of material presented here into the integrated general physical science offering.

Normally only a small percentage of the student body tends to enroll in a physics class. Even then it usually appeals only to those who have a need for physics as preparation for a specific field of study in higher education. In consequence, rather specialized aspects of health interests may be explored. Those phases of physics that once were regarded as purely theoretical or academic, but that now serve important uses, appeal especially to the impressionable youth whose interests are in science fields:

1. Light
2. Optics
3. Sound
4. Radioactivity
5. X-ray
6. Electron microscope
7. Electricity
8. Heat
9. Simple diffusion, dialysis, osmosis, and filtration
10. Composition of the atmosphere
11. Atmospheric pressure
12. Caisson disease and its prevention and treatment
13. Altitude sickness
14. Biophysics

All of these topics are important in health. Many of the recent discoveries in health science have been made possible by scientists who have applied the fundamental principles of physics. Special student reports on the application of physics to a health problem can be a fruitful source of investigation.

CHEMISTRY

The revival of interest in chemotherapy is an indication of the health implications in the field of chemistry:

1. Chemotherapy—sulfonamides, arsenic, and bismuth
2. Hormone chemistry
3. Antiseptics
4. Anesthetics

5. Insecticides
6. Detergents
7. Tracers in biochemistry
8. Fats, carbohydrates, and proteins
9. Industrial safety

Instructors in chemistry constantly seek motivating devices in the form of everyday applications. From the work of Paul Ehrlich to the present-day teams of chemists who are employed by pharmaceutical manufacturers or who work in clinics or college laboratories, chemotherapy has been a ray of hope for the conquest of tuberculosis and other diseases that thus far have defied the efforts of immunologists. A study of the recent use of radioactive tracers in research will encompass some of the principal health problems of today.

MATHEMATICS

Although at first glance it appears to be a field far removed from health, mathematics can nevertheless deal with problems of concern to human health. Applied mathematics can find a fruitful field in matters of human life, health, illness, and death. Especially challenging to the student is the attempt to project data into the future and to work out statistical probabilities. The future is a constant source of interest to idealistic youth:

1. Birth and death rates
2. Disease rates
3. School absence and illness
4. Cost of illness
5. Insurance problems
6. Population curves
7. Human growth curves
8. Life expectation

SUMMARY

Few instructors will exhaust all the possibilities for correlating their subject field with health. An awareness of the possibilities for correlation and a responsiveness to the health interests, needs, and questions of students assure a fair degree of correlation. Encouragement and assistance from the director of the health program are all important.

QUESTIONS AND EXERCISES

1. What is meant by the statement, "Education is a garment of seamless cloth?"
2. Why should all high school counselors have a fundamental knowledge of health?
3. How much health preparation should all members of a high school faculty have?
4. What in-service health program should be provided for all members of a high school faculty?
5. Why is it essential that all the faculty be included in the planning of the high school health program?
6. "The teaching staff composes the lookout team for health." Interpret this statement.
7. To have an assessment of a student's health status, what should the faculty members observe and interpret?
8. When a high school staff member has reason to believe a certain student's health is not up to par, what procedures should that staff member follow?
9. What are some questions students might ask that would indicate the students probably have specific health problems?
10. What school practices could have an adverse effect on the health of students?
11. If a mathematics instructor suspects that one of the students in the class may have a communicable disease, what procedures should the instructor follow?
12. What would be the indices of healthful living in any classroom in the high school?
13. South High School has an emergency building evacuation program entirely under faculty supervision. North High School has an emergency building evacuation program entirely under student supervision. What is your appraisal?
14. Evaluate the statement, "Correlation of health with other subject areas is surprisingly simple."
15. What are some of the possible undesirable aspects of correlation of health with other subject areas?
16. What are some health topics that could be used effectively for compositions in an English class?
17. What are some health issues that could be used as subjects for debate?
18. What subject area in the high school most implies health, and what is the basis for your selection?
19. "Practically all social problems have health overtones." Explain the quotation.
20. How can health be incorporated into a high school mathematics course?

REFERENCES AND SELECTED READINGS

Alberty, H. B., and Alberty, E. J.: Reorganizing the high school curriculum, ed. 3, New York, 1962, The Macmillan Co.

American Association of School Administrators: Health in schools, twentieth yearbook, ed. 2, Washington, D.C., 1951, National Education Association.

Clark, L.: Help yourself to health, New York, 1974, Pyramid Communications, Inc.

Clark, L.: Light on your health problems, New Canaan, Conn., 1972, Keats Publishing, Inc.

Crawford, C. D.: Health and the family, New York, 1971, The Macmillan Co.

Faunce, R. C., and Bossing, N. L.: Developing the core curriculum, ed. 2, New York, 1958, Prentice-Hall, Inc.

Goodlad, J. I.: Planning and organizing for teaching, Washington, D.C., 1963, National Education Association.

Grambs, J. D., and McClure, L. M.: Foundations of teaching today, New York, 1964, Holt, Rinehart & Winston, Inc.

Grout, R. E.: Health teaching in schools, ed. 5, Philadelphia, 1968, W. B. Saunders Co.

Haag, J. H.: School health program, ed. 3, New York, 1972, Holt, Rinehart & Winston.

Kilander, H. F.: School health education, ed. 2, New York, 1968, The Macmillan Co.

Kogan, B. A.: Health: man in a changing environment, New York, 1970, Harcourt Brace Jovanovich.

Koren, H.: Environmental health and safety, N.Y., 1974, Pergamon Press, Inc.

Lebowitz, G.: Exploring health careers: you and in health, New York, 1973, Fairchild Publications, Inc.

Mayshark, C., and Foster, R.: Health education in secondary schools, ed. 3, St. Louis, 1972, The C. V. Mosby Co.

Meier, F. A.: Opportunities in general science for health instruction, Research Quarterly 22:91, 1951.

Miller, R. I.: Education in a changing society, Washington, D.C., 1974, National Education Society.

Miller, R. I.: Evaluating faculty performance, New York, 1972, Irvington Books.

Miller, R. I.: Perspectives on educational change, New York, 1974, Irvington Books.

Podair, S.: The consumer's guide to good health, New York, 1974, Pyramid Communications, Inc.

Schneider, E., and McNeely, S. A.: Teachers contribute to child health, Washington, D.C., 1962, U.S. Government Printing Office.

Thut, I. N., and Adams, D. K.: Educational patterns in contemporary societies, New York, 1964, McGraw-Hill Book Co.

What should the high school teach? 1956 yearbook, Washington, D.C., 1956, Association for Supervision and Curriculum Development, National Education Association.

PART FIVE

Healthful school living

A man's dignity may be enhanced by the house he lives in.

Cicero

CHAPTER 16

Healthful school environment

For the student, school is a part of day-to-day living. Merely to erect an attractive, sanitary building is not enough. The important thing is the interaction of the environment and the student. Environment is here considered in the dynamic sense. The most important thing in that environment is people, and the most important person is the teacher. But the remainder of the environment is also important. The particular atmosphere created in a school conditions the behavior patterns of children either favorably or unfavorably. Their general school life is an effective learning experience. Whether that learning is a wholesome positive experience or an unwholesome negative one is important in terms of the child's health education and outlook on personal and community health.

Some children come from homes with a high level of healthful living. This standard should be further fortified by a high level of healthful living in the school. When a child has grown up respecting healthful family and public living conditions, as an adult he or she will more likely maintain an excellent home life and insist on a wholesome community environment. From such preparation community leaders are developed. Respect for high standards is the requisite of model citizens.

For children whose home life from the standpoint of healthful living is on a lesser plane, the school can serve both as an incentive and an experience in attaining a higher standard of healthful living. From their school experience many persons have received the incentive to establish living conditions in a home of their own that are vastly above those that they experienced in their own childhood. The influence of the school cannot always be measured by standard achievement tests or, indeed, in terms of dollars and cents.

Architectural, sanitary, esthetic, and social aspects of the school environment must be considered. Perhaps the health implications of school architecture have been overemphasized. Very wholesome living can be experienced in a school of rather poor architectural design. Yet a superbly designed school plant has a greater potential for healthful living than does the less well-designed one. Whether the esthetic, social, and functional possibilities are developed is the responsibility of those who "live" in the building.

Sanitation depends on adequate facilities that are properly utilized through sound housekeeping (or schoolkeeping) practices. All people living in the school should be active participants in schoolkeeping. It would be an injustice to the child to permit him or her to acquire the concept that the building is kept clean and orderly by someone else who is hired for the task. To recruit the youngster's interest and develop pride in this home away from home is a laudable educational objective. Each child must participate in the chore of keeping *our* school clean, orderly, and beautiful.

Esthetic and social appreciations and cultivated as by-products of a wholesome respect for beauty and our fellowman. A child acquires an understanding of what is worthwhile; it is not something he or she is crowned with. The achievement of wholesome relationships in attractive school surroundings is not an accident. It is a creation.

RESPONSIBILITY FOR HEALTHFUL SCHOOL ENVIRONMENT

Theoretically, responsibility for initiating and providing for the construction and maintenance of school buildings rests with the board of education. As a matter of practice such action originates with the superintendent, who is the professionally qualified expert on such problems.

Administrators. Full-time regularly employed school administrators are constantly appraising the needs of the school district. Classroom enrollments, age-group populations, migrations, consolidations, real estate developments, industrial changes, and other factors that affect present and future school needs are used as bases for constructing new school buildings or remodeling old ones. Knowledge of the present plant—its shortcomings and possibilities—is necessary to the administrator. The economics of building anew or rebuilding will loom as important.

Once administrators have agreed on the need for plant expansion, a tentative estimate and general plan are developed. The superintendent submits these recommendations to the board for its consideration.

Programs for maintaining the school plant are the responsibility of the superintendent and the administrators, especially the principals. General policies apply to the whole system, and each principal administers the policy to the best advantage for the particular building for which he or she is responsible. Although the superintendent does not intend to veto or even investigate particular problems or procedures of a particular school, he or she does need to be informed of unusual situations and circumstances.

Board of education. Sovereignty or ultimate authority rests with the people, but they delegate the exercise of it to the board of education. However, the board does not act on its own initiative in plant construction, but passes on the merits of recommendations made to it by the professional administrator. It is a wise board that asks a representative community committee to review the plans and make suggestions. This assures adequate study of the plan and community understanding of the proposal. When representative community leaders have approved the plans, the board of education can proceed in the knowledge that the community understands and supports the project.

If the plan is to go forward, an architect is engaged by the board to draw preliminary plans and to make preliminary estimates. The board then takes the necessary steps for financing—usually a bond issue for approval by the electors in a regular or special school district election. If the voters approve it, final plans are drawn, bids are called for and opened, and a construction contract is awarded. Because of better school architects, better engineers, illuminating specialists, ventilation experts, and a host of other specialists, school buildings today are a vast improvement over those of a generation ago.

Regulations governing maintenance of the school plant are approved by the board. Often certain board members have an extensive background in the needs and procedures of plant maintenance.

Architect. In recent years school architecture has become a specialty in the architectural profession. As a result, school districts are getting better plant designs. Yet even the most competent architect consults the school personnel who will "live" in the building. For effective school living the plan must be adapted to the recognized needs of the children. Who should know these needs better than the teachers? It is a wise architect who gets the composite judgment of all the people who may have something of value to suggest in the planning of the building. In addition to drawing plans, the architect has general supervision of construction.

Teachers. Once the structure is completed and furnished, it is the teacher's task to make the building serve the needs of healthful school living.

Student pride in the school is not difficult to develop, but it does require some planning and promotion. Loyalties to the school and what it stands for create a desirable atmosphere for wholesome living. Children do not always develop an appreciation of the meaning of the school in their lives. With the stimulation and guidance of an understanding teacher, students usually develop a desirable level of appreciation. This can be solidified by having the students assume responsibility for preserving and extending the attractiveness of their common home. Monitors may be designated for specific tasks, but all the children should feel that they have a responsibility. Procedures for the selection of monitors should be such that every youngster has a regular assignment. None should be excluded, even accidentally.

Within a classroom a wholesome respect for one another fostered by understanding courtesy creates a wonderful atmosphere for intellectual, emotional, physical, and social development. To rise above the common-

place requires a surprisingly small amount of extra effort.

Esthetic appreciation can be fostered through art, music, play, literature, and other creative activities. Recordings can be helpful, but it would be an error to introduce any such opportunity for esthetic appreciation to the exclusion of an appreciation of the beauties of the school and its surroundings. Not until years after they have left a school do some students appreciate the artistic grandeur of the school building, its landscaping, and its many aspects.

A teacher who is a one-person schoolkeeper lacks the vision and educational philosophy essential to the best interests of the pupils. The children gain nothing when the teacher assumes full responsibility. Indeed, they are the losers. They lose the opportunity for self-growth that comes only with participation.

Students. Insofar as is possible, students should assume the primary responsibility for the order and cleanliness of their school. On a cooperative basis some classes undertake to supply additional furnishings for the building. Pictures with a patriotic or story motif, vases, bowls, flowerpots, stands, lecterns, and a host of other furnishings have been contributed by classes at various times. On a group basis these projects have merit, but donations from individual pupils should be accepted only under unusual circumstances.

All-school organization for building cleanliness should be administered by a representative council or body under the supervision of a faculty adviser. In the elementary school the primary grades can have responsibility for the cleanliness of halls and stairways. The intermediate grades can supervise cleanliness of toilet rooms and rest rooms. An effective arrangement is to give each grade a month's assignment, with the class organizing for its task. In the high school the student council can assume responsibility for the organization and supervision of the cleanliness program.

Room organization is particularly important in the elementary school. A captain for each 2-week period, with necessary assistants, can be a simple form of organization. Division of labor is usually possible. Although the captains and assistants should lead the way, all the pupils should participate to some degree.

Special projects such as *Don't Be a Litterbug Week*, special pickup projects, locker cleanouts, rake-up campaigns, and other activities can add to the interest of the students in maintaining a healthful school environment.

Custodians. The nonskilled janitor has been replaced by the qualified custodian. Besides the mechanical skill needed for the assignment, the custodian should know sanitation, control of communicable diseases, and safety. In-service preparation, usually regional institutes, are provided in most states to assure the schools of well-qualified custodians. In addition to job know-how, the custodian should be in good health and be dependable. A competent custodian can care for 10 to 12 rooms properly. Some administrators supply the custodian with a printed list of duties and instructions.

A custodian has many miscellaneous duties, but certain of these duties are of specific health significance. These include heating and ventilating, dusting, gathering trash and waste paper and burning it, cleaning plumbing fixtures, filling soap dispensers, sweeping floors, mopping, cleaning steps, walls, and windows, cleaning chalkboards and erasers, taking care of the school grounds, checking playground apparatus, inspecting for safety, and eliminating hazards.

Custodian-staff cooperation is a two-way street. Insofar as is possible the custodian's schedule should be planned to avoid interference with the school routine. Time after school and on Saturday is used for dusting, washing walls, and doing other tasks in the classroom. When the students, teachers, and custodians cooperate, everyone's task is lighter, and the whole atmosphere of the school is refreshed.

Although the custodian should be friendly with the children, the role of a custodian is not the role of a teacher or counselor. Also, the custodian should not be regarded as a personal servant for any one teacher. When only a small special task for the custodian arises, the teacher may tactfully ask him or her to do the task. Otherwise such requests should be made to the principal, who will inform the custodian of the special assignment. A custodian has specified duties to carry out in the interest of order and cleanliness, but a healthful school environment is not solely the responsibility of the custodian.

The principal should make periodic inspections of the work that is the custodian's responsibility. Understanding on the part of the whole staff, plus tact on the part of the principal, will get the maximum service from the custodial force. An incompetent custodian, like an incompetent teacher, should not be retained in the school.

Lunchroom personnel. Sanitation is more important in the lunchroom than anywhere else in the school. A situation in which sanitation will prevent the spread of disease also provides an opportunity for the children to observe and understand proper conditions and procedures for food handling. Lunchroom experiences integrate health practices and instruction for the children.

The facilities and practices in school lunchrooms are those prescribed by public health departments for the regulation of sanitation in public food catering establishments. Observance of these regulations is doubly important in the school.

Lunchroom personnel should feel a special obligation to the children, which can be engendered by a feeling of pride in the importance of lunchroom work. Personal health habits should be exemplary. If the lunchroom workers suffer from a communicable disease, they should isolate themselves voluntarily. The worker who strives for perfection in sanitary measures is an important member of the health instruction team.

LOCATION AND PLAN OF SCHOOL BUILDING

Certain factors in the location and plan of a school building are of direct health significance. To these health factors the elementary classroom teacher and the secondary school health instructor should especially direct their attention. It is not suggested that other things about the building are unimportant, but for present purposes health factors alone will be considered.

Site. School sites should be considered from the standpoint of accessibility, safety, quietness, cleanliness of the air, adequate drainage, and recreation space. Distance to the school is not so important today as formerly because of means of transportation. Railroad areas, main highways, and through streets are physical hazards to be avoided. Taverns and similar establishments constitute moral hazards. However, city ordinances and state laws usually specify that no alcoholic beverages may be sold within a mile of a school building. For clean air and a quiet neighborhood, residential and rural areas are preferable to industrial or other congested areas. Either natural or installed drainage that will assure dry grounds is important. Adequate play and recreation space can be provided by setting a minimum of 5 acres for an elementary school, 12 acres for a junior high school, and 20 acres for a senior high school. A standard of 100 square feet of play space per child will be adequate for any situation.

For esthetic reasons the surrounding area should be attractive, and the school site itself should be properly landscaped.

Planning of the building. A school building should be located on an elevated part of the grounds. Window exposures should preferably be west or east for general classrooms; south or east for kindergarten, science classrooms, and laboratories; north or northwest for art and drafting rooms; and south or east for physical education needs.

Whenever possible, the open-type building plan should be employed. It has many good features:

1. Provides rapid horizontal traffic
2. Reduces fire and other hazards
3. Provides easy access to the ground for all parts of the building
4. Reduces disturbing noises and odors
5. Provides for better natural lighting and ventilation

Basement areas that provide poor natural light and ventilation should not be used as classrooms because of the unwholesome psychological effects. However, some well-lighted basement rooms are satisfactory for classroom purposes.

Corridors usually have a 12-foot unobstructed width. Corridor intersections should be reduced to a minimum. Stairs must be located to reduce corridor traffic. An auditorium should be reached by two nonconverging traffic channels.

A kindergarten room is usually 24 × 50 feet and should be a self-contained unit with cloakroom, work sink, fountain, and two toilet rooms. Other elementary school classrooms should be 24 × 40 feet, with work sink and clothes storage. In the high school, classrooms 24 × 36 feet are recommended. Corridor lockers are essential. All classrooms should have walls and ceilings that are treated to absorb noise.

HEATING AND VENTILATION

Proper heating and ventilation in the school are not life-or-death matters. Students will not be exposed to a classroom situation in which the oxygen content will be inadequate for survival. Yet for effective and enjoyable school living, heating and ventilation are important, and the instructor has an obligation to make every effort to provide a physical atmosphere that is comfortable. The only sound educational procedure is to enlist the students in the project.

In heating and ventilating schoolrooms, the entire emphasis must be on physical comfort. Body heat and moisture must be removed. When the elimination of heat and moisture are retarded, students experience drowsiness, lassitude, depression, headache, and loss of vigor. For an alert and stimulating class the room must have proper temperature, humidity, and movement of air.

Standards of physical comfort. For the usual school situation, established standards for physical comfort have been determined by scientific investigation and practical experience. These standards are expressed in terms of temperature, humidity, and movement of air. Properly all three should be discussed together, but practical considerations dictate that they be dealt with one at a time.

Temperature in the schoolroom should be held between 66° and 71° F. In the winter the lower half of this temperature range will feel comfortable. In the hotter seasons a room temperature of 71° F will feel comfortable.

Humidity or air moisture should be between 30% and 70% of the maximum amount of moisture the air will hold. A humidity of 50% and a temperature of 70° F are ideal. Several instruments, such as hygrometers and psychrometers, are used for a precise determination of humidity. In the absence of such a device a person may suspect a high degree of humidity when body moisture tends to cling to the body rather than evaporate rapidly. Without an air-conditioning unit it is difficult to affect the humidity of a classroom.

Air movement carries away body heat and moisture. To be effective, a current of air should be perceptible. The least perceptible current is spoken of as the threshold velocity. Under ordinary room conditions the movement of air should at least be of threshold velocity. A current perceptible at one moment may not be felt a few minutes later. As room temperature declines, the perceptible velocity rises. Since temperature and air movement vary, window ventilation is highly effective because it permits these variations to operate in producing comfortable sensations of the skin. Mechanical ventilating systems do not provide for variations; in this respect they are not so acceptable as the window-gravity method of ventilation.

Heating. Boiler and fuel rooms should be of fire-resistant construction. There is merit in building a brick boiler room separate from the school building.

Radiators and grilles should be so placed that warm air is uniformly distributed without noise or drafts. Heat for each room should be controlled individually. Radiators should be of the wall-hung type and placed beneath windows because this type of radiator is easy to clean.

A thermometer should be placed 5 feet above the floor in each room.

Ventilation. Ordinary window-gravity ventilation can be highly satisfactory if a glass deflector in the window starts the air current upward and an outlet high on the opposite wall permits circulation of the air. Glass deflectors are recommended only because they do not reduce the light from outdoors.

In practice, when there is window ventilation, several purposes are served if specific students are appointed to be responsible for proper ventilation. Someone is responsible for ventilation; the children develop a consciousness of the importance of ventilation; and student participation and responsibility are engendered. Third-grade pupils can assume this responsibility, although first- and second-grade children merely participate vicariously, since the teacher does the actual chore. If each child is appointed for a 2-week period, service opportunities for many pupils, girls as well as boys, are provided.

Mechanical ventilating systems are usually designed to provide 15 cubic feet of air per occupant per minute. Ventilation in one room does not depend on ventilation in another room. Zoned ventilation is necessary in large school buildings. The gymnasium, auditorium, shop, and cafeteria usually have independent ventilating units. Cloakrooms have separate ventilation. Toilet rooms have ventilating ducts and fans that are independent of the rest of the system. To remove objectionable fumes or odors, laboratories are provided with special means of ventilation. Chemistry laboratories are provided with fume hoods of acid-resisting construction.

Vent grilles are placed in the walls as far removed from the windows as possible. Neither floor nor ceiling grilles are approved. Fireproof exhaust ducts carry the air outside of the building. Ventilator heads protect the exhaust openings against back drafts and inclement weather.

Air conditioning. The objective of air conditioning is to control the temperature, humidity, movement, and purity of air. The air is filtered and washed to remove dust, smoke, obnoxious gases, and pollen. Temperature is maintained from 68° to 69° F during the winter and 70° to 71° F during hot weather. Humidity is maintained from 40% to 45% during winter and from 45% to 50% during hot weather. Air conditioning is used more widely in warmer climates than in colder climates. The primary purpose of air conditioning tends to be temperature control. Air conditioning has much to recommend it, but is not indispensable to good air control in the schoolroom. Air conditioning neither increases nor decreases the incidence of respiratory diseases. The expense is greater than the usual plenum system of ventilation, but in areas with badly polluted air or extremely high temperatures the expense may well be an investment in greater physical comfort and health protection.

ILLUMINATION

No one has ever become blind from poor schoolroom lighting, but proper lighting contributes to the effectiveness of students' work and, because it helps prevent fatigue, adds to the enjoyment of the school day. Efficiency and comfort of vision are the major considerations of illumination.

A distinction should be made between the terms *light, illumination,* and *brightness.* Light is the source, illumination is the effect, and brightness is the amount of light returned from a surface.

Intensity of visible light is measured in footcandles. A *footcandle* is the amount of light received at a point 1 foot removed from a source of a standard candle power. The universal standard unit of light is at the Bureau of Standards, Washington, D.C. Footcandle meters, adjusted to the standard unit, measure the intensity of illumination.

A *footlambert* is the brightness of any surface and is the product of the illumination in footcandles and the reflection factor of the surface. Thus if the light units on a task are recorded as 50 footcandles and the reflection factor of the task is 70%, the units reflected to the eye would be 35 footlamberts. The equation is $FC \times RF = FL$. The footlambert must be given major consideration when the environment is conditioned for visual efficiency and comfort.

Three factors in lighting are important— sufficient light, proper distribution of light, and absence of glare. The amount of needed light depends on the particular activity in which a person is engaged. A corridor requires less light than a reading area where speed of vision is a consideration. Distinctness of vision (visual acuity) attains its maximum effectiveness at about 5 footcandles.

Speed of vision attains its maximum effectiveness at about 20 footcandles. On a sunny day outdoor illumination may be up to 10,000 footcandles. In a schoolroom the illumination near a window may be above 200 footcandles.

Proper distribution of light demands that all areas of the visual field have the same approximate intensity. Recognition of the importance of brightness difference has led to the use of lighter-colored chalkboards, woodwork, floors, furniture, and equipment in schoolrooms. *Brightness difference* expresses the brightness of the task as compared with brightness of the surrounding area.

Brightness balance is essential to visual efficiency and comfort. This can be attained by maintaining low brightness differences between the task and the surrounding area. Absolute brightness balance in the classroom is not possible as a practical matter. However, the footlambert brightness of the best-lighted area in the room should not be as much as 10 times the footlambert brightness of the poorest-lighted task where tasks are being performed.

Glare is light that causes discomfort, annoyance, or distress to the eyes. It is annoying to face a window or an uncovered light bulb. Reflected light from a tabletop produces glare. Contrast in light is disturbing to vision. All these conditions produce glare and are much too common in schoolrooms.

Classroom factors. Satisfactory illumination in a classroom is more than just the necessary window space and light units. All surfaces should be dull or semiglossy to reduce glare. This means that the furniture must be a light color and have a dull finish. A highly reflective semiglossy paint should be used for the walls and ceiling. Reflective values indicate the colors that should be used in schoolrooms (Table 16-1).

It is apparent that the ceiling and the first 3 feet down on the wall should be painted white, ivory, or a light cream color. Attrac-

Table 16-1. Average reflective light of colors

Color	Percent of reflected light
Gloss mill white	75-80
Ivory	65-70
Cream	55-70
Yellow	55-65
Buff	45-60
Pastel green	45-60
Light varnish	40-45
Light pink	35-55
Pastel blue	35-55
Pastel gray	15-25
Green	15-25

tive pastel tints on the walls provide both attractiveness and good reflective value. Some architects recommend a buff color for the lowest portion of the wall. If this color is used up to the wainscoting, the usual appearance of finger marks will be prevented.

Chalkboards should be dull and light colored, but should never be located between windows. When they are placed in front of the room or on the wall opposite the windows, chalkboards may cause glare. Such glare can be prevented if the lower edge of the chalkboard is pulled out about 2 inches. If the board is tilted thus, the reflected rays are thrown above the heads of the children.

Seats should be placed so that no child faces the window light. By the same token, the teacher should not face the light or stand in front of the windows so that the children must face the windows in order to see the teacher.

Standards of light. Minimum intensity of light for different purposes has been determined by scientific study and practical experience (Table 16-2). Other standards have been set up in terms of footlamberts (Table 16-3).

Although sufficient light is important, contrasts should be avoided. The peripheral field

Table 16-2. Recommended lighting levels in schools*

Location	Minimum footcandles
Classrooms—on desks and chalkboards	30
Study halls, lecture rooms, art rooms, offices, libraries, shops, and laboratories	30
Classrooms for partially seeing pupils and those requiring lip reading—on desks and chalkboards	50
Drafting rooms and typing and sewing rooms	50
Reception rooms, gymnasiums, and swimming rooms	20
Auditoriums (not for study), cafeterias, locker rooms, washrooms, corridors containing lockers, and stairways	10
Open corridors and storerooms	5

*From American standard practice for school lighting, New York, 1948, Illuminating Engineering Society and American Institute of Architects (approved by Acoustical Society of America).

Table 16-3. Recommended footlamberts

Area	Foot-candles		Reflection factor		Foot-lamberts
Average task	30	×	70%	=	21
Desk top	30	×	50%	=	15
Floor	20	×	30%	=	6
Chalkboard	50	×	30%	=	15
Tackboard	50	×	50%	=	25
Walls	30	×	75%	=	22½

and background should be nearly as intensely illuminated as the field of work.

Natural light. Both for the psychological effect and for good visual conditions, natural light should be used to the fullest and most effective extent possible (Fig. 16-1). Window space should be one fifth of the floor area in rooms not more than 24 feet wide. Unilateral lighting or lighting from one side is recommended. The left side is preferred, but the right side is acceptable. Bilateral lighting from one side and the rear is satisfactory and even desirable in large rooms. Cross-lighting is condemned as unhygienic. A bank of windows on one side should cover the back four fifths of that wall, thus leaving the front fifth free of windows. Square-topped windows that extend as close to the ceiling as possible provide a good distribution of light.

Translucent shades diffuse direct sunlight, eliminate glare, and control illumination. If two rollers at the center of the window are used, both rollers can be drawn to allow a foot of clear window space at the top and bottom to remain. Shades should be wider than the windows. Venetian blinds, either horizontal or vertical, are satisfactory. Dark lower surfaces of the slats reduce glare. Venetian blinds are durable and do not flap, but are expensive, gather dust, and are hard to clean. Opaque shades can be placed above other shades for movie or other projection activities.

Artificial light. Regardless of the efficacy of the natural lighting in a school, artificial lighting should be planned as a separate system, sufficient within itself. The light source is called the luminaire. Incandescent lighting is usually semidirect, and the light bulbs are enclosed within Trojan glass units. Indirect lighting is excellent, but expensive. Units are concealed in the wall recesses, and light is projected to the ceiling, where it is reflected to the desks, walls, and other parts of the room. The light is uniformly distributed.

In semidirect lighting the units are dropped about 3 feet from the ceiling to provide more and better-distributed light. Units are spaced to given evenness of light. Six or eight units serve the normal-sized classroom. The enclosing units should be shaped to show a great deal of light on horizontal surfaces and should blend in with the ceiling to avoid pronounced contrast. Glass units should be cleaned frequently for maximum efficiency.

Fluorescent lights are more expensive to

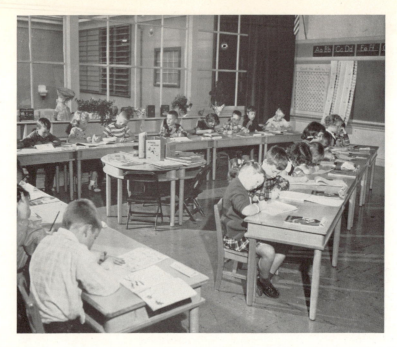

Fig. 16-1. Schoolroom lighting. A resourceful teacher planned a seating arrangement that eliminated the objectionable features of a single bank of windows for a small classroom.

install than incandescent lights, but are twice as efficient in converting electrical energy into light. Bare fluorescent lights must be shielded. Louvers, white plastic, and opal glass are most suitable for classroom purposes. White fluorescent lights are recommended for ordinary classroom and shop use, and daylight fluorescent lights for art rooms, sewing rooms, and other places where color discrimination is necessary. White fluorescent light gives off about 15% more light than daylight fluorescent light.

Local lighting units such as desk lamps should be used only in very special cases. General lighting should be adequate without the necessity for installing local units immediately over the field of vision.

Classroom illumination program. Insofar as is possible children should take an active role in the classroom illumination program. An awareness of lighting conditions is best developed through participation (Fig. 16-2). The National Society for the Prevention of Blindness has outlined such a program. Seeing conditions can be improved in the classroom if these procedures are observed:

1. Keeping upper portions of windows unshaded, except when the sun is shining directly on them
2. Drawing shades over the lower portions of the glass area only when necessary to diffuse direct sunlight or to reduce glare from snow, sky, or adjacent buildings
3. Checking illumination levels in all parts of the room periodically with a light meter
4. Making special seating arrangements for left-handed pupils so that light will fall over the right shoulder
5. Keeping windowsills free of all obstructions to light
6. Arranging seats and desks so that no pupil will face a window or work in his or her own shadow
7. Cleaning chalkboards frequently
8. Eliminating books, charts, maps, etc. that are so soiled they provide poor brightness contrast
9. Providing copyholders and easels to maintain good posture and optimum lighting for close eye tasks

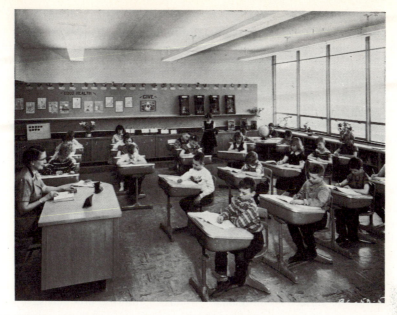

Fig. 16-2. Coordinated seating and lighting. Sufficient well-distributed light without glare contributes to more effective enjoyable living. The teacher's desk should be placed so that she does not face the light. (Courtesy American Seating Co., Grand Rapids, Mich.)

10. Making all board writing large and clear and placing it in the line of vision of the pupils
11. Planning the daily program to alternate periods of close eye work with activities less demanding visually
12. Switching on artificial lights whenever brightness levels fall below standard in any part of the room
13. Standing and sitting in positions that direct pupils' vision away from the windows
14. Planning for periodic adjustment of seats and desks to provide for best use of available light
15. Placing pupils with eye difficulties in the best-lighted places from the standpoint of their specific defects
16. Allowing pupils to change their seats whenever they desire more light or less light
17. Selecting work places to make best use of available light
18. Covering chalkboards not being used to conserve the available light
19. Covering glass doors on cabinets and removing pictures covered with glass
20. Selecting and using only those textbooks, maps, charts, posters, etc. that have nongloss surfaces, appropriate type size, and desirable contrast
21. Noting when lamps or tubes become blackened or

defective and calling for correction from the custodian
22. Developing in the child a sense of responsibility for assisting in the maintenance of good seeing conditions*

WATER SUPPLY

School authorities have the responsibility for providing a safe and adequate water supply for school use. When a municipal water supply is used, primary responsibility for its source and purity rests with the municipality and the public health department. Yet the school district is responsible for proper installation and maintenance of water facilities in the school. In addition to being free from contamination, water should be palatable and sufficiently abundant for normal school needs.

———

*From Classroom lighting, New York, 1950, National Society for the Prevention of Blindness, publication No. 498, p. 14.

Source. Most schools obtain their water from an established public water system. These supplies are under the surveillance of the health department, and the school properly can accept this supervision as adequate. Some schools provide their own water supply, usually by drilling wells.

A shallow well is one that is less than 30 feet deep. Whether dug or driven, shallow wells are unsatisfactory. Public health officials report that most troubles with rural water supplies are caused by shallow wells. A deep (more than 30 feet) drilled well is the recommended water source for a school when no public supply is available.

A well should be located so that it is above sources of contamination from groundwater flow. Groundwater usually runs toward lakes or rivers, whatever the surface contour may be.

The school district should engage experienced and competent well drillers. Drilled wells should go down at least 50 feet to a safe water-bearing stratum. This stratum is merely a gravel bed with water in the interstitial spaces. Several impervious layers will lie above the gravel bed and thus prevent contaminated surface water from reaching the groundwater stratum. Well casings should be sealed off so that surface water cannot trickle down to the water-bearing stratum. This means that there must be a tight concrete platform as well as sealed-off casing. Chlorination of a groundwater supply is usually not necessary, but a sample for bacteriological examination should be taken at least once a month. This test is for the coli-aerogenes group of bacteria. Their presence in water indicates that the water has been exposed to contamination from livestock or human beings and may be dangerous for drinking purposes. A positive test thus does not reveal the presence of disease organisms, but the possibility that they may now or later get into the water. One sample is not significant. A number of positive samples, supported by

the evidence of a sanitary survey, is the significant source of data. Health department personnel should be consulted. In the meantime water from another source should be used for drinking purposes, or the water should be boiled or chlorinated.

If there is no mechanical chlorinating device, as a temporary measure a bactericidal chlorine content of water can be obtained by adding 50 drops of 1% chlorine solution to 10 gallons of clear water or by adding 6 teaspoons of 1% chloride solution to 100 gallons of clear water. A silver spoon should not be used to measure the chlorine solution. The chlorinated water should be well stirred and permitted to stand for 30 minutes. Individual paper cups should be used for this supply. The labels on Clorox, Purex, and other commercial chlorine products give directions for obtaining a 1% chlorine solution.

Fountains. With running water, fountains provide the most sanitary drinking facilities for the school. One fountain per 75 pupils is an acceptable standard. To provide a strategic location, fountains sometimes are installed as an adjunct of a lavatory (Fig. 16-3). Recesses in corridor walls provide a safety factor (Fig. 16-4). The height of the nozzle should be adapted to the age of the students.

Grade level	Height of nozzle
Kindergarten	23 inches
Primary grades	25 inches
Intermediate grades	29 inches
Junior high school	32 inches
Senior high school	35 inches

The nozzle should be above the rim of the bowl and protected by guards. A foot-controlled jet may be more sanitary, but the hand-controlled type is satisfactory. A fountain should be equipped with a flow control valve so that the user merely turns the water off and on and the jet is always the same. The drainpipe should be trapped.

Children ought to have the responsibility for the cleanliness of the fountain and the immediate area surrounding it. A committee

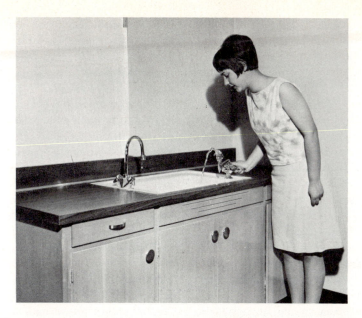

Fig. 16-3. Classroom fountain and lavatory. Located in the classroom, this fountain-lavatory is both convenient and economical. Students assume responsibility for proper care of the facility.

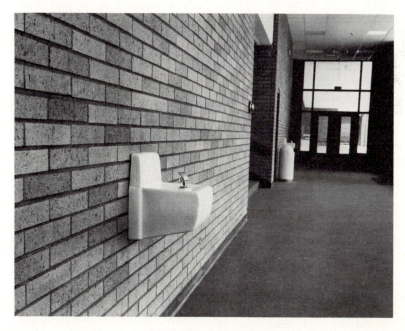

Fig. 16-4. Hazardous location for a fountain. To avoid possible injuries to students, a fountain should be set into the wall so that no part of the fountain protrudes.

responsibility for maintaining the fountain provides opportunities for group organization and discipline for training in citizenship.

GENERAL TOILET ROOM

When general toilet rooms are being located, an outside exposure with direct sunlight should be given preference. Accessibility is important. It is equally important that the girls' and boys' rooms be far removed from each other. Toilet rooms should not be located in the basement.

Ceilings, walls, and floors of toilet rooms should be of washable impervious materials. Uncoated cement floors are not suitable. Impregnated cement, terrazzo, and special tile make excellent floors. Proper drainage is essential, and both hot and cold hose outlets for flushing the floors should be provided. For ventilation, provision should be made for exhaust fans with a capacity to remove the room air every 10 minutes.

The students should be responsible for keeping the toilet rooms clean and orderly during the day. In the elementary school, the fourth, fifth, and sixth grades can take turns for a month each in being responsible for toilet room cleanliness. While one grade is responsible, other grades will respect its instructions. In junior and senior high schools the health council or student council can provide and administer a plan for orderliness of the toilet rooms. However, mopping, scouring, and other cleaning is the custodian's task.

Washbasins. One washbasin or lavatory for each 40 pupils is a recommended standard. Wash fountains can be substituted for washbasins. Height of the washbasins is important.

Grade level	Height to rim
Kindergarten	20 inches
Primary grades	22 inches
Intermediate grades	25 inches
Junior high school	28 inches
Senior high school	30 inches

Washbasins should have no stoppers so that students must wash their hands in running water. Each basin should have potable water that flows through one spigot with hot and cold water valves.

Liquid soap dispensers are preferred. A solution of equal parts of soap and water can be used, which will thus effect a saving. The diluted soap is not as harsh on hands, and students will use the same volume from the dispenser. Powdered soap is satisfactory. Bar soap is acceptable. No one has ever demonstrated that disease is spread by a bar of soap. The only real objection to bar soap is that it finds its way to the floor too easily.

Paper towels should be used. Roller towels are not as sanitary because there is no guarantee that a child will turn the roller. When the roll comes to the end, it truly becomes community property.

Wastepaper receptacles large enough to hold waste towels for a half day are *musts* if the toilet room is to be orderly. To empty the receptacles is the task of the custodian.

Water closets and urinals. The number of fixtures will vary for different age levels. Any suggested standard may be unsatisfactory for a specific situation.

Elementary school	Junior and senior high school
1 water closet to 30 girls	1 water closet to 45 girls
1 water closet to 60 boys	1 water closet to 90 boys
1 urinal to 30 boys	1 urinal to 30 boys

Water closets for elementary schools should be 13 inches to the rim—junior size. Standard size is proper for both junior and senior high schools. Construction should be of porcelain or vitreous china, with flush rim, siphon jet, extended lip or elongated bowl, and open-front seat without a cover. Flush valves and vacuum breakers are preferable to flush tanks. Indivdiual compartments with doors should be provided for each water closet.

Urinals of porcelain or vitreous china of

the individual bowl type that are automatically or individually flushed are recommended. Pedestal or wall-hung units are most sanitary. Trough or stall urinals are not acceptable.

Plumbing for sewage disposal. When a municipal sewage system is available for the disposal of school sewage, the problem that confronts the school is safe and adequate plumbing. Most states have a plumbing code that governs standards for new construction, but is not always applied to buildings already standing, whether they are public or private buildings. Yet older school buildings should be inspected for faulty plumbing.

Back siphonage is the greatest single hazard of faulty plumbing. Back siphonage may be due to cross-connections between water supply systems and sewers, breaks in sewers, or defective water and sewerage piping. Circulating and boosting pumps, water heaters, air compressors, and submerged water inlets

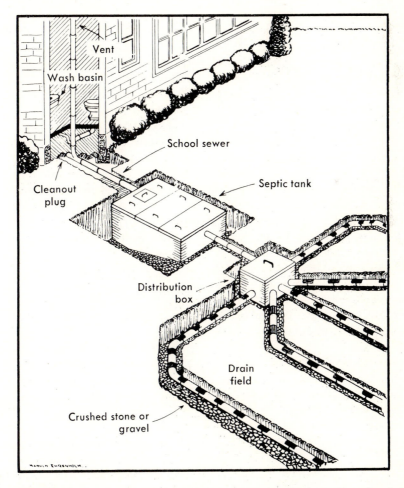

Fig. 16-5. Septic tank sewage disposal system. Facilities within the school are identical with those in schools connected to a municipal sewer. Wastes settle to the bottom of the tank, and liquid wastes soak into the ground by filtering out of spaces between tile.

in sinks may cause contaminated water to siphon back into the water main. If plumbing installation is not of recent vintage, it is an investment in health preservation to have a qualified plumber make a thorough inspection of the plumbing. His or her recommendations should not be neatly filed, but summarily carried out.

Septic tank. Schools without an available municipal sewerage system must provide their own sewage disposal system.

Chemical toilets are used when running water is not available. The vault may be a commercially produced metal one or constructed of concrete. Sodium hydroxide or some other caustic agent is added to the water in the tank. A bottom outlet permits the digested solid matter to be discharged into a soakage pit, where the liquid can seep into the soil. Chemical toilets are acceptable if running water is not available, but septic tanks are preferable if water can be provided.

A septic tank of adequate size that is properly designed and installed is entirely satisfactory for school use. Wastes are conducted into a concrete tank, which serves as a sedimentation and digestion chamber (Fig. 16-5). Liquids from the tank flow into a distribution box, which channels the effluent evenly to the three or four lines of tile buried about a foot under the surface of the ground. A space of ½ inch between the ends of 4-inch field tile permits the liquid to soak into the surrounding gravel and soil. The tank must be cleaned out every 2 or 3 years.

The size of septic tank depends on use. The usual formula is a tank capacity of 15 gallons per student. Most plumbing firms install septic tanks, and some firms make a specialty of their installation.

SPECIAL TOILET ROOMS

Kindergartens, locker rooms, faculty lounges, health service facilities, office suites, and other locations in a school building may have special toilet rooms. The number of fixtures in the kindergarten toilet room can follow the elementary school standards. In locker rooms the number of fixtures should be adequate for the enrollment of the largest physical education class. Other special toilet rooms should be equipped with fixtures to meet the maximum needs of the enrollment.

FOOD SERVICE

A food service unit is properly located on the ground floor and is conveniently accessible from the outside. It should be planned to facilitate the most direct route from corridor to serving line, to water cooler, to tables, to soiled-dish counter, and finally to corridor again. A large school will have a serving room, kitchen, and dining room (Fig. 16-6). In smaller schools the serving room is replaced by a serving counter between the kitchen and dining room. Some schools find it necessary to use the dining room for a classroom, for a study hall, and for student activities such as student council meetings. The dining room should be especially pleasant, should be well lighted, and should have smooth washable walls that are painted in attractive pastel shades.

Facilities. Expenditures on food service facilities represent a long-term investment in the health protection of schoolchildren. Dependable equipment costs very little more than inferior questionable equipment.

Storage rooms should be cool (50° to 60° F), well lighted, adequately ventilated, and vermin free. There should be adequate shelves and clean barrels, boxes, and bins for vegetable and fruit storage.

Refrigeration units should be spacious enough to allow ample room for all foods that need refrigeration. Temperatures must be below 50° F. Dairy products should be kept separate from meats or other foods from which they may absorb odors.

Dishwashing facilities must include an

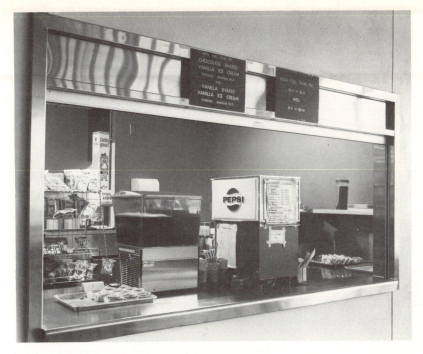

Fig. 16-6. Snack bar for high school students. As a supplement to the cafeteria, the snack bar has been especially valuable in serving students whose schedules are irregular. (Courtesy Corvallis Public Schools, Corvallis, Ore.)

adequate supply of hot water, a wash sink, a rinse sink, and a sanitizing sink that contains a decontaminant or water above 170° F. Use of baskets for the dishes will allow dipping, speed up handling, and make wiping unnecessary.

Dishes and trays should be of smooth nonporous material for easy cleaning. Rusted utensils and cracked or chipped dishes should be discarded.

Handwashing facilities should be available in the kitchen as well as in the toilet rooms. Hot and cold water, soap, and paper towels must be provided. Lockers for storing outdoor clothing and uniforms should be provided for the lunchroom workers.

Practices. The best facilities available would be of little value if the food service personnel did not carry out sound practices.

These are simple but important requirements:

1. Food service personnel should meet the same health standards as teachers.
2. The presence of symptoms of communicable disease or open sores should be sufficient cause to remove a worker from duty.
3. A susceptible worker who has been exposed to a communicable disease should have clearance from a physician before reporting for duty.
4. Workers should bathe and change clothing frequently.
5. Workers should wear light-colored washable uniforms while serving food, and aprons while preparing food.
6. Caps, bands, or hairnets should be worn.
7. Workers should wash the hands *before* beginning work, handling food, and serving food, and *after* coughing and sneezing, using a handkerchief, returning from the toilet, fixing the hair, and using objects handled by others; paper towels should be used for drying the hands.

8. Dishes and utensils should be scraped and pre-rinsed.
9. Dishes and utensils should be washed in hot water (100° to 120° F) containing a detergent, rinsed, then sanitized for 2 minutes in very hot water (170° F) or in water containing chlorine or other decontaminant.
10. Glasses and silverware should be wiped with clean dry towels; dishes should not be wiped.
11. "Tasting" spoons should be used for testing food.
12. Forks, tongs, or spoons should be used for serving.
13. Safety precautions should be taken to prevent the following:
    a. Burns, by using metal match containers, turning pot handles away from workers, using pot holders, opening oven door of gas range before lighting the burner, keeping inflammable materials away from the range, and preventing fat from getting too hot
    b. Cuts, by providing a holder for sharp implements and by requiring workers to cut away from themselves as well as to dispose of opened cans and broken dishes and glass immediately
    c. Falls, by keeping floors dry and free of rubbish, keeping passageways clear, requiring workers to wear low-heeled shoes, and disposing of opened cans and broken dishes and glass immediately
    d. Other hazards, by excluding all but workers from the kitchen, keeping poisons away from the kitchen, keeping shelves uncrowded, discarding broken equipment, following recognized practices in operating machines and disconnecting electrical appliances, and turning off gas when not in use
14. Good storage, including refrigeration, is both sanitary and economical.
15. Tight-covered garbage receptacles should be emptied daily.
16. Ample light in the kitchen and dining room is important.
17. Good ventilation is necessary.
18. Floors should be mopped daily.
19. Walls and ceilings should be clean and light in color.
20. A pleasant, moderately quiet atmosphere in the lunchroom during the lunch is desirable.

In any lunchroom the important factor is competent personnel; this is especially important for the person in charge. If every effort is made to familiarize the students and faculty with the needs and requirements of the lunchroom, understanding will lead to harmonious cooperation. The lunchroom is

there for the students and faculty. Respect by the students most likely comes from a realization that this is their lunchroom and they have a joint responsibility in making it a place of which they can be proud. Some noise in the lunchroom is inevitable, but it can be held within bounds without completely restraining the students.

Teachers should correlate the lunchroom experience with the health instruction program. Wash parades just before the lunch hour can establish the practice of washing the hands thoroughly before one eats. When lunch is eaten in the classroom, paper covers for the desks help to create desirable attitudes toward cleanliness at mealtime. Discussions on lunchroom practices and conduct can be fruitful.

Inspections. Administrators are responsible for the sanitation of the food services, and, although health department sanitarians may be asked to make periodic inspections and recommendations, school administrators should provide for in-school inspections. It is a common administrative practice to delegate the task to the director of the school health program. In the absence of a health director the health instructor may be assigned the duty. Such an inspection should be made constructively to improve conditions and to encourage lunchroom personnel in the performance of their duties. A concise, practical inspection form, developed jointly by the Oregon State Department of Education and the Oregon State Board of Health, has been highly satisfactory. (See accompanying form.)

Although this form is designed for use by an outside inspector, it is equally adaptable for use by school personnel.

GYMNASIUM AND ACTIVITY ROOM

The gymnasium in junior and senior high schools and the activity room in elementary schools should be clean, well lighted, adequately ventilated, and free of all possible

SANITATION REPORT

School and institution food-handling facilities

S Milk, cream _____   Name _____
O Ice cream _____   Location _____
U Cream-filled   No. served daily _____
R   pastry _____   Water supply _____
C Meats _____   Sewage system _____
E Shellfish _____
S Ice _____

All items are satisfactory unless otherwise indicated.

Superintendent's name _____   Mailing address _____

Physical plant	Items	Remarks

1. Floors _____
   Clean and good repair

2. Walls and ceilings _____
   Washable, clean, good repair

3. Doors and windows _____
   Clean screens if needed

4. Lighting _____
   Clean fixtures; adequate light

5. Ventilation _____
   Free from cooking odors (hoods or fans or forced ventilation)

6. Toilet facilities _____
   Clean, good repair; proper vestibules and signs; convenient

7. Lavatory _____
   Located in kitchen and/or toilet room; hot-cold water; soap; paper towels

8. Water supply _____
   Bacteriologically safe

9. Sewage disposal _____
   Adequate

10. Plumbing approved _____

11. Rodent, insect control _____
    Building free of rodent harborage

12. Employees' locker space _____
    Clean, adequate

Equipment

13. Cooking utensils _____
    Good construction; satisfactory condition

Continued.

SANITATION REPORT—cont'd

14. Worktables _____
                        Durable; easy to clean

15. Plates, silverware _____
                   Good condition; sufficient for size of operation

16. Refrigeration _____
                        Adequate; proper temperature

17. Protected display for exposed foods _____

18. Dishwashing equipment _____
        Approved construction for hand or machine dishwashing; sufficient hot water

19. Storage room _____
                Clean; dry; well-ventilated; vermin-free shelves; racks

20. Garbage cans _____
                        Cover; sufficient supply

Operation

21. Dishwashing _____
                     Proper washing and sanitizing

22. Food preparation _____
          Proper refrigeration (cream products, etc.); clean and minimum handling

23. Wholesomeness of food _____
          Free from spoilage and contamination; canned foods properly processed
                            from inspected sources

24. Equipment _____
                Power equipment; stoves, utensils, etc. kept clean

25. Storage _____
              Kept clean; food off floor; bulk food in tight containers

26. Employees _____
          Clean uniforms or aprons; hair confined; free from infectious disease; no
                        open or inflamed skin lesions

27. Garbage and refuse handling _____
              Cans kept covered and washed; proper disposal of garbage;
                            no trash accumulation

28. Premises _____
                Kept clean; free from rodents and insects

29. Storage of cleaning supplies _____
                        Separate from food storage

30. Cloths _____
                            Kept clean

Date of Inspection _____ Sanitarian _____

hazards. A hardwood floor with a nonslip finish, cleaned daily, keeps dust at a minimum. Windows are often more of a detriment than an asset in a gymnasium. Glass bricks should fill the window space when masonry is used in construction. High windows on both sides may not give adequate light because of the width of the gymnasium. Screens over the windows will reduce illumination, but may be necessary. Artificial lighting as the sole form of lighting can be entirely satisfactory. Forced ventilation is necessary when large crowds occupy the gymnasium. For classes of 30 to 40 students, window-gravity ventilation can be adequate. Regular inspections of conditions and practices are essential for the promotion of safety in the gymnasium.

LOCKER ROOMS

A well-lighted locker room is usually an attractive and sanitary locker room. Located adjacent to the gymnasium, the locker room should provide at least 12 square feet of floor space per student, based on the class with the largest number of students. Floors and walls constructed of nonporous material promote sanitation. Floors should have excellent drainage and should be cleaned daily. A clean, well-lighted locker room is usually a tidy one. Adequate heat and mechanical ventilation complete the picture of excellent sanitation.

SHOWER ROOMS

Nonslip tile flooring, slightly crowned in the center, is necessary for a satisfactory shower room. On the walls, tile wainscot to a height of 5 feet and nonporous material the rest of the way will complete the construction requirements. At least 10 square feet of floor space should be allowed for each shower head. The recognized standard is one shower head for every four students, based on the

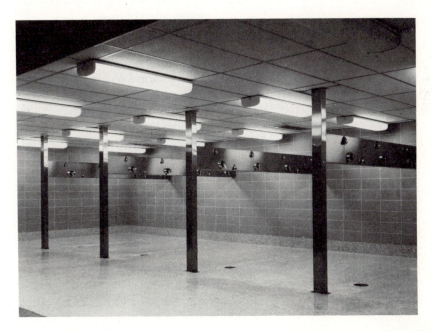

Fig. 16-7. Effective protection against ringworm (athlete's foot). Continuous light in shower and locker rooms destroys fungi that cannot tolerate light.

class with the largest number of students. Shower heads should be at chin height. Different levels of shower heads will provide for the height variation among students. Whether individual or gang showers are used, water-mixing chambers with wheel control valves are recommended. The control of water temperature is quicker and easier with this type of equipment. Compartments for individual showers have largely disappeared. However, drying rooms between the shower and locker rooms have found favor.

In practice, control of fungus infections of the feet is most effective if regular inspections of the feet are made and treatment of all students with the condition is required. Well-lighted locker rooms mopped daily with a detergent complete the picture of easy effective control of the spread of ringworm (Fig. 6-7). The footbath has many disadvantages and inconveniences and is not essential if other means of control are used.

SWIMMING POOL

Sanitation of the swimming pool is a special responsibility of the physical education staff. Two factors sum up the essence of a sanitary swimming pool—construction and regulation. A properly constructed pool provides for filtration, chlorination, and recirculation and straining of water. A chlorine content of 0.2 to 0.5 parts per million will inactivate all pathogenic organisms in the water. Daily samples are taken for determination of bacteriological and chlorine contents. Plans for swimming pools have become so well standardized that schools can now proceed in full confidence that the recommendations of architects and engineers will be totally reliable.

Regulation of a swimming pool has one essential—a qualified person to supervise the use of the pool. Standard regulations are posted governing the users of the pool. Personal cleanliness, freedom from communi-

cable disease, and proper conduct and personal habits in the pool are requisites. It is essential that everyone who uses the pool take a cleansing shower, wear a clean suit, and use clean towels. Water temperatures between 72° and 78° F and room temperatures between 75° and 82° F are maintained.

HOUSEKEEPING

The actual housekeeping of the school should be done by the custodial staff. However, the students should cooperate in all possible ways to make the task of the custodian easier and more effective.

It is the custodian's responsibility to clean the chalkboards and erasers, and it should be done when students are not present. If damp cloths for chalkboards and vacuum cleaners for erasers are used, dust in the school will be reduced. It is equally essential that furniture and fixtures be dusted with a treated cloth. Sweeping or any other activity of the custodian should be planned to cause a minimum of dust.

The key to good schoolkeeping is the work done during vacation periods. Schools in superb condition before the session for the year begins are easy to keep clean. Painted and washed walls and woodwork, refinished floors, renovated fixtures and furniture, general repair, and replacement of all defective equipment are the prelude to healthful school living.

HEALTHFUL MENTAL ENVIRONMENT

Important as the physical environment is, the mental environment is even more important because it is less tangible than the physical environment and thus more difficult to control. A healthy mental environment must be built up and maintained by recognizing the factors that favorably or unfavorably affect each child's adjustment.

Characteristics. There are certain attributes or characteristics of a healthy mental environment in the schoolroom that one can readily identify:

1. The children are relaxed and at ease.
2. They feel that the teacher and their classmates regard them highly. Their age-mates become their peer group, and approval of their peer group becomes progressively more important, even to such a degree that some high school students will rate peer approval to be more important than parental approval.
3. They have a high level of self-esteem.
4. They are challenged by the situation.
5. They are confident they can succeed.
6. They experience success.
7. They receive adequate personal gratification from their success.

To attain this atmosphere in the classroom, the school has certain responsibilities:

1. Recognize and identify in children those deviations in emotional adjustment that fall out of the normal range, and undertake reeducation
2. Provide all children with experiences that will stimulate the progressive development of desirable patterns of emotional behavior
3. Provide students with esthetic experiences that will develop an awareness of beauty in life and help them identify with cultural groups
4. Provide opportunities for the development of concepts of values and for practices in conduct arising from these concepts

Role of the teacher. Teachers must be realistic and deal objectively with student adjustment. They should know more about children than the children know about themselves. All school activities directly or indirectly contribute to the personality growth of the students. Because each child is unique, it is necessary to provide for all types and degrees of participation.

To create a hygienic mental environment,

a teacher can make many contributions to the adjustment of the student:

1. Adjust the difficulty of the curriculum to the mental capacity of the student
2. Adjust the curriculum to the educational maturity of the student
3. Make special provisions for specific deficiencies and thus fortify the weaknesses
4. Develop high ideals and good habits of conduct as by-products of reading, discussion, visual aids, and other procedures
5. Utilize the social influence of the group to aid in developing a child
6. Give students opportunities to make decisions
7. Develop responsibility and leadership
8. Develop a wholesome interest in law and order within the classroom, the school, and the community
9. Provide desirable social experiences
10. Create a desire in each child to participate in extracurricular activities
11. Instruct pupils in extracurricular activities
12. Restrict or extend extracurricular functions in keeping with the needs of each student
13. Give due encouragement and credit to each child for each accomplishment
14. Be an understanding listener
15. Make assistance as real as possible by helping pupils to help themselves
16. For the poorly adjusted child find the group and teacher to which he or she will best adjust
17. Help the parents know the child better
18. Help the parents develop a wholesome attitude toward a child's ability
19. Help the parents acquire a sensible attitude toward success in school
20. Help the parents give the child the most wholesome environment possible

21. Supplement the home environment as far as possible

Healthful school living is an environment in which students effectively and enjoyably carry out a self-gratifying program of activities in a school plant that provides for the highest possible level of physical health. A school provides healthful living when students can develop a high level of physical and emotional well-being in an atmosphere in which there develops a high level of self-esteem, growing out of self-gratification in accomplishment.

QUESTIONS AND EXERCISES

1. "A healthful school environment can motivate many students to aspire to a higher standard of home life than they now are accustomed to." Explain this statement.
2. "A lot of fine knowledge has been attained in old, unattractive school buildings." Interpret this contention.
3. What are the benefits that accrue from having the students assume responsibility for the cleanliness and attractiveness of their school?
4. When preliminary plans are being developed for a new school building, who should be consulted and have an opportunity to review plans and make suggestions?
5. Analyze the program of having student monitors responsible for various tasks in the school building.
6. How would you develop courtesy in an elementary school?
7. How would you develop courtesy in a secondary school?
8. Set up an organization to maintain order and cleanliness in the toilet rooms of an elementary school.
9. Why are public health officials greatly concerned about the possible spread of infectious hepatitis via the school lunchroom?
10. In selecting a school site, what undesirable social conditions should be avoided?
11. What is the primary purpose of school ventilation?
12. What are the advantages of air conditioning over window ventilation in a school?
13. Why do some school authorities prefer artificial lighting in schools?
14. Rate the illumination in the room in which your health class is held.
15. What would you rate as the number one essential in school sanitation?
16. Why should a kindergarten have special toilet facilities?
17. How frequently should the gymnasium, swimming pool, and outdoor physical education facilities be given a safety inspection?
18. How would you prevent "athlete's foot" from being spread in a school?
19. Compare the schoolroom having a mentally unhealthy atmosphere with the schoolroom having a mentally healthy atmosphere.
20. What can each teacher do to promote more healthful school living?

REFERENCES AND SELECTED READINGS

Aaron, J. E., and Bridges, A. F.: First aid and emergency care: prevention and protection of injuries, text ed., Chicago, 1972, The Macmillan Co.

Aaron, J. E., and Strasser, M. K.: Driver and traffic safety education, ed. 2, Chicago, 1977, The Macmillan Co.

American Academy of Pediatrics: School health: a guide to health professionals, Evanston, Ill., 1978, The Academy.

American Alliance for Health, Physical Education, and Recreation: Approaches to problems of public school administration in health, physical education, and recreation, Washington, D.C., 1969, The Alliance.

American Association for Health, Physical Education, and Recreation and National Education Association: Health aspects of the school lunch program, Washington, D.C., 1962, National Education Association.

American Association of School Administrators: American school buildings, twenty-seventh yearbook, Washington, D.C., 1949, National Education Association.

Arens, J.: Dangers to children and youth, Durham, N.C., 1970, Moore Publishing Co.

Boles, H. W.: Step by step to better school facilities, New York, 1965, Holt, Rinehart & Winston.

Brainerd, A. D.: Handbook for school custodians, ed. 5, Lincoln, Neb., 1961, University of Nebraska Press.

Fein, L. J.: Ecology of the public schools, Indianapolis, 1971, Bobbs-Merrill Co., Inc.

Haggerte, R. J., et al.: Child health and the community, New York, 1975, John Wiley & Sons, Inc.

Hamburg, M., and Hamburg, M. V.: Health and social problems in the school, Philadelphia, 1968, Lea & Febiger.

Hickols, J. E.: School building codes, New York, annual, American School Publishing Corp.

Hopkins, E. S., Bingley, W. M., and Schuker, G. W.: The practice of sanitation, ed. 4, Baltimore, 1970, The Williams & Wilkins Co.

Jefcoate, A.: Health and human values: an ecological

approach, New York, 1972, John Wiley & Sons, Inc.

Joint Committee on Health Problems in Education of the National Education Association and the American Medical Association: Healthful school environment, Washington, D.C., 1969, National Education Association.

Katz, A. H., and Felton, J. S.: Health and the community, New York, 1965, The Free Press.

National Council on Schoolhouse Construction: NCSC guide for planning school plants, East Lansing, Mich., 1964, National Council on Schoolhouse Construction, Michigan State University.

Roth, A.: The new schoolhouse, rev. ed., New York, 1966, Frederick A. Praeger, Ins.

School building research, Washington, D.C., 1963, Building Research Institute.

Spiegelman, M.: Introduction to demogra Philadelphia, 1974, Lea & Febiger.

Stack, H. J., and Elkow, J. D.: Education ed. 4, New York, 1966, Prentice-Hall, .

United States Department of Health, Education and Welfare, Public Health Service: Environmental engineering for the school: a manual of recommended practice, Public Health Service publication No. 856, Washington, D.C., 1961, U.S. Government Printing Office.

United States Department of Health, Education and Welfare, Public Health Service: School health programs—an outline for school and community, Washington, D.C., 1961, U.S. Government Printing Office.

Weeden, V.: Beware of the ides of April, Safety Education 40:entire issue, April, 1961.

PART SIX

Appraisal in school health practice

CHAPTER 17

Evaluation

How much has the school health program improved the health status of children? How effective is the school health program? Does it measure up to the recognized standards? Is the health instruction effective? Does the school meet standards for healthful living? All these are inevitable and logical questions for those who concern themselves with the school health program. To what extent the school health activities are meeting the general and specific objectives of the health program is of concern to the students, the parents, the community, the school administration, and, particularly, the health instructors.

Ideally, evaluation includes both objective measurements and the subjective judgments of experts. In school health, evaluation is a process of determining the effectiveness of the program and its several phases by measuring the degree to which the health objectives of the school are being achieved. It encompasses the purely subjective transient judgments incidental to health activities as well as the highly objective scientific measurement of factors affecting health. Thus evaluation is inherent in the teacher's observation of a child's attitude toward the dental examination and in the audiometrist's determination of a child's hearing acuity by means of a pure-tone audiometer. Evaluation includes a wide range of activities.

In appraising school health activities, a number of subjective judgments must be employed. Such judgments have particular value when they are made by specially trained and experienced personnel. Observations by teachers in daily contact with the student and by people outside of the school are also of special value. Proper interpretation and weighing of these judgments can make them highly meaningful. At the same time, there are some devices that provide objective data that could be standardized and used for measuring different aspects of school health. Although these are not necessarily instruments of precise measurement, they add objectivity to personal judgment. Their use is analogous to the use of a yardstick to measure the distance between two school buildings. The figure thus obtained will not be precisely correct, but will be more so than the estimate of some individual.

PURPOSES OF EVALUATION

In general terms, evaluation of the school health program is both an inventory of present status and an assessment of progress (Fig. 17-1). Moreover, a comprehensive approach includes two distinct aspects of evaluation, (1) the process or program, and (2) the product or pupil. In the area of program evaluation, the following purposes are served.

423

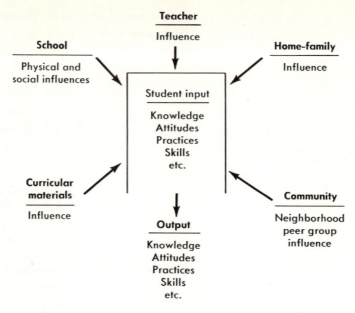

Fig. 17-1. Multiple factors affect health education outcomes.

1. To determine the present status of the school health program
2. To assess progress made toward achievement of program objectives
3. To provide information about program strengths and weaknesses
4. To provide data that can be used as justification for seeking additional support and funds for the program
5. To provide information about program activities such as health services and health instruction as a basis for modifying the program in order to improve it

Important purposes of pupil health evaluations are as follows:

1. To determine pupil health status as well as individual health education status
2. To provide information that will enable students to make self-evaluations and adjustments in their study programs in order to improve progress
3. To inform parents of their children's health status
4. To provide data on students' learning achievements from the health instruction program that can serve as a basis for grading students
5. To enable teachers and school officials to adapt school programs in order to meet the health and educational needs of children

Time of evaluation. Different conditions require different treatment, but a general pattern of evaluation suggests itself in almost all school health situations that merit measurement:

1. Pretest or a measurement before an activity begins, to establish a basis for future comparisons
2. Periodic tests during the program to determine the effects of a particular program or activity
3. Verification study when it is doubtful that the activity is effective or is producing the desired results
4. Special measures to determine possible effects of the program that were unintended
5. Posttest after the activity in order to

assess the final status or the full effect of the school health program

EVALUATION PROCEDURES

Because of the number of factors in the health program that must be evaluated and the variety of conditions and situations under which evaluation must be done, it is obviously not possible to set up a step-by-step procedure that will serve all purposes. Yet certain principles will apply. Some of these are as follows:

1. The general program objectives must be clearly stated
2. Specific objectives must be stated precisely in order to serve as measurable outcomes
3. All products, records, and by-products of the activity should be preserved, since they can be of value in assessing the effects of the program on participants
4. Methods and instruments used to collect program information must meet the standards of objectivitiy, reliability, and validity
5. Information about the program should be collected early enough to be useful in revising or modifying the program for improvement
6. Efforts should be made to determine whether students can transfer or apply what they have learned or to exhibit skills they have learned from the health instruction program
7. Evaluation of the school health program requires that information be collected from many different sources including the school, the home, the neighborhood, and the larger community
8. The final evaluation of the school health program involves first collecting valid data and then exercising expert judgment in arriving at decisions and program recommendations
9. The results of the evaluation must be applied to future situations by revising the program or perhaps modifying objectives to improve its effectiveness

Appraisers. The specific individual who evaluates any phase of the school program varies with the need and the situation. In one way or another, many people are evaluating the health program. Children, parents, and anyone coming in contact with the school can contribute useful information for the appraisal of the school health program. However, the final evaluation should be reserved for those persons most qualified by experience and training.

A system-wide or school-wide evaluation of the entire program may be conducted by outside specialists, the state department of education, the health education director of the school, an administrator, a committee of teachers, the school health council, or any combination of these. A special phase of the program may be appraised by one person or a small committee. In practice, evaluation of instruction is done for the most part by the teachers concerned. Occasionally comprehensive standardized health knowledge tests are administered. Testing is a specialty, but one that teachers can master by study and application. There are both advantages and disadvantages in evaluations that are made by those closest to the health program and most concerned with its success. Critical self-analysis on the part of the tester will help to eliminate the disadvantages of subjectivity and still retain the advantages of first-hand knowledge.

EVALUATION DEVICES

There are few things in life that can be said to be proved without qualification. The best that can be done is to present evidence one way or another. This should be kept in mind as a guide in the selection and use of any evaluation instrument, because the instrument is merely a device for obtaining evidence. Some human being must interpret and weigh the evidence. Some devices provide fairly precise data, whereas others yield only general tendencies or relative differences. Many evaluating devices that have recognized mechanical faults and qualitative shortcomings may nevertheless serve worthwhile purposes in certain situations. A critical analysis should be made of every measure used, but the device should also be appraised in terms of the service it performs and of the purpose for which it is used.

Statistical measures. Statistical methods have long been applied to measurement in education. Norms can be established and thus provide a standard for comparison. Numerical scores suggest precision and are objective and definite. Averages, variations, and consistencies can be determined with a high degree of accuracy. Tests of health knowledge are particularly amenable to statistical treatment. Raw scores can be made more meaningful if an analysis is made of the scores in specific sections of the test and of the types of errors that have been made. Statistical methods, when applicable in the measurement and evaluation of health outcomes such as knowledge and attitudes, should be given preference. However, care should be taken in the interpretation of statistical results as well as of other data. A high correlation does not establish a cause-and-effect relationship.

Clinical appraisals. Clinical evaluations are less precise and standardized than statistical evaluations. Yet clinical evaluation is the only means available for appraising some activities in health. The determination of the health status of a child does not lend itself readily to statistical treatment. The findings of the physician and dentist, the observations of the nurse and teacher, the personal history of the child, and the report of the parents can be adequate for clinically evaluating the health status of the child. Even though statistical precision may be lacking, the purpose

of health evaluation may be well served. To date, no satisfactory standardized test of health attitudes has been developed. Nevertheless, teachers can devise their own techniques for appraising attitudes by systematically observing children in situations that reflect their choices and atitudes toward health. Norms cannot be determined and perhaps are not necessary. Too many health activities and objectives are multiphased and involve too many intangible values to be gauged with objective test instruments. Until such measures are available, clinical appraisals will have to be utilized to attain a general evaluation of various health factors.

Types of instruments. A variety of devices is available for health evaluation purposes.

Observations. This is the most frequently used instrument in all school appraisal and can be both meaningful and valuable in health evaluation. To be most effective, observation must be critical and precise. By using self-discipline and self-direction in observation, a teacher can develop a highly accurate level of discrimination.

Interviews and conferences. These techniques reveal many things other devices cannot elicit. Conferences involving parents and friends who know a child are highly productive in disclosing health information.

Self-appraisal. Analysis by students of their own health discloses information and stimulates interest. A checklist combined with original comments will be highly meaningful.

Questionnaires. A series of specific questions can be helpful in obtaining information on health practices and problems of deepest personal concern. Several standard health questionnaires are in general use.

Checklist. Composed of objective items that usually consist of yes-or-no answers or descriptive lists, such lists are frequently used for studies of such things as sanitary conditions or health practices.

Surveys. Surveys relate to people, including sociological facts and psychological data, such as knowledge, attitudes, and practices as well as health status.

Records. Family and personal health records can be rewarding sources of data. School health records should be sufficiently complete to be a dependable source of information.

Reports. Accounts, descriptions, or statements, either incidental or developed for a special purpose, have value, especially when correlated with other data.

Achievement tests. The most commonly used form of measurement in the school is the written or oral test. Both are adaptable to health instruction and are particularly effective in revealing the nature and extent of student learning.

Criteria. The processes of evaluation, including procedures and instruments, should meet the criteria of objectivity, reliability, validity, and the practical considerations of usability.

Objectivity implies the elimination of personal bias, self-interest, or judgment. It is the converse of subjectivity, which denotes that personal interest colors the decision or choice. Certain laboratory tests that the physician uses in health examinations may be totally objective. An electrocardiograph gives an objective measure of the frequency and rhythm of the heartbeat and the nature of the action of the heart. Perhaps the recording of blood pressure is considered objective, although human judgment and a subsequent error can creep in. Whenever human judgment is involved, the evaluation cannot properly be termed totally objective.

Perhaps no test used by the teacher to measure learning is totally objective. Although the test items may be written in objective forms, such as a multiple-choice test, the selection of the item and judgment as to its quality is a subjective process. If a hundred specially trained people agree on the items, personal bias—and thus subjectivity—is reduced. The practical approach in evaluation is to reduce subjectivity to a minimum and use this approach only when no objective device is available.

Validity is the extent to which a test measures what it is designed to measure. When the busy teacher constructs tests, perhaps the best means for establishing a reasonable degree of validity is to depend on the collective judgment of several qualified people. Standard tests may also be used as a basis for comparison. Analysis of particular items will be of help. For example, selecting test items from the most relevant subject matter of the instruction program will help to strengthen the validity of the test, whereas the inclusion of any test items extraneous to the course will weaken it. Validity implies a balance in the test comparable to the weighing of the material (e.g., as used in a course) that is to be tested. In this regard certain test construction procedures help to establish the reliability and validity of a test, such as developing test items that have an acceptable level of difficulty and discrimination.

Care should be taken in the use of attitude tests. The results of such tests should not be used for grading. Under such circumstances the student is less likely to indicate his or her true attitude but instead may respond in terms of knowledge or what the individual believes to be the "desired" response.

Reliability is the consistency of measurement. Retesting, testing comparable groups, and treating the results statistically will yield a measure of group and individual consistency. If they are highly similar or correlated, two sets of scores obtained from two similar tests covering the same field indicate a high degree of reliability. The busy teacher hardly has the time needed to go through all the procedures necessary for establishing reliability. The standard procedure of the classroom teacher is to construct tests that personal experience indicates will obtain meaningful results and to supplement these with standardized tests.

EVALUATION OF CHANGE IN HEALTH STATUS OF CHILD

Since the present-day school health program places great emphasis on building up and maintaining the highest possible level of health in every child, a reliable means for measuring health status change would be extremely valuable. No single scale or measure has been devised, but a combination of several tests and methods can be used to obtain a workable profile of a student's health status.

A recent thorough health examination will obviously give the best indication of the child's health. Comparison with previous examinations will be relatively simple for children who have had defects corrected during the interim. However, for many youngsters no such corrections will have been necessary, and to make an evaluation of any change in health status commands the skills and expert judgment of the physician.

In the absence of a health examination the teacher's own assessment or appraisal of a child's level of health will be of value. Although highly subjective, the appraisal considers buoyancy, pleasure in activity, vigor, zest, endurance, capacity to recover from fatigue, ability to relax, steady weight increase, absence of defects, and social adjustment. The appraisal can be supplemented by the child's school health record. Dental corrections, vision tests and corrections, hearing tests, weight and height changes, and records of illnesses may be significant sources of information. The physical growth charts in Chapter 3 can be used to portray the child's developmental course.

If the teacher's appraisal is supplemented by the judgment of other teachers who have had ample opportunity to observe the child

and to obtain the assessment of the parents, the subjective factor will be reduced. Whether the evaluation will be of value is secondary to the importance of developing the child's interest in his or her own health status. If the child has had the benefit of good health guidance and instruction, a personal assessment of health status will be worthy of inclusion in the evaluation.

EVALUATION OF ADMINISTRATIVE PRACTICES

School health work is advanced or retarded in terms of administrative policies and practices that relate to the health program. An insight into the success or failure of the health program of a school may well be gained by a survey of administrative practices. The usual survey is made by means of a checklist of the widely accepted school health responsibilities of the administrator. Such a list should include the following:

1. Recognize health as a basic objective of education
2. Secure and budget adequate funds for the health program
3. Keep parents informed of the health program
4. Establish an appropriate cooperative relationship with community health agencies
5. Maintain communication with community organizations
6. Employ qualified school health service personnel
7. Become informed about health problems of the school-age group
8. Arrange the school day in accord with sound health practice
9. Establish an effective system for keeping health records
10. Establish a policy on school health examinations
11. Provide for health observations by the teachers
12. Establish a systematic referral program
13. Promote measures to ensure corrections for every child
14. Establish program policies aimed at control of communicable diseases
15. Procure necessary materials, facilities, and equipment for health instruction
16. Provide time and facilities for health instruction in the secondary school

17. Appoint only qualified teachers for health instruction
18. Provide a healthful physical environment
19. Participates in organized play at noon and recess
20. Establish a school safety program
21. Provide facilities, personnel, and an established plan to meet emergencies
22. Provide health services for professional personnel
23. Provide in-service health education for teachers
24. Provide for faculty sick leave

This checklist does not include all the health responsibilities of the administrator, but by specifying the essential minimum practices, it serves as a practical, realistic measure of the administration's contribution to the school health program.

EVALUATION OF THE SCHOOL HEALTH PROGRAM

Appraisal of the overall school health program is necessary as a measure of the completeness of the program, its function, and its effectiveness. A valid evaluation of the program would point up its strengths and weaknesses. Despite the recognized need for such an evaluation instrument, very few such appraisal forms are available. In consequence, most program assessments are either general surveys or evaluations of specific phases of the program, notably the health instruction phase.

Available standard forms differ in purpose, scope, and composition. They can be used to advantage, particularly if supplemented by other evaluative devices to serve specific situations and needs.

The following sources for use in evaluation are suggested:

1. Criteria for evaluating the junior college health program, Sacramento, Calif., 1962, State Department of Education (provides a good example of format, criteria, and rating scale that could be adopted for elementary and secondary school use).
2. Department of Health, Education and Welfare, Public Health Service: School health program: an outline for school and community, rev., Washington,

D.C., 1966, U.S. Government Printing Office, Public Health Service Publication No. 834.
3. Evaluative criteria, ed. 4, Washington, D.C., 1969, National Study of Secondary School Evaluation (sections on Health Education and Health Services).

A new school health program evaluation instrument is included in Appendix D. The self-appraisal checklist has been developed through a cooperative effort among representatives from state agencies and professional groups in the fields of education and health. It is published by the Ohio State Department of Education. The checklist contains an excellent set of standards pertaining to administration, health instruction, health services, and school health environment. Although the standards have been written specifically for the state of Ohio, school officials will find this checklist a very useful tool in evaluating their own programs.

Oregon State University developed a School Health Program Evaluation Scale in 1959. Perhaps ideally, a scale should measure the results of the health program, but the inherent difficulties are obvious. However, the use of inference tests in psychology has been highly successful, and this scale is based on the same principle. Studies have revealed that when school health programs attain their basic objectives, certain practices, procedures, standards, activities, and facilities are usually present. This scale was developed in terms of recognized procedures, practices, standard facilities, and activities. The inference is that if a school health program possesses certain attributes, the health objectives will be attained. Every effort has been exerted to make the scale applicable to urban and rural schools alike, and to small school systems as well as medium-sized and large school systems. A certain amount of subjectivity is inherent in some of the items; yet the total scale is reasonably objective. A member of the school staff may use the scale, or an independent outside person may rate the program with this instrument.

The scale appraises the various aspects of the health program and permits numerical scoring by providing for 1,000 possible points. Weighting is done by allocating 350 points to school health services, 400 points to health instruction, and 250 points to healthful school living. The scale has a two-fold purpose. First, it is of value to the teacher, health educator, and administrator in measuring the attainment and progress of the health program in terms of a recognized standard. It will indicate strengths and weaknesses. The second purpose is to furnish a means for comparing school health programs. The complete scale is given in Appendix D.

A review board of 24 experienced health educators critically analyzed all apsects of the original scale. Their independent criticisms and suggestions were incorporated into the next draft of the scale. The final form thus represents extended study, review, and experience. A scale must be a functional organ that undergoes constant growth and refinement in harmony with changes in the school health program.

Some health educators are apprehensive of any attempt to measure school health in terms that are too precise. Yet if we are to have tangible meaningful evaluations of school health work, our procedures must be well defined, clearly set forth, and definite. The field of school health has come of age sufficiently to accept discriminating, detailed examination rather than high-sounding generalities.

EVALUATION OF HEALTH SERVICES

Circumstances may make it desirable to evaluate health services independently of other phases of the health program. Such an evaluation would include the nature and frequency of health examinations, dental examinations; screening of vision, hearing, weight, and height; and the teacher's appraisal of the child's health. The follow-up program and correction of defects must be included. Prevention and control of diseases, emergency care, and first-aid provisions are part of the health services to be appraised.

Teachers and administrators can make effective use of two types of resources in evaluating school health services: (1) the evaluative checklist types of instruments, and (2) the published formal statements of standards from authoritative bodies. In this regard, the following references are suggested:

1. American Academy of Pediatrics: School health: a guide for physicians, Evanston, Ill., 1972, American Academy of Pediatrics, part III, pp. 81-112.
2. Joint Committee on Health Problems in Education of the National Education Association and the American Medical Association: Suggested school health policies, ed. 5, Chicago, 1966, American Medical Association, chap. 2, pp. 12-22.
3. School health program evaluation scale, part I, School health practices, Corvallis, Ore., 1959, Oregon State University. The section can be used independently of the remainder of the scale. In addition to weighting the different items, the section points up the different phases of health services that are recognized as essential.

EVALUATION OF HEALTHFUL SCHOOL LIVING

Any assessment of the school environment must extend beyond the mere static physical environment. It must encompass the activities and practices in the school that affect health promotion, disease prevention, safety, social adjustment, and esthetic appreciation. Evaluation must include factors affecting physical and mental health in terms of dynamic school living. The construction of the school plant and sanitation facilities are important, but an evaluation of healthful school living must be extended to the total school program and the people who are part of the child's environment.

No phase of the school health program is

as easy to appraise as the physical environment. Sanitary facilities are tangible, can be counted or tabulated, and involve relatively little analysis or subjective judgment. Even the safety elements of the school environment are amenable to easy identification and tabulation. Perhaps for these reasons sanitary surveys of schools have long been a common routine in school practice. Certainly these surveys should be continued but should be expanded into an evaluation of total healthful school living.

Most forms developed for use in making evaluations of the school environment are survey checklists that require yes or no answers, check marks, or × marks. Such survey forms have merit because of their directness, simplicity, and utility. Such a checklist is presented in Appendix D; it deals in definite terms, not relative ones. Either the school has 30 or more footcandles of light on working surfaces, or it does not. Either the fire extinguishers are properly distributed, or they are not. This type of survey has value in determining the status of the school environment and what should be done. It can serve as an incentive for improvement and, in subsequent appraisals, reveal improvement in conditions. Most state departments of education have similar checklist forms.

Perhaps a more functional evaluation of healthful school living can be made if part III in Appendix C is used. In this section the school is visualized in action as a dynamic community of students and school personnel. The various forces and factors that affect the well-being of the child are included and evaluated in terms of their influence on the student's total health. In addition to its appraisal of school life in action, this scale can serve as a stimulating instructional instrument. The students can benefit from the opportunity to participate in the evaluation if a scale of this type is used.

EVALUATION AND HEALTH INSTRUCTION

Two aspects of evaluation are applied to health instruction. An evaluation *of* the health instruction program differs from evaluation *in* health instruction, although the former carries a connotation of the measurement of the effectiveness of the health instruction activities.

Evaluation of the health instruction program. What should be included in a health instruction program? What subject areas should be included? What objectives should be recognized? What time allotment is made? What facilities, equipment, and materials are available? What methods are being used? To what extent do integration and correlation take place? What preparation should teachers have in health education? These are questions that must be answered in an evaluation of the school health instruction program.

Because schools vary markedly in their perception of the cardinal aims of health instruction, developing a universally applicable scale would be difficult. Any form broad enough to encompass all purposes and situations would be so all-inclusive as to be virtually impractical. The problem is to determine the essentials of health instruction and to construct a scale to evaluation such a program. Each school can rate itself in terms of these basics and then supplement the rating with an evaluation of the special features of its own program.

In part II, Health Instruction, of the School Health Program Evaluation Scale in Appendix C, the recognized essentials of school health instruction are presented. An individual health instructor can use part II as a suggested approach to health instruction. It can indicate strengths in the present program and possibilities for improvement. This scale can also be used in a time series study or as a pretest—posttest measure in order to assess progress or changes that may have occurred during a specific period.

An evaluation of a specific health course can be done by use of a checklist that includes the important criteria of classroom practice applied to health.

Inventory of the health course

A. Objectives of health instruction
  1. Are there both general and specific objectives?
  2. Are the objectives stated in terms of student behaviors?
  3. Do the statements of objectives specify the type of behavior and the content or subject matter to be learned?
  4. Are the objectives related to the health needs and interests of both students and society?
  5. Are objectives stated in terms of attitudes, skills, and practices as well as knowledge?
B. Course organization and content
  1. Is there use of conceptual statements or generalizations to facilitate organization and understanding of health content?
  2. Is there a logical order of health content?
  3. Is there a logical sequence of topics to be covered?
  4. Is the content or subject matter scientifically accurate?
  5. Are health topics correlated and/or integrated with other school subjects?
C. Learning activities and materials of instruction
  1. Do class activities relate to student interests?
  2. Are a variety of methods used in teaching?
  3. Are there a variety of materials and instructional aids used in teaching?
  4. Are provisions made for individual differences and for individualized instruction?
  5. Are materials current and scientifically accurate?
  6. Are students given frequent reviews of instruction?
D. Evaluation of instruction
  1. Is the classroom atmosphere conducive to learning?
  2. Do students appear alert and interested in the health instruction?
  3. Are students given ample opportunity for class participation?
  4. Are student objectives, content, learning activities, and materials effectively related?
  5. Is student progress effectively measured in terms of course objectives?
  6. Is the course of curriculum regularly evaluated and revised?

Evaluation in health instruction. The development of instruments for evaluating the effectiveness of health instruction requires an understanding of the subject field, a grasp of the outcomes toward which health instruction is directed, competency in test construction, and a willingness to put forth the effort that creativeness demands. Whether a teacher needs a simple survey of health practices or a complex objective test to measure students' understanding and appreciation of health values, demands on time, patience, ingenuity, and energy are involved.

Test construction and testing are competencies that every classroom teacher should strive to master. Standard tests have their place and value, but constant reliance on such tests indicates a limited classroom testing program. Standard tests cannot replace teacher-made tests. A rich, meaningful evaluation program means tests and testing that are integrated with the objectives, procedures, activities, experiences, techniques, concomitant learning, skills, and values developed in the class. Like other teaching competencies, testing is not something mysterious and beyond the ability of the typical health teacher. Testing can be mastered by study and practice. A teacher need not attain the competence of a specialist to do an acceptable job of testing. In addition to its contribution to the instructional program, competency in testing is a source of personal professional gratification to the teacher.

Tests are used for diagnostic purposes, to determine progress, and to measure final achievement. In all cases, tests should reveal the nature and extent of learning. They can be tailor-made to fit each situation and can be both enjoyable and stimulating. Tests should be considered a means to facilitate learning. Students should be encouraged to think of tests as an opportunity to demonstrate knowledge and skill. Student fear of tests can be overcome by using tests frequently as another method of teaching. Instead of invariably using tests results for the purpose of grading, they can be used as a means of review and of stimulating learning. By developing tests of high quality and by making proper use of them, teachers can help students develop positive attitudes toward testing. In all testing, teachers should make an effort to put students in a proper frame of mind before the test.

The steps in test construction should follow a fairly well-developed set of procedures such as the following:

1. Prepare a list of the major objectives
2. Develop a content outline of topics to be covered
3. Develop a comprehensive list of specific objectives
4. Classify the objectives into categories, such as
   a. Cognitive or knowledge facts, terminology, application, analysis interpretation, synthesis, and evaluation
   b. Affective interests, attitudes, appreciations, and values
   c. Psychomotor skills, practices, and technical performances
5. Devise test situations that will reveal what students have learned in relation to the specific objectives
6. Prepare test items appropriate to the different types (domains) of objectives
7. Try out the test in order to determine
   a. The degree of difficulty of items
   b. The discrimination index of items
   c. General usability of the test
8. Revise the test to overcome weaknesses revealed in pretesting

Health practices tests should do more than measure the pupils' knowledge of health practices. Such tests have decidedly limited value, for the pertinent question is whether or not this knowledge is being applied.

Since health practices are stressed in the primary grades, adequate evaluation of the health instruction program at this level must be concerned with the extent to which health practices are established. Daily observation by the teacher is an acceptable, although not completely satisfactory, means of determining child health practices. The health practices of the children can be surveyed by

---

THINGS OUR CHILDREN DO FOR HEALTH

Our first grade is working hard to do the things that will mean better health. Would you help us by checking the practices of your first-grade child?

My child _____

Check here

_____ 1. Washes carefully before each meal
_____ 2. Keeps fingernails clean
_____ 3. Helps with own grooming
_____ 4. Bathes frequently
_____ 5. Has milk each breakfast
_____ 6. Has fruit daily
_____ 7. Has breakfast cereal at least four times a week
_____ 8. Eats an adequate evening meal

_____ 9. Avoids eating candy between meals
_____ 10. Brushes teeth thoroughly after each meal
_____ 11. Keeps all possessions in good order
_____ 12. Helps with tasks about the home
_____ 13. Is considerate of others
_____ 14. Has a happy disposition
_____ 15. Goes to bed early
_____ 16. Is improving in health practices

_____
parent
_____
date

querying the class as to how many drank milk for breakfast, how many brushed their teeth after breakfast, and how many carried out other health practices. Group discussion should logically follow the tally, and group motivation can be utilized advantageously. Successive surveys will reveal group progress. Opportunities are present for teaching honesty, self-discipline, and self-reliance.

Some teachers have developed a short *health practices questionnaire* for parents, which asks them to indicate their child's health practices. A brief form, as shown on p. 433, indicates the nature of this type of questionnaire.

The questionnaire is obviously slanted to interest the parent in the child's health practices and in the school health program. Items are relatively simple and easily scored. If a scoring is done after the class program has been in operation for 2 or 3 months, it will not preclude a follow-up survey with the same form several months later.

A *health practices inventory* is a satisfactory instrument for calling the teacher's attention to the progress of the program in general and specific practices in particular. It depends on the teacher's observation, but it is a directed observation on an item-to-item basis. In practice this type of evaluating device has served its intended purposes.

Health practices inventory

1. Comes to school rested
2. Comes with hair combed
3. Has clean face, ears, and neck
4. Has clean hands and nails
5. Brushes teeth
6. Has neat and clean clothing
7. Removes and hangs up outdoor wraps when indoors
8. Takes off rubbers indoors
9. Keeps all possessions orderly
10. Uses a clean handkerchief properly
11. Covers coughs and sneezes
12. Keeps fingers and other objects away from mouth
13. Washes hands before eating
14. Is cheerful and orderly at lunchtime

15. Has a good appetite for school lunch
16. Eats fruit with lunch
17. Refrains from eating candy at school
18. Brushes teeth after lunch
19. Participates in organized play at noon and recess
20. Washes hands after lunch and recess
21. Maintains a posture that reveals a sense of poise and well-being
22. Works in good light
23. Holds work in correct position
24. Wears glasses when prescribed
25. Follows good work practices
26. Displays ability to accomplish tasks
27. Displays cheerfulness and vitality
28. Adjusts well to others
29. Experiences and enjoys success
30. Is at ease in the classroom

Several health practices inventories are available from which the teacher may select the forms needed rather than construct an original form. The following source is suggested:

1. Solleder, M. K.: Evaluation instruments in health education, Washington, D.C., 1969, American Alliance for Health, Physical Education, and Recreation.

Health attitudes tests in the affective domain, such as those designated to measure interests, attitudes, appreciation, and values, are difficult to measure directly. A number of test developers in this area agree that assessing student achievement of such objectives or deciding whether a person holds a particular attitude is something that is inferred from his or her overt behavior. For example, if a student consistently *obeys* pedestrian traffic signs, the inference can be made that this student has a "good" attitude toward traffic safety.

When evaluating students' status or progress in the area of affective objectives, teachers are cautioned against using such results for the purpose of assigning grades. Should the students suspect that they are being graded, the issue then becomes not how one feels about a health practice such as dieting but what is the "desired" answer. Once teachers have gained the confidence of students and assured them that they will not be penalized or punished for their feelings, attitudes, or values about health, the reliability and validity of these data are greatly improved. There are two principal techniques that can be used in evaluating outcomes in the affective domain: (1) teacher observation and (2) self-reports using such techniques as rating scales, checklists, personal inventories, and student reports. In areas that may be personally or socially sensitive, the anonymity of students should be protected and the results used for group or class evaluations rather than for individual students.

In actual practice the teacher's own evaluation, subjective as it is, can adequately serve to indicate the predispositions of children to react to health situations and values. The evaluation of several teachers has additional significance.

Health knowledge and understanding tests constitute the health teacher's principal evaluation instruments. Knowledge as a recognized objective of health is amenable to fairly precise measurement, and many test forms can serve this purpose. Understanding is equally important as an objective and, although more difficult to measure than knowledge, can be evaluated by means of tests built on recognized principles of test construction.

Certain forms and criteria are recognized in test item construction. They are helpful guides in aiding the health teacher to develop classroom tests that are challenging to the students and that truly evaluate aspects of health education.

Essay tests. The essay examination has considerable merit. It can reveal the students' general grasp of a subject and their ability to organize and express understanding of the subject. These are skills or attitudes that the whole school program seeks to develop. The essay test is especially valuable for diagnostic purposes. An essay question should call for a sequence of ideas, for the development of logical thinking, or for support for an idea.

Some suggestions for the construction, use, and scoring of essay tests can be channeled into the needs of the teacher of health. Questions might be structured as follows:

1. Elicit reactions to a situation, not merely a description of it.
2. Base items on how, why, or of what significance rather than merely restating facts. "How can you help to protect the health of others?" is a better question than "When should the health department isolate a child?"
3. Call for definite, precise points and ask that the most important points in the answers be underlined.
4. Work out several model answers for use in grading and set up certain pertinent points.
5. Read the first question on all papers, then the second on all papers, and on through the last in order to give uniformity to grading; subjectivity can be reduced by taking the average score of several qualified graders, but there is not likely to be such a luxury as several graders in the usual school situation.
6. Use either the positive approach in scoring by adding points for each contributing statement or the negative approach of starting the reading by giving the question an arbitrary value (e.g., 20) and then deducting from the maximum score as the answer is deficient in meeting the model or standard answer.
7. Read selected answers in class in order to help students to evaluate their own performance and understand what a topflight answer is.

True-false test. To many people an objective test means only one thing—a true-false test. Most widely used, most abused, and most maligned, the true-false test can be a useful testing technique. It is easy to construct, is useful in testing for misconceptions, is especially suitable for situations involving just two alternatives (such as infectious or noninfectious), provides for wide sampling, and is easy to score.

Testing as well as teaching should discourage rote learning without understanding. For this reason, if the number of wrong answers are subtracted from the number of right ones (R − W = S) in obtaining the score, both rote memorizing and guessing will be discouraged. For a single test, correction for guessing (R − W = S) quite likely will produce a different distribution of letter grades than when no penalty is received for an incorrect answer.

R equals number of right answers
W equals number of wrong answers, not counting omissions
S equals score corrected for guessing

As Julian C. Stanley contends, the best scoring procedure for objective tests is to give the same credit for each correct answer and to provide a correction for questions omitted. Correcting for omissions is in effect a correction-for-chance, as shown by the following example. On a 100-item true-false test, student A had 60 correct answers and 40 incorrect answers. Thus he received a score of 20. Student B, on the same test, also had 60 correct answers but he had only 20 incorrect answers with 20 items omitted. Therefore student B received a higher score of 40 (60 − 20 = 40). However, over a period of time (e.g., a semester) in which several tests are involved, the final distribution of letter grades will be much the same under either plan.

A good test uses new terms and phrases, cast in a new mold, and avoids common word associations and textbook statements. A good test will favor the student whose preparation has been thorough and who understands the material. It will penalize and confuse the student whose preparation has been superficial and who tries to get by through cleverness and outguessing the tester. A few suggestions may be helpful.

1. Use true and false statements approximately in equal proportions.
2. Make the important factor in the statement apparent to the student.
3. Use straightforward statements, not confusing or trick statements.
4. State exactly what is meant and avoid ambiguity.
5. Use quantitative rather than qualitative terms.
6. Do not depend on recalling a precise figure or word to determine whether the statement is true or false.
7. Exercise caution in the use of the following terms:
   a. Absolute words, such as *only, never, always,* and *all* are usually found in false statements.
   b. Qualifying words, such as *usually, frequently,* and *almost* are more often employed in true statements.
   c. The longer the statement, the more likely it is to be true.

Thus although all these terms can be used, care must be exercised in constructing statements that contain them.

A modified true-false item is an item in which one or more key words are underlined. If the statement is correct, it is marked true. If it is incorrect, the underlined term is crossed out and a correct substitute term is written in the blank space.

Other variations of the true-false test include the alternate response tests, which permit only two possible responses such as yes-no, correct-incorrect, and same-opposite. Still other forms of this test include the use of S and U for satisfactory and unsatisfactory or the use of A, D, and U to designate agree, disagree, and undecided.

Sample true-false items will illustrate some of the enumerated suggestions:

Items 1 to 10 are true-false questions. If the statement is true, circle the T; if false, circle the F.

T F   1. Health means more than being out of a sick bed.

T F   2. There is no single index of the quality of a child's health.

T F   3. Large persons always have good health.

T F   4. A person who inherits a good constitution will usually have good health.

T F   5. A mentally healthy person never gets angry.

T F   6. Fatigue and hunger can affect a person's mental health because they tend to be upsetting.

T F   7. A balanced diet is one having the same number of calories each meal of the day.

T F   8. Overweight is primarily caused by a glandular condition.

T F   9. The best position in which to sleep is the most comfortable one.

T F 10. Toothpaste is better for bleeding gums (pink toothbrush) than oranges.

11. Alcohol is always a <u>stimulant</u> to the human body.   narcotic

12. The most harmful substances in cigarette smoke are the *irritants*.   <u> T </u>

Some common errors in item construction have been purposely included.

Material that lends itself to modified true-false items can usually be converted to simple true-false or short-answer items.

Multiple-choice tests. Superficially all multiple-choice questions appear to be similar, but a wide variety of items is included. In general, multiple-choice items should contain at least four responses, and five responses are preferred if each of the options can be made to appear plausible.

The first type is a direct question followed by five possible responses, one of which is correct or the best answer. Some examples will illustrate:

*Items 13 to 35 are multiple-choice questions. From the key select the best answer to each item. Place the letter of the best answer in front of the number of the item.**

_____13. The statement, "In solving one problem we often create a new problem," is best illustrated by which of the following?
   A. The discovery of penicillin put the producers of tincture of iodine out of business.
   B. Controlling infectious diseases has made new immunization methods necessary.

_____
*If machine-scored, numbers may be used for responses in place of letters.

   C. Prolonging the length of life has resulted in new economic and social needs.
   D. The decline of infectious disease has created the problem of an oversupply of physicians.
   E. The discovery of the electron microscope has added new diseases to be conquered.

_____14. Which of the following statements has no scientific basis?
   A. Smoking irritates the respiratory tract.
   B. Smoking has a stimulating effect on some people.
   C. Smoking has a soothing effect on some people.
   D. Smoking stunts growth.
   E. Smoking is usually a release mechanism.

_____15. What tends to promote drowsiness?
   A. Reading while lying down
   B. Warm lunch
   C. Lack of air movement
   D. Lukewarm bath
   E. All of the above

In the second type of multiple-choice test, the items are stated as incomplete sentences; there are five proposed completions, one of which is the best:

_____16. The expression, "Nature grants biological function without social favor," means
   A. Reproduction is solely a function of socially well-adjusted people
   B. Only responsible people should have children
   C. Some people, capable of being fathers and mothers, are incapable of being proper parents
   D. The ability to reproduce is independent of economic or educational level
   E. Sterility does not occur among the more socially fortunate

_____17. With recent health advances we can now logically abandon
   A. Sanitary measures
   B. Program to prevent childhood diseases
   C. Immunization programs
   D. Health research programs
   E. None of the above

_____18. The usual sequence to chronic alcoholism is
   A. Week-end drinking, solitary drinking, alcoholism
   B. First drink from curiosity, alcoholism, social drinking

C. Curiosity, social drinking, to relieve tensions, alcoholism
D. To relieve tensions, social drinking, alcoholism
E. Curiosity, aggressive drinking, social drinking, alcoholism

In the third type of multiple-choice test, one key with five responses for a series of statements is used:

Key for items 19 to 23
A. *Favorable for prevention of respiratory infection*
B. *Unfavorable for prevention of respiratory infection*
C. *Not related to prevention of respiratory infection*
D. *Favorable for prevention of respiratory infection only when a person is under 10 years of age*

_____19. Vigorous exercise
_____20. Avoiding crowds
_____21. Avoiding night air
_____22. Fatigue
_____23. Taking a laxative

Another example of the same type of multiple-choice test that has some characteristics of a matching test is as follows:

Key for items 24 to 30
A. *An A level of mental health*
B. *A B level of mental health*
C. *A C level of mental health*
D. *All of the above levels*
E. *None of the first three*

_____24. Improvement in mental health possible
_____25. Alcoholism
_____26. Never gets angry
_____27. Minimum of friction; maximum of enjoyment
_____28. Uninspired, everyday boredom
_____29. Perfect mental health
_____30. Constructive, effective adjustment

Another design of multiple-choice test may stimulate analytical thinking:

Key for items 31 to 35
A. *Statement is correct; reason is correct.*
B. *Statement is correct; reason is incorrect.*
C. *Statement is incorrect; reason is correct.*
D. *Statement is incorrect; reason is incorrect.*

_____31. All overweight people should exercise vigorously because exercise increases metabolism.
_____32. Drinking fluids before or during a meal will stop digestion because water will dilute stomach acid.
_____33. Regularity is favorable to good digestion be-cause it permits a cycle or rhythm in the function of the digestive system.
_____34. Dentifrices should be used in brushing teeth because dentifrices are antiseptics.
_____35. Fluoride prevents decay for adults because it destroys bacteria.

Another variation in multiple-choice tests is a chart on which designations are used as the key and the items refer to the designations on the chart.

In the construction, use, and scoring of multiple-choice items, certain safeguards are suggested:

1. There should be only one correct or best answer.
2. The position of the correct response should be changed from item to item. There is a tendency to make the second response the correct one more frequently than the other four positions.
3. Skill in constructing foils is the key to good multiple-choice test construction.
4. Foils should be attractive and vary in degree of plausibility.
5. One item may ask the student to select the exception to the other four items.
6. Direct statements are preferable to incomplete sentences.
7. If incomplete sentences are used, the responses should come at the end of the sentence.
8. All responses to incomplete sentences should be grammatical completions of the sentence.
9. Responses should be as homogeneous as possible.
10. When multiple-choice items are placed in a block, the student is aided and scoring is more simple.
11. Avoid words in the response that repeat words in the sentence, except when inserted as foils to counter attempts to outguess the test.
12. Correct responses should not be conspicuous by being long or short.
13. Avoid the use of direct phrases from the text.
14. If the five response items are well constructed, deducting ¼ point for each error ($R - \frac{1}{4}W = S$) will spread the scores and reduce guessing.
15. The multiple-choice test lends itself to the effective measurement of understanding.

Matching tests. Matching tests are a modification of the multiple-choice test. Two columns are used; one is either incomplete statements or a list of questions, and the other column is a list of responses. Another form of matching test consists of parallel columns.

From the key at the right, select the best response to each statement in the column to the left. Place the letter of that response in front of the number of the statement.

_____36. Health of the gums	A. Vitamin A
_____37. Important for thyroxin production	B. Vitamin B
_____38. Elevates a schoolchild's intelligence	C. Vitamin C
_____39. Necessary mineral for red corpuscles	D. Vitamin D
_____40. Helps prevent infection	E. Fat
_____41. Bone growth and development	F. Iodine
_____42. Growth and repair of tissues	G. Iron
_____43. Citrus fruits	H. Protein
	I. None of the above

Statements in items 44 to 47 are to be compared quantitatively.

Key for items 44 to 47
A. *Statement M is* greater than *statement N.*
B. *Statement M is* less than *statement N.*
C. *Statement M is* the same as *statement N.*

Statement M	Statement N
_____44. Number of chromosomes in a sperm	Number of chromosomes in a mature ovum
_____45. Number of ova in newborn girl	Number of sperms in newborn boy
_____46. Rate of maturation in the male	Rate of maturation in the female
_____47. Action of progesterone before ovulation	Action of estrone before ovulation

Matching tests are quickly constructed and require little space. For large subject areas they are satisfactory, but they are not readily adaptable to small subject areas. Matching tests are excellent for testing knowledge and association, but have limited value for testing analysis and interpretation.

In the construction, use, and scoring of matching tests, certain suggestions are helpful:

1. Using the same number of terms in each column should be avoided.
2. Statements should be in the left column and responses in the right column.
3. The same response may be used more than once.
4. Each statement should have at least two plausible answers that serve as foils in addition to the correct response.
5. A single block should contain only homogeneous material from a single area.
6. Sentence structure and the form of the responses should be consistent.
7. The students should understand the mechanics of the test.

Deduction for errors presents a problem. If a deduction is to be made, the number of possible choices must be considered. An arbitrary formula of $R - \frac{1}{4}W = S$ serves in most instances, since usually no more than four foils would likely apply to the statement.

Completion tests. Incomplete statements are given, and the student either selects the correct responses from a list or writes in the appropriate terms. This test is not satisfactory for grading purposes, but has diagnostic value. It is used almost to excess largely because it is easy to construct. It is convenient for small areas of subject matter and can be objective if terminology is not a major consideration. Completion tests are used frequently to test student recall of sheer factual material. Care should be taken in sentence structure in order to prevent confusion.

For items 48 to 59 in each blank space place the letter of the term that best completes the statement.

Key for items 48 to 59.

A. *Age*	G. *Organic*
B. *Building*	H. *Protein*
C. *Carbohydrate*	I. *Regulation*
D. *Energy*	J. *Sex*
E. *Fat*	K. *Upkeep*
F. *Height*	L. *Weight*

A food is any substance that provides cells with (48)_____, materials for (49)_____ and (50)_____, or that provides for the (51)_____ of functions. Only (52)_____ foods are digested and these are of three classes, (53)_____ the sugars and starches, (54)_____ which contains nitrogen, and (55)_____. Placed in alphabetical order, four factors are important in determining a person's basal metabolic rate: (56)_____, (57)_____, (58)_____, and (59)_____.

There is merit in using more responses than blanks. However, that style was not followed in this example. This type of test can be challenging and even takes on some of the aspects of a puzzle. Deduction for errors is difficult to determine.

A simple type of completion test is one in which a short key applies throughout:

Key for items 60 to 64
A. *Increase (increased)*
B. *Decrease (decreased)*
C. *Not change (not changed)*

Regular exercise may (60)_____ one's resistance to disease and (61)_____ one's immunity to infection. Regular exercise will (62)_____ one's predisposition to a particular disease. Regular exercise will (63)_____ the output of the thyroid. According to present studies, an athlete's life expectancy will (64)_____ as a result of athletics.

Short-answer tests. In these tests, the student completes the statement by writing a short answer in the space provided. Credit should be given for reasonably correct responses. Textbook sentences should not be used in the items, and care should be taken to avoid revealing the correct response. Sentence structure is highly important. The shorter the answer required, the less the subjective judgment of the grader will enter into the scoring. A few examples of short-answer items, shown in the following section, illustrate this type of test.

Items 65 to 70 are short-answer questions.
In your words complete the following sentences with a brief statement:

65. A food is any substance that _____
66. The most nearly perfect food is _____
67. The best way for a person to lose weight is _____
_____
68. Infection is _____
69. As a cause of death in the United States, communicable diseases are _____
_____
70. Three of the five leading causes of death in the United States are _____
_____

Limitations inherent in the short-answer tests are obvious, but tests of this type can be used to some advantage. They can be constructed quickly, which is especially helpful when a limited area of material is to be tested. Because of the limited area of subject matter that can be tested, the reliability of test results is reduced.

SUMMARY

Individual instructors find certain types of tests preferable to others. Doubtless the particular skill of the instructor is reflected in the preference. Practical considerations of a busy teacher frequently determine the type of test developed. Ideally, test results should be analyzed statistically, but the health teacher has neither the time nor the inclination for such an analysis. For that reason the occasional use of a standard health knowledge test may be advisable. Several standard health knowledge tests are available.

To ask for perfection in a health test is to ask for the impossible. These tests depend on words, and although words are our best tools for conveying ideas, they themselves are the biggest obstacle to understanding. Different connotations and shades of meaning are an ever-present difficulty. Health tests need not be perfect to be valuable. A precise measure to the most minute increment is not necessary in the practical affairs of life.

A health test is not the end of health education; it is a record of the past and a barometer for the future. In health evaluation as well as in all other aspects of the school health program, the instructor should keep in mind that the important thing is to plant a seed of health interest, water it with understanding, and nourish it with confidence in its value. Evaluation in health is continuous and never-ending.

QUESTIONS AND EXERCISES

1. In the final analysis, what is the true measure of the effectiveness of a school health program?
2. Distinguish between subjective and objective evaluation.
3. What are the advantages of using a standardized test instrument in evaluation in the school health program?
4. Why does not an evaluation device in school health need to have the precision of a micrometer in order to be highly satisfactory?
5. To what extent is health evaluation a measure of progress?
6. How can a health evaluation be an inventory?
7. Why are objectives of a program necessary as a guide in developing evaluation instruments?
8. When subjective judgments are necessary, how can subjectivity be reduced?
9. To what extent is testing a specialty?
10. "The greatest shortcoming in American education today is evaluation." Analyze the statement.
11. A healthful school environment is relatively easy to evaluate, but not so healthful living. Why the difference in degree of difficulty?
12. A youngster's health status may decline so little each day that it will be imperceptible to the teacher. How then can we identify the youngster whose health is declining?
13. Distinguish between the validity and the reliability of a test.
14. Employing a School Health Program Evaluation Scale for appraising an entire health program, what uses can be made of the results of the appraisal?
15. What is your appraisal of the practice of involving the parents of pupils by sending home health practices questionnaires for parents to check off?
16. How valid are health attitude tests with which you are familiar?
17. "Essay tests are not outmoded and can be highly valuable for certain evaluation purposes." Explain.
18. Make an appraisal of true-false tests.
19. In multiple-choice tests why is the const. foils the critical skill demanded?
20. Interpret the statement, "A student who do on one type of test usually does well on any type of test."

REFERENCES AND SELECTED READINGS

Anderson, S. B., et al.: Encyclopedia of education evaluation, San Francisco, 1975, Jossey-Bass, Inc., Publishers.

Crawford, M.: Madison health knowledge test (college), Harrisburg, Va., 1964, Madison College.

Criteria for evaluating the elementary school health programs, Sacramento, 1962, California State Department of Education.

Criteria for evaluating the high school health programs, Sacramento, 1962, California State Department of Education.

Criteria for evaluating the junior college health programs, Sacramento, 1962, California State Department of Education.

Eiss, A. F., and Harbeck, M. B.: Behavioral objectives in the affective domain, Washington, D.C., 1969, National Education Association Publications, NSTA.

Kapfer, M. B.: Behavioral objectives in curriculum development, Englewood Cliffs, N.J., 1971, Educational Technology Publications.

Kilander, H. F.: Health knowledge test, ed. 6, East Orange, N.J., 1966, The Author.

Kilander, H. F.: Information test on biological aspects of human reproduction (junior high, senior high, college), Staten Island, N.Y., 1968, Wagner College.

Kilander, H. F.: Nutrition information test, ed. 5, Staten Island, N.Y., 1968, Wagner College.

LeMaistre, E. H., and Pollock, M. B.: Health behavior inventory (senior high), Monterey, Calif., 1963, California Test Bureau.

Meise, W. C.: A scale for the measurement of attitudes toward healthful living, Slippery Rock, Pa., 1962, Slippery Rock State College.

Pollock, M. B.: Mood altering substances: a behavior inventory, Los Angeles, 1968, Tinnon-Brown Publishing Co.

School health education evaluation study (E. B. Johns, Director), Los Angeles, 1957, Los Angeles County Tuberculosis and Health Association.

Solleder, M. K., editor: Evaluation instruments in health education, Washington, D.C., 1969, American Alliance for Health, Physical Education, and Recreation.

Stanley, J. C.: Measurement in today's schools, ed. 4, Englewood Cliffs, N.J., 1964, Prentice-Hall, Inc.

Willgoose, C. E.: Evaluation in health education and physical education, New York, 1961, McGraw-Hill Book Co.

Appendices

APPENDIX A

Resources in health instruction

TEXTBOOKS
Elementary school

1. *Health for Young America Series:* Wilson, C., and
   Wilson, E. A.: Indianapolis, The Bobbs-Merrill Co.,
   Inc.
   Grade
   1   Health at school, 1968
   2   Health day by day, 1968
   3   Health and fun, 1968
   4   Health and growth, 1968
   5   Health and living, 1968
   6   Health and happiness, 1968
   7   Men, science and health, 1968
   8   Health, fitness and safety, 1968
2. *Laidlaw Health Series:* Byrd, O. E., Nielson, E. A.,
   and Moore, V.: River Forest, Ill., Laidlaw Brothers.
   Grade
   1   Health 1, 1970
   2   Health 2, 1970
   3   Health 3, 1970
   4   Health 4, 1970
   5   Health 5, 1970
   6   Health 6, 1970
3. *Health For All Series:* Bauer, W. W., et al.: Glenview, Ill., Scott, Foresman & Co.
   Grade
   1   Junior Primer—Health for all, 1965
   1   Book 1—Health for all, 1965
   2   Book 2—Health for all, 1965
   3   Book 3—Health for all, 1965
   4   Book 4—Health for all, 1965
   5   Book 5—Health for all, 1965
   6   Book 6—Health for all, 1965
4. *Healthful Living Program:* Fodor, J. T., et al.: River
   Forest, Ill., Laidlaw Brothers.

Grade
1   Your health
2   Being healthy
3   Your health and you
4   Keeping healthy
5   Growing up healthy
6   Health for living
7   Healthier you
8   Your health and your future

5. *You and Your Health:* Richmond, J. B., Pounds, E.
   T., and Sanders, L. P.: Glenview, Ill., 1977, Scott,
   Foresman & Co.
   Grade
   K   You and your health, kindergarten activity
        booklet; Bueno ysano, Spanish transla-
        tion of kindergarten activity
   1   You and your health
   2   You and your health
   3   You and your health
   4   You and your health
   5   You and your health
   6   You and your health
   7   You and your health
6. *Basic Concepts Booklets:* River Forest, Ill., Laidlaw
   Brothers.
   Book
   1   Needle, R. H., and Hill, A. E.: Basic con-
        cepts of alcohol
   2   Sumner, E. D., Needle, R. H., and Hill,
        A. E.: Basic concepts of drugs
   3   Needle, R. H.: Basic concepts of tobacco
        and smoking
   4   Harlin, V. K., and Shuly, E. D.: Basic con-
        cepts of human life

Book

5   Boyer, D. A., and Brandt, E. R.: Human growth and reproduction, grades 5 to 8

6   Boyer, D. A.: For youth to know, grades 7 to 10

7. *Health: decisions for growth:* Collins, D. A., New York, 1978-1979, Harcourt Brace Jovanovich, Inc.
   Grade
   1   Health: decisions for growth
   2   Health: decisions for growth (sound film-strips)
   3   Health: Decisions for growth (study prints)
   4   Your health and safety for better living
   5   Your health and safety in a changing environment
   6   Toward your future
   7   Heredity: what is DNA?
   8   The brain: how it works for you

Junior high school

1. *Health and Growth Program:* Richmond, J. B., et al.: Glenview, Ill., 1974, Scott, Foresman & Co.
   Grade
   7   Book 7—Health and growth
   8   Book 8—Health and growth
   9-10   The new health and safety
2. *Health for Young America Series:* Wilson, C., and Wilson, E. A.: Indianapolis, The Bobbs-Merrill Co., Inc.
   Grade
   7   Men, science and health, 1968
   8   Health, fitness and safety, 1968
3. *Laidlaw Health Series:* Byrd, O. E., Nielson, E. A., and Moore, V.: River Forest, Ill., Laidlaw Brothers.
   Grade
   7   Health 7, 1970
   8   Health 8, 1970
4. Byrd, O. E., et al.: Health—today and tomorrow, level 9 to 12, River Forest, Ill., 1975, Laidlaw Brothers.
5. Blanzaco, A.: V.D.: facts you should know, Glenview, Ill., 1975, Scott, Foresman & Co.
6. *Health for All Series:* Bauer, W. W., et al.: Glenview, Ill., Scott, Foresman & Co.
   Grade
   7   Book 7—Health for all, 1965
   8   Book 8—Health for all, 1965
7. Jenkins, G., et al.: Health and safety for teenagers, Glenview, Ill., 1966, Scott, Foresman & Co.
8. Williams, D. M.: Health science I, Philadelphia, 1967, J. B. Lippincott Co.
9. Williams, D. M.: Health science II, Philadelphia, 1967, J. B. Lippincott Co.
10. McClendon, E. J., et al.: Healthful living for today and tomorrow, River Forest, Ill., 1978, Laidlaw Brothers.
11. McClendon, E. J., et al.: Healthful living in your environment, River Forest, Ill., 1978, Laidlaw Brothers.
12. Pickett, R., et al.: Human factors in health care, Lexington, Mass., 1975, Lexington Books.

Senior high school

1. Diehl, H. S., Laton, A., and Vaughn, F. C.: Health and safety for you, ed. 3, rev., New York, 1969, McGraw-Hill Book Co.
2. Gallagher, J. R., Goldberger, I. H., and Hallock, G. T.: Health for life, Boston, 1964, Ginn & Co.
3. Haag, J. H.: Health education for young adults, Austin, Tex., 1965, Steck-Vaughn Co.
4. Neilson, B., Bland, H. B., and Hill, A. E.: Healthful living in your environment, River Forest, Ill., 1975, Laidlaw Brothers.
5. Stresser, M. K., Eales, J. R., and Aaron, J. E.: Driver education, River Forest, Ill., 1975, Laidlaw Brothers.
6. Wilson, C. C., Cracken, J. C., and Almack, J. C.: Life and health, Indianapolis, 1974, The Bobbs-Merrill Co., Inc.
7. Neilson, A. E., et al.: Healthful living in your environment, River Forest, Ill., 1975, Laidlaw Brothers.
8. Lawrence, T. G., Clemenson, J. W., and Burnett, R. W.: Your health and safety, ed. 5, Chicago, 1963, Harcourt Brace Jovanovich, Inc.
9. Meredith, F. L., Irwin, L. W., and Staton, W. M.: Health and fitness, ed. 4, Boston, 1966, D. C. Heath & Co.
10. Nicoll, J. S., Foster, J. C., and Bolton, W. W.: Health today and tomorrow, River Forest, Ill., 1966, Laidlaw Brothers.
11. Otto, J. H., Julian, C. J., and Tether, J. E.: Modern health, New York, 1967, Holt, Rinehart & Winston, Inc.

Family living

1. *Family Life Education Program:* Cogan, T., et al.: Chicago, Follett Publishing Co.
   Grade
   1   Families live together
   2   World of living things
   3   How new lives begin
   4   Living things and their young
   5   How we are born
   6   Men and women
2. Christensen, H. T., editor: Handbook of marriage and the family, Skokie, Ill., 1964, Rand McNally & Co.

3. Clemens, A. G.: A design for successful marriage, Englewood Cliffs, N.J., 1964, Prentice-Hall, Inc.

4. Crawley, L. Q., Malfetti, J. F., and Stewart, E. I.: Reproduction, sex and preparation for marriage, Englewood Cliffs, N.J., 1964, Prentice-Hall, Inc.

5. Duvall, E. M.: Family living, New York, 1961, The Macmillan Co.

6. Home Economics Education Association: Family life education, Washington, D.C., 1975, The Association.

7. Kirkendall, L. A., and Adams, W. J.: The students' guide to marriage and family life literature, Du-buque, Iowa, 1976, William C. Brown Co., Publishers.

8. Landis, J. T., and Landis, M. G.: Personal adjustment, marriage, and family living, ed. 5, Englewood Cliffs, N.J., 1966, Prentice-Hall, Inc.

9. Osborne, E. G.: Understanding your parents, New York, 1962, Association Press.

10. Schulz, E. D., and Williams, S. R.: Family life and sex education, New York, 1969, Harcourt Brace Jovanovich, Inc.

11. Petersen, M. E.: Guide to a happy marriage, ed. 2, Englewood Cliffs, N.J., 1964, Prentice-Hall, Inc.

Record and report forms

HEALTH EXAMINATION

To be filled in by parent or guardian before the time of the examination.
(please print plainly with ink)

Pupil's name _____ Birth _____ Sex M __ F __
         (last)   (first)   (middle)   (month) (day) (year)

Address_____ Phone _____ Parent or guardian _____
    (street or route) (city)

Family physician's name_____ Phone _____
         (last)   (first)   (initial)

Infancy and preschool history: Record unusual problems, e.g., convulsions, accidents, operations, exposure to tuberculosis, behavior difficulties _____

_____

_____

Past history of illnesses; state the year in which the child had any of the following:

Communicable diseases		Other diseases		Other conditions	
Chickenpox	19___	Asthma	19___	Constant cough	19___
Diphtheria	19___	Diabetes	19___	Fainting spells	19___
German measles	19___	Hay fever	19___	Frequent colds	19___
Measles	19___	Heart trouble	19___	Frequent sore throat	19___
Mumps	19___	Kidney trouble	19___	Frequent urination	19___
Poliomyelitis	19___	Pneumonia	19___	Hearing difficulty	19___
Scarlet fever	19___	Rheumatic fever	19___	Tire easily	19___
Whooping cough	19___	Tonsilitis	19___	Vision difficulty	19___

History of immunization and tests

	Completed	booster dose		Completed	booster dose		Completed	booster dose
Diphtheria	19__	19__	Poliomyelitis	19__	19__	Smallpox	19__	19__
Tetanus	19__	19__	Whooping			Measles	19__	19__
Other	19__	19__	cough	19__	19__			

	Date	Result			Date	Result
Chest x-ray	19___	___		Other test	19___	___

Other information of value to the teacher _____

_____

_____

Front

HEALTH EXAMINATION

To be completed by examining physician

Vision, without glasses, right eye 20/____, left eye 20/____

with glasses, right eye 20/____, left eye 20/____

Color vision_____, test used_____

Hearing, right ear_____, left ear_____

Eyes	____	Normal	____	Defect _____
Ears	____	Normal	____	Defect _____
Nose	____	Normal	____	Defect _____
Throat	____	Normal	____	Defect _____
Thyroid	____	Normal	____	Defect _____
Lymph nodes	____	Normal	____	Defect _____
Heart	____	Normal	____	Defect _____
Lungs	____	Normal	____	Defect _____
Blood pressure	____	Systolic	____	Diastolic _____
Abdomen	____	Normal	____	Defect _____
Genitals	____	Normal	____	Defect _____
Posture	____	Normal	____	Defect _____
Extremities	____	Normal	____	Defect _____
Nervous system	____	Normal	____	Defect _____
Skin	____	Normal	____	Defect _____
Nutrition	____	Normal	____	Defect _____
Musculature	____	Normal	____	Defect _____
Other	____	Normal	____	Defect _____

Laboratory tests _____

Findings and recommendations _____

_____

_____

_____

Immediate medical referral Yes _____ No _____ Dental referral Yes _____ No _____

Unlimited activity _____ Limited activity _____

_____

Parent present Yes____ No____

_____ M.D. _____
(examining physician)   *(date)*

Back

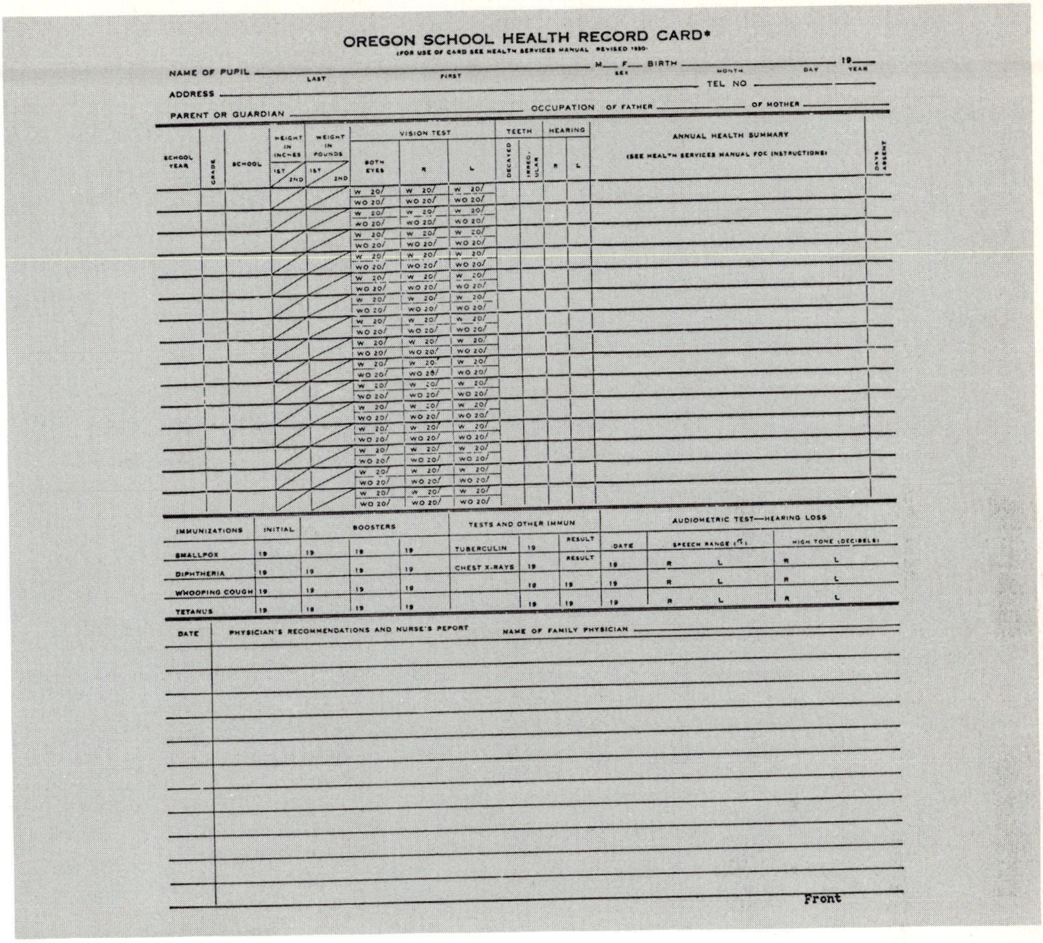

OREGON SCHOOL HEALTH RECORD CARD*
(FOR USE OF CARD SEE HEALTH SERVICES MANUAL REVISED 1950)

NAME OF PUPIL ______ LAST ______ FIRST ______ M___ F___ SEX BIRTH ______ MONTH ______ DAY 19___ YEAR

ADDRESS ______ TEL NO ______

PARENT OR GUARDIAN ______ OCCUPATION OF FATHER ______ OF MOTHER ______

SCHOOL YEAR	GRADE	SCHOOL	HEIGHT IN INCHES 1ST / 2ND	WEIGHT IN POUNDS 1ST / 2ND	VISION TEST BOTH EYES	R	L	TEETH DECAYED	IRREG-ULAR	HEARING R	L	ANNUAL HEALTH SUMMARY (SEE HEALTH SERVICES MANUAL FOR INSTRUCTIONS)	DAYS ABSENT
					W 20/ WO 20/	W 20/ WO 20/	W 20/ WO 20/						
					W 20/ WO 20/	W 20/ WO 20/	W 20/ WO 20/						
					W 20/ WO 20/	W 20/ WO 20/	W 20/ WO 20/						
					W 20/ WO 20/	W 20/ WO 20/	W 20/ WO 20/						
					W 20/ WO 20/	W 20/ WO 20/	W 20/ WO 20/						
					W 20/ WO 20/	W 20/ WO 20/	W 20/ WO 20/						
					W 20/ WO 20/	W 20/ WO 20/	W 20/ WO 20/						
					W 20/ WO 20/	W 20/ WO 20/	W 20/ WO 20/						
					W 20/ WO 20/	W 20/ WO 20/	W 20/ WO 20/						
					W 20/ WO 20/	W 20/ WO 20/	W 20/ WO 20/						
					W 20/ WO 20/	W 20/ WO 20/	W 20/ WO 20/						
					W 20/ WO 20/	W 20/ WO 20/	W 20/ WO 20/						
					W 20/ WO 20/	W 20/ WO 20/	W 20/ WO 20/						
					W 20/ WO 20/	W 20/ WO 20/	W 20/ WO 20/						
					W 20/ WO 20/	W 20/ WO 20/	W 20/ WO 20/						

IMMUNIZATIONS	INITIAL	BOOSTERS			TESTS AND OTHER IMMUN		
SMALLPOX	19	19	19	19	TUBERCULIN	19	RESULT
DIPHTHERIA	19	19	19	19	CHEST X-RAYS	19	RESULT
WHOOPING COUGH	19	19	19	19		19	19
TETANUS	19	19	19	19		19	19

AUDIOMETRIC TEST—HEARING LOSS				
DATE	SPEECH RANGE (%)		HIGH TONE (DECIBELS)	
19	R	L	R	L
19	R	L	R	L
19	R	L	R	L

DATE	PHYSICIAN'S RECOMMENDATIONS AND NURSE'S REPORT NAME OF FAMILY PHYSICIAN ______

Front

REPORT OF SCHOOL DENTAL EXAMINATION

To: ______________________________ Parent or guardian

A dental examination of your child ______________________________
has been made by the school dentist. This examination shows:

☐ 1. Need for dental service. You are advised to consult your family dentist as soon as possible.

☐ 2. No apparent defects.

Signed ______________________________ Date ______

Front

HISTORY OF PAST AND CURRENT ILLNESS, ACCIDENT, DISABILITY, AND ABSENCE

OBSERVATIONS BY TEACHER

SCHOOL YEAR		19	19	19	19	19	19	19	19	19	19	19	19
GRADE IN SCHOOL													
EYES	STYES OR CRUSTED LIDS												
	INFLAMED EYES												
	CROSSED EYES												
	FREQUENT HEADACHES												
	SQUINTING AT BOOK OR BLACKBOARD												
EARS	DISCHARGE FROM EARS												
	EARACHES												
	FAILURE TO HEAR QUESTIONS												
ORAL CAVITY	INFLAMED GUMS												
	INFLAM. OF LIPS, CHEEKS, PALATE												
	FAULTY ORAL HYGIENE												
NOSE AND THROAT	PERSISTENT MOUTH BREATHING												
	FREQUENT SORE THROAT												
	FREQUENT COLDS												
GENERAL CONDITION AND APPEARANCE	FAILURE TO GAIN WEIGHT												
	EXCESSIVE GAIN IN WEIGHT												
	DOES NOT APPEAR WELL												
	TIRES EASILY												
	POOR MUSCLE COORDINATION												
	POOR POSTURE												
BEHAVIOR	EMOTIONAL DISTURBANCES												
	SPEECH DEFECT												
	TWITCHING MOVEMENTS												
	UNDUE RESTLESSNESS												
	SHYNESS												
	NAIL BITING												
	EXCESSIVE USE OF LAVATORY												
	EXCESSIVE DROWSINESS												
	POOR FOOD HABITS												

CODE   V = DEFECT   T = UNDER TREATMENT   C = CORRECTED   R = REFERRAL   NT = NO TREATMENT NEEDED

STATE PRINTING DEPT.

Back

REPORT OF DENTAL WORK

This is to report that _____

☐ 1. Needs no dental work at present.
☐ 2. Has all necessary dental work completed.
☐ 3. Is receiving dental treatment.

Recommendation _____

___ _____

Signed _____ Date _____

(child should return this card to the teacher)

Back

REPORT OF FAMILY DENTIST'S EXAMINATION

Dear Parents: In the interest of better health for your children, the school urges you have them visit their family dentist at least twice a year. After the family dentist has filled out this card, will you have your child return it to the school?

Sincerely,

_____ Principal

Front

REPORT OF FAMILY DENTIST'S EXAMINATION

_____ has had a dental examination and

☐ 1. Needs no dental work.
☐ 2. Has all necessary dental work completed.
☐ 3. Is receiving dental treatment.

Recommendation _____

_____

Signed _____ Date _____

(child should return this card to the teacher)

Back

REFERRAL CARD*

Recommended medical or dental consultation

School _____ Date _____

Dear _____

Observation of _____ indicates

_____

_____

The school urges that you consult your physician or dentist.

Sincerely,

_____

Vision screening report

School _____ Date _____

Dear _____
Results of the school vision screening test reveal the possibility that your child
_____ may be having some difficulty in
seeing properly. The school urges you to consult a doctor for a professional examination of
your child's vision.

Sincerely,

_____

*Reported after teacher-nurse conference when nurse is available. If there is no nurse, teachers make the report.

STUDENT ACCIDENT REPORT—SHORT FORM   No. _____

Name of student _____ Age _____ Grade _____

Time and date of accident _____ Place of accident _____

Cause and nature of accident _____

_____ Injury _____

First aid by _____ Medical care by _____ M.D.

How could accident have been prevented? _____

_____

Reported by _____ Signed _____
               (signed)   (principal)

STUDENT ACCIDENT REPORT   No. ___

Name of student _____ Age _____ Grade _____

Time and date of accident _____ Place of accident _____

Staff member in charge at time of accident _____

Where was staff member at time of accident? _____

Cause and nature of accident _____

_____

_____

Nature of injury _____

_____

First aid by _____ Nature of first aid _____

_____ Medical care by _____ M.D.

Nature of medical care _____

Where was student taken? _____ by _____

_____ Parent or guardian notified by _____

Via phone _____ message _____

Witnesses: _____   _____

How could this accident have been prevented? _____

_____

To be added when student returns to school: Days absent _____ Recovery _____

Reported by _____ Signed _____
               (signed)   (principal)

State Department of Education
Instruction Division
Curriculum and Instructional Services
Salem, Oregon

REQUEST FOR PHYSICIAN'S RECOMMENDATIONS ON
PHYSICAL EDUCATION ACTIVITY

_____ 19 ____

Dear Parent:
We have your request that your child _____

of _____ School, be excused from physical education.
The activity portion is but a part of the larger health and physical education program.
The health and physical education program is, however, flexible, since it involves various
forms of activities. In order to comply with your request and in order to serve best the interests
of the child, we ask that you have your physician complete the following statement and
return it to the school.

_____   _____
(signature of person requesting information)   _(position or title)_

_____ 19 ____

Physician's report
Nature of disability _____
Recommendations:

☐ 1. Unlimited activity
    Comment _____
☐ 2. Limited activity
    Comment _____
☐ 3. No activity
    Comment _____
☐ 4. Special recommendations:

_____

_____

I recommend reexamination in _____ weeks.

This statement is valid until _____ and does not
extend beyond the current school year.

_____
(physician's signature)

PHYSICIAN'S RECOMMENDATIONS ON PHYSICAL EDUCATION ACTIVITY

Medford Public Schools
Medford, Oregon

Dear _____ :
(teacher)

_____ , a patient under my care,
(student's name)

should participate in physical education activities to the following extent:

☐ 1. Full activity except for _____

☐ 2. Limited activity
    Recommendations _____

_____

☐ 3. Special remedial class (high school only)

    Recommendations _____

_____

_____

☐ 4. No activity
I (will) (will not) reexamine the patient in _____ weeks.

_____
(physician's signature)

Date _____

Front

DESCRIPTION OF PHYSICAL EDUCATION PROGRAM
Medford Public Schools
Medford, Oregon

1. *Full program*

Grades 1-2-3	*Grades 4-5-6*	*Junior high school*	*High school*
Basic rhythms	Folk dance	Folk dance	Track and field°
Active games°	Square dance	Square dance	Field hockey°
Quiet games	Active games°	Exercises°	Touch football†
Basic skills	Relays°	Gymnastics°	Wrestling†
Self-testing°	Sports skills	Trampoline°	Trampoline
Exercises	Tumbling°	Wrestling†	Gymnastics
Fitness tests°	Exercises°	Track°	Weight training†
	Fitness tests°	Basketball°	Swimming°
		Touch football†	Volleyball°
		Softball	Badminton
		Volleyball°	Basketball°
		Soccer°	Softball
		Speedball°	Archery
		Fitness tests°	Tennis
			Exercises°
			Fitness tests°

2. *Limited program*

   Many times the disability is localized and of a nature that permits the use of other parts of the body without detriment. The physician's recommendation in such cases will be faithfully followed.

3. *Special remedial class (high school only)*

   Special classes are scheduled at the high school for students who have problems that require a more individual approach than is possible in the regular class. No medical cases are included in these classes without the recommendation of the physician. The exercises and activities prescribed by the physician will be closely supervised by the physical education teacher.

°Strenuous for the grade level.
†Boys' activity only.
Underlined: girls' activity only.

Back

School health program evaluation scale

PART I. SCHOOL HEALTH SERVICES   **(350 points)** _____

A. Health appraisal
   1. Frequency of health examinations
      a. Entering pupils examined: 90%-100%, 15 pts; 80%-89%, 12 pts; 70%-79%,
        9 pts; 50%-69%, 6 pts; 20%-49%, 3 pts ------------------------------- (15 pts) _____
      b. New pupils entering the school system examined: 90%-100%, 5 pts; 80%-89%,
        4 pts; 70%-79%, 3 pts; 50%-69%, 2 pts; 20%-49%, 1 pt ------------------ (5 pts) _____
      c. Pupils examined at least once through grades 3 to 10: 90%-100%, 5 pts; 80%-
        89%, 4 pts; 70%-79%, 3 pts; 50%-69%, 2 pts; 20%-49%, 1 pt -------------- (5 pts) _____
      d. Pupils referred by teacher or examined by nurse: 90%-100%, 10 pts; 80%-
        89%, 8 pts; 70%-79%, 6 pts; 50%-69%, 4 pts; 20%-49%, 2 pts ----------- (10 pts) _____
      e. Interscholastic athletic participants examined: 90%-100%, 5 pts; 80%-89%,
        4 pts; 70%-79%, 3 pts; 50%-69%, 2 pts; 20%-49%, 1 pt ------------------ (5 pts) _____
      f. Pupils sustaining injuries at school or serious illness necessitating absence of
        5 days or more from school examined: 90%-100%, 5 pts; 80%-89%, 4 pts; 70%-
        79%, 3 pts; 50%-69%, 2 pts; 20%-49%, 1 pt ---------------------------- (5 pts) _____
      g. Pupils tested with audiometer every 3 years or more often (elementary schools
        only): 90%-100%, 5 pts; 80%-89%, 4 pts; 70%-79%, 3 pts; 50%-69%, 2 pts;
        20%-49%, 1 pt --- (5 pts) _____
   2. Dental examinations
      Pupils examined by dentist during the year: 90%-100%, 5 pts; 80%-89%, 4 pts;
      70%-79%, 3 pts; 50%-69%, 2 pts; 20%-49%, 1 pt ------------------------- (5 pts) _____
   3. Screening
      a. Pupils whose height and weight are recorded at least twice a year (elementary
        school only): 90%-100%, 5 pts; 80%-89%, 4 pts; 70%-79%, 3 pts; 50%-69%,
        2 pts; 20%-49%, 1 pt --- (5 pts) _____
      b. Pupils whose vision and hearing were tested during first 2 months of school
        year (elementary school only): 90%-100%, 5 pts; 80%-89%, 4 pts; 70%-79%,
        3 pts; 50%-69%, 2 pts; 20%-49%, 1 pt --------------------------------- (5 pts) _____
B. Activities of health appraisal personnel
   1. Physician's examination rated according to time used per child: 10 minutes or
      more, 10 pts; 7-9 minutes, 8 pts; 5-6 minutes, 6 pts; 3-4 minutes, 4 pts; 1-2 min-
      utes, 2 pts -- (10 pts) _____

2. Nurse's procedures
   a. Obtaining health history* of children examined: 75%-100%, 3 pts; 50%-74%, 2 pts; 1%-49%, 1 pt ------------------------------------ (3 pts) _____
   b. Making health assessment† of students as requested by teachers ---------- (3 pts) _____
3. Teacher's activities
   a. Elementary school teacher
     (1) Reviewing and using records relating to child's health status ---------- (5 pts) _____
     (2) Recognizing outward indices of child health -------------------------- (3 pts) _____
     (3) Making continuous observations of child's health status and recording appraisal at least twice a year -- (3 pts) _____
     (4) Making continuous observations of child's attitudes and social behavior and recording them at least twice a year -------------------------- (3 pts) _____
     (5) Making referrals promptly through available channels
       (a) Child not making satisfactory weight and height gains -------------- (2 pts) _____
       (b) Excessively overweight child --- (2 pts) _____
       (c) Child with defective posture or body mechanics ------------------ (2 pts) _____
       (d) Pupil with emotional or personality problems ------------------- (3 pts) _____
       (e) Child with apparent hearing difficulties ------------------------ (2 pts) _____
       (g) Child with speech difficulties --------------------------------- (2 pts) _____
       (h) Child with abnormal skin conditions ------------------------- (2 pts) _____
       (i) Child with low vitality ------------------------------------- (2 pts) _____
       (j) Child with other symptoms of illness ------------------------ (3 pts) _____
     (6) Preparing pupils for examination through discussion, 1 pt; review of experience, 1 pt; evaluation of the examination, 1 pt --------------------- (3 pts) _____
   b. Secondary school classroom teachers
     (1) Recognizing outward indices of student health ---------------------- (3 pts) _____
     (2) Making continuous observation of student's health status with referral to health educator or nurse --- (3 pts) _____
     (3) Making continuous observation of student's attitudes and social behavior, with referral to health educator or nurse -------------------------- (3 pts) _____
   c. Secondary school health educator
     (1) Reviewing and using records relating to student's health status -------- (3 pts) _____
     (2) Providing for adequate screening of students with emotional or personality problems --- (3 pts) _____
     (3) Making referrals promptly through teacher-nurse conference regularly scheduled at least once a week ----------------------------------- (3 pts) _____
4. Parent's participation
   a. Making written report of observed practices of child on personal history form (2 pts) _____
   b. Accepting opportunity to confer with physician or nurse ------------------ (2 pts) _____
5. Child's participation
   a. Discussing health problems with teacher, nurse, or physician ------------ (3 pts) _____
   b. Reevaluating health status in terms recommended by physician, nurse, or teacher -- (3 pts) _____
C. Follow-up and counseling procedures
1. Counseling pupils regarding health status -------------------------------- (3 pts) _____
2. Giving parents adequate information on health status of child within 2 weeks after examination --- (3 pts) _____
3. Giving parents information or other aid in implementing physician's findings and recommendations --- (3 pts) _____
4. For teachers, interpreting the physician's findings and recommendations ------ (3 pts) _____

---

*May be obtained by teacher.
†May be made by health director or other qualified personnel.

    5. Adapting the school program to meet the needs of handicapped children: 100%, 10 pts; 75%-99%, 8 pts; 50%-75%, 6 pts; 25%-49%, 4 pts; 1%-24%, 2 pts ----   (10 pts) _____

    6. Making effective use of state and community resources

       a. Consultants: hearing, 2 pts; vision, 2 pts; mental health, 2 pts; dental health, 2 pts; nutrition, 2 pts; sanitation, 2 pts -----------------------------------   (12 pts) _____

       b. Social workers -----------------------------------   (4 pts) _____

    7. Aiding in obtaining professional services for children needing corrections but unable to pay: 90%-100%, 10 pts; 80%-89%, 8 pts; 70%-79%, 6 pts; 50%-69%, 4 pts; 20%-49%, 2 pts -----------------------------------   (10 pts) _____

    8. Making follow-up survey to determine which corrections have been made: after 2 months, 5 pts; after 4 months, 3 pts; after 6 months, 1 pt -----------   (9 pts) _____

    9. Recording corrections on student's health record form --------------------   (3 pts) _____

    10. Obtaining dental certificates: 80%-100% of pupils, 5 pts; 60%-79%, 4 pts; 40%-59%, 3 pts; 20%-39%, 2 pts; 1%-19%, 1 pt -----------------------------------   (5 pts) _____

D. Prevention and control of communicable disease

    1. Tuberculosis tests for children exposed to tuberculosis: annually, 10 pts; biennially, 5 pts -----------------------------------   (10 pts) _____

    2. Tuberculosis tests available for all high school students: annually, 6 pts; biennially, 4 pts; every 3 years, 2 pts; every 4 years, 1 pt -----------------------------------   (6 pts) _____

    3. Spot x-ray surveys: annually, 3 pts; biennially, 2 pts; every 3 years, 1 pt ------   (3 pts) _____

    4. Tuberculosis tests required of all school personnel: annually, 3 pts; biennially, 2 pts; only before entry, 1 pt -----------------------------------   (3 pts) _____

    5. Children immunized (elementary school)

       a. For diphtheria: 80%-100%, 5 pts; 60%-79%, 4 pts; 40%-59%, 3 pts; 20%-39%, 2 pts; 1%-19%, 1 pt -----------------------------------   (5 pts) _____

       b. For smallpox: 80%-100%, 5 pts; 60%-79%, 4 pts; 40%-59%, 3 pts; 20%-39%, 2 pts; 1%-19%, 1 pt -----------------------------------   (5 pts) _____

       c. For poliomyelitis: 80%-100%, 5 pts; 60%-79%, 4 pts; 40%-59%, 3 pts; 20%-39%, 2 pts; 1%-19%, 1 pt -----------------------------------   (5 pts) _____

    6. Children with suspected communicable disease reported to the health department -----------------------------------   (5 pts) _____

    7. Children with symptoms of communicable disease isolated (exclusion of child based on appearance, behavior, and complaints) -------------------------   (3 pts) _____

    8. Parents notified when child appears to be ill -----------------------------   (3 pts) _____

    9. Teachers provided with list of characteristics of common illnesses of schoolchildren -----------------------------------   (2 pts) _____

    10. Pupils inspected in early morning and before noon during epidemics --------   (5 pts) _____

    11. Teacher observation made for symptoms of illness when no epidemic exists   (3 pts) _____

    12. Pupils absent less than 5 days checked by nurse or teacher for communicability of disease on readmission -----------------------------------   (3 pts) _____

    13. Pupils and school personnel absent from school 5 days or more because of illness with no official isolation, readmitted to school only on presentation of statement of noncommunicability signed by health department or licensed physician ----   (5 pts) _____

    14. Pupils readmitted to school after official isolation for communicable disease only on release by health department -------------------------------------   (4 pts) _____

    15. Pupils returning to school after serious illness permitted to participate in strenuous activities only by approval of physician or nurse --------------------   (3 pts) _____

    16. Perfect school attendance not emphasized ----------------------------   (2 pts) _____

    17. Teacher illness reported to principal and recommended control procedures followed -----------------------------------   (3 pts) _____

E. Emergency and first-aid provisions

    1. First-aid training required of every teacher -----------------------------   (3 pts) _____

    2. Responsibility for care of serious cases assigned to at least one specially qualified person in each building -----------------------------------   (3 pts) _____

3. Well-planned written procedures giving instructions to follow in case of emergency or disaster reviewed and understood by all school employees _____ (3 pts) _____
4. Emergency and disaster plans rehearsed: six times or more per year, 5 pts; five times, 4 pts; four times, 3 pts; three times, 2 pts; twice, 1 pt _____ (5 pts) _____
5. Accidents reported, investigated, and report filed _____ (4 pts) _____
6. Record of family physician of each child kept available _____ (2 pts) _____
7. Adequate first-aid supplies made readily available _____ (5 pts) _____
8. Telephone made easily available _____ (3 pts) _____
9. Important numbers posted at telephone, e.g., nearest physician, ambulance, police, and fire department _____ (2 pts) _____
10. Fire and emergency alarm systems working efficiently _____ (3 pts) _____
11. Transportation home provided for ill children _____ (3 pts) _____
12. Rest rooms provided for ill or injured children
    a. Separate rooms for boys and girls _____ (3 pts) _____
    b. At least two cots for boys and two for girls _____ (3 pts) _____
    c. Rooms partially darkened _____ (2 pts) _____
    d. Room temperature and ventilation controlled _____ (2 pts) _____
    e. Responsible person in attendance _____ (2 pts) _____

F. Health room equipment for clinics, conferences, and examinations (table, chairs, good light and ventilation, window shades, scales, measuring rod, and eye charts) (5 pts) _____

G. Records
1. Cumulative health records kept up-to-date, transferrable with other school records (3 pts) _____
2. Cumulative health records made available to administrators, teachers, and medical advisers _____ (3 pts) _____

PART II. HEALTH INSTRUCTION   (400 points) _____

A. Direct health instruction
1. A general plan of progressive health instruction for all grades used _____ (10 pts) _____
2. Subject areas included in health instruction
    a. Structure and function _____ (5 pts) _____
    b. Personal health _____ (5 pts) _____
    c. Sex education _____ (5 pts) _____
    d. Nutrition _____ (5 pts) _____
    e. First-aid and safety _____ (5 pts) _____
    f. Mental health _____ (5 pts) _____
    g. Control of disease (communicable and noncommunicable) _____ (5 pts) _____
    h. Narcotics and other poisons _____ (5 pts) _____
    i. Community health and sanitation _____ (5 pts) _____
    j. Choice and use of health services and products _____ (5 pts) _____
3. Organized course of study for each grade kept on file in principal's office (including aims, objective, and methods of teaching) _____ (5 pts) _____
4. Course of study reviewed and revised annually _____ (5 pts) _____
5. Health practices, attitudes, and information included in aims and objectives of instruction _____ (5 pts) _____
6. Planned instruction in grades 1 to 8: three or more times a week, 5 pts; two times a week, 3 pts; once a week, 1 pt _____ (5 pts) _____
7. Graduating seniors who had taken high school health instruction: all students, 10 pts; 80%-99%, 8 pts; 60%-79%, 6 pts; 40%-59%, 4 pts; 20%-39%, 2 pts; 10%-19%, 1 pt _____ (10 pts) _____
8. Scheduled health classes in secondary schools: two semesters during grades 9 through 12, 10 pts; four quarter years during 9 through 12, 10 pts; alternating during week with another subject for 1 year (at any grade), 5 pts; one semester during grades 9 through 12, 5 pts _____ (10 pts) _____

9. Health classes held in standard classroom ------------------------------- (3 pts) _____
10. Instruction based on needs and interests of children (as revealed by surveys of their health histories, records, interests, and practices) -------------------- (3 pts) _____
11. Up-to-date readers or textbooks in health instruction available; all children in health classes, 10 pts; 80%-99%, 8 pts; 60%-79%, 6 pts; 40%-59%, 4 pts; 20%-39%, 2 pts; less than 20%, 0 pts -- (10 pts) _____
12. Methods used in teaching health
    a. Discussion (group, buzz sessions, or panels) ---------------------------- (2 pts) _____
    b. Reading and study assignments ------------------------------------- (2 pts) _____
    c. Oral and written reports --- (2 pts) _____
    d. Lectures -- (2 pts) _____
    e. Demonstrations -- (2 pts) _____
    f. Conferences -- (2 pts) _____
    g. Projects -- (2 pts) _____
    h. Problem solving -- (2 pts) _____
    i. Field trips -- (2 pts) _____
    j. Supplementary aids
        (1) Models, charts, and posters ------------------------------------- (2 pts) _____
        (2) Lantern slides and motion pictures -------------------------------- (2 pts) _____
    k. Plays and role playing --- (2 pts) _____
    l. Health surveys (practices, illness, medical treatment, immunizations, etc.) (2 pts) _____
    m. Experiments -- (2 pts) _____
13. Both official and voluntary agencies used in health instruction (literature and speakers), etc. -- (5 pts) _____
14. Health instruction evaluated by
    a. Conferences -- (2 pts) _____
    b. Objective tests --- (2 pts) _____
    c. Surveys of health practices ------------------------------------- (2 pts) _____
    d. Surveys of health attitude -------------------------------------- (2 pts) _____
    e. Surveys of health knowledge ------------------------------------ (2 pts) _____
15. Handicapped children provided with appropriate learning activities ---------- (3 pts) _____
16. Students encouraged to evaluate own health behavior and to assume responsibility for improvement -- (5 pts) _____
17. Supplementary health materials available for student use ------------------- (3 pts) _____
18. Sufficient facilities provided for adequate health instruction --------------- (5 pts) _____
19. Only materials from reliable sources used ------------------------------- (5 pts) _____
20. Adult health education program offered --------------------------------- (3 pts) _____

B. Correlated health instruction
    1. With art --- (10 pts) _____
    2. With biological science -- (10 pts) _____
    3. With physical science -- (10 pts) _____
    4. With home economics -- (10 pts) _____
    5. With physical education -- (10 pts) _____
    6. With social studies -- (10 pts) _____
    7. With other subject fields --- (10 pts) _____

C. Integrated health instruction
    1. Health education made functional in classroom activities
        a. Control of heat --- (5 pts) _____
        b. Control of ventilation -- (5 pts) _____
        c. Practice of cleanliness -------------------------------------- (5 pts) _____
    2. Health education made functional in nonclassroom activities
        a. Recreation
            (1) Use of safety precautions ------------------------------------- (5 pts) _____
            (2) Emphasis on personal adjustment -------------------------------- (5 pts) _____

  b. Lunch program
   (1) Selection of food -- (5 pts) _____
   (2) Adequate time for eating -- (5 pts) _____
   (3) Time for washing before meals -------------------------------------- (5 pts) _____
   (4) Favorable lunchroom atmosphere ----------------------------------- (5 pts) _____
  c. Safety program
   (1) Safety patrol -- (5 pts) _____
   (2) Traffic patrol --- (5 pts) _____
 3. Pupils given individualized guidance in evaluating daily health ------------- (3 pts) _____
 4. Medical and dental examinations utilized as learning experiences ----------- (2 pts) _____
 5. Health instruction integrated with other worthwhile experiences (field trips, projects, clubs, home and family experiences, etc.) --------------------------- (5 pts) _____

D. Preparation of teachers
 1. Areas included in training elementary teacher
  a. Personal health -- (5 pts) _____
  b. School health services -- (5 pts) _____
  c. School health instruction -- (5 pts) _____
  d. Healthful school living -- (5 pts) _____
  e. Community health --- (5 pts) _____
 2. Training for secondary school health educator
  a. Health teaching major -- (20 pts) _____
  b. Health teaching minor -- (10 pts) _____
  c. Ten to 20 quarter hours in health courses ---------------------------------- (5 pts) _____
  d. Six to 10 quarter hours in health courses ----------------------------------- (2 pts) _____
 3. Health education included in in-service program for teachers and principal
  a. Instruction and illustrations of recognizable signs and symptoms of communicable disease given by qualified person ---------------------------- (3 pts) _____
  b. Policies and recommendations of health department interpreted to teachers (5 pts) _____
  c. Health information presented through
   (1) Library --- (2 pts) _____
   (2) Bulletin boards -- (2 pts) _____
   (3) Faculty meetings -- (2 pts) _____
   (4) PTA meetings -- (2 pts) _____
   (5) Radio programs -- (2 pts) _____
   (6) Newspapers -- (2 pts) _____

PART III. HEALTHFUL SCHOOL LIVING   **(250 points)** _____

A. Safe and sanitary school facilities
 1. School site
  a. Easily accessible
   (1) Elementary schools not more than one-half mile walking distance or 30 minutes riding distance --- (3 pts) _____
   (2) Junior high schools not more than one mile walking or 1 hour riding distance -- (3 pts) _____
   (3) Senior high schools not more than two miles walking or 1 hour riding distance --- (3 pts) _____
  b. Free from disturbances
   (1) No distracting noises -- (2 pts) _____
   (2) No irritating dust -- (2 pts) _____
   (3) No noticeable odors -- (2 pts) _____
   (4) No objectionable odors --- (2 pts) _____
  c. Well-drained -- (2 pts) _____

    d. Adequate size
      (1) Elementary school grounds: 4 or more acres, 4 pts; 3 acres, 3 pts; 2 acres, 2 pts; less than 2 acres, 1 pt ------------------------------------- (4 pts) _____
      (2) Secondary school grounds: 6 acres or more, 4 pts; 5 acres, 3 pts; 4 acres, 2 pts; less than 4 acres, 1 pt ----------------------------------- (4 pts) _____

2. Water supply
    a. Ample -- (3 pts) _____
    b. Clear and cool -- (2 pts) _____
    c. Free from undesirable flavors and odors --------------------------- (2 pts) _____
    d. Free from contamination and pollution --------------------------- (3 pts) _____
    e. Adequate in fluorine content ------------------------------------- (2 pts) _____

3. Waste disposal
    a. Safe and sanitary garbage disposal ------------------------------- (3 pts) _____
    b. Sewage disposal meets state standards --------------------------- (5 pts) _____

4. Building
    a. Fire protection
      (1) Building construction of fire-resistant material ----------------- (4 pts) _____
      (2) Fire extinguishers placed conveniently to all parts of the building ------ (2 pts) _____
      (3) Fire alarms and extinguishers kept in working order --------------- (2 pts) _____
      (4) Fire alarms and extinguishers tested: twice a year or more often, 2 pts; once a year, 1 pt --- (2 pts) _____
      (5) Fire doors at all stairs --- (2 pts) _____
      (6) Outside doors open by inside bar --------------------------------- (2 pts) _____
      (7) Doors to exits unlocked or chutes open at all times building is in use -- (2 pts) _____
      (8) Exits and fire escapes sufficient to empty building in 2 minutes ------ (3 pts) _____
      (9) At least two exits from each floor -------------------------------- (2 pts) _____
      (10) Exits well marked and lighted ----------------------------------- (2 pts) _____
      (11) Last section of fire escape stairs left down ----------------------- (2 pts) _____
    b. Ventilation
      (1) Controllable in each room --------------------------------------- (1 pt) _____
      (2) Comfortable circulation of fresh air ----------------------------- (2 pts) _____
    c. Heating
      (1) Facilities inspected for safety weekly ---------------------------- (3 pts) _____
      (2) Classroom temperature range 68° to 72° F ----------------------- (2 pts) _____
    d. Lighting
      (1) Inspection and approval of electrical wiring at least once a year -------- (3 pts) _____
      (2) Footcandles of light available at desk level: 25 or more, 3 pts; 15-24, 2 pts; 5-14, 1 pt --- (3 pts) _____
      (3) Uniform light in each room -------------------------------------- (2 pts) _____
      (4) Absence of glare
        (a) Chalkboards of dull finish not beside windows -------------------- (2 pts) _____
        (b) Desks and tables of dull finish ---------------------------------- (2 pts) _____
        (c) Shades adjustable for maximum light control ---------------------- (2 pts) _____
      (5) Walls and ceiling of good light-reflecting colors: white or ivory, 4 pts; yellow, 3 pts; light buff, 2 pts; light gray, 1 pt ------------------- (4 pts) _____
      (6) Stairways, entrances, and corridors well lighted: more than 15 footcandles, 3 pts; 10-14, 2 pts; 5-9, 1 pt ------------------------------------- (3 pts) _____
    e. Seating
      (1) Individual seats --- (1 pt) _____
      (2) Movable seats -- (1 pt) _____
      (3) Regular adjustments to meet the needs of children: two or more times a year, 2 pts; once a year, 1 pt ----------------------------------- (2 pts) _____

(4) Seat arrangement
    (a) No child facing window --- (3 pts) _____
    (b) Teacher's desk not facing window ----------------------------- (2 pts) _____
(5) Provision for left-handed pupils ------------------------------------- (3 pts) _____
f. Drinking fountains
  (1) Type approved by board of health ---------------------------------- (2 pts) _____
  (2) Adequate number: one or more for 50 children, 3 pts; one for 60, 2 pts; one for 70 or more, 1 pt --- (3 pts) _____
g. Handwashing facilities
  (1) Type of basin approved by board of health ------------------------- (2 pts) _____
  (2) Adequate number of washbasins
    (a) Elementary school: one for each 20 pupils, 3 pts; one for each 30, 2 pts; one for each 40 or more, 1 pt ------------------------ (3 pts) _____
    (b) Secondary schools: one for 50 pupils, 3 pts; one for 60, 2 pts; one for 70 or more, 1 pt -------------------------------------- (3 pts) _____
  (3) Hot and cold water available ------------------------------------- (2 pts) _____
  (4) Paper or roller towels available ---------------------------------- (2 pts) _____
  (5) Liquid or powdered soap available --------------------------------- (2 pts) _____
  (6) Wastebasket available --- (1 pt) _____
h. Toilet facilities
  (1) Rooms clean, well lighted, and ventilated ------------------------- (3 pts) _____
  (2) Toilets
    (a) Type meeting state board of health standards ----------------- (2 pts) _____
    (b) Number
      i. For elementary girls: one for 20, 3 pts; one for 25, 2 pts; one for 30, 1 pt --- (3 pts) _____
      ii. For elementary boys (toilets and urinals): one for 20, 3 pts; one for 25, 2 pts; one for 30, 1 pt --------------------------- (3 pts) _____
      iii. For girls in grades 9 through 12: one for 45, 3 pts; one for 50, 2 pts; one for 55, 1 pt --------------------------------- (3 pts) _____
      iv. For boys in grades 9 through 12 (toilets and urinals): one for 60, 3 pts; one for 65, 2 pts; one for 70 or more, 1 pt -------------- (3 pts) _____
    (c) Plumbing conforming to state plumbing code -------------------- (3 pts) _____
5. Custodial service
  a. Cleaning practices
    (1) Floors cleaned daily with dust-preventive material --------------- (2 pts) _____
    (2) Light fixtures and windows cleaned at least three times a year ------- (2 pts) _____
    (3) Toilet room care
      (a) Swept daily --- (1 pt) _____
      (b) Scrubbed at least twice a week ----------------------------- (2 pts) _____
      (c) Towels, soap, and toilet paper kept available --------------- (2 pts) _____
  b. Building and equipment kept in good repair --------------------------- (2 pts) _____
  c. Building kept free from accumulations of rubbish --------------------- (2 pts) _____
  d. Inflammable material kept only in tight metal containers -------------- (2 pts) _____
  e. Custodian having special training for work --------------------------- (2 pts) _____
6. Lunchroom service
  a. School lunch facilities conforming to standards of state board of health ------ (3 pts) _____
  b. Serving designated to promote good eating practices ----------------- (2 pts) _____
  c. Sale of carbonated beverages, gum, and candy: prohibited, 2 pts; restricted, 1 pt --- (2 pts) _____
  d. All milk pasteurized --- (2 pts) _____
  e. All food handlers instructed in sanitary food handling and personal health practices --- (3 pts) _____
  f. Dishes cleaned and stored in manner approved by board of health ------- (3 pts) _____

   g. Metal garbage cans watertight and rodentproof ------------------------- (1 pt) _____
   h. Kitchen well lighted, well ventilated, clean, and attractive --------------- (2 pts) _____
   i. Dining room well lighted, well ventilated, clean, and attractive ----------- (2 pts) _____
 7. Play facilities and practices
   a. Play areas and equipment inspected for accident hazards and such conditions
       promptly corrected: weekly, 3 pts; monthly, 1 pt ----------------------- (3 pts) _____
   b. Adequate indoor play areas with nonslip floors ----------------------- (2 pts) _____
   c. Adequate outdoor play areas with nonslip surfaces --------------------- (2 pts) _____
   d. Pupils instructed and supervised in proper use and care of classroom, gym-
       nasium, and playground facilities ------------------------------------- (2 pts) _____
 8. Safety program
   a. Planned program --- (2 pts) _____
   b. Responsible supervisor -- (2 pts) _____
   c. Weekly safety inspections --- (2 pts) _____
   d. Traffic problems are adequately supervised and controlled --------------- (3 pts) _____
B. Healthful school program
 1. Teaching methods that promote both physical and mental health
   a. Frequent success experienced by all pupils --------------------------- (2 pts) _____
   b. Mental health of child considered in school discipline -------------------- (2 pts) _____
   c. Excessive fatigue avoided --- (3 pts) _____
   d. Length of school day and frequency and length of recess periods adjusted to
       age levels -- (2 pts) _____
   e. Each child encouraged in special interest ----------------------------- (3 pts) _____
   f. Each pupil given opportunity to lead and follow ----------------------- (3 pts) _____
   g. Each child assisted in development of self-confidence, self-judgment, and good
       social attitudes --- (3 pts) _____
 2. Good rapport between pupils and teacher
   a. Children feel free to express themselves ----------------------------- (2 pts) _____
   b. Pupils are relaxed --- (3 pts) _____
   c. Pupils feel they are held in esteem by teacher and associates ------------- (3 pts) _____
 3. Emotional effect on pupils taken into consideration in making decisions ------ (3 pts) _____
 4. Teaching staff emotionally well adjusted ------------------------------- (3 pts) _____
 5. Established standards of health required of all school personnel ------------- (3 pts) _____
 6. General health examination required of all school personnel; annually, 3 pts;
     biennially, 2 pts; only before entry to school system, 1 pt ------------------ (3 pts) _____
 7. Teaching load: total work load limited to 40 hours or less per week, 3 pts; 41-44,
     2 pts; 45-48, 1 pt --- (2 pts) _____
 8. One week sick leave granted to school personnel ------------------------- (2 pts) _____

SUMMARY

Part I. School health services --- (350 points) _____
Part II. Health instruction --- (400 points) _____
Part III. Healthful school living -- (250 points) _____
COMPOSITE SCORE _____

Self-appraisal checklist for school health programs*

FOREWORD

In 1966, The Ohio Association for Health, Physical Education and Recreation, in cooperation with the State Department of Education, the State Department of Health, and The State Planning Committee for Health Education in Ohio, developed and distributed the Evaluative Criteria manual for use in Ohio's schools.

This instrument was useful in surveying and comparing actual practice with ideal practice. It included the three major areas:

School Health Services
Healthful School Environment
Health Instruction

This appraisal checklist was well received. In answer to the many and continuing requests for the "Self-Appraisal Checklist," this new revised edition has been developed.

Additional copies may be requested by writing to:

---

*From Ohio Department of Education, Health, Physical Education and Recreation Section: Self-appraisal checklist, Columbus, Ohio 43215.

Ohio Department of Education
Health, Physical Education and Recreation Section
65 South Front Street
Columbus OH 43215
   or
Ohio Department of Health
Health Education
P.O. Box 118
Columbus OH 43216

INTRODUCTION

The School Health Program is designed to maintain and enhance the health of students, school personnel, and the community. It should be a foundation for action programs in the community by providing a health oriented school population. Students will be equipped to deal wisely with their own and their families' health problems and should provide a potential source of adult leadership for future community health problems. The program supplements and reinforces home and community programs. It utilizes the resources of official agencies, professional associations, voluntary organizations, and other community groups, including civic clubs.

Four inter-related parts make up the

School Health Program: (**I**) **Administration of the School Health Program, (II) School Health Services** which strive to determine the total health status of the student and seek remedial action for health problems, (**III**) **Healthful School Living** which designates the plans, procedures and activities which provide a school environment conducive to optimum physical, mental and social health and safety, and (**IV**) **Health Education** which provides formal classroom experiences for favorably influencing knowledge, attitudes, habits, values and skills and behavior pertaining to individual and group health.

This guide can be useful in surveying what a school is doing in terms of health and comparing this to what is considered good practice. As a result, desirable changes can be undertaken to improve the school health program as the needs are indicated.

HOW TO USE THIS GUIDE

It is recommended that an evaluation team be organized which include representatives from school administration, teaching staff, medical and dental professions, nursing, health departments, parents, community groups, etc.

The team should review and discuss the guide prior to its utilization and formulate a plan of action to help insure that techniques and resources are available to appropriately complete the study. The team can then proceed to evaluate its health program by answering the questions and comparing the existing program with the recommended practices.

The third column of the form provides space for comments, priorities, proposed plans and time schedules.

Shortcomings should be prioritized upon consideration of how critical they are and what resources are needed to correct them. A thorough plan of action will include deficiencies subject to immediate and easy correction as well as a timetable and methodology for the correction of problems requiring larger amounts of resources and time (may take one to two years). Follow-up is encouraged to see that corrections are being made according to the specified plan of action.

The study group should not hesitate to request help from specialists or consultants from agencies listed, in addition to local community resources.

Also, this checklist could serve as a valuable tool to school personnel to point out strengths and weaknesses of their respective areas or responsibilities.

PART I. ADMINISTRATION OF THE SCHOOL HEALTH PROGRAM

A successful school health program involves understanding and leadership by the School Administrator in his role as top-ranking coordinator and liaison with the Board of Education, his staff members and the community. He must be able to present school health needs to his board and utilize all resources and facilities in the community for fostering the health of the school children. He is responsible for the enforcement of the state laws regarding school health, including immunizations. The school experiences of students in our school health programs will largely determine their knowledge and their attitudes about health, and it is the responsibility of every school to offer a comprehensive and effective health education program taught by adequately prepared instructors. This effort should be supported by all groups in the community. The administrator sets the keynote for effective working relationships with school personnel, students and the community. A school should be responsive to and involve the community in planning, developing, implementing and evaluating programs in a variety of ways, including the establishment of and/or the participation in school-community health committees.

Text continued on p. 477.

Standards and recommended practices	What are we doing	Comments, priorities, proposed plans, time schedule
Program organization and administration		
A. A well organized school health program should be planned jointly by the schools, the health department, educational and health professional associations and other responsible community groups.	A. What methods are used to provide for joint planning of the school health program? 1. on a community-wide basis? 2. on an individual school basis?	
B. Both the Board of Health and Board of Education may be charged with specific responsibilities. If this is so, the administration of the duties should be the result of joint planning, and roles and responsibilities of personnel clearly defined.	B. List the responsibilities of the: 1. School 2. Department of health	
C. A school health program is best integrated when a well qualified school person is appointed to coordinate it.	C. 1. The person responsible for the coordination and administration of the school health program is: a. Superintendent ☐ b. Health coordinator ☐ c. Principal ☐ d. School medical advisor ☐ e. School dental advisor ☐ f. School nurse ☐ g. Other (list): ☐ 2. The person responsible for the development of the health curriculum is: a. Superintendent ☐ b. Curriculum director ☐ c. Health coordinator ☐ d. Principal ☐ e. Nurse ☐ f. Supervisor, Health, physical education and recreation ☐ g. Other (list):	

a. Superintendent ☐
b. Health coordinator ☐
c. Nurse ☐
d. Supervisor, Health, physical
   education and recreation ☐

D. Administrative objectives are:

1. To develop sound school health practices and to facilitate and make more effective the work of teachers, school health service personnel, and other related non-teaching staff (cafeteria workers, bus drivers, custodians).

2. To provide for special in-service education programs to be conducted for the personnel directly involved in the school health program.

3. To provide for periodic evaluation and improvement to help keep the program in step with changing needs and trends.

4. To define and develop sound and effective working relationships among agencies directly concerned with the school health program, and to communicate school health concerns to the community-at-large.

D. 1. Does the school have written policies that:
   a. Clearly define agency responsibility including legal. Yes ☐ No ☐
   b. Clearly define roles of personnel, e.g., nurses, administrators, teachers, etc. Yes ☐ No ☐
   c. When were the policies last reviewed?

2. Special in-service education programs are conducted for these personnel? Yes ☐ No ☐
   How often?
   These in-service education programs are evaluated to determine their effectiveness? Yes ☐ No ☐

3. Periodic evaluations and improvements are provided in the program?
   In what ways?
   How often?

4. There are sound and effective working relationships between those involved in the school health program and agencies? Yes ☐ No ☐
   If not, what plans are being made to improve these relationships?
   Check ways the school health concerns are communicated to the community:
   PTA or PTO ☐
   School health committee ☐
   School communications ☐
   Official agencies ☐
   Voluntary health agencies ☐

Continued.

Standards and recommended practices	What are we doing	Comments, priorities, proposed plans, time schedule
Program organization and administration — cont'd		
	The person responsible for helping to insure sound and effective working relationships is:	
	a. Superintendent ☐	
	b. Principal ☐	
	c. Health coordinator ☐	
	d. School nurse ☐	
	e. Supervisor, Health, physical education ☐	
	f. Other (list): ☐	
E. Well prepared personnel, in all phases of the school health program are essential for its effective and successful implementation.	E. Qualifications of school health personnel.	
	1. Check the qualifications and experience of the school health coordinator:	
	a. Certificated ☐	
	b. 3 to 5 years experience in health education or school health programs ☐	
	c. Recent courses or workshops related to school health ☐	
	d. Other (list):	
	2. What percent of the school nurses are:	
	a. Registered in the state of Ohio? ☐	
	b. Certificated? ☐	
	c. Have had post-baccalaureate courses in school health? ☐	
	3. How many elementary teachers have background (a minimum of three semester hours) in health education and/or health science? ☐	
	4. Are the secondary teachers assigned to teach health certificated in health education? Yes ☐ No ☐	
	5. The school provides an in-service education program for:	
	a. Teachers? Yes ☐ No ☐	
	Date:	
	One-half day or less ☐	
	One day or more ☐	

Continued.

b. Nurses? Yes ☐ No ☐
   Date:
      One-half day or less ☐
      One day or more ☐
      College credit ☐

c. Administrative personnel?
   Guidance counselors, social workers, etc.
   Yes ☐ No ☐
   Date:
      One-half day or less ☐
      One day or more ☐
      College credit ☐

d. Non-teaching (non-certified) personnel?
   Yes ☐ No ☐
   Date:
      One-half day or less ☐
      One day or more ☐
      College credit ☐

F. The school administration promotes the integration of health and safety in all curricular and extra curricular activities of the school by:
   Leaving to individual teachers ☐
   Combined efforts of teachers/coordinators ☐
   Suggestions in teachers guides ☐
   Written policies and procedures ☐

G. The director is readily available to all school personnel?   Yes ☐ No ☐

H. The school utilizes the following community resources:
   Health department ☐
   Other official agencies ☐
   Medical society/auxiliary ☐
   Dental society/auxiliary ☐
   Voluntary agencies ☐
   Civic groups ☐
   Other (list): ☐

F. The school administration promotes the integration of health and safety in all curricular and extra curricular activities of the school.

G. If available, schools utilize their community directory of health services.

H. Schools should know what health resources are available in the community and how they can be utilized effectively.

Standards and recommended practices	What are we doing	Comments, priorities, proposed plans, time schedule
First aid for sudden illness and accidents:		
A. State law (Sec. 3313.712) requires that an emergency medical treatment authorization form be annually filled out on each student by his parent or legal guardian before October of each year. This form is to be kept on file in the school.	A. Emergency medical treatment authorization forms for all students are filled out annually and are on file in each school? Yes ☐ No ☐	
B. First aid and sudden illness procedures agreed upon by administrator and staff are written and disseminated to all staff.	B. 1. Are policies agreed upon by administrators and staff? Yes ☐ No ☐ 2. Are written copies of first aid and sudden illness policies made available to all staff? Yes ☐ No ☐	
C. Persons (other than nurses) trained in first aid procedures should be available for administering first aid or providing direction in cases of sudden illness.	C. 1. How many persons with current first aid preparation are available? _____ 2. Are all teachers working in high risk areas qualified in first aid, such as: Science labs ☐ Shops ☐ Home economics ☐ Physical education ☐	
D. First aid procedures should be briefly written for quick reference and posted in special areas, such as science labs, shops, home economics rooms, school health clinic, and physical education areas.	D. Check areas posted: Science labs ☐ Shops ☐ Home economics room ☐ Health clinic ☐ Physical education ☐	

E. First aid equipment/supplies should be kept in stock and readily accessible. All medicines, compounds, bandaging materials should be clearly labeled for use. A designated person should be responsible for ordering supplies.

E. 1. In what locations are first aid supplies stored?
   2. All supplies clearly labeled?
     Yes □ No □
   3. Check the person responsible for ordering and restocking supplies?
     Superintendent □
     Principal □
     Nurse □
     Supervisor, Health, physical education and recreation □
     Health coordinator □

Accident reporting system

A. Written policies and procedures (developed by administration and faculty, outlining a system for reporting school accidents) should be available to all school personnel.

A. Policies are written and made available to all staff?
   Yes □ No □

B. The Ohio Department of Health has an Accident Reporting Form, No. 4966.32. They may be utilized if the schools will report the statistical data to the accident prevention program at the end of the year.

B. Does your school use the Ohio Department of Health Accident Reporting Form?
   Yes □ No □

C. The reporting system should:
   1. define a "reportable accident"
   2. indicate the time lapse in reporting the accident
   3. record information to include: who, what, where, when, why
   4. include follow-through on treatment or referral
   5. indicate who is responsible for recording and reporting accidents

C. Does the reporting system include:
   1. definition of a reportable accident □
   2. time lapse in reporting accident □
   3. who-what-where-when-why □
   4. follow-up—
     a. number of days lost from school □
     b. possible action in future to avoid or eliminate future occurrences □
   5. who is responsible for recording accidents? □

Continued.

Standards and recommended practices	What are we doing	Comments, priorities, proposed plans, time schedule
Accident reporting system — cont'd		
D. School personnel should be familiar with school accident forms and should complete or use them uniformly.	D. School personnel are informed regarding the use of accident forms by: 1. Staff conferences ☐ 2. News bulletin ☐ 3. Teacher handbooks ☐ 4. Other (list):	
E. At the end of each school year, all accident data should be reviewed, analyzed, and compared with last year's records to determine the needs for next year's program.	E. List recommendations as a result of reviewing this year's records.	
F. A safety committee is recommended to provide leadership for planning a comprehensive safety education program. It should include such people as: administrator, safety specialist, teacher, driver education teacher, physician, school nurse, sanitarian, custodian, student, parent, etc.	F. 1. Do you have a safety committee? Yes ☐ No ☐ 2. Who is on the committee? 3. List the name of the Specialist in Safety.	

PART II. SCHOOL HEALTH SERVICES

In order to meet the educational and health needs of students, it is essential to secure data concerning their physical, mental and emotional condition. Thus, school health services are an important part of the school health programs. These services are planned to protect the health of the students and to help each pupil reach and maintain good health. Also, the school health service program serves as a learning experience for students, teachers, and parents, thereby helping to insure positive health practices.

The school health program is influenced by local customs, the types of professional manpower, the resources available, the understanding and cooperation of the community.

Text continued on p. 487.

Standards and recommended practices	What are we doing	Comments, priorities, proposed plans, time schedule
Teacher observation A. To teach effectively it is important that the teacher keep informed of the health needs of all her pupils. 1. Teachers should receive in-service education in the health observation of school children so that they may refer children who they suspect as having a health problem to appropriate health service personnel. This should be a year round program. 2. "A Teacher Worksheet for Student Health Observation" would be useful to familiarize teachers with signs and symptoms of health and emotional problems. This may be ordered from the Ohio Department of Health. (No. 3611.13)	A. What type of in-service education is provided teachers to improve their skills of observation and referral procedures? 1. Teacher/nurse conferences Yes ☐ No ☐ Health education workshops Yes ☐ No ☐ College/university credit courses Yes ☐ No ☐ Other (list): 2. Do teachers use "A Teacher Worksheet for Student Health Observation"? Yes ☐ No ☐	

Continued.

Standards and recommended practices	What are we doing	Comments, priorities, proposed plans, time schedule
Health screening *Hearing* A. The following should be screened annually: (1) all children in grades K through 3 (2) all teacher referrals (3) all children new to the school system (4) all children in grades 6 and 9 These tests should be administered with the individual pure tone audiometer.	A. Check grades you are screening with the pure tone audiometer:	

A. (table below)

	No. screened	No. failed 1st screening	No. failed 2nd screening	Failed threshold test and referred
K				
1st				
2nd				
3rd				
Other grades				
Referrals				
New students				
Total				

Standards and recommended practices	What are we doing
B. All students failing the first screening should be re-screened within two weeks.	B. The number of children who failed to pass threshold screening tests represents ———— percent of all children screened.
C. Refer all children who fail to pass the threshold screening test to appropriate resources as: medical or audiological.	C. What percentage of the children referred for follow-up care are known to have received it? ————
D. Assure that follow-up care has been obtained for each person referred for care.	D. Procedures used to secure follow-up care ☐ Visit to home ☐ Telephone call (by teacher or nurse) ☐ Note sent home ☐ Other (list):

Vision

E. Ideally, all children (kindergarten through grade 12 and all teacher referrals) should be screened annually with a Snellen chart. Minimum: K and grades 1, 3, 5, 7, 9.

F. Screen all children for ocular muscle imbalance, excessive farsightedness, and near acuity in grades one or three, and screen for color deficiency in either elementary or junior high grade.

E. Check grades you are screening with the Snellen eye chart:

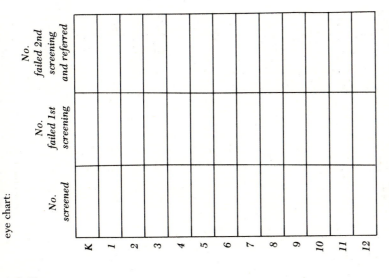

	No. screened	*No. failed 1st screening*	*No. failed 2nd screening and referred*
K			
1			
2			
3			
4			
5			
6			
7			
8			
9			
10			
11			
12			

F. Are you screening all children in grades 1 or 3 for:

Ocular muscle imbalance	Yes ☐	No ☐
Excessive farsightedness	Yes ☐	No ☐
Near acuity	Yes ☐	No ☐
Color deficiency	Yes ☐	No ☐

(elementary or jr. high grade. Please indicate which grade_____).

Continued.

Standards and recommended practices	What are we doing	Comments, priorities, proposed plans, time schedule
Health screening—cont'd *Vision—cont'd* G. Refer all children who fail a screening test to a vision specialist. H. Determine that follow-up care has been obtained for each child referred for eye care.	G. How many children were referred for eye care after last screening? This represents _____ percent of the children screened. H. What percentage of the children referred are known to have received follow-up care? _____ %	
Health room (clinic) A. A health room or clinic should be provided and adequately equipped to carry on essential school health services: examinations, tests for vision, hearing, speech, psychological, and private conferences.	A. Does your school have a room where the school physician, school nurse and other specialists can perform: Examination Yes ☐ No ☐ Vision testing Yes ☐ No ☐ Hearing testing Yes ☐ No ☐ Psychological testing Yes ☐ No ☐ Speech therapy Yes ☐ No ☐ Private conferences Yes ☐ No ☐ 1. Does it have a place where pupils who are injured or who become suddenly ill can wait until someone can transport them home? Yes ☐ No ☐ 2. Does it have space for use by health service personnel for individual or small group conferences? Yes ☐ No ☐ 3. Is there adequate space for storing first aid supplies, school health records, etc.? Yes ☐ No ☐	

Continued.

Medical examinations

A. "School Health: A Guide for Physicians," American Academy of Pediatrics, suggests that the priority of medical appraisal should be:

(1) children identified as having problems

(2) children entering school

(3) children in mid-school (6-7 grades)

(4) children before leaving school (11-12 grades)

Medical examinations should be done by a physician in his office or in a clinic. Parents of elementary children should be present. These examinations should be comprehensive and any abnormal findings of the school screening tests should be provided to the physician. The results of the physician's examination should be reported to school personnel.

B. Arrangements should be made for children of low income families to receive examinations. Plans should be formulated whereby school and physicians share necessary information.

C. Medical examinations should be given to students enrolled in athletic programs. Consideration should be given to students enrolled in other groups, such as, marching bands, intramural and inter-scholastic sports, etc.

A. Do pupils receive a medical examination upon entrance to school? Yes ☐ No ☐
  1. Are they examined at mid-school?
     Yes ☐ No ☐
  2. Are referrals with special problems examined?
     Yes ☐ No ☐
  3. Are they examined at senior high school?
     Yes ☐ No ☐

B. Is this examination done by:
  Health department   Yes ☐ No ☐
  School health service   Yes ☐ No ☐
  Other (list):
  If there are no arrangements for this examination, give reason:

C. Are boys and girls in the athletic program provided medical examinations?
  Boys   Yes ☐ No ☐
  Girls   Yes ☐ No ☐
  By whom?
  When?
  Other groups such as:
  Marching band members   Yes ☐ No ☐
  Drill teams   Yes ☐ No ☐
  Intra-mural sports   Yes ☐ No ☐
  Inter-scholastic sports   Yes ☐ No ☐

Standards and recommended practices	What are we doing	Comments, priorities, proposed plans, time schedule
Medical examinations — cont'd		
D. All families receiving ADC, should be enrolled in the Early Periodic Screening Diagnosis and Treatment (EPSDT) Program.	D. How many children are enrolled in EPSDT Programs in: Elementary _____ Secondary _____	
E. Plans should be developed with Department of Welfare to share this information as needed by professional personnel planning health services for the child.	E. Check the method the Welfare Department utilizes to share EPSDT screening information on students: Phone Yes ☐ No ☐ Written form Yes ☐ No ☐ Other (list):	
Health records		
A. A health record should be started when the child enters school and should follow the student as he moves from grade to grade and from school to school. Confidentiality of all health and mental health records should be respected. All personnel should be very careful of sharing any information that might prove speculative or damaging to any student.	A. Does each pupil have a health record on file? Yes ☐ No ☐ Does your school use School Health Records, form 3613.13 Rev. 1974, from the Ohio Department of Health? Yes ☐ No ☐ If not, what form is used: Is the permanent health record transferred when a child changes schools? Yes ☐ No ☐	
Health counseling		
A. A definite plan of continuous follow-up should be established. The school nurse should be a liaison with school, parents and community resources.	A. Has your school established a plan of referral and follow-up? Yes ☐ No ☐	
B. Health counseling is one of the main functions of the school nurse, and important information should be shared with and utilized by school counselors, psychologists, teachers, etc.	B. Is the nurse given time for counseling? Yes ☐ No ☐	

C. The school nurse follows through to help the parent with remedial action. Upon discovering a health defect in a student, the school nurse should follow-up by assisting parents with a plan of remedial action. This could involve a team, such as: physician, psychologist, public health nurse, visiting teacher, speech therapist, school counselor, etc.

D. The school nurse should have some training in mental health counseling. The school nurse and counseling psychologist should have agreed upon procedures for mutual referral and collaboration on students with significantly overlapping physical (somatic) and mental health problems.

Teacher-nurse conferences

A. A teacher-nurse conference should be held at least once a year or as often as needed.

Children with special problems

A. Identification of and special provision for handicapped children; deaf and hard of hearing, crippled, visually impaired, neurologically and emotionally, educable mentally retarded, etc., is an important aspect of school health services.
The school should make special provisions for handicapped pupils in regular classes when this is the most appropriate placement.

C. Does the nurse communicate with parents regarding child health defects and remedial action by:

Written note	Yes ☐	No ☐
Telephone	Yes ☐	No ☐
Home visit	Yes ☐	No ☐
Conference at school	Yes ☐	No ☐

D. Has the school nurse had any courses in mental health?
Yes ☐ No ☐
Are there mutually agreed procedures for referral by school nurse and by psychologist?
Yes ☐ No ☐

A. Is time provided for the nurse to schedule conferences with teachers?
1. Once a year   Yes ☐ No ☐
2. As often as necessary Yes ☐ No ☐

A. Number of children with special problems in:
Elementary _____
Secondary _____
List types of handicaps:

Continued.

Standards and recommended practices	What are we doing	Comments, priorities, proposed plans, time schedule

Children with special problems—cont'd
Special facilities and/or programs should be made available to the children with any handicapping conditions.
	What provision is made for children with special problems? Check:
	1. Special facilities:
	   Ramps ☐
	   Special toilets ☐
	   Rest areas ☐
	2. Special services:
	   Occupational therapy ☐
	   Physical therapy ☐
	   Speech therapy ☐
	   Psychological ☐
	3. In-service education for teachers ☐
	4. In-service education for auxiliary personnel ☐
	   Types:
	5. Transportation provided ☐
	6. Other (list):	

Dental examinations
A. Examinations by a dentist for school purposes should be given to all pupils entering the system and at the beginning of the secondary school level.
	A. Do pupils receive a dental examination upon entrance to school? Yes ☐ No ☐
	   If yes, what percent? _____ %
	   1. Do pupils receive a dental examination at the secondary level? Yes ☐ No ☐
	      If yes, what percent? _____ %	

B. These examinations should be done by a dentist in his office or clinic with the parents of elementary children accompanying them.	B. Outline your plan for making a concentrated effort to have all students visit their dentist regularly
	   1. Check reasons why students are not receiving dental care:
	      Lack of dental manpower ☐
	      Lack of funds ☐
	      Lack of transportation ☐
	      Other (list):	

C. The school or the community should provide for the dental examinations of indigent pupils. The local dental society working with the school and community should formulate a program to provide services for indigent students.

D. All students involved in inter-scholastic contact athletics should be provided with mouth protectors. The local dental society should be contacted for assistance.

E. The community water supply should be fluoridated.

F. In a good school health program, oral hygiene should be observed by the teacher, school nurse and other personnel involved in the health of the student. Pertinent information should be recorded on the cumulative health record. Evidence of dental neglect should be reported by the school nurse or teacher to parents. Follow-up of this referral should ·be done by the responsible person.

G. Dentists, dental auxiliaries or affiliated groups are resources that can be utilized in a dental health education program.

C. What dental services are provided for children whose parents cannot afford such services?
1. What arrangements are made for the examination of indigent children?

D. What arrangements are made for mouth protectors for students involved in inter-scholastic contact athletics?

Provided by student   Yes ☐ No ☐
Provided by schools   Yes ☐ No ☐
Provided by local dental society Yes ☐ No ☐
Provided by other (list):

E. Is your community water supply fluoridated?
Yes ☐ No ☐
1. If not, why?

F. Pertinent dental health information is filed in the cumulative health folder?
Yes ☐ No ☐
Referrals from dentists   Yes ☐ No ☐
Recorded by nurse   Yes ☐ No ☐
Other (list):

G. Check the resources listed below which have been utilized in your dental program in the past.
Dentists   Yes ☐ No ☐
Dental hygienists   Yes ☐ No ☐
Dental auxiliaries   Yes ☐ No ☐
PTA or PTO   Yes ☐ No ☐
Others (list):
Future plans:

Continued.

Standards and recommended practices	What are we doing	Comments, priorities, proposed plans, time schedule
Health of school personnel		
A. Pre-employment health examinations should be required of all school personnel.	A. Pre-employment examinations are required for all school personnel? Yes ☐ No ☐	
B. Periodic medical examinations of school personnel are recommended.	B. If periodic medical examinations are required, state the time intervals:	
Communicable disease control		
A. There should be well defined school health policies developed in cooperation with local health departments and/or with School Health Services and approved by the Board of Education.	A. Does your school have written school health policies? Yes ☐ No ☐	
B. School personnel and parents should be informed regarding these policies.	B. Parents and teachers are informed regarding these policies by: Meetings Yes ☐ No ☐ Newsletters Yes ☐ No ☐ Other (list):	
C. School nurses should report cases of communicable diseases, including pediculosis and scabies, to local health department.	C. Check the method the school nurses use in reporting communicable diseases to the local health department: Phone ☐ Written form ☐	
D. All students should comply with the law of Ohio regarding immunizations as stated in Section 3313.671 of the Ohio Revised Code. This law requires a pupil to be or in the process of being immunized against polio, rubeola, diphtheria, rubella, pertussis and tetanus. This is the responsibility of the administrator.	D. Does your school have a formal plan for enforcement of this law? Yes ☐ No ☐	

PART III. HEALTHFUL SCHOOL LIVING

The health of the students and school personnel is affected by the environment in which they work and play. Environment influences the health, the habits, the attitudes, the comfort, the safety and the working efficiency of school personnel. The environment is the responsibility of the school administration; helping to maintain it is the responsibility of all school personnel, and inspecting for environmental deficiencies is the statutory responsibility of the local department of health.

Text continued on p. 494.

Standards and recommended practices	What are we doing	Comments, priorities, proposed plans, time schedule
Inspection		
A. Semi-annual inspections of the school facilities are made by the local health department sanitarians and school health personnel (custodial staff—school administrators). A copy of the School Environment Inspection Form is on page 493.*	A. Date of school inspection: School official Name and title: _____ 1. Progress of inspection recommendations:	

*Copy of "Sanitation in The School Environment" No. 2116.32 is available from the Ohio Department of Health.

Continued.

Standards and recommended practices	What are we doing	Comments, priorities, proposed plans, time schedule
Inspection — cont'd		
B. Semi-annual inspections of the school food service operation (if provided) are made by the local health department's sanitarian and school personnel (cafeteria supervisor—school administrators).	B. Date of food service inspection: School official _____ Name and title: _____ 1. Progress in correcting (remedying) inspection violations:	
C. Procedure has been established to insure that inspection reports are properly interpreted to school authorities.	C. The inspection results are reviewed and explained with recommendations to the school officials at the time of the inspection. School officials consulted: 1. Superintendent or principal ☐ 2. School administrator ☐ 3. Custodial supervisor ☐ 4. Cafeteria supervisor ☐ 5. Others ☐	
D. Copies of the inspection reports are sent to the appropriate persons.	D. Copies of the inspection reports are sent to: 1. Board of Education ☐ 2. School administrator ☐ 3. Health supervisor/coordinator ☐ 4. Custodial supervisor ☐ 5. Cafeteria supervisor ☐ 6. Others ☐	
E. Plans for any new physical structure, (including all major improvements) are submitted to the appropriate agencies prior to construction.	E. Plans are submitted to: 1. State Department of Industrial Relations ☐ 2. State Plumbing Unit, Ohio Department of Health ☐ 3. Local health department ☐ 4. Others as required ☐	

F. Periodic in-service education programs sponsored jointly by the health department and the school system for custodial and food service employees are recommended.

G. The school environment should stimulate learning and the development of good sanitation practices such as:
1. Food handling instructions for students assisting in the lunch room.
2. Students to learn and appreciate good food handling practices.
3. Maintaining a more attractive lunch room.
4. Proper storage of food.

F. Check the in-service education programs for custodial and food service employees during the last 12 months.
1. A program conducted by the Health Department for custodial and food service employees. Yes □ No □
2. Personnel attended workshop in Columbus conducted by the Department of Education.
Yes □ No □
List future plans for in-service education programs for the next 12 months.

G. Check any activities initiated by school officials which serve to motivate environmental sanitation practices.
1. Enlists the help of student patrols to make inspections of the environment to check for good sanitation and safety practices.
Yes □ No □
2. Food handling class conducted for students assisting in the lunch room.
Yes □ No □
3. Group of students works with lunch room personnel in improving attractiveness of lunch room. Yes □ No □
4. Invites local sanitarian to discuss sanitation and safety practices to school personnel and/or health classes. Yes □ No □
5. Others (list):

Safe school environment

Accident prevention is a vital part of semiannual inspections conducted by local health sanitarians and school health personnel. These inspections place considerable emphasis on maintaining, planning and developing safety practices within the school environment and especially at specific locations.

Continued.

Standards and recommended practices	What are we doing	Comments, priorities, proposed plans, time schedule

Safe school environment — cont'd

A. The sanitarian's inspection of safety of the environment should include the following major areas:

School grounds
Parking area
Playground and equipment
Athletic field and equipment
Floor areas, stairs, ramps
Classrooms
Dressing/shower rooms
Gymnasium
Vocational areas/chem labs/home economics rooms
School cafeteria/kitchens
Restrooms
Fire fighting equipment/exits
First aid emergency rooms

A. 1. Parking kept away from playground equipment? Yes ☐ No ☐
2. Playground equipment maintained in good repairs? Yes ☐ No ☐
3. Has soft, absorbent surface been provided around playground equipment? Yes ☐ No ☐
4. Are floor surfaces kept clean, free of tripping, slipping hazards? Yes ☐ No ☐
5. Classrooms arranged for best traffic pattern, least amount of congestion? Yes ☐ No ☐
6. Classroom furniture kept in good repair, adequate lighting provided? Yes ☐ No ☐
7. Adequate supervision provided for organized/unorganized activity on the school grounds and in the gymnasium? Yes ☐ No ☐
8. Necessary safety precautions taken in vocational shop, chem labs, home economics areas, i.e.:
   Protective eyeware provided Yes ☐ No ☐
   Faucet for eye lavage if chemically burned Yes ☐ No ☐
   Fire extinguisher close to heating elements Yes ☐ No ☐
9. In-service safety programs presented for food service personnel in school kitchen? Yes ☐ No ☐
   Date of last in-service workshop?
   Projected date for next food safety program?
10. Restroom floors kept dry, free of debris? Yes ☐ No ☐
11. Fire extinguishers checked monthly to determine operability? Yes ☐ No ☐
    Date of last fire extinguisher check?

Continued.

12. Proper class of extinguishers provided according to type of fire hazard, i.e., electrical, paper, chemical, etc.?
Yes □ No □

13. Health department sanitarian meets with school personnel or safety committee to discuss findings of the school inspection and needed or recommended corrections?
Yes □ No □
Comments:

B. An effective school safety program encompasses many areas within the school system:
1. Constant awareness to potential hazards of new products being introduced into the school environment.
2. Special training, and drills of school bus drivers and children in school bus safety practices along with regular school vehicle inspections.
3. School safety concerns integrated into appropriate curriculum designs.
4. Fire drills
5. Safety education

B. Check any special safety in-service education programs during the past school year for:

Bus drivers	Yes □	No □
Lunch room personnel	Yes □	No □
Teachers	Yes □	No □
Custodians	Yes □	No □
Safety patrol	Yes □	No □

C. Safety concerns should be integrated into the health education curriculum.

C. Check safety concerns that have been integrated into the curriculum this past year, such as:

1. Accident etiology	Yes □	No □
2. Bicycle	Yes □	No □
3. Home (urban/suburban)	Yes □	No □
4. Home (rural)	Yes □	No □
5. Toy safety	Yes □	No □
6. Pedestrian safety	Yes □	No □
7. Vacation	Yes □	No □
8. Poisons	Yes □	No □
9. Firearms and hunting	Yes □	No □
10. Automobile and seat belt	Yes □	No □
11. Pets	Yes □	No □
12. Fires	Yes □	No □
13. Athletic and playground	Yes □	No □
14. Water and boating	Yes □	No □

Standards and recommended practices	What are we doing	Comments, priorities, proposed plans, time schedule
School nutrition program		
A. There is a food service provided in the school and all pupils are encouraged to participate.	A. Is there a food service program in your school? Yes ☐ No ☐	
B. The lunch served meets the National "Type A" Standard.	B. Does it meet National "Type A" Standard? Yes ☐ No ☐	
C. Even though it is legal to sell candy and sweetened beverages in the school, it is recommended that this practice not be permitted during school or lunch hours. Sale of such items is in direct competition with a good lunch program.	C. Does your school sell: 1. Candy — Yes ☐ No ☐ 2. Soft drinks — Yes ☐ No ☐ 3. Chocolate milk or drink — Yes ☐ No ☐ 4. Other snack items — Yes ☐ No ☐	
D. The school lunch program should be utilized as a learning laboratory for good nutrition in a child's life.	D. Check any of these activities related to lunch room and nutrition that are utilized in the health education program. 1. Classroom units — Yes ☐ No ☐ 2. Pupils given an opportunity to evaluate menus to determine if they meet "Type A" school lunch requirements. — Yes ☐ No ☐ 3. Pupils or art classes make posters for the lunch room. — Yes ☐ No ☐ 4. Classes plan menus and solicit the assistance of head cook in serving it to students. — Yes ☐ No ☐ 5. A class makes a survey of eating habits of students in lunch room to see foods rejected or wasted. — Yes ☐ No ☐ 6. Class tours the kitchen to observe dish washing, storage of food, etc. and to discuss why certain practices are necessary. — Yes ☐ No ☐	
E. School food service personnel should be required (expenses to be paid by the Board of Education) to attend workshops and conferences sponsored by the State Department of Education for the lunch room workers.	E. In this school year, how many school lunch personnel attended the workshops and conferences sponsored by the State Department of Education? 1. How many attended local workshops?	

SCHOOL ENVIRONMENT INSPECTION FORM

_____
(health district)

Name of school _____ Address _____

Clerk, Board of Education _____ Address _____

Superintendent or principal _____ Address _____

Custodians _____

☐ Elementary   No. classrooms _____   ☐ Municipal sewage
☐ Junior high   Food service ☐ Yes ☐ No   ☐ Public sewage
☐ Senior high   Swimming pool ☐ Yes ☐ No   ☐ Municipal water
Enrollment _____   ☐ Public water

Items marked by (x) are explained below with recommendations.

I. Surroundings
   A. Location ☐
   B. Grounds, walkways and driveways ☐
   C. Playground equipment ☐

II. Building
   A. Structure ☐
   B. Floor cleaning and repair ☐
   C. Walls and ceiling—cleaning
     and repair ☐
   D. Doors and windows ☐

III. Heating and ventilation
   A. Thermostat and thermometer
     each classroom ☐
   B. Temperature and humidity ☐
   C. Ventilation and dust control ☐

IV. Lighting
   A. Adequate artificial lighting ☐
   B. Maintenance of fixtures ☐
   C. Quality and proper use of lighting ☐

V. Water supply
   A. Source, development and treatment ☐
   B. Pressure and chemical quality ☐
   C. Plumbing, maintenance and design ☐
   D. Drinking fountains ☐

VI. Toilet and locker room facilities
   A. Cleaning, repair and adequacy of
     1. Rooms ☐
     2. Showers and toilet fixtures ☐
     3. Lockers and modesty equipment ☐
     4. Handwashing facilities ☐
   B. Ventilation ☐
   C. Rest room supplies ☐

VII. Waste disposal
   A. Sewage system operation ☐
   B. Sewage system maintenance ☐
   C. Refuse and garbage disposal ☐
   D. Refuse and garbage storage ☐

VIII. School room facilities
   A. Adequate equipment and
     furnishings ☐
   B. Maintenance of equipment and
     furnishings ☐
   C. Room population (overcrowding) ☐

IX. Accident prevention
   A. Traffic safety ☐
   B. Fire exits marked, adequate ☐
   C. Fire fighting equipment ☐
   D. Rooms and halls free of hazards ☐
   E. Stairways and playgrounds free
     of hazards ☐
   F. Properly equipped emergency room ☐

X. Insect and rodent control
   A. No evidence of insect infestation ☐
   B. No evidence of rodent infestation ☐
   C. Proper control procedures used ☐

Recommendations: _____

_____

_____

_____

_____

_____   _____
       Date   Sanitarian

PART IV. HEALTH EDUCATION

Schools are the official community agencies for the education of children. They have the major responsibility for the health instruction of children, grades K through 12. Health education instruction should be organized to provide learning experiences which favorably influence understandings, attitudes, and behavior in respect to individual and community health. In addition, the program should be designed to teach the individual to assume an ever increasing responsibility for his own health status.

Careful and continuous planning on the part of the school is necessary for an effective health instruction program. Objectives must be established; a sequential curriculum K-12 must be developed or adopted; content should be appropriate to the needs, interests and intellectual ability of the pupils; adequate time and credit must be allotted; and, most important, well qualified, certificated and enthusiastic teachers must be assigned to teach the health classes.

Text continued on p. 503.

Standards and recommended practices	What are we doing	Comments, priorities, proposed plans, time schedule
Administration		
A. Authorities recommend that health be taught 15-30 minutes daily at the elementary level; a full year course taught daily at the 7th, 8th, or 9th grade; and a full year course on a daily basis at the 10th, 11th or 12th grade. In the elementary schools, the Ohio State Department of Education requires a minimum of two 40 minute periods per week in grades 3 through 6, and two 45 minute periods per week in grades 7 and 8. The Ohio State Department of Education requires a semester course or its equivalent be taught at the high school level (9-12).	A. 1. Time allotted/week *Grade* K _____ 1 _____ 2 _____ 3 _____ 4 _____ 5 _____ 6 _____ 2. Health is taught as a separate course at the junior high level? (Circle grade(s): 7, 8, 9) Yes ☐ No ☐ 3. Health is taught as a separate course at the high school level? (Circle grade(s): 10, 11, 12) Yes ☐ No ☐	

4. How often do the classes meet?
   Junior high _____
   Senior high _____

5. How much time is allotted per class period?

B. The number of pupils assigned to health classes should be no greater than those assigned to other classes.

1. Average number of students per health class is _____.

2. Average number of students per all other classes is _____.

C. Most authorities recommend that health be taught in a natural setting and that the sexes should only be separated if they are separated for other courses.

1. Which of the following is typical in your school?
   Separate classes, boys and girls   Yes ☐ No ☐
   Coed classes   Yes ☐ No ☐
   Usually coed, but separated for some classes
   Yes ☐ No ☐
   If yes, which topics:
   Human sexuality   Yes ☐ No ☐
   Feminine hygiene   Yes ☐ No ☐
   Other (list):

D. Scheduling for health instruction should be like all other disciplines.

Health receives the same status on scheduling as other disciplines?   Yes ☐ No ☐

E. A staff member, specialized in health education (major in health education) should be designated health chairman of coordinator and assigned the responsibility for coordinating the entire health program.

A health chairman is designated?
Yes ☐ No ☐

1. If yes, is the health chairman a specialist in health education by professional preparation?
   Yes ☐ No ☐

2. If chairman is not a specialist in health education, check any of the following that apply:
   a. Has taken some health education courses and had experience in teaching health?
      Yes ☐ No ☐
   b. Has attended a school health workshop at a college or university?
      Yes ☐ No ☐

Continued.

Standards and recommended practices	What are we doing	Comments, priorities, proposed plans, time schedule
Administration — cont'd		
F. An interdisciplinary committee of persons should be appointed to plan and evaluate the health program cooperatively. The health coordinator should chair this group.	F. A health committee is appointed? Yes ☐ No ☐ 1. How often does the committee meet? 2. The health coordinator chairs this committee? Yes ☐ No ☐ 3. The local health committee is represented by the following (check appropriate ones): Teachers ☐ Parents ☐ Administrators ☐ Physicians ☐ Nurses ☐ Guidance counselor ☐ Psychologist ☐ Students ☐ Others (list):	
G. The school administration should provide a setting conducive to health instruction, including an equipped classroom, moveable furniture, supplies and materials and tables for demonstrations.	G. Our school utilizes: Regular sized classroom ☐ Moveable furniture ☐ Materials and supplies ☐ Tables for experiments and demonstrations ☐	
H. The school should provide in-service education programs for teachers to assist them in conducting health instruction in an interesting and sequential manner.	H. How many in-service programs on health education were offered during the past year? 1. How many faculty attended each program? 2. List the grades represented by teachers attending: 3. Were the in-service programs evaluated? Yes ☐ No ☐	

4. Topics covered (check appropriate ones):
   - General health knowledge ☐
   - New materials reviewed ☐
   - Teaching ideas shared ☐
   - Organization and curriculum development planning of program by grade level ☐
   - Demonstration of use of audio-visual and other equipment ☐
   - Other topics (please indicate):

5. Were resource persons from universities, state and/or local health agencies utilized?
   Yes ☐ No ☐

6. If yes, name participating agencies.

I. The school administration should provide textbooks, charts, filmstrips, resource books, models, pamphlets, transparencies, and other aids which are authoritative, up to date, interesting and appropriate for the grade level in which they are used.

I. List source of textbooks?

1. When were the health textbooks printed?

2. Have resources been reviewed by health committee? Yes ☐ No ☐

3. Which of the following are readily available?
   - Textbooks ☐
   - Charts ☐
   - Filmstrips ☐
   - Resource books ☐
   - Models ☐
   - Pamphlets ☐
   - Transparencies ☐
   - Others (list): ☐

Curriculum planning

A. The health instruction program should be based on the problem solving conceptual approach to studying and meeting the health needs, interests and problems of the students.

A. 1. Check ways students were surveyed to find their needs and interests:
   - Questionnaires ☐
   - Tests ☐
   - Checklists ☐
   - Personal essays ☐

2. List ways the community has been utilized to find local needs and interests:

3. Are morbidity and mortality statistics for the community studied and utilized?
   Yes ☐ No ☐

Continued.

Standards and recommended practices	What are we doing	Comments, priorities, proposed plans, time schedule
Curriculum planning—cont'd		
B. Curriculum planning should be carried out by the interdisciplinary committee responsible for the school health program.	B. Is the interdisciplinary committee assigned the task of writing the health education curriculum? Yes ☐ No ☐ 1. If not, who is responsible for the curriculum?	
C. The health instruction program should utilize the conceptual approach such as: School Health Education Study, "A Conceptual Approach to Curriculum Design," the ASHA Curriculum, the Ohio Department of Education Comprehensive Drug Education Curriculum.	C. Is the conceptual approach utilized? Yes ☐ No ☐ 1. Of the following, check those which have been reviewed by the health committee: School Health Education Study, "A Conceptual Approach to Curriculum Design" ☐ American School Health Association's Curriculum ☐ Ohio Department of Education Comprehensive Drug Education Curriculum, K-12 ☐ 2. If none of the above are utilized, name others that have been used as references: 3. Check the grade levels in which the conceptual approach is used: 1-3 ☐ 4-6 ☐ 7-9 ☐ 10-12 ☐	

D. The school system provides for use in the school a teaching guide, which contains:

1. A statement of philosophy upon which the school health education program is based.

2. Health education instructional content which includes a developmental scope and sequence approach to curriculum design, including the following:

   a. Concept emphasis
   b. Content
   c. Suggested teacher methods and techniques
   d. Student learning activities
   e. Evaluation
   f. Student/teacher resources and materials

E. A long range plan should be developed for implementing the health instruction program outlined in the teaching guide. A definite time plan should be included.

D. A health instruction guide is available and used in the school? Yes ☐ No ☐

1. Is a statement of philosophy included in the guide? Yes ☐ No ☐

2. Of the areas recommended in column 1, for inclusion in the guide, check those which are presently available:

	K-3	4-5-6	7-8-9	10-11-12
a.				
b.				
c.				
d.				
e.				
f.				

E. Is a plan available? Yes ☐ No ☐
   Three years _____
   Five years _____

Continued.

Standards and recommended practices	What are we doing	Comments, priorities, proposed plans, time schedule

Curriculum content

A. In general, the health instruction program for the school includes the following large areas with careful consideration being given to proper grade placement and sequence.

1. Nutrition
2. Dental health
3. Physical activity, sleep, rest and relaxation, recreation
4. Personal cleanliness and appearance
5. Body structure and operation
6. Prevention and control of disease
7. Safety and first aid
8. Drugs, alcohol and tobacco
9. Community health
10. Consumer health
11. Health careers
12. Mental, emotional and social health, including aggressive behavior
13. Sex and family life education
14. Environmental health

A. Indicate in which grades each subject is taught by placing a check in the appropriate square. Please write in the grade level.

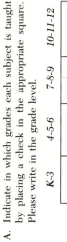
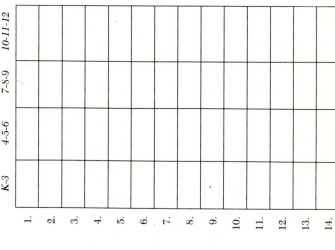

	K-3	4-5-6	7-8-9	10-11-12
1.				
2.				
3.				
4.				
5.				
6.				
7.				
8.				
9.				
10.				
11.				
12.				
13.				
14.				

(Note: the above data should be analyzed and plans made for removing duplication and adding omitted topics to the curriculum.)

Continued.

Methods and instructional aids

A. The students whenever possible should be actively involved in planning the health education program.

A. Of the following student related activities, check those which are used:
- Role-playing ☐
- Group discussions ☐
- Dyad (interaction between 2 students) ☐
- Debates ☐
- Panels ☐
- Case study ☐
- Independent studies and reports ☐

B. The health instruction program should include a variety of teaching techniques. Instruction should be geared towards skill development in seeking information, analyzing it carefully, drawing conclusions, and making behavioral decisions.

B. Of the following methods, check those which are used:
- Lecture ☐
- Field trips ☐
- Resource speakers ☐
- Demonstrations and experiments ☐
- Surveys ☐
- Problem solving discussion ☐

C. The school library should contain current periodicals and other reading matter as resource material for health classes.

C. Of the following, check the ones available to the students and staff:
- "School Safety" ☐
- "Today's Health" ☐
- "Journal of School Health" ☐
- Public affairs pamphlets ☐
- Science Research Associates booklets ☐
- Materials from American Medical Association ☐
- Ohio Department of Education Media Centers ☐
- "Ohio's Health" ☐
- Materials from Drug/Health Education Curriculum Center ☐
- Materials from AAHPER ☐
- Materials from the Ohio Department of Health ☐
- Materials from voluntary health agencies (heart, lung, cancer, etc.) ☐
- Supplementary texts ☐
- Others (list): ☐

Standards and recommended practices	What are we doing	Comments, priorities, proposed plans, time schedule
Methods and instructional aids — cont'd		
D. Projection equipment, tape recorders, and record players should be available for use in the classroom.	D. The following are available within the school for use in the classroom: 16 mm projectors ☐ Record players ☐ Tape recorders ☐ Slide projectors ☐ Filmstrip projectors ☐ Transparencies ☐	
E. Educational media is utilized in the teaching of health education.	E. Which of the following instructional television and/or film series are available: "Inside Out" NIT-AIT ☐ "Self-Incorporated" NIT-AIT ☐ "Knowing About Growing" BGSU ☐ "Feeling Good" NIT-AIT PBS ☐	
Evaluation		
A. The school makes periodic evaluation of the health instruction program to determine if behavioral objectives for pupils are being met. This includes an appraisal of knowledge gained, interests and values modified and behavior changed.	A. The health instruction program has been evaluated within the last three years? Yes ☐ No ☐	
B. Evaluation of the school physical and emotional climate is also included.	B. An effort has been made to appraise the school atmosphere? Yes ☐ No ☐	
C. The evaluation includes the interdisciplinary committee or program for health, the combined efforts of classroom teachers, health educators, administrators and, where appropriate, pupils.	C. The team approach has been used in the program evaluation? Yes ☐ No ☐ 1. A north Central or similar team has evaluated the health program in the last five years? Yes ☐ No ☐	
D. The results of the evaluation are used as a basis for curriculum revision and program improvement.	D. The results of evaluations are being used? Yes ☐ No ☐	

SOME RESOURCES FOR MATERIALS IN SCHOOL HEALTH PROGRAMS*

Ohio State Medical Association
600 South High Street
Columbus OH 43215
"Suggested Procedures for School Emergencies"

American Medical Association
535 North Dearborn Street
Chicago, Illinois 60610
"Health Appraisal of School Children"
"Suggested School Health Policies"
Prepared by Joint Committee on Health Problems in Education of the NEA and the AMA

American Academy of Pediatrics
P.O. Box 1034
Evanston, Illinois 60204
"School Health: A Guide for Physicians"

American School Health Association
ASHA National Office Building
Kent OH 44240

American Alliance for Health, Physical Education and Recreation
1201 Sixteenth Street, N.W.
Washington, D.C. 20036

Mental Health Materials Center
419 Park Avenue South
New York, New York 10016

Ohio Department of Education
Division of Elementary and Secondary Education
65 South Front Street
Columbus OH 43215

---

*Recognized National, State and Local Voluntary Health Agencies Addresses and phone numbers are available in local telephone listings or directors of health agencies.

and
Ohio Department of Education
Division of Special Education
933 High Street
Worthington OH 43085

Ohio Department of Mental Health and Mental Retardation
Office of Communications
2929 Kenny Road
Building A, Room 101
Columbus OH 43221

The following materials are available from the:
Ohio Department of Health
P.O. Box 118
Columbus OH 43216

1100 Hours—Film
15 minutes, 16mm, sound—showing aspects of sanitation in the school environment. Suited for school officials and interested adult groups.
Health Education Section

"School Accident Report Form" 4966.32
"Summary Form for School Accident Report Form" 4965.32
Accident Prevention and Product Safety Unit

"Sanitation in the School Environment" 2116.32
"Food Service Operation" 2231.32
Bureau of Environmental Health

"Communicable Disease Information—A Guide for Schools" 0945.11
Division of Communicable Diseases

"School Health Record Form" 3613.13 Rev. 1974
"Teacher Worksheet for Student Health Observation" 3611.13 Rev. 1967
Division of Maternal and Child Health

Index

A

Abrasions, 210
Abscess, 90
Accidents, school, 192-194, 195
Activity room, 412-415
Adaptability, 30
Administration
    school, 132, 153
    of school health program, self-appraisal checklist for, 469-476
Administrator, 275, 396
    health, 113
Adolescence, 45-50
Age
    biological, 39, 49
    chronological, 40, 41, 48
    skeletal, 39, 41, 48
Air conditioning, 401
Air movement, 40
Ajzen, I., 259, 260-261
Alcohol, 336-339
Allergy, 89
Amblyopia, 91-92, 132, 144
American College of Preventive Medicine, 245
American Dental Association, 294, 295
American Health Foundation, 320, 321, 357
American School Health Association, 14
Amphetamines, 97
Androgens, 284
Anemia, 86
Antibodies, 41, 166
Appraisal; *see* Evaluation; Health, appraisal
Appraisers, 245
Arches, weak, 234
Architects, 397
Arithmetic, 310-312
Art, 310

Artificial respiration, 205-207
Asphyxiation, 205-207
Assessment, health, 142, 144
Asthma, 33
Astigmatism, 91, 145
Attitudes, health, 338, 341, 347
Audiogram, 151
Audiometer, 132, 153
Audiometrist, 132
Auditorium, 196
Autonomic neuron system, 67

B

Bacillus fusiformis, 90
Bacteriological phase, 4
Bandura, A., 257, 258, 265
Barbiturates, 341
Behavior modification, 257-259, 265-267
Behavioral objective, 266
Berkeley Project, 267-271
Biological science, 388
    health education incorporated into, 352-353
Blood pressure, 61-63
Blum, H., 245
Board of education, 105, 106, 128, 136, 396
Boils, 164
Borrelia vincentii, 90
Brightness balance, 402
Brightness difference, 402
Bugelski, B. R., 247
Burns, 212-213
Bursitis, achilles, 234

C

Califano, J., 241
Callus, plantar, 233
Cardiovascular disorders, 84-86, 226

Caries, 90, 119, 140
Causative agents, 162
Cavities, 90, 139-140
Cerebral palsy, 224-225
Chadwick, E., 6
Checklist, 426
Chemistry, 389-390
Chickenpox, 163, 167
Child
    elementary school, 43-45, 69-70, 129
    healthy, 27
    highly nervous, 228
    hyperkinetic, 96-97
    junior high school, 70-71, 129
    preschool, 42-43, 69
    senior high school, 72-76
Child study movement, 7
Chlorination, 405-408
Chlorosis, 86
Chorea, 93, 228
Classroom, 128, 196, 399
    illumination in, 402
Cleft palate, 224
Code of ethics for health educators, 244
Cold, head, 163, 168
Communicable diseases, 162-164, 181-184, 305-309
Communication, 372, 387
Competition, 74
Conditions
    cardiovascular, 226
    foot, 223, 224
    general, 205-210
    localized, 210-214
Conference, pupil-teacher, 309
Confidence, 30
Congeniality, 31
Congestion, nasal, 88-89
Consumer health education, 14
    activities, 245-246
    task force on, 245-246
Contamination, 162
Contusions, 210
Convalescence, 167
Convulsions, epileptic, 208
Cooperation, custodian-staff, 398
Coordinator, 117-118
    health resource, 275
Corn, 234
Corrective measures, 219-221
Correlation, 20, 277, 310-312, 350-351, 384-385
Cortin, 39
Coryza, 163, 168
Council, school safety, 200
Counseling, 19, 155-156, 157, 158

Courage, 30
Course, health
    full-year, 320, 353
    half-year, 320, 353-354
    quarter-year, 319-320, 353
CPR, 204
Cretinism, 83
Criteria, 427
Cross-eye, 92, 227
Curriculum
    health major, 354-356
    health minor, 354-356
Custodian, 122, 398

D

Darwin, C., 247
Dating, 373
Daydreaming, 31
DDST; *see* Denver Developmental Screening Test
Deafness, 92-93
Death, 370-371
Death rate, among school population, 191-192
Decontamination, 162
Defection, 167
Defects, 223-224
    congenital, 223
    congenital heart, 84-85
    dental, 228
    noncorrectable, 221-222
    orthopedic, 223-226
    posture, 231-232
    speech, 234-235
    vision, 226-227
Defervescence, 167
Deficiency disease, 230
Dehydration, 162
Dental disease, 140
Dental health education; *see* Oral Health Teaching-Learning Guide
Dental hygienist, 118-119, 132, 140-141
Dentist, 139-142
Denver Developmental Screening Test, 56
Desiccation, 162
Development
    personality, 369-372
    role, 370
Deviations
    mental health, 94-97
    respiratory system, 88-90
Diabetes mellitus, 33, 82-83
Dieting, 229-231
Differences
    intellectual, 370
    male-female, 50-53

Differences—cont'd
  psychosexual, 370
Diphtheria, 136, 163, 168, 177-178, 179, 224
Director
  health, 274, 382
  of school, 114-116
Disability, 221
  hearing, 92-93
Disease
  control of, 165, 174-177
  detection of, 181-184
  infections, transmission of, 164
Disinfection, 161-162
Dislocations, 213
Disorders
  cardiovascular, 84-86, 226
  neurological, 93
  oral cavity, 90-91
  personality, 370
  physical, 218
  vision, 91-92
Dispensers, liquid soap, 408
Disturbances
  digestive system, 81-82
  endocrine, 82-83
Drugs, 336-342
  and sexual behavior, 373
DTP, 179, 180
Dwarfism, 54
Dysentery, 163

E

Early Periodic Screening Diagnosis and Treatment,
  135-136
Education
  department of, 105
  drug abuse, 339
  health, 19
  physical, 8
  sex, 284-290
Educator
  health, 25-26
  physical, 121
  secondary school health, 121-122
Egocentricity, 69
Emergency care, 202-203, 384
Emotions, 66-69, 70, 71, 73, 96
  control of, 31
English, 387
Environment, 49
  healthful mental, 416-417
  healthful school, 20, 384, 395-418, 430
Epidemics, 187
Epilepsy, 33, 93, 208-209
Epiphyses, 45, 54

EPSDT; *see* Early Periodic Screening Diagnosis and
  Treatment
Equal rights movement, 50
Escherichia coli, 162
Esotropia, 227
Estrogen, 46, 284
Evaluation, 107, 156, 284, 342, 343, 378-379
  administrative practices in, 428-429
  clinical, 426
  devices for, 425-428
  health, 156
    change in, 428
  health instruction program and, 383-392
  health services, 430
  healthful school living, 430-431
  height and weight, 152-153
  procedures of, 425
  purposes of, 423-424
  resources for, 430
  scale of, 459-467
  school health program, 429-430
Examination
  clinical, 131-133
  dental, 136, 139-142
  health, 9, 128-139, 158
  multiphasic, 132-133
  speech, 234-235
Exclusions, 185-186
Experiences
  community, 280
  disturbing, 31
  school, 279

F

Facilities
  emergency care, 202
  food service, 410-412
  handwashing, 408
  health services, 110
Failure, fear of, 75
Fainting, 209
Family, 373-374
Family Education Rights and Privacy Act, 137
Family planning, 373-374
Farsightedness, 91, 144-145
Fastigium, 167
Feet, tender, 234
Fire chief, 199
Fire protection, 196
First aid, 203, 214
Fishbein, M., 259, 260, 261
  behavioral intension model, 261
  conceptual framework, 260
Fluoridation, 119
Fogarty International Center, 245

Follow-up programs, 142, 147, 152, 218-219
Food service, 410-412
Foot, Morton's painful, 233
Footcandle, 401-403
Footlambert, 401-403
Forward Plan for Health, 13, 241, 245
  dental, 451-453
  evaluation record, 142-143
  examination record, 139, 141-142
  health examination, 449-450
  physical education activity, 449-450
  referral, 454
  student accident, 455
Fountains, 406-408
Fractures, 213
Frank, J. P., 6
Furunculosis, 164

G

General science, health education as part of, 318-319
Genetics, 373
Geography, 312
German mealses, 163, 169, 179-180, 224
Gigantism, 54
Gingivitis, 90
Glare, 402
Glycosuria, 82
Golaszewski, T., 265
Gonadotropins, 45
Gonorrhea, 164
Goodladd, J., 264
Governor's Steering Committee, 12
Grade level
  primary, 281-304
  junior high, middle school, 305-312, 314-344
  secondary, 314-379
Graphs and tables, usefulness of, 58-61
Gravity method, 232
Green, L., 252
Group A beta-hemolytic streptococcus, 83
Growth
  abnormal, 54
  accelerated, 94
  adolescent, 50-53
  biological, 39
  cellular, 37-39
  delayed, 94
  emotional, 370, 388-389
  environmental, factors of, 40
  physical, 56-60
  social, 388-389
Guidance, 19
  health, 109, 153-156
  school health services, 107-110
Guidelines, health instruction program, 271

Guides, curriculum, 349-350
Gym itch, 164, 172-173
Gymnasiums, 196, 412-415

H

Halls, safety in, 196
Handedness, 144
Harelip, 224
Harvey, W., 3
Health, 18; *see also* Course, health
  appraisal, 109, 127-159
  behavior goals, 253
  community, 316
  environmental, 111
  levels of, 31-32
  mental, 30-31, 316, 342-343
  physical, 27-29, 315
  public, 135
  student appraisal of personal, 156-158
Health Belief Model, 254-256
Health code, Hebrew, 1-2
Health department, 131, 133
  county, 132
Health education
  bureau of, 12, 13
  contribution to health, 244
  current legislative developments in, 12
  definitions of, 242-244
  local, 290
  purpose of, 242
  self-appraisal checklist for, 494-503
  teacher preparation for, 15
  theories and models of, 252
Health Education Act of 1978, 14
Health esteem, 137
Health practices, 16
Health problems, 383
Health record card, 138
Health status, 382-383
Health teacher preparation, 354-356
Healthful school living, 17-18, 106, 111-112, 116
  evaluation scale for, 464-467
  self-appraisal checklist for, 487-493
Hearing, conservation of, 148-152
Hearing impairment, 149, 227-228
Hearing loss, prevention of, 148-149
Heart, 52, 61-62
Heating, 399-400
Height, 46-49, 54-55, 152-153
Hemoglobin, 136
Hepatitis, 170
  infectious, 169-170
  viral, 163
Heroin, 341
Heterosexuality, 72

HGH; *see* Human growth hormone
Hill, W., 248, 249, 262, 263
Hilleboe, H., 241
Hillgard, E., 248
History, 312
   medical, 132
Holmes, T., 375
Home economics, 389
Hormones; *see* specific hormones
Housekeeping, 416
Human growth hormone, 45
Human needs, 369-370
Humidity, 400
Humor, perception of, 31
Hydrolysis, 162
Hyperglycemia, 82
Hyperkinetic child, 96-97
Hyperopia, 91, 144-145
Hypertension, 85, 226
Hyperthyroidism, 68, 83
Hypochondria, 96
Hypocrisy, 75
Hypoglycemia, 83
Hypothyroidism, 68, 83
Hysteria, 95

I

Illness
   major, 202
   minor, 202-203
Illumination, 401-405
Immunity
   active, 166
   infantile, 40, 166
   passive, 166
Immunization schedule, 179-180
Impetigo contagiosa, 164, 172-173
Incubation, 166
Individuality, 54
Infant
   full-term, 40
   premature, 40-41
Infantile paralysis, 136, 163, 171, 178-179, 224
Infection, 161-162
   skin, 172-173
Influenza, 163
Inheritance, 39, 54, 55-56
Injury
   accidental, 225
   ear, 212
   eye, 212
   general, 205-210
   head, 214
   localized, 210-214
   neck and back, 214

In loco parentis, 15
Inspection, food services, 410-414
Instruction, health, 16, 106, 110-111, 113
   classroom, 276-277
   correlated, 271
   elementary school, 267, 274-312; *see also* School Health Curriculum Project
   evaluation scale for, 462-464
   framework for, 14
   incidental, 309-310, 316
   integrated living, 277-280
   junior high school, 267
   middle school, 314-344; *see also* School Health Curriculum Project
   organizing, 274-276, 316-320
   planned direct, 280-309
   senior high school, 346-379
   separate subject, 353-354
Instructor; *see* Teacher
Instruments of evaluation, 425-428
Integration of instruction, 16-17
Intermediate host, 164
Interview, 426
Inventory, health practices, 434
Isolation, 185
Itch, 173

J

Janitor, 122, 398
Jenner, E., 3

K

Kindergarten, 281-286
Knowledge, health, 279-280
Know Your Body Program, 320-335, 356-369
Koch, R., 4
Koplik spots, 170
Kreuter, M., 252
Kwashiorkor, 229
Kyphosis, 224

L

LA; *see Lactobacillus acidophilus*
Laboratory, 196
Lactobacillus acidophilus, 90
Language arts, 310
Learning, health, 316, 351
Learning theories, 248-252
   cognitive, 250
   connections, 248-252
   field, 250, 251
   Gestalt, 250
Legal aspects, 128, 194-195
Lewin, K., 251, 254, 255
Li, C. H., 39

Liability, 194-195
Light
   artificial, 403, 404
   natural, 403
   standards for, 402, 403
Locker room, 196, 415
Loner, 94-95
Lordosis, 224
Lousiness, 173
Loyalty
   group, 71, 314
   school, 397
LSD-25; *see* Lysergic acid diethylamide
Lunchroom, 398
Lysergic acid diethylamide, 340-341

M

Mager, R., 249
Malaria, 164
Malnutrition, 42, 80-82, 229
Malocclusion, 91, 228
Mann, H., 8
Marihuana, 340
Marriage, 373
   troubled, 374
Materials for health instruction, 283-284
Mathematics, 390
Maturation, 38, 48-50, 289-290
   accelerated, 94
   delayed, 94
   emotional, 69-70
Measles, 136, 163, 169, 170, 179, 180
Medicaid, 131, 135
Meningococcus meningitis, 163, 171
Method, 282-283
   teaching, 320, 375-378
Miasma phase, 4
Mononucleosis, 171
Moodiness, 96
Morphine, 341
Motivation, 282
Movies, 75
Mumps, 163, 171, 180
Muscular dystrophy, 225
Music, 310
Myocarditis, 85
Myopia, 91, 144-145

N

Narcotics, 292, 338-339
National Cancer Institute, 13
National Committee on Health Education, 12, 13
National Health Council, 13
National Heart, Lung, and Blood Institute, 13
Nature study, 312

Nearsightedness, 91, 144-145
Negligence, 194-195
Neurosis, 372
Normal, concepts of, 18-19, 26
Nosebleed, 211-212
Nurse
   public health, 117
   school, 116-117, 129
Nutrition, 49

O

Obesity, 80-81
Objectives
   health instruction, 314-315, 346-347
   unit, 285
Objectivity, 427
Observation, 144, 147, 426
Ophthalmologist, 132, 227
Oral Health Teaching-Learning Guide, 294-305
   basic concepts, 295
   dentist and helpers, 303
   diet and dental health, 299
   keeping teeth safe, 304
   teeth, 300
   plaque control, 296
Orderliness, 30
   all-school, 397, 398
   room, 398
   school safety, 197-200
Orthoptics, 227
Ossification, 38
Osteomyelitis, 225
Oxidation, 161
Ozena, 87

P

Parotitis, 163, 171, 180
Pasteur, L., 4
Pathogens, in transmission of infectious disease, 164-165
Patrol
   building and grounds, 199-200
   fire, 199
   school safety, 197-199
Payment, 136
Pediatrician, 133
Pediculosis, 173
Pep pills, 97
Pericarditis, 85
Permissiveness, 75
Personality structure, 370
Personality, troubled, 372
Personnel
   instructional, 320
   lunchroom, 398
   public health, 174-175

Personnel—cont'd
  school, 175-177
Pertussis, 163, 177-178, 224
Pes cavus, 234
Pes planus, 234
Petersen, H. E., 154
Phagocytosis, 166
Phonocardioscan screen, 134
Physical education, 387
Physical education, health education alternated with, 319
Physician
  health department, 131
  private, 130-131, 175
  school, 113-114, 132
Physics, 389
Playground, 196
Plumbing, 409, 410
Poisoning, 209-210
Policies, school, 187
Poliomyelitis, 136, 163, 171, 178-179, 224
Polyp, 87
Positive health phase, 4
Practices
  administrative, evaluation of, 428, 429
  desirable, 76
  food services personnel, 411, 412
  health, 1-6, 338, 347, 348
  nutritional, 290
  school, 383, 384
Pride
  personal, 276-277
  student, 396
Procedures
  measuring, 152
  test
    hearing, 150-152
    vision, 145-147
Profile, developmental, 56-58
Progesterone, 43
Program
  auditory screening, 149
  dental examination, 139-142
  diet, 229-231
  follow-up, 218-223
  health appraisal, 127-128, 135-136
  immunization, 136, 177-181
  modified, for handicapped, 235, 236
  public health, 19
  school health; see School health program
  school safety, 190-202
Projects, 398
Promotion, mental health, 97-99
Pseudohysteria, 95
Psychosis, 374

Ptosis, 92
Puberty, 45-50, 71-72
Pubescence, 45
Pyorrhea, 90

Q

Questionnaire, health practices, 434

R

Rabies, 164
Readers, health, 310
Readmissions, 186-187
Records, health, 427
Refrigeration, 410
Rehabilitation, 222, 223
Relationship
  interpersonal, 372, 373
  pupil-teacher, 278, 279
Reliability, 427-428
Remedial measures, 109-110
Report, student, 427
Requirements, legal, 128, 194-195
Resistance, 165-166
Resources
  evaluation, 430
  health instruction, 445-447
  human, 33-34
Respiratory disease, 103-104, 166-173
Responsibility
  of administrator, 396
  of architect, 397
  of board of education, 396
  of custodian, 398
  of lunchroom personnel, 398, 399
  parental, 131, 155
  of school, 78-79, 219-223
  of school health program, 153-158
  of student, 397
  of teacher, 382, 397
Restlessness, 95
Resuscitation, 207
Retardation, growth, 41
Rheumatic fever, 33, 83-84, 163, 171
Rheumatic heart disease, 85
Richmond, J., 241-242
Ringworm, 173
Risk Factor Teaching
  Level I, 320-335
  Level II, 356-369
Rocky Mountain spotted fever, 164, 180
Rosenstock, I., 254
Rubella, 163, 169, 179-180, 224
Rubeola, 136, 163, 169, 170, 179, 180

S

Safeguards, 385-387
Safety, 190
St. Vitus' dance, 93, 228
Salmonellosis, 163
Sanitation, 20, 395, 396
    report, 413, 414
Scabies, 173
Scald, 212
Scarlet fever, 163, 171, 224
Schedule
    examination, 128-130
    test
        hearing, 149-150
        vision, 145
School building, 395-418
School Health Curriculum Project, 267-271
School health developments, 14
    Committee on School and College Health, 10
    Joint Committee NEA-AMA, 10, 242-243
    Kellogg project, 11
    National Conference on Cooperation, 10
    policies, 10
    professional preparation, 11
School Health Education Study, 14, 262-264
School health movement, 6
School health program, 15-18, 19
    evaluation scale for, 459-467
    objectives of, 17-18
    philosophy of, 15-16
    self-appraisal checklist for, 468-503
School health services, 19, 107-110, 113, 116
    appraisal aspects of, 109, 127-159
    evaluation scale for, 459-462
    facilities for, 110
    prevention aspects of, 161-187
    remedial aspects of, 109-110
Screening, 109, 127-159
Security, 30
Self-appraisal, 426
Self-discipline, 30
Self-esteem, 30
Self-gratification, 30
Selfishness, 96
Self-reliance, 30-31
Septic tank, 410
Septum, deviated, 89
Serum, 166
Services
    guidance, 19
    school health; see School health services
Sex differences, 50-53
Sexual behavior
    drugs and, 373
    premarital, 373

Sexual feelings, 373
Shattuck, L., 7
Shock, 207-208
Shops, safety of, 196
Shower room, 415, 416
Shyness, 94
Sickle cell abnormality, 136
Sincerity, 31
Sinusitis, 89
Skinner, B., 249, 250, 265
Sleeping pills, 341
Smallpox, 163, 172
Smoking, 293-294; see also Tobacco
Social conflict, 72-73
Social development activities, 286-290
Social engineering phase, 5
Social Security Act, 131, 135
Social studies, 388
    health education as part of, 319
Society, 75
Society for Public Health Education, 244
Somatotropin, 39, 54
SOPHE; see Society for Public Health Education
Spermatozoa, 45
Spina bifida, 224
Sprains, 213
Stability, 30
Staff, secondary school, 381-382
Stairs, 196
Standards
    light, 402, 403
    physical comfort, 400
Stanford Heart Disease Prevention Program, 259
Stanley, J. C., 436
Stigmata, 224
Storage room, 410
Strabismus, 92, 227
Strain, foot, 233
Streptococcal throat infection, 163, 171-172
Streptococcus albus, 161
Stress, 370-372
    dealing with, 371
    ineffective reactions to, 371, 372
Subject areas and health education, 348-350
Subject fields, 387-390
Subjectivity, 427
Sullivan, D., 243
Supervision, health, 153
Supplies, first aid, 215
Surgeon General's Report, 14
Surveys, 427
Suspiciousness, 96
Swimming pool, 196, 416
Sydenham's chorea, 93, 228
Syphilis, 164

T

Talipes, 223
Tanner, J. M., 45-47
Teacher, 129, 397
  classroom, 275-276
  elementary, 119, 142
  secondary, 119-121
  health of, 158-159
Television, 75
Temperament, 67
Temperature, 400
Tensions
  national, 75
  world, 74-75
Tests
  construction of, 432-433
  intellectual
    completion, 439, 440
    essay, 435
    health attitudes, 434
    health practices, 433-434
    matching, 438, 439
    multiple-choice, 437, 438
    short-answer, 440
    true-false, 435, 436
  physical
    achievement, 427
    Denver Development Screening, 56
    hearing, 149-152
    laboratory, 133, 134
    Schick, 178
    Snellen vision, 144, 146-147
    tuberculosis, 136
    vision screening, 144-148
Testosterone, 46
Tetanus, 136
Textbooks, 283, 284
  elementary school, 445, 446
  family living, 446, 447
  junior high school, 446
  senior high school, 446
Therapist, speech, 132, 133
Thompson, B., 6
Thorndike, E., 249, 250, 265
Thyroxin, 49, 54, 67
Tic, 228
Tinea, 173
Title V, 131
Title XIX, 131, 135
Tobacco, 336-338
Toilet, chemical, 410

Toilet room, 408, 409, 410
Torticollis, 224, 226
Toxin, 161, 177
Trauma, 225
Travers, R., 247, 248, 250
Trench mouth, 90
Tuberculosis, 163, 172, 180
Tularemia, 164
Turbinate bones, enlarged, 89
Turner, C. E., 9
Tyler, R., 248, 249
Typhoid, fever, 163, 180

U

Unit, teaching, 285-309, 320-343, 356-378
  aim of, 285
  health education, 369-378
  resource, 284-294, 336-343
Urinals, 408-409

V

Vaccine, 133, 179
Validity, 427
Variola, 163, 171, 224
Ventilation, 399, 400, 401, 408
Vincent's disease, 90
Vision, 44, 132, 144
Vitality, low, 79, 231

W

Wart, plantar, 234
Washbasin, 408
Water closet, 408
Water supply, 405-408
Watson, J., 250, 265
Weight, 55-56, 152-153
Well as water supply, 406
White House Conference on Child Health Protection, 8, 10
Whooping cough, 163, 177-178, 224
Winslow, C. E. A., 19
Women's liberation, 370
Wounds, 210-211
Wryneck, 224, 226

Y

Yellow fever, 164

Z

Zais, R., 255, 263